PUBLIC HEALTH
RESEARCH METHODS

PUBLIC HEALTH
RESEARCH METHODS

Greg Guest

FHI 360, Social Research Solutions

Emily E. Namey

FHI 360, Social Research Solutions

Editors

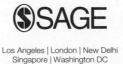

Los Angeles | London | New Delhi
Singapore | Washington DC

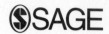

Los Angeles | London | New Delhi
Singapore | Washington DC

FOR INFORMATION:

SAGE Publications, Inc.
2455 Teller Road
Thousand Oaks, California 91320
E-mail: order@sagepub.com

SAGE Publications Ltd.
1 Oliver's Yard
55 City Road
London EC1Y 1SP
United Kingdom

SAGE Publications India Pvt. Ltd.
B 1/I 1 Mohan Cooperative Industrial Area
Mathura Road, New Delhi 110 044
India

SAGE Publications Asia-Pacific Pte. Ltd.
3 Church Street
#10-04 Samsung Hub
Singapore 049483

Acquisitions Editor: Vicki Knight
Assistant Editor: Katie Guarino
Editorial Assistant: Jessica Miller
Production Editor: Libby Larson
Copy Editor: Sarah J. Duffy
Typesetter: C&M Digitals (P) Ltd.
Proofreader: Dennis W. Webb
Indexer: Sheila Bodell
Cover Designer: Karine Hovsepian
Marketing Manager: Nicole Elliott

Printed in the United States of America

Library of Congress Cataloging-in-Publication Data

Public health research methods / [edited by] Greg Guest, Emily E. Namey.

p. ; cm.
Includes bibliographical references and index.

ISBN 978-1-4522-4133-3 (hardcover : alk. paper)
ISBN 978-1-4833-1142-5 (web PDF)

I. Guest, Greg, 1963- editor of compilation.
II. Namey, Emily E., editor of compilation. [DNLM: 1. Public Health—methods. 2. Research Design. 3. Epidemiologic Methods. 4. Health Services Research—methods. WA 20.5]
RA425

362.1—dc23   2013040638

This book is printed on acid-free paper.

14 15 16 17 18 10 9 8 7 6 5 4 3 2 1

BRIEF CONTENTS

DETAILED CONTENTS

PREFACE

Russ Bernard once wrote a book chapter titled "Methods Belong to All of Us." This conviction is the central theme underlying this book. With this volume, we aim to provide researchers, and future researchers, with an up-to-date and comprehensive set of tools to investigate public health issues and problems, to ultimately better inform public health policy and practice. The range and diversity of research methods currently used in public health is vast and continues to expand. Public health research is no longer confined to traditional epidemiological designs. The new methodological landscape includes research methods from a myriad of research disciplines, and new technology continues to advance this constantly changing terrain.

We believe that the more methodological tools researchers have in their repertoire, the better equipped they are to successfully accomplish their research objectives and build on the existing evidence base. A primary motivation for creating this book, therefore, is to convey a diverse and contemporary view of public health research methods. In this spirit, the contents of this book go beyond traditional epidemiologic approaches and cover the various research methods and technologies that define the public health landscape. We also believe that the successful conduct of research requires good planning, including the ability to translate research findings into action, which is why we've included the sections Planning and Preparing for Research (Part I) and Applying Research Findings (Part VI).

The order of chapters in this volume reflects two chronological trajectories. One is the overall research process, moving from planning and preparation (Part I) to implementation (Parts II–V) to application of findings (Part VI). The other temporal dimension guiding the order of chapters (albeit imprecisely) is the historical development of epidemiologic and public health research methods, outlined in Chapter 1.

The internal structure within each chapter necessarily varies, due to the diversity in subject matter across chapters. However, a certain degree of structural consistency is maintained with the inclusion of several general content areas in each chapter—a definition of the topic area, the relevance of the chapter topic to public health, a discussion of practical dimensions (i.e., the how-to of the approach), current issues and future directions, and additional resources. Where applicable, chapters also contain sections that present the subject matter in the context of global health. The diverse examples contained in the chapters of this book demonstrate how a public health research problem can be viewed from a number of different methodological perspectives and likewise addressed with a number of possible research methods.

Creativity and resourcefulness, combined with rigor and transparency, are the cornerstones of good research and have led to many of the major milestones in public health research. As eloquently expressed by John Dewey, "Every great advance in science has issued from a new audacity of the imagination." We hope that you find in this book new ideas and methods to inspire your own creative thinking about the research process in the field of public health.

Online instructional resources to accompany the book are available at www.sagepub.com/guestph.

Greg and Emily

Durham, NC

September 10, 2013

ACKNOWLEDGMENTS

This book is the result of the cumulative efforts of many talented contributors. We are extremely grateful to all of them and the hard work they put into the chapters that constitute this book. Thank you!

Multiple thanks are also due to everyone at SAGE, particularly Vicki Knight and Jessica Miller. Their support throughout the entire process was vital in transforming an amorphous idea into a 700+ page book. As always, Sage has been a true collaborator.

On a more personal level, Greg wishes to thank his family (Gretel, Hunter, and Aaron) for tolerating his evening and weekend absences while (co)putting this book together.

Emily extends gratitude to her family as well: to her husband, Jason, whose moral and parenting support made her contributions to this volume possible, and to her daughters, Isabelle and Lucia, whose hugs and laughter were the perfect antidote to hours of "screen time."

SAGE Publications and the authors would also like to express their gratitude to the following reviewers for their thoughtful and constructive comments:

Tracey Barnfather, University of Northampton

Peter Benson, Washington University in St. Louis

Mary Lou Bost, Carlow University

Pamela J. Bretschneider, PhD, Massachusetts College of Pharmacy and Health Sciences

Sandra Minor Bulmer, Southern Connecticut State University

Rosemary M. Caron, PhD, MPH, University of New Hampshire

Beverly A. Cigler, Penn State Harrisburg

Joan E. Cowdery, Eastern Michigan University

Cynthia Fowler, Wofford College

Peggy Gallup, Southern Connecticut State University

Roya Ghiaseddin, University of Notre Dame

Linda Highfield, PhD, MS, University of Texas School of Public Health

Scott Kahan, MD, MPH, Johns Hopkins University School of Public Health

Allyson Kelley, University of North Carolina at Greensboro

Russell S. Kirby, College of Public Health, University of South Florida, Tampa

Frederick J. Kviz, PhD, School of Public Health, University of Illinois at Chicago

Michele Morrone, Ohio University

Willie H. Oglesby, PhD, MSPH, FACHE, Kent State University

Josh Packard, Midwestern State University

Dhitinut Ratnapradipa, PhD, Southern Illinois University–Carbondale

Kerry J. Redican, MPH, PhD, Virginia Tech

Karen Rich, PhD, RN, University of Southern Mississippi

Dr. Monika Sawhney, PhD, Mercer University

Linda Agustin Simunek, RN, PhD, JD, Abraham S. Fischler School of Education, Nova Southeastern University

Sheryl Strasser, PhD, Georgia State University Institute of Public Health

Fabienne Williams MS, APRN, PMHCNS-BC, Chicago State University

ABOUT THE EDITORS

Greg Guest received his PhD in anthropology from the University of Georgia. Over the past 15 years, he has designed and managed public health research studies in more than 15 countries. Greg is currently the director of research and evaluation in the Economic Development and Livelihoods Department at FHI 360. In this capacity he oversees multisite, mixed methods, research and evaluation activities across multiple fields of public health. His other books include two edited volumes—*Globalization, Health and the Environment: An Integrated Perspective* (AltaMira, 2005) and *Handbook for Team-Based Qualitative Research* (AltaMira, 2008)—and two coauthored textbooks, *Applied Thematic Analysis* (Sage, 2012) and *Collecting Qualitative Data: A Field Manual for Applied Research* (Sage, 2013). He has published articles in journals such as *Field Methods, Journal of Mixed Methods Research, American Journal of Public Health, JAIDS, AIDS Care, AIDS Education and Prevention, African Journal of AIDS Research, AIDS and Behavior, Journal of Family Planning and Reproductive Health Care,* and *Journal of Health Communication.* Greg is also owner of the research consulting firm Social Research Solutions, which specializes in methodological training and consultation (www.social-researchsolutions.com).

Emily E. Namey has nearly 15 years' experience applying skills in project management and knowledge of research methods to the design, implementation, conduct, monitoring, and dissemination of public health research. Emily has spent half her career at FHI 360, where she manages domestic and international qualitative and mixed methods projects related to health disparities and HIV prevention in the Social and Behavioral Health Sciences Department. She also spent several years at Duke University, splitting time among the Institute for Genome Sciences and Policy, the Department of Obstetrics and Gynecology, and the Trent Center for Bioethics. At Duke, Emily implemented qualitative research on subjects ranging from maternity care to vaccine trial participation to ethical approaches for genomic research recruitment. Emily serves as a consultant and instructor for Social Research Solutions, has designed and led qualitative research training courses in more than a dozen countries, and has coauthored several methodological publications, including *Collecting Qualitative Data*: *A Field Manual for Applied Research* (Sage, 2013), *Applied Thematic Analysis* (Sage, 2012), *Qualitative Research Methods: A Data Collector's Field Guide* (Family Health International, 2005), and "Data Reduction Techniques for Large Qualitative Datasets" in *Handbook for Team-Based Qualitative Research* (AltaMira, 2008). Her publications also include articles in *Social Science & Medicine, Fertility and Sterility, AIDS Care, IRB,* and the *Journal of Empirical Research on Human Research Ethics.* Emily received her MA in applied anthropology from Northern Arizona University.

ABOUT THE CONTRIBUTORS

Jeanne Bertolli is associate chief for science, Behavioral and Clinical Surveillance Branch, in the Division of HIV/AIDS Prevention at the U.S. Centers for Disease Control and Prevention. She holds master's and doctoral degrees in epidemiology from the University of California, Los Angeles. Jeanne has led and collaborated on surveys in the United States and internationally, and has most recently served as principle investigator on a multisite survey to characterize barriers and facilitators to accessing medical care among HIV-infected individuals. She currently advises on the planning and design of research and public health surveillance activities.

Lyndal Bond, PhD, is the principal research officer at the Centre of Excellence in Intervention and Prevention Science (CEIPS). Prior to her appointment at CEIPS, Lyndal was the associate director at the MRC/CSO Social and Public Health Sciences Unit, in Glasgow, Scotland, and honorary professor in the Faculty of Medicine at the University of Glasgow. While in the UK she led a program of research evaluating the effects on health of social interventions. Her research interests include understanding the effects of social interventions on health and health inequalities, researching the implementation and sustainability of complex interventions, and evaluating the implementation of evidence-based policy into practice.

David Borasky received his MPH from the University of North Carolina at Chapel Hill. He has over 15 years of experience managing institutional review boards (IRBs) as well as facilitating training activities on basic research ethics and IRB operations and function for research staff and their collaborators worldwide. David is currently the deputy director of the Office of Human Research Ethics at the University of North Carolina at Chapel Hill. In this role he oversees the operations of five IRBs that together are responsible for the ethical oversight of the entire research portfolio of the university. David is a coauthor of the award-winning *Research Ethics Training Curriculum* and the *Research Ethics Training Curriculum for Community Representatives*, which together have been used to train individuals in over 70 countries. He is a contributing author of *Institutional Review Board: Management and Function*. He has served as a consultant for the Office of Human Research Protections, the U.S. Department of Energy, the World Health Organization, and numerous other institutions. David is a Certified IRB Professional and member of the Board of Directors for Public Responsibility in Medicine and Research.

Sarah Boslaugh earned her PhD from the City University of New York and her MPH from St. Louis University. She has 20 years of experience in educational, public health, and medical research and is currently a data journalist and grant writer for the Center for Sustainable Journalism at Kennesaw State University, in Georgia. Her fifth book, *Health Care Systems Around the World: A Comparative Guide,* was published in 2013. She served as the editor-in-chief for the *Encyclopedia of Epidemiology* (Sage, 2007) and previously published *An Intermediate Guide to SPSS Programming: Using Syntax for Data Analysis* (Sage, 2004), *Secondary Data Sources for Public Health: A Practice Guide* (Cambridge University Press, 2007), and *Statistics in a Nutshell* (2nd ed., O'Reilly, 2012). In addition she has published numerous professional articles on everything from GLBT athletes in documentary film to the influence of neighborhood perceptions on adult physical activity.

Raymond Buck has over 25 years of experience providing statistical and regulatory support in the design, analysis, programming, reporting, and review for preclinical and clinical pharmaceutical drug and device research and development. He has proficiency in writing the statistical sections of protocols and data safety monitoring charters, statistical analysis plans, results sections of study reports, and integrative summaries of marketing applications for the United States and Europe. Raymond has served on data monitoring committees for medical devices, drugs, and biologics for NIH- and FDA-regulated research. He has supported federally sponsored university research grants at the University of North Carolina at Greensboro (UNC-G) and is an author on over 20 publications. Raymond cotaught Development and Clinical Investigations of Drugs at the University of North Carolina at Chapel Hill (UNC-CH) Eshelman School of Pharmacy and taught statistical applications courses in the UNC-G PhD Nursing Research program. He held senior positions in the pharmaceutical and contract research industries and has operated his own consulting firm for the past 8 years. Raymond has a PhD in Biostatistics from UNC-CH.

Holly McClain Burke, PhD, MPH, is a behavioral scientist at FHI 360 with over a decade of experience designing and managing international reproductive health research studies. She has expertise in conducting studies incorporating both qualitative and quantitative research methods to expand understanding of complex contraceptive and HIV prevention behaviors. Recently Holly served as the principal investigator for three research projects studying contraceptive behavior in East and West Africa. Previously she studied the social and contextual factors triggering HIV risk behavior among men in Ghana and Tanzania. She has also served on research teams evaluating MTV's global HIV prevention campaign, community-based HIV prevention peer education programs in the Dominican Republic and Zambia, and a national sex education curriculum in Jamaican middle schools. Holly earned an MPH in health behavior/health education with a minor in epidemiology, and a PhD in maternal and child health with a minor in quantitative psychology, both from the School of Public Health at the University of North Carolina at Chapel Hill.

Mary Cavanaugh, PhD, is an associate professor in the Silberman School of Social Work at Hunter College, City University of New York. Her primary research focuses on examining the origins of violent behavior in male and female offenders and in designing and testing preventative interventions that may decrease the potential risk for violence in intimate relationships. She has been a practitioner in the field of family violence, facilitating batterers' intervention programs in cooperation with Adult Probation and Parole Departments and victim service agencies. In addition to numerous journal articles, she coauthored *Randomized Controlled Trials: Design and Implementation for Community-Based Psychosocial Interventions* (Oxford University Press, 2009)

Sruthi Chandrasekaran, a research associate at J-PAL, works on randomized control trials to evaluate health projects. A Felix scholar, she holds an integrated master's degree in economics from the Indian Institute of Technology, Madras and an MSc in comparative social policy from the University of Oxford. She has interned on projects at the Indian Institute of Management-Ahmedabad, Max Planck Institute for Human Development (Berlin), and Kenya Education Partnerships. She is interested in understanding the use of behavioral economics tools to tackle policy issues.

Rachna Nag Chowdhuri works at J-PAL on evaluations of education and health programs across India. She completed her master's degree in development economics from the University of Sussex in 2009. Before joining J-PAL, Rachna worked as a graduate intern economist at a nonprofit in Vietnam, where she was involved in conducting a baseline survey in Lao PDR to analyze the impact of bamboo sector interventions in the region.

Amy Corneli is a social scientist at FHI 360. She has a PhD in health behavior and health education from the University of North Carolina at Chapel Hill and an MPH in international health from Emory University. Over the past 18 years, Amy has conducted social science research in multiple countries in Africa, the Middle East, Asia, and North America focusing on HIV prevention, the prevention of micronutrient malnutrition, and research ethics, including research on the comprehension of informed consent, acceptability of informed assent, and functioning of research ethics committees. Amy has also been involved in IRB capacity-building activities in Africa and has published ethics-related research in the *Journal of Medical Ethics, AIDS and Behavior, Journal of the International AIDS Society, Journal of Empirical Research on Human Research Ethics,* and *Contemporary Clinical Trials*. She also served as an investigator of research on pre-exposure prophylaxis (PrEP) for HIV prevention, including FEM-PrEP, a USAID-funded phase 3, placebo-controlled, clinical trial of oral Truvada as PrEP for HIV prevention in women in sub-Saharan Africa; and an NIH-funded study on PrEP and risk compensation, also among women in sub-Saharan Africa.

Elizabeth Costenbader, PhD, is a social scientist in the Department of Social and Behavioral Health Research at FHI 360. Her research has focused on understanding the social context of risk for HCV, HIV, and other STIs among injecting drug users, sex workers, men who have sex with men, and other high-risk populations both in the United States and in international settings, and she has often found social network analysis (SNA) to be useful in this type of research. Her experience with SNA includes working with sociometric as well as egocentric data and ranges from secondary analyses and mathematical modeling to designing and collecting empirical data on social, sexual, and drug-using networks. Betsy received her MS from the Harvard School of Public Health and her PhD from the Johns Hopkins School of Public Health.

Johnnie Daniel earned a PhD degree from the University of Michigan and a JD from the Georgetown University Law Center. He teaches courses in research methods and statistics at Howard University, where he is a full professor in the Department of Sociology and Criminology. He has also taught at Loyola University (Chicago), the University of Wisconsin-Milwaukee, Tuskegee University, and the University of Michigan. He has recently published *Sampling Essentials: Practical Guidelines for Making Sampling Choices*, a textbook written for the nontechnical researcher. He presents workshops on evaluation research, survey research, and proposal writing for researchers and others in government and private industry. Johnnie has served as a scholar in residence for the Health Care Financing Administration and as editor of the *Journal of Social and Behavioral Sciences*. Throughout his career he has conducted national and community surveys and other research across a wide range of topics for such private and public organizations as the National Science Foundation, U.S. Department of Transportation, U.S. Department of Treasury, U.S. Census Bureau, U.S. Department of the Army, U.S. Department of the Navy, U.S. District Court for the District of Columbia, District of Columbia Public Schools, DuPont Chemicals, Martin Marietta Corporation, the Institute for College Research Development and Support, and the Washington Urban League.

Deborah Dee is the Senior Scientist for the Applied Sciences Branch in the Division of Reproductive Health at the Centers for Disease Control and Prevention (CDC) and a commissioned officer in the U.S. Public Health Service. Deborah earned her undergraduate degree in psychology, and her MPH and PhD in maternal and child health, with a minor in epidemiology, from the University of North Carolina at Chapel Hill. She began her career at CDC in 2007 as an Epidemic Intelligence Service officer in the Division of Nutrition, Physical Activity, and Obesity, where she conducted research on breastfeeding, maternity care, foodborne-related outbreaks, pandemic influenza, and assessments of childhood obesity prevention programs. She also was involved in helping to establish the nation's Healthy People 2020 breastfeeding objectives, and was a key member of the federal interagency workgroup that developed the 2011 *Surgeon General's Call to Action to Support Breastfeeding*. She has collaborated on publications related to breastfeeding, health disparities, pandemic A (H1N1) influenza, and maternal and child health in general. She is a recognized expert on breastfeeding and provides related assistance to health professional and nonprofit organizations in programmatic and policy development.

Dázon Dixon Diallo received her MPH in maternal and child health from the University of Alabama at Birmingham. For more than 28 years, she has created, designed, and implemented community- and evidence-based strategies to address challenges to women's reproductive health, especially HIV and AIDS. Dázon is the founder and currently the president/CEO of SisterLove, a not-for-profit organization based in Atlanta, Georgia, and eMalahleni, Mpumalanga, South Africa. She also serves as adjunct faculty at Morehouse School of Medicine in the Master of Public Health Program. Dázon has over 20 years of experience as a community partner in behavioral, public health, and academic research, and nearly 30 years in nonprofit community-based health services. She has published articles in a diversity of journals, including *American Journal of Health Studies; Emory*

University International Law Review; Meridians: Feminism, Race and Transnationalism; AIDS and Behavior; Prevention Science; Journal of Acquired Immune Deficiency Syndrome; and *Emerging Infectious Diseases.*

Cam Donaldson holds the Yunus Chair in Social Business and Health at Glasgow Caledonian University. He is a leading health economist who has also held chairs at the Universities of Newcastle, Calgary, and Aberdeen and won £25m (£10m as PI) in research funding during his 30-year career. He is renowned for his methodological and practical research on economic evaluation and health care priority setting, having published over 200 refereed journal articles in economics, medical, health policy, and health management journals. Cam has coauthored or edited several books on various aspects of health economics and public service delivery, his latest offering being *Credit Crunch Health Care* (Policy Press, 2011). Cam's work has attracted several competitive personal awards, including senior investigatorships from the Canadian Institutes of Health Research and the National Institute for Health Research, and the Health Foundation Chair in Health Economics. Since taking up the Yunus Chair in 2010, his main focus has been in assessing impacts of microcredit and social business on health and wellbeing.

Paul Fleming is completing a PhD at the University of North Carolina in Chapel Hill in the Department of Health Behavior. He is currently a predoctoral trainee at the Carolina Population Center, where he conducts HIV prevention research in the Dominican Republic focusing on the role of male gender norms in men's sexual behaviors. Previously, he was a public health research fellow at FHI 360, where he worked on global sexual and reproductive health projects in Ghana, Tanzania, and India. His research uses both quantitative and qualitative research methods to identify new and innovative culturally appropriate strategies for promoting sexual and reproductive health. He received his BA from the University of Illinois in Urbana-Champaign and MPH from Emory University.

Paula M. Frew is currently assistant professor of medicine in the Division of Infectious Diseases at the Emory University School of Medicine, and she holds a secondary appointment at the same rank in the Department of Behavioral Sciences and Health Education at the Emory Rollins School of Public Health. She currently serves as the director of applied community research at the Hope Clinic of the Emory Vaccine Research Center, Emory University School of Medicine. Her work has focused on engaging Black churches in the Hope in Our Soul and Dose of Hope community-based clinical research intervention projects. She served as co-principal investigator at the Atlanta site on the HIV Prevention Trials Network women's HIV seroincidence estimation study and served as a qualitative research leader on its companion study, Understanding Women's HIV Risk in the United States. She has also been an active investigator with the Women's Interagency HIV Study, the HIV Vaccine Trials Network, the "Involvement" study, and EnhanceLink. Paula has authored several peer-reviewed journal articles on health communication practices, HIV/AIDS clinical trial and prevention product acceptability issues, and the role of community engagement in prevention research. She holds an undergraduate degree from the University of California at San Diego, an MA in liberal arts: health, culture, and society from San Diego State University, an MPH from Emory University, and a PhD in health promotion and behavior from the University of Georgia. She recently was awarded the Gerald Ludd Lifetime Achievement Award for HIV/AIDS Community Service from the National AIDS Education and Services for Minorities and the Outstanding Early Career Research Award from Emory University Department of Medicine.

Angie M. Funaiole is pursuing a degree in prevention science with an emphasis in health communication. Her research focuses on the utilization of participatory research models to advance understanding of health inequities. Specifically, she examines how to develop practical, evidence-based strategies at the community level to address the social, economic, political, and environmental conditions that contribute to health outcomes. Prior to pursuing her doctoral degree, Angie worked for a nonprofit organization in Connecticut, where she devised communication plans to enhance the delivery of public health services across the state. Primarily, she supported a healthy equity initiative funded by the W. K. Kellogg Foundation.

Theresa Gamble received her PhD in biophysics from the University of California, San Francisco. Subsequent to earning her degree, she completed two postdoctoral fellowships, one at the University of Utah conducting basic laboratory research in HIV and the other at Cato Research, gaining experience in clinical research, drug development, and regulatory affairs. For the past 11 years, she has worked as a clinical research scientist at FHI 360, designing and managing international and domestic clinical trials in the area of HIV and AIDS prevention, treatment, and vaccine development. She has published articles in journals such as *Sexually Transmitted Diseases, Current Opinion in HIV & AIDS, Contemporary Clinical Trials, The Open AIDS Journal, New England Journal of Medicine, JAIDS, Science,* and *Cell.*

Glenn Gamst received his doctorate in experimental psychology from the University of Arkansas. He is professor and chair of the Psychology Department at the University of La Verne, where he teaches the doctoral advanced statistics sequence. He also teaches undergraduate courses in cognitive psychology and the introductory course. He has coauthored the following statistics texts: *Applied Multivariate Research: Design and Interpretation* (2nd ed., Sage, 2013), *Performing Data Analysis Using IBM SPSS* (Wiley, 2013), *Data Analysis Using SAS Enterprise Guide* (Cambridge, 2009), and *Analysis of Variance Designs* (Cambridge, 2008). He also coauthored *Handbook of Multicultural Measures* (Sage, 2011) and *CBMCS Multicultural Training Program* (Sage, 2008). His current research program examines the effects of multicultural variables on clinical outcome and client service satisfaction.

A. J. Guarino received his bachelor's degree from the University of California, Berkeley, and a PhD from the University of Southern California in educational psychology with an emphasis in statistics and research methodologies. Currently, he is professor of biostatistics at Massachusetts General Hospital, Institute of Health Professions, where he serves as the methodologist for graduate students' capstones and dissertations and teaches the advanced biostatistics courses. He is the statistician on numerous NIH grants and coauthor of several statistical textbooks.

Karen Hacker is the director of the Allegheny County Health Department in Pennsylvania. She previously held the position of executive director of the Institute for Community Health, in Cambridge, Massachusetts. She was also an associate professor of medicine at the Harvard Medical School and Harvard School of Public Health, where she taught Community-Based Participatory Action Research. Additionally, she served as the senior medical director for public and community health at the Cambridge Health Alliance and provided leadership for population health initiatives as well as practicing as a primary care physician. She received her MD from Northwestern University, her adolescent medicine fellowship from Children's Hospital of Los Angeles, and her master's from Boston University. She has extensive experience with community-based participatory research (CPBR) and has worked with diverse community partners on topics that include child mental health, immigrant health, obesity prevention, and school health centers. Karen is the author of *Community-Based Participatory Research* (Sage) and numerous journal articles and research reports. She has also served on many state and national committees and led CBPR efforts for the Harvard Clinical Translational Science Award-Harvard Catalyst.

Kathy Hageman is a behavioral scientist for the Behavioral Surveillance Team, Division of HIV/AIDS Prevention (DHAP), at the U.S. Centers for Disease Control and Prevention, which conducts the National HIV Behavioral Surveillance System (NHBS) among populations at risk for HIV (men who have sex with men, injection drug users, and heterosexuals at increased risk). She received her MPH and PhD in behavioral science and health education at the Rollins School of Public Health at Emory University with a primary focus on HIV among serodiscordant couples in sub-Saharan Africa. While at CDC, she has designed and implemented qualitative, formative, and evaluation research; assisted in the design, implementation, and analyses of NHBS; and provided technical support to DHAP's Open Label Study for pre-exposure prophylaxis in Botswana to monitor sexual behavior and adherence.

Danielle Haley received her MPH from the University of North Carolina at Chapel Hill, Department of Health Behavior, and at the time of publication is a doctoral student at Emory University's Laney Graduate School in the Department of Behavioral Sciences and Health Education. She has over 11 years of experience working in HIV/AIDS prevention, care, and support both in the United States and abroad. Danielle's areas of expertise include a focus on women at risk, substance-using and incarcerated populations, with a special interest in social and structural determinants of health. She has published articles in journals such as *Annals of Internal Medicine, JAIDS,* and *Journal of Offender Rehabilitation.*

Douglas H. Hamilton received both his PhD in microbiology and his MD from Vanderbilt University. He completed residencies in family practice (University of Minnesota) and preventive medicine (Centers for Disease Control and Prevention) and is board certified in family practice and a fellow in the American Academy of Family

Physicians. In addition to his CDC position, he holds an adjunct assistant professor appointment at the Rollins School of Public Health, Emory University, in Atlanta. In 2010, Douglas was recognized as the U.S. Public Health Service Applied Public Health Physician of the Year. He has extensive experience in organizing and teaching epidemiology courses both domestically and in field epidemiology training programs in many countries around the globe. In his position at CDC, Douglas is responsible for the day-to-day operation and management of the Epidemic Intelligence Service (EIS) program, as well as providing the leadership necessary for the program to adapt to changing public health needs. With a current enrollment of approximately 160, the EIS officers serve as the frontline troops in CDC's response to public health emergencies, both domestic and international.

Rick Homan is a health economist with over 15 years of experience in operations research of health service delivery, including family planning, STI prevention and treatment services, HIV/AIDS programs, primary care, and prenatal care. In addition to program evaluation activities, Rick has been actively engaged in capacity building among service providers and researchers in techniques of applied health economics. He has extensive experience in the evaluation of clinical and community-based service delivery initiatives, assessing the cost-effectiveness of interventions, and assessing the cost of program scale-up. Currently Rick works with governmental and NGO service providers in South Asia and in East and Southern Africa. Prior to joining FHI 360, Rick worked with the Department of Veterans Affairs to assess the efficiency of primary care services within the VA system. He has a PhD from the University of Michigan and is an adjunct professor in the Department of Health Policy and Management in the Gillings School of Public Health at the University of North Carolina at Chapel Hill.

Andrea Kim, PhD, MPH is the chief of surveillance and epidemiology at CDC's Division of Global HIV/AIDS (DGHA) in Kenya. Prior to this, Andrea joined the DGHA Kenya team as a senior epidemiologist to provide direct technical advice to the National AIDS and STD Control Programme (NASCOP) on CDC-supported HIV surveillance initiatives. In this role, she focused on building the technical and scientific capacity within NASCOP and other Government of Kenya divisions in the design, implementation, analysis, dissemination, and use of surveillance and epidemiologic data. Andrea has served as a CDC epidemic intelligence service officer (2004–2006) and epidemiologist (2006–2011) on the HIV surveillance team at DGHA in Atlanta. From 2001 to 2004, Andrea was an epidemiologist at the University of California San Francisco, where she led several HIV prevention studies among high-risk women in Cambodia. She has served as a reviewer for numerous publications and conference proceedings, presented over 50 abstracts in international and domestic conferences, and authored over 40 publications in peer-reviewed journals. Andrea holds a PhD in epidemiology from the University of California at Berkley (2003), an MPH in the epidemiology of microbial diseases from Yale University (1998), and a BS in microbiology and molecular genetics from the University of California Los Angeles (1996).

Kenny Lawson is an economist focused on the economic evaluation of social and public health interventions and the translation of evidence into policy. He is part of the Health

Economics and Health Technology Assessment team at the University of Glasgow and is 50% funded by the Medical Research Council's Social and Public Health Sciences Unit. He has a wide range of experience prior to academia as an applied economist in the government, international development, banking, and consultancy.

Temina Madon is executive director of the Center for Effective Global Action (CEGA), a research network headquartered at the University of California, Berkeley. CEGA focuses on rigorous evaluation of anti-poverty programs and economic development interventions, primarily in low-income countries. Her interests include scientific capacity in developing countries, research incentives for challenges neglected by the private sector, and the emerging field of implementation science. She has served as an advisor to the World Health Organization on implementation research and teaches a course at Berkeley on global health disparities. Earlier, Temina served as founding executive director of the Center for Emerging and Neglected Diseases at UC Berkeley. From 2006 to 2008, she was the science policy analyst for the Fogarty International Center at the National Institutes of Health. Prior to this, she led a portfolio of global health initiatives for the U.S. Senate HELP Committee (under the leadership of the late Senator Edward Kennedy), serving as an AAAS Congressional fellow. She received her PhD in 2004 from UC Berkeley and her BS in 1998 from MIT.

Helen Mason is a lecturer in health economics at Glasgow Caledonian University, working primarily in the area of economic evaluation. Helen's main research interest is in the development and use of methodologies to measure the benefits of health care. In 2007 she was awarded a PhD from Newcastle University, in which she developed methods to estimate the monetary value of quality-adjusted life years (QALYs).

Dr. **Emma McIntosh** has an MSc in health economics from York University and a PhD in economics. Emma is a Reader in Health Economics and program leader on the Economics of Population Health program at the University of Glasgow. Emma's methodological interests are in the area of economic evaluation methods, stated preference methods, and cost benefit analysis more generally. She recently co-authored a book titled *Applied Methods of Cost-Benefit Analysis in Health Care* as part of Oxford University Press's Handbooks in Health Economic Evaluation series. Emma also holds a senior research fellowship with Parkinson's UK. The title of the fellowship is The Economics of Parkinson's: Advancing the Scope of Costs and Benefits. She is on the editorial board of *The Patient* and is associate editor of *BMC Medical Research Methodology*.

Lawrence S. Meyers received his doctorate from Adelphi University and worked on a National Science Foundation postdoctoral fellowship at the University of Texas, Austin, and Purdue University. The rest of his academic career has been spent at California State University, Sacramento, where he is currently a full professor of psychology. He teaches undergraduate and graduate courses in research design, data analysis, and data interpretation; testing and measurement; and history and systems of psychology. He was a coauthor of a textbook in research methods in the 1970s. More recently, he coauthored the second edition of *Applied Multivariate Research: Design and Interpretation* (Sage, 2013). He also coauthored *Analysis of Variance Designs* (Cambridge, 2008), *Data Analysis*

Using SAS Enterprise Guide (Cambridge, 2009), and *Performing Data Analysis Using IBM SPSS* (Wiley, 2013). He has over three dozen publications; some of his relatively recent work has been in such areas as measurement/testing and positive psychology. He has also offered expert consulting in test validation, development, and evaluation; employment promotion/selection procedures; adverse impact analysis; organizational and consumer survey design and analysis; and research design and data analysis.

Candace Nykiforuk, is an associate professor in the School of Public Health, University of Alberta, and is a health geographer and health promotion researcher with a strong interest in the role of built and social environments on health and well-being. She also has expertise in the development and diffusion of healthy public policies, particularly in how these create the settings-based conditions for health. The work undertaken in her Place Research Lab employs geographic information systems (GIS) and spatial analysis in the areas of community environments and health, prevention of cancer and other chronic diseases, tobacco control, and health program evaluation. Candace's research has involved children, youth, adult, and senior populations across multiple settings and is grounded in social-ecological theory and community-based participatory research perspectives. Most of her studies over the past 15 years have employed mixed methods, involving both quantitative and qualitative techniques, as well as the use of GIS for data analysis and sharing findings with researchers, practitioners, and decision-makers. Candace was the recipient of the 2009 CAFA Distinguished Academic Early Career Award for her scholarly contributions to the community beyond the university.

Hans C. Ossebaard studied clinical and developmental psychology at Utrecht University and received his PhD in social sciences from the University of Twente, in the Netherlands. His primary interest is on how information and communication technologies can support and improve (public) health and healthcare. He is a product manager and researcher at the Dutch National Institute for Public Health and the Environment, where he specializes in consumer health informatics, eHealth, and ePublic Health. As a lecturer and researcher he is also affiliated with the Center for eHealth Research and Disease Management, the Institute for Governance and Innovation Studies, and the Department of Psychology, Health and Technology of the University of Twente. Hans is a member of the Board of the Netherlands Society for Research on Internet Interventions and a fellow of eTELEMED, International Academy, Research and Industry Association. As an eHealth advisor he currently works at the Dutch Institute for Health Care Quality. He has recently published articles in the *Journal of Medical Internet Research, Bulletin of the World Health Organization, Policy & Internet, International Journal of Medical Informatics,* and *Journal of Telemedicine and Telecare* and coedited the book *Improving eHealth* (2013).

Jeffery Chaichana Peterson is an Associate Professor of Communication at Washington State University where his research and teaching focus on issues related to culture, communication, and health. He has investigated the creation, utilization, and dissemination of both science-based research and habit-based public health practice created *for, with,* and *by* vulnerable communities (e.g., Hispanic farm workers, American Indians, the formerly homeless). He received his PhD from the University of New Mexico where he also served as a Research Associate at the Center for Health Promotion and Disease

Prevention (CHPDP). He is a former Minority Doctoral Fellow from the U.S. Associated Schools of Public Health/Centers for Disease Control and Prevention/Prevention Research Centers. He has published in such journals as the *American Journal of Preventive Medicine, Health Education & Behavior, Health Communication,* and the *Journal of International and Intercultural Communication,* among others.

Heidi W. Reynolds is the deputy director for HIV/AIDS and Other Infectious Diseases for the MEASURE Evaluation Project, based in the Carolina Population Center, and an adjunct assistant professor in the Department of Maternal and Child Health at the University of North Carolina at Chapel Hill (UNC-CH). MEASURE Evaluation is the U.S. Agency for International Development (USAID) Global Health Bureau's primary vehicle for supporting improvements in monitoring and evaluation in population, health, and nutrition worldwide. As deputy director she provides leadership, technical direction, and management of HIV and AIDS activities; liaises with USAID and other global partners; and provides oversight of activities in other infectious diseases and emerging public health priorities. Heidi's areas of expertise include health service integration, health services research, and evaluation. Prior to joining UNC, she worked for 7 years at Family Health International (now FHI 360), leading HIV and family planning health service research studies. She has worked professionally in Cote d'Ivoire, Ethiopia, Ghana, Haiti, Kenya, Senegal, Uganda and Zambia. She was a Fulbright Doctoral Scholar in France and lived in Gabon for 2 years as a Peace Corps volunteer. Heidi holds a PhD in maternal and child health from UNC-CH and an MPH in health behavior and health education from UNC-CH.

Travis Sanchez received a doctorate of veterinary medicine from the University of Georgia in 1994. After a veterinary internship at North Carolina State University, he practiced as an emergency veterinarian in the Metro Atlanta area until he returned to the Rollins School of Public Health at Emory University and received his MPH in international health and epidemiology in 2000. Travis began his public health career working for the Georgia Division of Public Health in the notifiable diseases epidemiology section and coordinated the state's district epidemiologist program. He came to CDC in 2001 and worked for the Surveillance Branch in the Division of HIV/AIDS Prevention and later for the newly created Behavioral and Clinical Surveillance Branch (BCSB) as a project officer for the National HIV Behavioral Surveillance System. In 2005, he became BCSB's associate chief for science and served for extended periods as an acting team leader and the acting branch chief for BCSB. Travis participated in CDC's IETA program in Vietnam in 2005 and worked closely with CDC's associate director for science in 2007 during a training detail. From 2008 to 2009 he was the chief of the Epidemiology and Strategic Information Branch of the CDC-South Africa office. From 2009 to 2011, Travis served as the associate chief for science in the HIV Epidemiology Branch at CDC. In 2011 he took an associate professor appointment with the Rollins School of Public Health in the Department of Epidemiology. His current projects include a web-based HIV behavioral surveillance among men who have sex with men; InvolveMENt, an Atlanta prospective cohort study of men who have sex with men to explain differences in HIV and STI prevalence and incidence between black and white MSM; and AIDSVu, an online resource with continually updated information about HIV infections in the United States.

Nirupama Sista received her PhD in microbiology from the University of Tennessee, Knoxville. She started her professional career as a research assistant professor at the University of North Carolina at Chapel Hill, after her postdoctoral fellowship there. Niru is a career researcher with more than 20 years of experience in the academic, pharmaceutical, and nonprofit sectors. She served as a medical team leader for a novel antiretroviral molecule at Triangle Pharmaceuticals (which was acquired by Gilead Sciences), and in that capacity collaborated with regulatory authorities, physician and community advisory boards, and others. She currently serves as the Director of the Leadership and Operations Center for HPTN, at FHI 360, where she oversees the development and implementation of all ongoing clinical research studies in the United States and internationally. Her role also focuses on strategic partnerships with funding agencies and all the collaborative partners. In this capacity, she has served on workshops hosted by WHO and other organizations focusing on HIV prevention. She has published articles in journals such as *Clinical Investigations, JAIDS, Proceedings of National Academy of Sciences, Nucleic Acids Research, Molecular and Cell Biology,* and *Journal of Virology* as well as book chapters.

C. Kay Smith, MEd, has more than 30 years' experience in scientific writing and editing, publishing, and adult instruction. She is the lead health communication specialist in the Science Office of the Division of Scientific Education and Professional Development (DESPD) at the Centers for Disease Control and Prevention (CDC). Kay came to CDC in 1997 from the Indian Health Service, where she had served as the environmental protection specialist for 23 federally recognized Indian tribes located throughout the eastern United States. After transferring to CDC, she became a lead technical writer-editor with the *Morbidity and Mortality Weekly Report* serial publications, and in 2005 she became the lead health communication specialist in the Science Office of the newly formed Office of Workforce and Career Development under the directorship of Dr. Stephen B. Thacker. That CDC program office eventually evolved into DESPD, but through the various reincarnations of the organization, Kay has continued to work closely with CDC's premiere disease detectives, the Epidemic Intelligence Service Officers.

Phyllis Solomon, PhD, is a professor in the School of Social Policy and Practice, a professor of social work in psychiatry, Department of Psychiatry, and senior fellow, Center for Public Health Initiatives, University of Pennsylvania. In 2013, she was the Moses Distinguished Visiting Professor at the Silberman School of social Work, Hunter College. She has conducted a number of psychosocial randomized controlled trials (RCTs), mainly in public mental health, as well as on the Internet. Phyllis coauthored *Randomized Controlled Trials: Design and Implementation for Community-Based Psychosocial Interventions.* One of her articles, reporting on the results of an RCT, received the first place award from the Society of Social Work and Research. She has received a number of awards for her work in mental health and psychiatric rehabilitation, including the Knee/ Wittman Outstanding Lifetime Achievement Award in Mental Health Policy and Practice from NASW Foundation, Outstanding Non-Psychiatrist Community Achievement Award from American Association of Community Psychiatrists, and Armin Loeb award for Research in Psychosocial Rehabilitation from the International association of Psychosocial

Rehabilitation Services. In 2014, Dr. Solomon received the Distinguished Career Achievement Award from the Society of Social Work and Research.

Michael Stalker, MPH, has more than 20 years' experience working with sexual and reproductive health programs, including the design, implementation, and evaluation of sexual and reproductive health interventions; more than 10 years' experience working with government officials, local implementation partners, and scientific and technical staff on HIV/AIDS prevention; and 5 years' experience coordinating epidemiological and behavioral research. Michael has also worked with research professionals and program managers/implementers to translate findings into policies and programs, ensuring evidence-based best practices inform expended services. His experience in service delivery has provided insight into the challenges in delivering quality services. That experience, combined with a natural curiosity on the role of attitudes and beliefs in health behaviors, led to the exploration of vignettes as an optimal approach to identify possible sources of variation in the provider-patient interaction.

Donna F. Stroup, PhD, MSc, has over 20 years of international experience in building high-performing research teams, spearheading epidemiology programs, and impacting public health worldwide. She is currently the founding director of Data for Solutions, a scientific research firms with clients throughout the United States and internationally. She is a senior consultant for UNAIDS and WHO on estimating the sizes of populations at risk of HIV and AIDS in Southeast Asia, Eastern Europe, the Middle East and Africa, and the Caribbean. Prior to establishing her firm, Donna was a senior scientist at the Centers for Disease Control and Prevention, where she directed critical scientific and program activities in infectious diseases, including HIV and AIDS, and chronic disease prevention and health promotion. As part of her duties, she orchestrated national public health surveillance activities, including initiating surveillance for HIV and AIDS in the 1980s. Donna has served on the faculties of Emory University, the University of Georgia, St. George's University, the University of Texas-Austin, Rider University, and Temple University. She is a fellow of the American Statistical Association, an elected member of the American Epidemiologic Association, and an honorary member of the Epidemic Intelligence Service. Donna holds an MS in community medicine (Cambridge University), PhD in statistics (Princeton University), an MSc in mathematical statistics (University of North Carolina, Chapel Hill), and BA in mathematics (Magna Cum Laude, Vanderbilt University). She serves on numerous editorial boards and scientific review committees and is the author or coauthor of more than 200 publications.

Stephen B. Thacker, MD, MSc, RADM/ASG (ret.), U.S. Public Health Service, passed away in February 2013. Throughout his 37 years at CDC, Dr. Thacker was a leader of public health science and the professionals who practice that science. He served as the director of the Office of Surveillance, Epidemiology, and Laboratory Services (2010–2012), director of the Office of Workforce and Career Development (2004–2010), and director of the Epidemiology Program Office (1989–2004), as well as acting director of multiple centers. As a committed steward of CDC's programs, Dr. Thacker ensured their viability, credibility, and scientific rigor. For more than 20 years, he reviewed articles to be published in

CDC's *Morbidity and Mortality Weekly Report.* He was instrumental in the development of Epi Info and the Guide to Community Preventive Services. Programs developed or expanded under his leadership include the EIS Program, the Public Health Informatics Fellowship Program, the Public Health Prevention Service, and the Prevention Effectiveness Fellowship. He also was instrumental in launching the Field Epidemiology Training Programs in more than 35 countries. Dr. Thacker held an undergraduate degree from Princeton University (1969), a medical degree from Mount Sinai School of Medicine (1973), and a master of science from the London School of Hygiene and Tropical Medicine (1984). His accomplishments were recognized through more than 40 major awards and commendations. Among his greatest honors were the Philip S. Brachman Friend of EIS Award (2002), the Charles C. Shepard Lifetime Scientific Achievement Award (2009), and the Surgeon General's Medallion (2013). Through more than 240 publications on public health surveillance, meta-analyses, infectious diseases, environmental public health, injury prevention, sports medicine, and other topics, his influence on public health practice will continue well into the future.

Mitesh Thakkar is the co-founder of Fieldata.org. He has worked globally on development initiatives with organizations like Pratham (India), the World Bank (United States), Altai Consulting (Afghanistan), and Ministry of Education (Vietnam). He holds a BA in astronomy from the University of Texas, Austin; an EdM in education policy from Harvard University; and an MBA from INSEAD.

Robert T. Trotter II is a Regents' Professor, and Associate Vice President for Research (Translational Health Research Initiative), Northern Arizona University. His research and applied anthropology interests include the confluences among cross-cultural health care delivery systems, traditional healing, organizational research, ethnographic methods, social network analysis, ethics, alcohol and drug abuse, evaluation research, community-based participatory research, rapid ethnographic assessment, HIV/AIDS prevention, cancer disparities, cardio/pulmonary transitional care, culturally competent interventions, and cultural models research. He has worked on collaborative projects with the National Institutes of Health (NIDA, NIMH, NCI), the Centers for Disease Control and Prevention, and the World Health Organization. He has more than 140 publications, and his most recent books are *Ethics in Anthropological Research and Practice* (with Linda Whiteford; Wadsworth, 2008), *Partnering for Performance: Collaboration and Culture From the Inside Out* (with Elizabeth K. Briody; Rowman and Littlefield, 2008), and *Transforming Culture: Creating a Better Manufacturing Organization* (with Elizabeth K. Briody and Tracy L. Meerwarth; Palgrave-Macmillan, 2010).

Thomas W. Valente, PhD, is a professor in the Department of Preventive Medicine, Institute for Prevention Research, Keck School of Medicine, University of Southern California. He is author of *Social Networks and Health: Models, Methods, and Applications* (Oxford University Press, 2010); *Evaluating Health Promotion Programs* (Oxford University Press, 2002); *Network Models of the Diffusion of Innovations* (Hampton Press, 1995); and over 125 articles and chapters on social networks, behavior change, and program evaluation. Tom uses social network analysis, health communication, and mathematical models to implement and evaluate health promotion programs designed to prevent tobacco and substance abuse, unintended fertility, and STD/HIV infections. He is also engaged in mapping community coalitions and collaborations to improve health care delivery and reduce healthcare disparities. He received his BS in mathematics from the University of Mary Washington, his MS in mass communication from San Diego State University, and his PhD from the Annenberg School for Communication at the University of Southern California. In 2008 he was a visiting senior scientist at National Institutes of Health for 6 months, and in 2010–2011 he was a visiting professor at the École des Haute Études en Santé Publique (Paris/Rennes).

Lisette van Gemert-Pijnen received her PhD in communication sciences from the University of Twente, in the Netherlands. Today she is associate professor at the University of Twente, for design and adherence to eHealth interventions, at the University Medical Center Groningen, and adjunct professor at the University of Waterloo, in Canada. Lisette founded and is the director of the first Center for eHealth Research and Disease Management (www.ehealthresearchcenter.nl). Her research group's program focusses on persuasive designs (people-driven) and business modeling (value-driven) for interactive eHealth interventions, in particular on how persuasive designs can increase trust, engagement, and adherence to eHealth interventions aimed at safe care and self-care. Lisette is the chief editor of the book *Improving eHealth*, which provides mixed methods for developing and implementing eHealth interventions aimed at behavior change. She has published in several high-impact journals on eHealth (*Journal of Medical Internet Research*) and health informatics (*Journal of Medical Informatics*), and she contributes as keynote to several international eHealth conferences. Lisette is chief editor of the *International Journal on Advances Life Sciences*. She is part of the scientific board of eTelemed conferences and the association for Health Informatics (NIHI) Canada. She received an award for outstanding research (IARIA, 2011). Lisette collaborates with the University of Groningen (UMCG, EurSafetyHealthnet) and with the National Institute for Public Health and Environment) to enhance compliance with safety precautions and with the University of Toronto in PhD projects about eHealth interventions for chronic care.

Lee Warner, PhD, MPH, is currently Associate Director for Science for the Division of Reproductive Health at the Centers for Disease Control and Prevention. He received his undergraduate degree in business administration from the University of North Carolina at Chapel Hill and his doctoral degree in epidemiology from the Rollins School of Public Health of Emory University. He joined the CDC in 1996 with the Division of HIV/AIDS Prevention and previously worked with the Office of Perinatal Epidemiology at the Georgia Division of Public Health and the Department of Gynecology and Obstetrics at Emory University. He also is an adjunct associate professor with the College of Public Health at the University of Georgia. During his 20-year career, Lee has published numerous research articles and book chapters in various areas related to reproductive health, including the use and effectiveness of contraception, adolescent pregnancy, HIV counseling and testing, STD/HIV prevention interventions, congenital syphilis prevention, infertility, and male circumcision. He is a nationally recognized expert in the evaluation of barrier method effectiveness and was recently a member of the FDA's Advisory Panel for Obstetrics and Gynecologic Devices. Lee was the recipient of the 2006 CDC Charles

C. Shepard Science Award for Scientific Excellence in Assessment and Epidemiology, in recognition of his methodologic work examining the effectiveness of condoms for STD prevention.

Mark A. Weaver received his PhD in biostatistics from the University of North Carolina at Chapel Hill (UNC-CH). He is currently a faculty member in the Departments of Medicine and Biostatistics at UNC-CH, where he primarily supports the career development of junior faculty in Medicine and Public Health as part of the NC Translational and Clinical Sciences Institute. Prior to returning to academia, Mark spent almost 8 years at Family Health International (now FHI 360), where he helped to design, analyze, and interpret the results of numerous randomized, cluster-randomized, and observational global health studies with clinical, behavioral, and health services research outcomes.

Nikhil Wilmink, is a policy and training associate for CLEAR/J-PAL South Asia at IFMR. He has worked on randomized evaluations assessing the impact of education programs of Pratham, the largest education focused NGO in India. He has been working with the J-PAL Policy and Training team in Delhi, as well as working with the CLEAR initiative to strengthen monitoring and evaluation capacity in South Asia. He holds an honors degree in international development studies from McGill University.

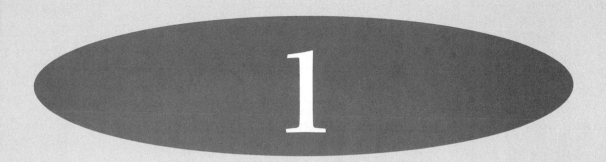

Introduction to Public Health Research Methods

Greg Guest

Governments will always play a huge part in solving big problems. They set public policy and are uniquely able to provide the resources to make sure solutions reach everyone who needs them. They also fund basic research, which is a crucial component of the innovation that improves life for everyone.

Bill Gates

Public health practice aims to protect and improve the health of a community or population. Improvements can be achieved through preventive medicine, health education, control of communicable diseases, and the application of policy or infrastructural change, among other activities. Governmental will and public policy play a critical role in the well-being of a nation's citizens. But as Bill Gates observes above, research is an integral part of this process. In short, good policy and practice rely on good research to inform them.

The word *research* derives from the Middle French *recherche*, which means "to go about seeking." Research is the process of seeking out, collecting, and analyzing data to advance the collective knowledge about a particular theory, topic, or problem. Research provides the foundational knowledge upon which health policy and practice are—or at least should be—formulated and revised as new evidence emerges.

Contemporary public health research is incredibly diverse and multidisciplinary in nature, reflecting the complex interaction among human biology and behavior, environmental factors, and disease. The outcomes of this research, when put into practice, can result in dramatic improvements in the health of individuals, communities, and populations. The chapters in this book describe the diverse array of public health research designs and methods used today. Some of these methods seem so well integrated with, and so much a part of, contemporary public health practice that we often forget many of these methods are recent developments, the majority of them adapted to

CHOLERA AND THE BROAD STREET PUMP

In the late summer of 1854, a major outbreak of cholera struck the Soho district of London. Over the course of just three days, 127 people on or near Broad Street died. Through various investigative techniques (which are described in this book), Dr. John Snow identified the public water pump on Broad Street (now Broadwick Street) as the source of the contaminated water causing the outbreak (see Chapters 6 and 7 for additional detail on his methods). Snow subsequently took his findings to the local parish authorities. They (reluctantly) agreed to close the pump, and the spread of cholera stopped abruptly as a result. This quasi-experiment provided the first real evidence of a water-borne vector for cholera.

Figure 1.1   "Death's Dispensary," by John Pinwell. Published in *Fun* magazine, a British satirical journal, in 1866

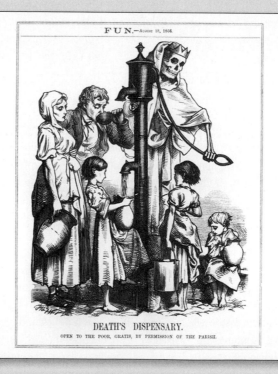

public health after World War II. These designs and methods also evolved from a series of discoveries, events, and innovations and the diffusion of knowledge across a range of academic fields. This history is briefly outlined below.

A BRIEF HISTORY OF PUBLIC HEALTH RESEARCH

Public health research has come a long way since John Snow's cholera investigation and the iconic removal of London's Broad Street water pump handle in 1854 (see text box). Health in the industrialized cities of mid-19th century Europe suffered as the industrial revolution expanded. Living conditions in the rapidly growing urban centers deteriorated, with poorly built houses rendering damp and unsafe conditions. This, combined with poor ventilation and crowded quarters, created a ripe environment for the spread of disease. Low standards of sanitation and a corresponding lack of potable water compounded the situation, leading to frequent outbreaks of water-borne diseases such as cholera and typhoid. Working conditions in factories and coal mines (particularly grueling for young children) also contributed to the urban syndemic, as did malnutrition and other afflictions associated with poverty and overcrowding. The prominent diseases of the time (Table 1.1) are a testament to these conditions.

Table 1.1   Top 10 Causes of Death in London—1850 (contemporary terminology)

1. Tuberculosis	6. Pneumonia
2. Dysentery/diarrhea	7. Diphtheria
3. Cholera	8. Scarlet Fever
4. Malaria	9. Meningitis
5. Typhoid Fever	10. Whooping Cough

Based on a growing body of knowledge about disease transmission and a burgeoning advocacy for workers' rights and the well-being of the poor, several bold public measures in the United Kingdom laid the foundation for healthier British cities, and the country as a whole:

- Child labor laws were passed in 1833, which began the progressive move toward increasing occupational safety.
- In 1848 the first Public Health Act established a Board of Health and gave towns the right to appoint a Medical Officer of Health. One of the first things medical officers did was to order the improvement of drainage systems and construction practices for houses and streets (though these took a long time to implement).

- In 1853 vaccination against smallpox was made compulsory; many other countries followed suit, leading to eventual worldwide eradication of the disease in 1979.
- In 1854 improvements in hospital hygiene were initiated, and over time these reduced the number of deaths caused by infection contracted during surgery.
- In 1875 a Public Health Act strengthened the enforcement of laws about slum clearance and provision of sewers.

Similar measures were taken in other industrial nations in due course, and by the turn of the 20th century, many of the worst public health problems of the 1800s had been eradicated or were in decline. Better living and working conditions coupled with public health and medical advances, such as development of vaccines and routine use of disinfectants, led to a rise in life expectancy and a decrease in both child and infant mortality in most industrial nations during the early 1900s.

PUBLIC HEALTH: THE EARLY, EARLY YEARS

When we think of the formative years of public health, most of us likely think of British scientists such as John Snow, Edwin Chadwick, and William Farr. And indeed these individuals, and other scientists of 19th century, can be credited with many of the concepts that have led to the research methods and practice we see in public health today. Their contributions to the field are indisputable. But we must also acknowledge that an earlier public health exists, beginning with the earliest civilizations and emergence of cities. Archaeological evidence of bathrooms and sanitation drains, for example, dates as far back as 4,000 years ago in regions such as Northern India, Egypt, and Crete (Rosen, 1958/1993). The Romans took water management to entirely new levels some 1,500 years later, building massive aqueducts (to supply potable water) and drainage facilities for their growing urban populations.

Systematic disease surveillance can be traced back to at least the ancient Greeks in the 5th century BC, who tracked the prevalence of malaria and observed the association between the disease, the seasons, and the presence of swamps (though discovery of the real causal vector eluded them).

Immunization provides another example from antiquity. According to Temple (1986), smallpox inoculation was practiced as early as the 10th century in China, preceding the first vaccines of the early 1800s by more than 800 years. These early inoculations took the form of inhaling powdered smallpox scabs through one's nose, or scratching material from smallpox lesions into one's skin (a process known as variolation).

These are just a few notable examples of public health practices that have been documented in antiquity.

Figure 1.2   Public "Toilets" in Ephesus, Turkey (circa 1st century AD)

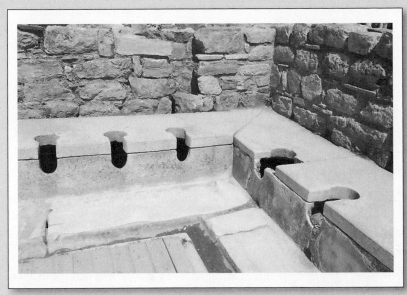

Source: Photo courtesy of ScheckTrek Travel. http://schecktrek.blogspot .com/2011/06/day-9-ephesus-turkey-oceania-cruise.html

The Emergence of Observational and Quasi-Experimental Designs

Trends in public health research methodology parallel both the trajectory of contemporary health issues of the times and methodological advances made in fields outside of public health. Ecological studies, which focused on populations rather than individuals, and registry studies (using government data on causes of death) were common practice in the 1800s, particularly in the United Kingdom. Snow, however, an innovator for his time, went beyond these types of research and employed observational and quasi-experimental designs. He went door to door in various districts of London, collecting data about cholera and sources of drinking water (among other methods). Once he had enough observational data to develop a hypothesis, he employed a quasi-experimental design by removing the water pump handle from Broad Street and observing the effect.

During the latter part of the 19th century, the identification of, and understanding behind, disease agents and vectors progressed. Robert Koch, a German bacteriologist, isolated and identified the tubercle bacillus (*Mycobacterium tuberculosis*) in 1882 and the bacterium that causes cholera (*Vibrio cholerae*) in 1883. Alphonse Laveren, a French army surgeon, discovered the parasite responsible for malaria in humans (*Plasmodium*) in 1880. It took another army surgeon, in the Indian Medical Services, Ronald Ross, to identify the vector behind the transmission of the parasite. Following up on the mosquito vector theory of malaria proposed by Patrick Manson in 1894, Ross looked for, and found, the *Plasmodium* parasite in the stomach wall of an *Anopheles* mosquito in 1897 (Rosen, 1958/1993).

KEY TERMS

Public Health—the science and practice of protecting and improving the health of a community or population. Public health includes preventive medicine, health education, control of communicable diseases, policy development and application, and infrastructural improvements.

Epidemiology—the study of the distribution and determinants of disease frequency in populations. Epidemiology focuses on the incidence and prevalence of disease in populations and the sources and causes of epidemics (Part II).

Behavioral Epidemiology—the study of human behavior and social structures and processes as they relate to health outcomes.

Surveillance—the ongoing systematic collection, analysis, interpretation, and dissemination of data pertaining to a health-related event in a community or population. Data are used to monitor trends in diseases and health-related behavior (Chapter 5).

Ecological Study—examines the relationship between exposure to a particular condition, or set of conditions, and disease with population-level rather than individual-level data.

Registry Study—uses data from an existing patient registry to understand trends in health and disease. A registry is an organized database containing uniform health information about individuals within a population.

Cohort Study—type of epidemiologic study design that compares disease incidence between individuals who have an exposure (exposed group) and comparable individuals who do not (unexposed group). Individuals within the cohort are defined according to their exposure levels and followed over time for disease occurrence (Chapter 7).

Case-Control Study—a type of epidemiologic study design that identifies individuals who develop a particular health condition (cases) and comparable individuals who do not (controls). Data on exposure history are compared between the groups to look for factors associated with development of the condition (Chapter 7).

Life-Course Perspective—a multidisciplinary approach to understanding the psychological, physical, and social health of individuals. The approach incorporates both life span and life stage concepts that determine an individual's health trajectory.

Multi-Causation Model (of Health)—a public health framework that views health and disease development as being dependent on multiple variables and levels of analysis.

Probability Theory—one of the foundational mathematical theories behind inferential statistics. Probability theory provides a quantitative estimation of the likelihood that an observed event or relationship is beyond random occurrence (Chapter 18).

Observational Research—a form of research in which no events or conditions are manipulated by the researcher, but rather passively observed as the natural occurrence of events unfolds (Chapter 2).

Quasi-Experimental Research Design—an observational study in which the individuals to be observed are not randomly assigned to a control or treatment group. Assignment is based on criteria determined by the investigator or conditions beyond the investigator's control. Pretest-posttest designs are quasi-experimental (Chapter 2).

Experimental Design—subjects are randomly assigned to one or more control groups and one or more treatment groups (Chapter 2).

Randomized Controlled Trial (RCT)—a type of experimental design, involving randomization, that is used in health research to test the efficacy and/or effectiveness of various types of health interventions (Chapters 8 and 16).

Clinical Trial—biomedical research study with human subjects designed to assess the safety, efficacy, or effectiveness of a biomedical intervention (e.g., drugs, treatments, devices; Chapter 8).

Qualitative Research—research that generates, collects, and/or analyzes data that are non-numerical in nature. In public health, qualitative data are typically in the form of words and narratives, from interview and focus groups, but also include images and unstructured observation (Chapter 15).

Quantitative Research—research that collects data in a structured format and in which the outcome is typically analyzed through statistical methods. Most biomedical and survey research is quantitative in nature.

Mixed Methods Research—research in which qualitative and quantitative methods are integrated within a single project or study (Chapter 19).

Vectors and agents became better understood through more sophisticated theories of disease and laboratory research, while at the same time the use of observational and quasi-experimental research increased in prevalence to become the predominant research paradigm by the early 1900s. Once a causal pathway between a vector and disease became suspected or demonstrated in a laboratory setting, interventions were developed to eradicate the vector, if feasible, and the prevalence of that disease was tracked. Time and good surveillance would tell whether an intervention was effective. In these formative years of modern epidemiology, a large number of lives were saved, particularly in urban centers, due to the epidemiological insights gained. Note that insight does not always immediately translate into action and better health outcomes. Application of knowledge and implementation of policy, no matter how scientifically sound, can be extremely difficult. A good example is the amount of effort and time it took to get good diphtheria vaccine coverage in New York City, as chronicled by Evelyn Hammonds (1999). Even with a proven vaccine, a massive media campaign and extensive community outreach efforts were required to achieve the desired coverage (Figure 1.3).

Figure 1.3 Diphtheria Mailer From the New York Immunization Campaigns of the 1920s

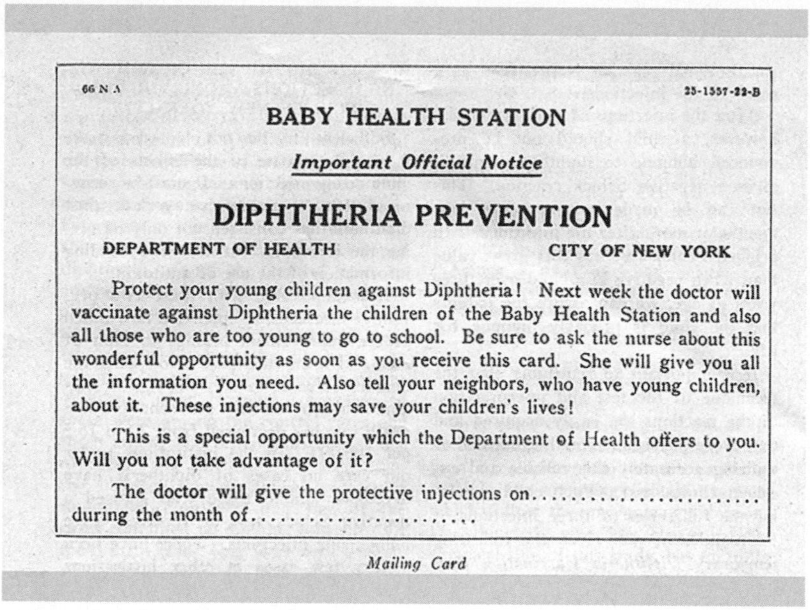
66 N A 25-1557-22-B

BABY HEALTH STATION

Important Official Notice

DIPHTHERIA PREVENTION

DEPARTMENT OF HEALTH CITY OF NEW YORK

Protect your young children against Diphtheria! Next week the doctor will vaccinate against Diphtheria the children of the Baby Health Station and also all those who are too young to go to school. Be sure to ask the nurse about this wonderful opportunity as soon as you receive this card. She will give you all the information you need. Also tell your neighbors, who have young children, about it. These injections may save your children's lives!

This is a special opportunity which the Department of Health offers to you. Will you not take advantage of it?

The doctor will give the protective injections on........................ during the month of........................

Mailing Card

Source: http://www.historyofvaccines.org/content/diphtheria-mailer

Chronic Disease and the Rise of Case-Control and Cohort Studies

As the deadly infectious and nutritional diseases that once plagued urban dwellers were expunged through better living conditions, vaccines, and other public health and

Table 1.2   Leading Causes of Death in London—1950

1. Heart disease	6. Influenza/pneumonia
2. Cancer	7. Tuberculosis
3. Stroke	8. Arteriosclerosis
4. Accidents	9. Kidney disease
5. Infant death	10. Diabetes

medical advancements, the epidemiological landscape (at least in developed countries) changed. By 1950, many of these diseases in industrialized countries had been virtually wiped out. New diseases began to dominate, with heart disease, cancer (predominantly lung), and stroke heading up the list (Table 1.2).

With the decline in infectious disease and the rise of noncommunicable diseases, a new epidemiologic paradigm emerged in the middle of the 20th century. The primary object of study shifted from the population to the individual level, and the role of multiple causes gained more prominence in epidemiologic thinking (Pearce, 1996). New study designs, data collection techniques, and analytic methods were developed and/or incorporated into public health research to accommodate the foci of the "new epidemiology" (Susser, 1985). Two notable advancements were the refinement and use of case-control and cohort study designs (Chapter 7), both employed in the pursuit of demonstrating the causal relationship between smoking and lung cancer.

Prior to the 1950s, statistical associations based on observational data did not constitute enough evidence to change public policy on smoking (which turned out to be a long and arduous process), so public health researchers needed improved research designs that could more convincingly document the causal connection between behavior and disease. Researchers responded with more rigorous case-control and cohort studies, and in 1950 results of three separate case-control studies connecting smoking and lung cancer were published (Doll & Hill, 1950; Levin, Goldstein, & Gerhardt, 1950; Wynder & Graham, 1950). A host of cohort and other case-control studies ensued, and in 1964 Doll and Hill published the results of a 10-year cohort study on the subject, known as the British Doctors Study (Doll & Hill, 1964). Doll and colleagues presented a another report on the same cohort 20 years into the study (Doll & Peto, 1976), another 40 years later (Doll, Peto, Wheatley, Gray, & Sutherland, 1994), and another representing the 50-year cohort (Doll, Peto, Boreham, & Sutherland, 2004).

The post-WWII era also ushered in birth and pregnancy cohort studies (Power & Elliot, 2006). This increased emphasis on the relationship between developmental processes and health outcomes ultimately led to the emergence of the *life-course perspective* in the 1960s (Lynch & Davey Smith, 2005), which views human development and health across the life span, from the prenatal period through senescence. The life-course approach has since become one of the prevailing conceptual frameworks in contemporary epidemiology and public health.

Randomized Controlled Trials

Another major research design type to emerge in public health during this period was the randomized control trial (RCT), which had its roots in experimental psychology (Peirce & Jastrow, 1885), education (see Stigler, 1992), and agriculture (Neyman, 1923).[1] The methodological works of Ronald Fisher (1925, 1935), an agricultural researcher, and Austin Bradford Hill (1937), a medical statistician, have often been credited as the impetus behind the popularization of randomized experiments. One of the first published RCTs appeared in the *British Medical Journal,* presenting the results of the effects of streptomycin treatments on pulmonary tuberculosis (Streptomycin in Tuberculosis Trials Committee, 1948). Treatment trials such as this, and clinical trials for disease prevention products, have become vanguards of medical and public health research in the post-WWII era. The history of RCTs also features Archie Cochrane, a Scottish physician who wrote the influential *Effectiveness and Efficiency: Random Reflections on Health Services,* first published in 1972. Cochrane's book and his general advocacy of randomized controlled trials were eventually taken up by others and led to the development of the Cochrane Library. The core of its collection is the Cochrane Reviews, a database of systematic reviews and meta-analyses which summarize and make readily available the results of health research, particularly RCTs. At the time of writing, the Cochrane Library held data on more than 600,000 RCTs (www.cochrane.org/cochrane-reviews).

RANDOMIZED CONTROLLED TRIALS: THE GOLD STANDARD?

The RCT is considered by many researchers as the apotheosis of evidence in the health sciences. The ability to minimize confounding forces and maximize internal validity—the quintessential feature of experimental designs—certainly provides credence to this view. Yet not all researchers agree that the RCT deserves an unequivocal position at the top of the evidentiary ladder. For some research contexts, like assessing individual-level interventions or testing new drugs, many researchers agree that RCTs are indeed the gold standard; however, they simultaneously argue that for population-level studies RCTs are generally not the best approach (Sanson-Fisher, Bonevski, Green, & D'Este, 2007).

Common criticisms of RCTs include poor generalizability to real-world contexts, high costs, potential for contamination between treatment and control groups, insufficient time for long-term follow up, and the ethicality of withholding potentially beneficial interventions from control population(s) (English, Schellenberg, & Todd, 2011; Golden, 2012; Kaplan, Giesbrecht, Shannon, & McLeod, 2011). And in some cases, RCTs are simply not necessary. Smith and Pell (2003), in their satirical article "Parachute Use to Prevent Death and Major Trauma Related to Gravitational Challenge: Systematic Review of Randomised Controlled Trials," present a humorous, fictional, case study to make this point: An RCT isn't necessary to know, with certainty, that parachutes save lives!

It's doubtful that the RCT will relinquish its top spot in the scientific pecking order any time soon. However, other methods, such as meta-analyses, are becoming increasingly employed and respected across many areas of public health. Meta-analysis uses a statistical approach to combine and analyze the results from multiple studies, rendering results that are typically generalizable to a larger population. For more information on meta-analysis refer to Stegenga (2011), Pigott (2012), Cooper, Hedges, and Valentine (2009), Borenstein, Hedges, Higgins, and Rothstein (2009), and the PRISMA Statement (prisma-statement.org).

The research designs and methods described above form the methodological foundation of modern epidemiology, which has long been considered the central research arm of public health. Observational disease surveillance and analysis, case-control and cohort studies, and randomized control trials together constitute the primary methodological toolset for the discipline. Not surprisingly, each method receives significant coverage in epidemiology textbooks and courses, from the first epidemiology textbook published in 1960 by McMahon & Pugh to those more recently published (e.g., Friis, 2009; Merrill, 2013; Rothman, Greenland, & Lash, 2008; Szklo & Nieto, 2012). The first methodological section in this book (Part II—Traditional Epidemiologic Methods and Designs) reflects this classic epidemiologic perspective. The section's four chapters cover, respectively, epidemiologic surveillance (Chapter 5), outbreak investigation (Chapter 6), cohort and case-control studies (Chapter 7), and randomized control trials (Chapter 8).

Structural Determinants, Multi-Causality, and the "New Epidemiology"

The shift in epidemiologic focus midway through the 20th century was not limited to the types of diseases studied or the use of more rigorous study designs. The "new epidemiology" also recognized the multi-causal and biopsychosocial nature of disease, adopting a more holistic approach to public health (Anderson, 2007; Pearce, 1996). Since many of the world's worst pathogens had been identified, researchers began to study the social and structural determinants of health, such as race, socioeconomic status, and access to health care. Key indicators of this changing landscape were the establishment of the fields of social epidemiology and social medicine in academic institutions during the middle of the 20th century (Honjo, 2004) and the entrance of the multi-causality concept into mainstream epidemiology (Susser & Watson, 1962). Inclusion of the *web of causation* in McMahon and Pugh's (1960) classic epidemiology textbook is an example of the latter.

Commensurate with these theoretical developments was the expansion and refinement of research methods in other fields. By the middle of the 20th century, sophisticated sampling and survey methods were increasingly employed in government censuses,[2] social psychology (Stouffer, Lumsdaine, et al. 1949; Stouffer, Suchman, et al., 1949), public opinion polling (Converse, 1987; Lazarsfeld, 1948), and psychiatric epidemiology. For example, the Manhattan Midtown Study (Srole, 1962) sought to examine the relationship between mental health and sociodemographic factors through a survey administered to 1,660 randomly selected respondents in midtown New York City.

During this period, statisticians had also begun developing multilevel modeling and other regression techniques that could deal with more complex data sets with multiple variables and outcomes. An important public health milestone during this period was the initiation of the National Health Interview Survey (NHIS) in 1957 (Powell-Griner & Madans, 2007). The NHIS is a large-scale household interview administered annually to a large sample from the general American population. Survey content includes a core set of sociodemographic and health questions (little changed over the past 50 years) and sets of supplemental questions that change from year to year.

The focus on demographic and structural variables and their interwoven relationship to population-level disease has retained an important place in contemporary public health research and practice. Part III (Structural and Operational Research) contains chapters on some of the key methods and subfields within this area of public health. The first chapter in this section, on using secondary data, covers one of the core data retrieval and analysis techniques used in public health, particularly in the area of chronic disease. Although many branches of epidemiology, or scientific inquiry in general, use secondary data in some capacity or another, it is often in a formative or supplementary capacity. As demonstrated in Chapter 9, secondary data analysis as a primary method is a much more rigorous and complicated endeavor.

Part III also includes a chapter on health economics, a branch of economics concerned with issues of efficiency and cost-benefit analyses in the context of health, healthcare, and health policy. Kenneth Arrow's (1963) article "Uncertainty and the Welfare Economics of Medical Care" is viewed by some scholars as the official birth of health economics as a discipline. The field has grown substantially in the past 50 years, and as McIntosh and colleagues note in Chapter 10, its scope and impact in public health have broadened considerably.

Chapter 11 describes the principles and methods within the field of health services research. Originating in the 1960s, health services research "examines how people get access to health care, how much health care costs, and what happens to patients as a result of this care" (Shi, 2008, p. 21). The focus of analysis is the nexus of interaction between health care services, health behavior, and health outcomes. As described in the chapter, health services research is really a suite of techniques that are employed to address research questions specific to the provision of, and access to, health services. One of these techniques is the mystery client method, a type of participant observation technique, used to document and assess health service provision.

The Rise of Behavioral Epidemiology

Part IV (Behavioral and Social Science Research) represents a slightly different focus of research than the demographic and structural emphasis in Part III. While founded on a similar multi-causal perspective, and the view that an individual's environment is a key factor in the distribution of health outcomes, behavioral epidemiology examines behavior and social structures and processes as they relate to the well-being of populations. Mason and Powell (1985) demarcate the field into two main types of inquiry. The first, more traditional, aspect is concerned with identifying specific behaviors that are linked to disease and other health outcomes. Probably the most notable example of this approach is the link researchers established between cigarette smoking and lung cancer.

As the body of knowledge in the traditional vein of behavioral epidemiology continues to grow, more behavioral risk factors have been, and continue to be, identified and documented for a large number of diseases and health conditions. Much like the bacteriological identification of pathogens paved the way for the refocusing of public health efforts on structural determinants of health, identification of behavioral risk factors has directed more research to understanding what drives (un)healthy behavior. This focus on the distribution and determinants (psychosocial, environmental, and cultural) of health-related behavior constitutes the other half of Mason and Powell's behavioral epidemiology. Sallis, Owen, and Fotheringham (2000) operationalize the field into a five-phase framework, with mature research areas expected to have more studies in the latter phases:

1. Establish links between behaviors and health.

2. Develop measures of the behavior.

3. Identify influences on the behavior.

4. Evaluate interventions to change the behavior.

5. Translate research into practice.

In his 1989 article on behavioral epidemiology and health promotion, Jonathon Raymond expressed the hope that this new focus would advance public health promotion by "pushing beyond the conventional borders of behavioral risk factors research to the excitement of discovering the antecedents of health in the social contexts of behavior" (p. 286). The past two decades have indeed witnessed major developments in the application of behavioral and social science concepts and methods to the field of public health. This growth in social-behavioral epidemiology has been supported by theoretical and methodological developments within behavioral and social science disciplines. Growth in this field has also been driven by the emergence of global pandemics—HIV/AIDS in particular—which has created the need for such research to fill the gap left by the lack of biomedical prevention methods.[3] Concomitantly, the post-WWII period ushered in various health-related academic subfields—medical anthropology, medical sociology, and medical/health geography—each bringing new ideas and methods to bear on public health problems.

This trend toward increasing acknowledgment and inclusion of social, cultural, and behavioral factors in public health can be observed in practice as well. The 1957 version of the National Health Interview Survey included only one behavioral component—smoking—which was in a supplement. In 1997, however, the Centers for Disease Control and Prevention (CDC) added an entire set of behavioral questions (adult health behavior) to the core NHIS instrument. CDC also established the Behavioral Risk Factor Surveillance System in 1984, designed to track health conditions and risk behaviors across the entire United States and its territories. The system is based on a large number of ongoing telephone surveys, the results of which are reported annually. In 1991 the CDC implemented a similar system for youth (Youth Risk Behavior Surveillance System).

The behavioral and social science methods described in Part IV have played substantial roles in the advancement of social and behavioral epidemiology and our understanding of health and illness. And each method, or set of methods, arises from a unique historical trajectory. As mentioned earlier, modern survey methods stem from the combined work of political pollsters, sociologists, and statisticians, and today surveys are the most commonly used data collection method in behavioral and social epidemiology. The structured nature of the typical survey instrument, combined with probability sampling and inferential statistics, lends itself well to studying variability within and between populations. That the structured survey is, and has been, used so widely in public health research is a testament to its utility. In Chapter 12 Hageman and colleagues discuss the practical aspects of planning and conducting surveys, the various forms that they can take, and their application to public health problems.

Rating scales—consisting of a battery of interrelated questions—are often included as part of a larger survey, but their historical roots and methods for development and validation are unique. Rating scales originated within the field of clinical psychology, where they have been used to assess specific personality traits (e.g., introvert vs. extrovert, propensity for risk) or emotional states (e.g., depression, anxiety). The early large-scale use of scales in epidemiology—surveys of mental health—can be observed in various disciplines such as epidemiological psychiatry, medical sociology, and medical anthropology. Over the past several decades, the development and use of rating scales has expanded to measure different types of constructs related to behavioral, social, or structural attributes. Rating scales come in all shapes and sizes, and many are readily attainable, but the degree to which any one has been validated, especially in a particular cultural context, will vary. In Chapter 13, the authors explain the concept of validation and other key dimensions associated with developing and using rating scales in public health research.

The Incorporation of 'New' Social and Behavioral Research Methods

Over the decades, traditional surveys and scales have proven to be invaluable tools in public health research and practice. They are limited, however, in their ability to describe and quantify interaction between two or more individuals, which is a particularly important concept in epidemiology. Social network analysis (SNA) is designed to do just that—characterize social ties between individual items (usually, but not always, people) within the context of a larger network. As a focus of research, the notion of social ties dates back to the 1920s, in the field of educational psychology (Freeman, 1996), but one of the key historical events in the development of modern social network analysis was Moreno's (1934) creation of the *sociogram*. The sociogram is a way of visually representing relationships. It includes points, or nodes (depicting people), connected by lines (indicating interpersonal relationships) and is a central concept in contemporary SNA. Moreno later founded the first social network journal, *Sociometry*, in 1937.

In the decades that followed, the field of modern social network analysis blossomed, with significant theoretical and methodological contributions from a diverse range of fields, including sociology, anthropology, psychology, political science, communication, business, computer science, statistics, physics, and mathematics (Luke & Harris, 2007). One of the earliest uses of SNA in health sciences was a study carried out by Coleman, Katz, and Menzel (1957) that examined the relationship between interpersonal communication among physicians and the diffusion of new drugs. In the decades since, researchers have increasingly utilized SNA to examine a broad range of public health issues. Of particular note are SNA's contributions to the areas of transmission networks (disease, communication, and information), social networks (social support, health behavior), and the more recent focus on organizational networks (Luke & Harris, 2007). These applications, as well as the concepts and procedures behind SNA methodology, are discussed in detail in Chapter 14.

Structured surveys, rating scales, and SNA are excellent tools for comparing variability of measures within and between populations; however, they are not well equipped to document complex processes, dig deeper into emergent concepts, or investigate topics that are poorly understood. In contrast, qualitative research methods—in-depth interviews, focus groups, participant observation—are ideal for these types of objectives. The less structured and inductive nature of qualitative inquiry facilitates probing into concepts as they emerge. What qualitative data lack in statistical generalizability, they make up for in their capacity to explain complex phenomena, provide rich and meaningful descriptions, and capture information not anticipated by the researcher (Guest, Namey, & Mitchell, 2013).

Qualitative research methods were first incorporated into academia at the turn of the 20th century, under the wing of early anthropologists such as Bronislaw Malinowski and Franz Boas. Their use expanded into sociology and other social sciences in the second half of the 20th century. Although semistructured/unstructured interviews and other qualitative techniques were no doubt employed in the earliest epidemiologic investigations, their systematic and more formal use in the field of public health became evident in the 1980s, as behavioral epidemiology began to take hold. Qualitative research continues to gain greater acceptance in public health. While still accounting for only a relatively small portion of published articles in medical journals overall (4.1% in 2007), this number represents a 3.4-fold increase between 1998 and 2007 (Shuval et al., 2011). Since their emergence on the public health stage, qualitative research methods have made significant discoveries and contributed to public health practice and policy. Namey and Trotter discuss these contributions in Chapter 15, describing the basics of qualitative methods and giving examples of how various approaches have been applied in public health.

Chapter 16 rounds out Part IV, looking at how randomized control trials are used to test nonbiomedical (i.e., psychosocial) interventions in the field, and provides strategies for dealing with the challenges associated with this enterprise. Logistical and methodological challenges associated with carrying out experimental designs with a behavioral or social "treatment" have tended to discourage the use of such designs in field settings. Despite these challenges, RCTs have been, and continue to be, employed to test the effectiveness of behavioral interventions in public health. It is noteworthy that, since 2001, the Office of Behavioral and Social Sciences Research at the National Institutes of Health has run an annual 2-week Summer Training Institute for the Design and Conduct of Randomized Clinical Trials Involving Behavioral Interventions.

Foundational Elements of Public Health Research

The organization of this book's contents is partially designed to reflect different research paradigms within the field of public health. However, the complexity and interrelated nature of research methods and approaches, and the substantive topics to which they are applied, makes it impossible to neatly fit every topic into a section. Conceptually, some methods and approaches would easily be at home in two or more sections. Part V contains these "cross-cutting" topics. The section begins with a chapter on one of the most critical components of research—sampling. The degree of generalizability (or not) of research findings and the degree to which they represent the larger population. Sampling is the most often critiqued component of research studies. Chapter 17 covers the two major approaches to sampling (as well as censuses)—probabilistic and nonprobabilistic—and the various sampling strategies within each approach. Included in this chapter are descriptions of each sampling strategy, reasons for using it (or not), and instructions on how to execute it. The chapter also provides guidance on choosing appropriate sample sizes.

Another key component of the research process is data analysis. For quantitatively oriented studies this means statistics, which is the topic of Chapter 18. The development of modern inferential statistics can be traced back to the origins of probability theory, created in the mid-1600s by French mathematicians Blaise Pascal and Pierre de Fermat. The list of contributions to the field throughout the subsequent 350 years is too lengthy to cover here, but a few milestones in the context of public health stand out. Regression and ANOVA techniques, for example, were founded on the method of "least squares" developed by Carl Gauss, but first published by Adrien-Marie Legendre in 1805 (Gauss, 1809, 1821; Legendre 1805). The term *regression* itself was coined by Francis Galton later in the 19th century to describe how the heights of descendants of tall ancestors tend to "regress" down toward a normal average (Galton, 1890), a phenomenon often referred to as *regression toward the mean*. At the turn of the 20th century, work by Karl Pearson introduced the chi square statistic (Pearson, 1900) and what is now known as Pearson's r correlation coefficient.

The early part of the 20th century witnessed significant developments in statistical theory and practice. Ronald Fisher, for example, was one of the first researchers to formally write about *analysis of variance*, in a 1918 article, and shortly thereafter published another paper describing the application of the technique (Fisher, 1921). Publication of Fisher's book *Statistical Methods for Research Workers* in 1925 expanded the usage of both the term *ANOVA* and the statistical technique. The following decade, Jerzy Neyman (1937) introduced the concept of *confidence intervals* in statistical testing. From these and other fundamental developments in statistics, the field expanded rapidly over the second half of the 20th century. Statistics are now an inextricable part of public health methodology. Chapter 18 describes the main statistical concepts used today in public health research and provides examples of their application. The author, however, moves beyond commonly used statistical methods and discusses some of the more recently developed techniques for the analysis of nonrandomized data such as survival analysis and structural equation modeling.

More Recent Methodological Approaches

For decades the conceptual and practical divide between quantitative and qualitative approaches has been propagated in literature across many research fields, positioning qualitative and quantitative approaches as diametrically opposed to one another. In some fields, such as anthropology, this perceived divide has led to innumerable heated debates and, in some cases, the reconfiguration of entire academic departments. The formal emergence of the field of mixed methods has calmed some of the epistemological fires that have fueled these debates.

Although researchers in several fields, including public health, have been integrating qualitative and quantitative methods and data for at least a century, the formal field of mixed methods is a more recent phenomenon. It was not until the late 1980s and early 1990s that researchers began to explicitly operationalize data integration and develop mixed methods design typologies to denote various forms of qualitative and quantitative data integration (Greene, Caracelli, & Graham, 1989; Morse, 1991). In the decades that have ensued, mixed methods research has become increasingly common and continues to expand, both theoretically and in practice. The field now boasts a number of textbooks and handbooks (e.g., Bergman, 2008;

Creswell & Plano Clark, 2011, Greene, 2007; Morse & Niehaus, 2009; Tashakkori & Teddlie, 2003, 2010; Teddlie & Tashakkori, 2009), and a flagship journal, *Journal of Mixed Methods Research*, founded in 2007.

The basic premise behind the mixed methods paradigm is that the combination of qualitative and quantitative approaches provides a better understanding of a research problem than either approach could alone (Creswell & Plano Clark, 2011). Guest and Fleming, in Chapter 19, provide various examples of how this integrative approach has been used in public health research. They also describe some of the major typologies in the field, the mechanics of data integration, and current issues being discussed in the discipline.

Geographic Information Systems (GIS) is another recent methodological development. Mapping itself is certainly not a new technique, nor is its application in public health. Snow's landmark research that led to the discovery of the source of cholera in 19th century London included the creation and use of maps. But modern GIS, which is defined as a set of tools and technologies, is only 50 years old. It wasn't until the 1960s, when computer and remote sensing technologies were sophisticated enough, that GIS was possible. One of the first operational GIS was developed by the Department of Forestry and Rural Development in Canada in 1960. The system was used to store and analyze data to determine land capability in rural Canada (Longley, Goodchild, Maguire, & Rhind, 1999).

Modern GIS technologies use digital information, for which various data creation methods are used. The most common method of data creation is digitization, where a hard copy map or survey plan is transferred into a digital medium through the use of a computer-aided design (CAD) program. With this technology, researchers and users of research can map locations of key areas, map quantities and densities of attributes of interest (e.g., disease, health outcomes, sociodemographic variables), examine relationships between space and other attributes, and map changes in spatial data over time. The power of GIS is twofold—its capacity to visually convey complex spatial information (i.e., maps) and the ability to incorporate geographic variables into statistical analyses. The potential benefit of the technology and methods for public health, as Krieger (2003, p. 384) observes, is that GIS "makes it ever easier to connect spatially referenced physical and social phenomena to population patterns of health, disease, and well-being."

Despite its potential, application of GIS to public health research and practice is a recent phenomenon. As Richards, Croner, Rushton, Brown, and Fowler (1999) noted more than a decade ago, while the local government use of GIS increased across the United States during the 1990s, geocoded public health data like vital statistics were in "short supply." Scholars have also pointed out issues with accuracy of geocoding and misinterpretation of GIS data (Krieger, 2003; Ricketts 2003). Notwithstanding, GIS has made a foray into the public health sector and has been used in disease surveillance, risk analysis, health access and planning, and community health profiling (Nykiforuk & Flaman, 2011). These uses, among others, and the potential future of GIS application in public health are the focus of Chapter 20.

Some of the methods and approaches in public health and epidemiology have been around for a long time. Others, such as GIS, are more recent entrants into public health's repertoire of research methods. The final chapter in Part V (Public Health 2.0) discusses a burgeoning movement in public health practice and research. Public health 2.0[4] is essentially an extension of the participatory and collaborative principles behind Web 2.0.

MONITORING AND EVALUATION

Monitoring and evaluation, or M&E, can mean different things to different audiences. Typically, though, practitioners define monitoring as an ongoing process of checking progress or quality and evaluation as a systematic appraisal of something:

Monitoring is a continuous function that uses the systematic collection of data on specified indicators to provide management and the main stakeholders of an ongoing intervention with indications of the extent or progress and achievement of objectives in the use of allocated of funds.

Evaluation is the systematic and objective assessment of an ongoing or completed project, program, or policy, including its design, implementation, and results. The aim is to determine the relevance and fulfillment of objectives, intervention efficiency, effectiveness, impact, and sustainability. (Gorgens & Zall Kusek, 2009, p. 2)

The field and practice of M&E is often considered distinct from research in public health (and other fields), and numerous textbooks are available on the topic (e.g., Gorgens & Zall Kusek, 2009; Harris, 2010; Patton, 2008; Wholey, Hatry, & Newcomer, 2010). However, M&E practice often uses many of the research methods described in this book. Program process evaluations, for example, frequently use qualitative research methods to obtain information. A rigorous impact evaluation may employ a randomized controlled research design. The demarcation between research and evaluation is blurry at best (see Chapter 3). The one distinction that can be made is that evaluation *always* assesses a program, intervention, or policy. Research may or may not embody this characteristic.

The term Web 2.0 was coined over a decade ago by Darcy DiNucci (1999) in her article "Fragmented Future." The term's entrance into mainstream vocabulary, however, is attributed to the O'Reilly Media and MediaLive conference hosted in 2004. Examples of Web 2.0 technologies include blogs, social networking sites, social bookmarking, mobile applications, virtual meetings, wikis, podcasts, and media sharing sites. Researchers are increasingly employing these technologies across a range of public health research endeavors (e.g., Blumenthal, Mayman, & Allee, 2009; Frost, Massagli, Wicks, & Heywood, 2008; Lombardi & Baum, 2011; Ossebaard, Van Gemert-Pijnen, & Seydel, 2011; Spring, 2011; Van De Belt, Engelen, Berben, & Schoonhoven, 2010; van der Vaart, Drossaert, de Heus, Taal, & van de Laar, 2013), with the number of published examples growing each year. Chapter 21 is about the research potential that the Internet and Web 2.0 technologies hold for public health. It describes some existing research examples in public health and some of the Internet-based methods, as well as the potential these methods hold for the future.

Figure 1.4 Selected Events From the History of Public Health in the Western World

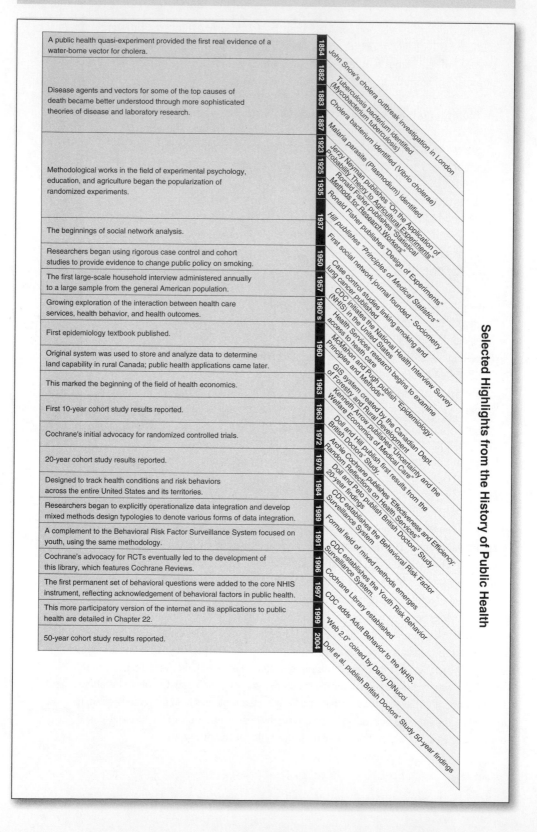

Description	Year	Event
A public health quasi-experiment provided the first real evidence of a water-borne vector for cholera.	1854	John Snow's cholera outbreak investigation in London
Disease agents and vectors for some of the top causes of death became better understood through more sophisticated theories of disease and laboratory research.	1882	Tuberculosis bacterium identified (Mycobacterium tuberculosis)
	1883	Cholera bacterium identified (Vibrio cholerae)
	1887	Malaria parasite (Plasmodium) identified
Methodological works in the field of experimental psychology, education, and agriculture began the popularization of randomized experiments.	1923	Jerzy Neyman publishes "On the Application of Probability Theory to Agricultural Experiments"
	1925	Ronald Fisher publishes "Statistical Methods for Research Workers"
	1935	Ronald Fisher publishes "Design of Experiments"
The beginnings of social network analysis.	1937	Hill publishes "Principles of Medical Statistics"
Researchers began using rigorous case control and cohort studies to provide evidence to change public policy on smoking.	1950	First social network journal founded - Sociometry
The first large-scale household interview administered annually to a large sample from the general American population.	1957	Case control studies linking smoking and lung cancer published
Growing exploration of the interaction between health care services, health behavior, and health outcomes.	1960's	CDC initiates the National Health Interview Survey (NHIS) in the United States
First epidemiology textbook published.	1960	Health Services research begins to examine access to health care
Original system was used to store and analyze data to determine land capability in rural Canada; public health applications came later.		McMahon and Pugh publish "Epidemiology: Principles and Methods"
This marked the beginning of the field of health economics.	1963	GIS system created by the Canadian Dept. of Forestry and Rural Development
First 10-year cohort study results reported.	1963	Kenneth Arrow publishes "Uncertainty and the Welfare Economics of Medical Care"
Cochrane's initial advocacy for randomized controlled trials.	1972	Doll and Hill publish first results from the British Doctors Study
20-year cohort study results reported.	1976	Archie Cochrane publishes "Effectiveness and Efficiency: Random Reflections on Health Services"
Designed to track health conditions and risk behaviors across the entire United States and its territories.	1984	Doll and Peto publish British Doctors' Study 20-year findings
Researchers began to explicitly operationalize data integration and develop mixed methods design typologies to denote various forms of data integration.	1989	CDC establishes the Behavioral Risk Factor Surveillance System
A complement to the Behavioral Risk Factor Surveillance System focused on youth, using the same methodology.	1991	Formal field of mixed methods emerges
Cochrane's advocacy for RCTs eventually led to the development of this library, which features Cochrane Reviews.	1996	CDC establishes the Youth Risk Behavior Surveillance System.
The first permanent set of behavioral questions were added to the core NHIS instrument, reflecting acknowledgement of behavioral factors in public health.	1997	Cochrane Library established
This more participatory version of the internet and its applications to public health are detailed in Chapter 22.	1999	CDC adds Adult Behavior to the NHIS.
50-year cohort study results reported.	2004	"Web 2.0" coined by Darcy DiNucci
		Doll et al. publish British Doctors' Study 50-year findings

Selected Highlights from the History of Public Health

FROM RESEARCH TO POLICY AND PRACTICE

The goal of most public health research is to inform policy and/or to improve health outcomes. Yet, unfortunately, findings from many well-executed and potentially informative research studies never get beyond the readership of academic journals. Or if they do, policymakers may ignore the findings or may be unable to implement the findings in a meaningful way. Even in cases where findings are delivered to the appropriate stakeholders who are able to implement them in the form of a policy change and/or intervention, multiple barriers often exist that prevent realization of anticipated change. The focus of Part VI is on these all-too-common gaps between research, practice, and outcomes. Chapter 22 starts the section off by providing insights and useful techniques for enhancing the utilization of research findings and creating linkages between research and appropriate audiences.

The uneven and relatively limited uptake of research findings spawned a new field of research—implementation science—which is the subject of Chapter 23. Eccles and Mittman (2006), the founding editors of the journal *Implementation Science,* define the field as "the scientific study of methods to promote the systematic uptake of research findings and other evidence-based practices into routine practice, and, hence, to improve the quality and effectiveness of health services and care" (p. 1). Though a relatively new area of study, it is growing rapidly in all fields of public health. In Chapter 23, Madon describes this growth and diversity, the predominant methods and frameworks within the field, and the contributions that implementation science has made to public health outcomes over the past decade.

COMING FULL CIRCLE: PREPARING FOR RESEARCH

The discussion so far has focused on unique research methodologies and approaches, as well as the application of research to public health policy and practice. But a lot of planning and preparation are required before the first piece of data is even collected, especially in field research where most data are collected directly from people. Complicating the research planning phase is the highly politicized and regulated research environment in which contemporary researchers work. Indeed, a lot has changed in this regard since the formative years of epidemiology and the social and behavioral sciences. Part I (Planning and Preparing for Research) navigates the reader through the general research design process, as well as the regulatory and political environment within which public health researchers operate. This section begins with Chapter 2, by Reynolds and Guest, on the research design process. The authors discuss the major components of research design and planning, such as literature reviews and developing research questions, and describe some of the major types of research designs. This chapter is intended to serve as a basic foundation for the remaining chapters in the book, including Chapter 3, which deals with the ethical dimensions of doing research with human subjects.

One of biggest changes in the research regulatory environment is in the field of research ethics. Prior to World War II, research ethics review committees—or Institutional Review Boards (IRBs)—were nonexistent. Institutional review boards are committees that have been formally created to approve, monitor, and review research involving humans. Members of IRBs often have a diverse range of backgrounds and can include subject matter experts, community representatives, religious leaders, local health officials, and attorneys, among others. The primary function of an IRB is to safeguard the rights and well-being of individuals and communities that are the subject of research studies. Nowadays most countries in the world have some form of a national-level IRB, and larger, more developed countries can have hundreds of IRBs connected with academic, governmental, and nonprofit organizations.

Since World War II, various guidelines, codes, and regulations have also been created to guide research with human subjects. Their creation and refinement have been driven in large part by historical events, the first of which was the set of horrific events associated with the holocaust, specifically the Nazi treatment of prisoners as "research subjects." The Nuremburg Code of 1947, an outcome of the Nuremburg trials, includes a set of 10 points centered on protecting the rights of research subjects. These points embody many of the foundational principles of contemporary research ethics, such as informed consent, the absence of coercion, proper scientific design, and beneficence toward research participants. While not a legally binding entity, the Nuremburg Code brought ethics to the foreground of research discourse and paved the road for the creation of subsequent international research organizations and guidelines (e.g., Declaration of Helsinki, Council for International Organizations of Medical Sciences Guidelines, International Conference on Harmonization, Nuffield Council on Bioethics).

In terms of U.S. regulations, a key event in research ethics was the public disclosure of the Tuskegee study that took place in the southern United States from 1932 to 1972. The government-sponsored study included more than 400 African American men with latent syphilis. Despite the discovery of penicillin in the 1940s—a known cure for syphilis—these men were denied treatment for over 30 years. Once exposed, this study was the impetus for the creation of the National Commission for the Protection of Human Subjects of Biomedical and Behavioral Research in 1974. Four years later the commission published *The Belmont Report: Ethical Principles and Guidelines for the Protection of Human Subjects of Research*, outlining fundamental ethical principles underlying research involving human subjects. The report also served as the foundation for the U.S. Code of Federal Regulations, a policy adopted in 1991 by 16 federal agencies that conduct, support, or regulate human participant research.

Today, IRB approval is required for virtually all research involving human participants. Chapter 3 provides a detailed accounting of research ethics, IRB processes, and practical considerations associated with IRB submissions. Included in this chapter are discussions on what constitutes "research," types of exemptions, and some of the current issues in the field of international research ethics.

Democratization of research is another recent trend in public health. From the increasing use of participatory research methods to the establishment of the Global Health Initiative in 2009, more and more research is being put in the hands of local communities. Chapter 4 outlines many of the processes involved in engaging communities and local stakeholders in the research process, as well as the challenges associated with these activities and relationships. Based on years of experience, the authors offer useful insights and practical steps designed to involve local communities and stakeholders in proposed research efforts and to ultimately increase the probability of successful and ethical research outcomes.

GLOBAL HEALTH

With a few exceptions, the brief history presented above is admittedly ethnocentric, focusing on the development of modern epidemiology and public health in developed regions of the world, such as Europe and the United States. Certainly, this history is brimming with public health success stories, but it is also evident that this history is not necessarily shared with other regions of the world. Distribution of disease and illness varies dramatically between countries and geographic regions (including *within* countries). Table 1.3 compares the top 10 causes of death between high- and low-income countries in the year 2008. Note that some of the deadliest illnesses in developing countries, such as diarrhea and tuberculosis, rarely cause death in developed areas of the world.

Table 1.3   Comparative List of Leading Causes of Death in 2008: High- vs. Low-Income Countries (WHO, 2013)[5]

High-Income Countries	Low-Income Countries
Ischemic heart disease	Lower respiratory infections
Stroke and other cerebrovascular disease	Diarrheal diseases
Trachea, bronchus, lung cancers	HIV/AIDS
Alzheimer's and other dementias	Ischemic heart disease
Lower respiratory infections	Malaria
Chronic obstructive pulmonary disease	Stroke and other cerebrovascular disease
Colon and rectum cancers	Tuberculosis
Diabetes mellitus	Prematurity and low birth weight
Hypertensive heart disease	Birth asphyxia and birth trauma
Breast cancer	Neonatal infections

Huge disparities also exist with respect to infant mortality rates and overall life expectancy between wealthy and less wealthy nations. Infant mortality in some of the poorest countries of the world is higher than 100 deaths per 1,000, whereas that figure drops to less than 5 per 1,000—a twentyfold difference—in most developed countries. Similarly, the estimated life expectancy in 29 of the world's healthiest countries (the top 13%) is over 80 years of age, contrasted with a life expectancy of less than 60 years (and as low as 38.8 years) for the majority of African nations (*The World Fact Book*, 2013). The fields of international and global health are a response to these disparities and ultimately aim to improve health outcomes for all of the world's citizens. The work of prominent public health scholars, such as Paul Farmer (1999, 2004) and Michael Marmot (Marmot, 2005, Marmot, Friel, Bell, Houweling, & Taylor, 2008; Marmot & Wilkinson, 2005), as well as the tireless efforts of political activists, have played a major role in propelling the field of global health forward. The AIDS pandemic has been another important catalyst.

Global health is concerned with the health of populations in a global context and transcends the focus at the level of individual nations (Brown, Cueto, & Fee, 2006). Koplan et al. (2009) define the field as "the area of study, research and practice that places a priority on improving health and achieving equity in health for all people worldwide" (p. 1995). Like many of the major developments in public health, the roots of modern global health have their origin in the post-WWII era, with the establishment of international organizations such as the United Nations (1945) and the World Bank Group (1945). Three years after its own creation, the United Nations founded the World Health Organization in 1948. Two subsequent milestones in the global research sphere were the establishment of the International Epidemiological Association in 1956 and the demographic and health survey in 1984. Demographic and health surveys are nationally representative household surveys that provide data for a wide range of monitoring and impact evaluation indicators in the areas of population, health, and nutrition. As of 2009, more than 260 surveys had been conducted in over 90 countries (Zuehike, 2011).

Global health is a rapidly growing field (the term itself replacing the older terminology of "international health"; Brown et al., 2006). The number of global health programs and departments in academic institutions is burgeoning, as is the number of global health textbooks. The same is true at the policy level. Multiple global health initiatives have been launched since the turn of the 20th century, such as the globally endorsed Millennium Development Goals, the U.S. government's President's Emergency Plan for AIDS Relief (PEPFAR), and the Global Health Initiative. New funding mechanisms have also been established, such as the Global Fund to Fight AIDS, Tuberculosis and Malaria (2002); the World Bank's Multi-Country HIV/AIDS Program (1999); and private foundations led by individual philanthropists such as Bill Gates, Warren Buffett, Ted Turner, and Bill Clinton.

Globalization is a permanent feature of the current sociodemographic, political, and economic landscape. So too is global health and the international concern for the well-being of all of the world's people. This concern is embedded in the majority of chapters in this book. Most chapters contain a section on global health that connects the chapter's contents with current trends in the expanding field of global health. The section also includes a practical side. Conducting research domestically is wrought with many challenges, but these are often amplified, and supplemented with other challenges, when implementing research in other cultures and countries. To help cope with these challenges, many chapters provide practical and logistical insights into preparing for and carrying out research in an international context.

How successful global (and domestic) public health activities will eventually be is unknown. Numerous political, economic, and environmental barriers exist that can thwart the best of intentions. One thing is certain, however. When public health policies and practices are informed by good research, and political will drives these policies forward, major achievements can be made. Lives can be saved and lengthened, and their quality significantly improved. Rigorous and well-designed research is, and will continue to be, a foundational element in fulfilling public health's goals of protecting and improving the health of communities and populations, both domestically and globally.

ADDITIONAL RESOURCES

Honjo, K. (2004). Social epidemiology: Definition, history, and research examples. *Environmental Health and Medicine, 9,* 193–199.

Krieger, N. (2011). *Epidemiology and the people's health: Theory and context.* New York, NY: Oxford University Press.

Morabia, A. (2006). *A history of epidemiologic methods and concepts.* Basel, Switzerland: Birkhäuser.

Raymond, J. (1989). Behavioral epidemiology: The science of health promotion. *Health Promotion, 4,* 281–286.

Rosen, G. (1993). *A history of public health.* Baltimore, MD: John Hopkins University Press. (Original work published 1958)

Susser, M., & Stein, Z. (2009). *Eras in epidemiology: The evolution of ideas.* New York, NY: Oxford University Press.

REFERENCES

Abdool Karim, Q., Abdool Karim, S., Frohlich, J., Grobler, A., Baxter, C., Mansoor, L., . . . Taylor, D. (2010). Effectiveness and safety of tenofovir gel, an antiretroviral microbicide, for the prevention of HIV infection in women. *Science, 329,* 1168–1174.

Anderson, H. (2007, October). *History and philosophy of modern epidemiology.* Paper presented at History and Philosophy of Science Conference, Pittsburgh, PA.

Arrow, K. (1963). Uncertainty and the welfare economics of medical care. *American Economic Review, 53,* 941–973.

Auvert, B., Taljaard, D., Lagarde, E., Sobngwi-Tambekow, J., Sitta, R., & Puren, A. (2005). Randomized, controlled intervention trial of male circumcision for reduction of HIV infection risk: The ANRS 1265 trial. *PloS Medicine, 2,* e298.

Baeten, J. M., Donnell, D., Ndase, P., Mugo, N. R., Campbell, J. D., Wangisi, J., . . . Celum, C. (2012). Antiretroviral prophylaxis for HIV prevention in heterosexual men and women. *New England Journal of Medicine, 367,* 399–410.

Bailey, R. C., Moses, S., Parker, C. B., Agot, K., Maclean, I., Krieger, J. N., . . . Ndinya-Achola, J. O. (2007). Male circumcision for HIV prevention in young men in Kisumu, Kenya: A randomised controlled trial. *Lancet, 369,* 643–656.

Bergman, M. (Ed.). (2008). *Advances in mixed methods research.* Thousand Oaks, CA. Sage.

Bernard, H. R. (1993). Methods belong to all of us. In R. Borofsky (Ed.), *Assessing cultural anthropology* (pp. 168–178). New York, NY: McGraw-Hill.

Bickman, L., & Rog, D. (2009). Applied research design: A practical approach. In L. Bickman & D. Rog (Eds.), *Handbook of applied social research methods* (2nd ed., pp. 3–43). Thousand Oaks, CA: Sage.

Blumenthal, J., Mayman, G., & Allee, N. (2009, August–September). *Public health 2.0: Collaborative partnerships for integrating social technologies into the practice community.* Paper presented at the International Congress on Medical Librarianship, Brisbane, Australia.

Borenstein, M., Hedges, L., Higgins, J., & Rothstein, H. (2009). *Introduction to meta-analysis.* Chichester, UK: Wiley.

Brown, T., Cueto, M., & Fee, E. (2006). The World Health Organization and the transition from "international" to "global" health. *American Journal of Public Health, 96,* 62–72.

Cochrane, A. (1990). *Effectiveness and efficiency: Random reflections on health services* (2nd ed.). London, UK: Nuffield Provincial Hospitals Trust. (Original work published 1989)

Coleman, J., Katz, E., & Menzel, H. (1957). The diffusion of innovations among physicians. *Sociometry, 20,* 253–270.

Converse, J. M. (1987). *Survey research in the United States: Roots and emergence 1890–1960.* New Brunswick, NJ: Transaction.

Cooper, H., Hedges, L., & Valentine, J. (Eds.). (2009). *The handbook of research synthesis and meta-analysis* (2nd ed.). New York, NY: Russell Sage Foundation.

Creswell, J., & Plano Clark, V. (2011). *Designing and conducting mixed methods research* (2nd ed.). Thousand Oaks, CA. Sage.

DiNucci, D. (1999). Fragmented future. *Print, 53*(4), 32.

Doll, R., & Hill, A. (1950). Smoking and carcinoma of the lung: Preliminary report. *British Medical Journal, 2*(4682), 739–748.

Doll, R., & Hill, A. (1964). Mortality in relation to smoking: Ten year's observation of British doctors. *British Medical Journal, 1*(5396), 1460–1467.

Doll, R., & Peto, R. (1976). Mortality in relation to smoking: 20 years' observations on male British doctors. *British Medical Journal, 2*(6051), 1525–1536.

Doll, R., Peto, R., Boreham, J., & Sutherland, I. (2004). Mortality in relation to smoking: 50 years' observation on male British doctors. *British Medical Journal, 328*(7455), 1519–1533.

Doll, R., Peto, R., Wheatley, K., Gray, R., & Sutherland, I. (1994). Mortality in relation to smoking: 40 years' observations on male British doctors. *British Medical Journal, 309*(6959), 901–911.

Eccles, M., & Mittman, B. (2006). Welcome to implementation science. *Implementation Science, 1,* 1–3.

English, M., Schellenberg, J., & Todd, J. (2011). Assessing health system interventions: Key points when considering the value of randomization. *Bulletin of the World Health Organization, 89,* 907–912.

Farmer, P. (1999). *Infections and inequalities: The modern plagues.* Berkeley: University of California Press.

Farmer, P. (2004). *Pathologies of power: Health, human rights, and the new war on the poor.* Berkeley: University of California Press.

Fisher, R. (1918). The correlation between relatives on the supposition of Mendelian inheritance. *Philosophical Transactions of the Royal Society of Edinburgh, 52,* 399–433.

Fisher, R. (1921). On the "probable error" of a coefficient of correlation deduced from a small sample. *Metron, 1,* 3–32.

Fisher, R. (1925). *Statistical methods for research workers.* London, UK: Oliver & Boyd.

Fisher, R. (1935). *Design of experiments.* Oxford, UK: Oliver & Boyd.

Freeman, L. (1996). Some antecedents of social network analysis. *Connections, 19,* 39–42.

Friedman, L., Furberg, C., & DeMets, D. (2010). *Fundamentals of clinical trials* (4th ed.). New York, NY: Springer.

Friis R. (2009). *Epidemiology 101.* Burlington, MA: Jones and Bartlett.

Frost, J., Massagli, M., Wicks, P., & Heywood, J. (2008). How the social web supports patient experimentation with a new therapy: The demand for patient-controlled and patient-centered informatics. *American Medical Informatics Association Annual Symposium Proceedings, 6,* 217–21.

Galton, F. (1890). Kinship and correlation. *North American Review, 150,* 419–431.

Gauss, C. (1809). *Theoria motus corporum coelestium in sectionibus conicis solem ambientum.* Hamburg, Germany: Friedrich Perthes and I. H. Besser.

Gauss, C. (1821). *Theoria combinationis observationum erroribus minimis obnoxiae.* Göttingen, Germany: Societati Regiae Scientiarum Exhibita.

Golden, I. (2012). Beyond randomized controlled trials: Evidence in complementary medicine. *Journal of Evidence-Based Complementary & Alternative Medicine, 17,* 72–75.

Gorgens,, M., & Zall Kusek, J. (2009). *Making monitoring and evaluation systems work.* Washington, DC: World Bank.

Grant, R., Lama, J., Anderson, P., McMahan, V., Liu, A., Vargas, L., . . . Glidden, D. V. (2010). Preexposure chemoprophylaxis for HIV prevention in men who have sex with men. *New England Journal of Medicine, 363,* 2587–2599.

Gray, R. H., Kigozi, G., Serwadda, D., Makumbi, F., Watya, S., Nalugoda, F., . . . Wawer, M. J. (2007). Male circumcision for HIV prevention in men in Rakai, Uganda: A randomised trial. *Lancet, 369,* 657–666.

Greene, J. (2007). *Mixed methods in social inquiry.* San Francisco, CA: Jossey-Bass.

Greene, J. C., Caracelli, V. J., & Graham, W. F. (1989). Toward a conceptual framework for mixed-method evaluation design. *Educational Evaluation and Policy Analysis, 11,* 255–274.

Guest, G., Namey, E., & Mitchell, M. (2013). *Collecting qualitative data: A field manual for applied research.* Thousand Oaks, CA: Sage.

Hammonds, E. (1999). *Childhood's deadly scourge: The campaign to control diphtheria in New York City, 1880–1930.* Baltimore, MD: John Hopkins University Press.

Harris, M. (2010). *Evaluating public and community health programs.* San Francisco, CA: Jossey-Bass.

Hill, A. B. (1937). *Principles of medical statistics.* London, UK: Lancet.

Honjo, K. (2004). Social epidemiology: Definition, history, and research examples. *Environmental Health and Medicine, 9,* 193–199.

Kaplan, B., Giesbrecht, G., Shannon, S., & McLeod, K. (2011). Evaluating treatments in health care: The instability of a one-legged stool. *BMC Medical Research Methodology, 11,* 65.

Koplan, J., Bond, C., Merson, M., Reddy, K., Rodriguez, M., Sewankambo, N., & Wasserheit, J. (2009). Towards a common definition of global health. *Lancet, 373,* 1993–1995.

Krieger, N. (2003). Place, space, and health: GIS and epidemiology. *Epidemiology, 14,* 384–385.

Lazarsfeld, P. (1948). *The people's choice.* New York, NY: Columbia University Press.

Legendre, A. (1805). *Nouvelles méthodes pour la détermination des orbites des comètes.* Paris, France: Firmin Didot.

Levin, M., Goldstein, H., & Gerhardt, P. (1950). Cancer and tobacco smoking: A preliminary report. *Journal of the American Medical Association, 143,* 336–338.

Lombardi, G., & Baum, N. (2011). Health 2.0: How interactive web sites are changing the healthcare industry. *Journal of Medical Practice Management, 26,* 242–244.

Longley, P., Goodchild, M., Maguire, D., & Rhind, D. (1999). Introduction. In M. Goodchild, D. Maguire, & D. Rhind (Eds.), *Geographical information systems: Principles and technical issues, Vol. 1* (2nd ed., pp. 1–27). New York, NY: Wiley.

Luke, D., & Harris, J. (2007). Network analysis in public health: History, methods, and applications. *Annual Review of Public Health, 28,* 69–93.

Lynch, J., & Davey Smith, G. (2005). A life course approach to chronic disease epidemiology. *Annual Review of Public Health, 26,* 1–35.

Marmot, M. (2005). *The status syndrome: How social standing affects our health and longevity.* New York, NY: Holt.

Marmot, M., Friel, S., Bell, R., Houweling, T., & Taylor, S. (2008). Closing the gap in a generation: Health equity through action on the social determinants of health. *Lancet, 372,* 1661–1669.

Marmot, M., & Wilkinson, R. (2005). *Social determinants of health.* Oxford, UK: Oxford University Press.

Mason, J., & Powell, K. (1985). Physical activity, behavioral epidemiology, and public health. *Public Health Reports, 100,* 113–115.

McMahon, B., & Pugh, T. (1960). *Epidemiology: Principles and methods.* London, UK: Little, Brown.

Merrill, R. (2013). *Introduction to epidemiology* (6th ed.). Burlington, MA: Jones and Bartlett.

Moreno, J. (1934). *Who shall survive?* New York, NY: Beacon.

Morse, J. (1991). Approaches to qualitative-quantitative methodological triangulation. *Nursing Research, 40,* 120–123.

Morse, J., & Niehaus, L. (2009). *Mixed method design: Principles and procedures.* Walnut Creek, CA. Left Coast Press.

National Commission for the Protection of Human Subjects of Biomedical and Behavioral Research. (1978). *The Belmont Report: Ethical principles and guidelines for the protection of human subjects of research.* Washington, DC: U.S. Government Printing Office.

Neyman, J. (1923). On the application of probability theory to agricultural experiments. *Statistical Science, 5,* 465–472.

Neyman, J. (1937). Outline of a theory of statistical estimation based on the classical theory of probability. *Philosophical Transactions of the Royal Society of London. Series A, Mathematical and Physical Sciences, 236*(767), 333–380.

Nykiforuk, C., & Flaman, L. (2011). Geographic information systems (GIS) for health promotion and public health: A review. *Health Promotion Practice, 12,* 63–73.

Ossebaard, H. C., Van Gemert-Pijnen, J., & Seydel, E. (2011). ePublic health: Fresh approaches to infection prevention and control. In J. Van Gemert-Pijnen, H. C. Ossebaard, & P. Hämäläinen (Eds.), *Proceedings 3rd International Conference on eHealth, Telemedicine, and Social Medicine eTELEMED 2011* (pp. 27–36). Red Hook, NY: Curran Associates.

Patton, M. (2008). *Utilization-focused evaluation* (4th ed.). Thousand Oaks, CA: Sage.

Pearce, N. (1996). Traditional epidemiology, modern epidemiology, and public health. *American Journal of Public Health, 86,* 678–683.

Pearson, K. (1900). On the criterion that a given system of deviations from the probable in the case of a correlated system of variables is such that it can be reasonably supposed to have arisen from random sampling. *Philosophical Magazine, Series 5, 50*(302), 157–175.

Peirce, C., & Jastrow, J. (1885). On small differences in sensation. *Memoirs of the National Academy of Sciences, 3,* 73–83.

Pigott, T. (2012). *Advances in meta-analysis.* New York, NY: Springer.

Powell-Griner, E., & Madans, J. (2007, July–August). *History of the national health interview survey.* Paper presented at the meeting of the American Statistical Association Salt Lake City, UT.

Power, C., & Elliott, J. (2006). Cohort profile: 1958 British birth cohort (National Child Development Study). *International Journal of Epidemiology, 35*(1), 34–41.

Raymond, J. (1989). Behavioral epidemiology: The science of health promotion. *Health Promotion, 4,* 281–286.

Richards, T., Croner, C., Rushton, G., Brown, C., & Fowler, L. (1999). Geographic information systems and public health: Mapping the future. *Public Health Reports, 114,* 359–373.

Ricketts, T. (2003). Geographic information systems and public health. *Annual Review of Public Health, 24,* 1–6.

Rosen, G. (1993). *A history of public health.* Baltimore, MD: John Hopkins University Press. (Original work published 1958)

Rothman, K., Greenland, S., & Lash, T. (2008). *Modern epidemiology* (3rd ed.). Philadelphia, PA: Lippincott Williams & Wilkins.

Sallis, J., Owen, N., & Fotheringham, M. (2000). Behavioral epidemiology: A systematic framework to classify phases of research on health promotion and diseases prevention. *Annals of Behavioral Medicine, 22,* 294–298.

Sanson-Fisher, R., Bonevski, B., Green, L., & D'Este, C. (2007). Limitations of the randomized controlled trial in evaluating population-based health interventions. *American Journal of Preventive Medicine, 33,* 155–161.

Shi, L. (2008). *Health services research methods* (2nd ed.). Clifton Park, NY: Delmar Learning.

Shuval, K., Harker, K., Roudsari, B., Groce, N., Mills, B., Siddiqi, Z., & Shachak, A. (2011). Is qualitative research second class science? A quantitative longitudinal examination of qualitative research in medical journals. *PLoS One, 6*(2), e16937.

Smith, G., & Pell, J. (2003). Parachute use to prevent death and major trauma related to gravitational challenge: Systematic review of randomised controlled trials. *British Medical Journal, 327,* 1459–1461.

Spring, H. (2011). If you cannot beat them, join them! Using Health 2.0 and popular Internet applications to improve information literacy. *Health Information and Libraries Journal, 28*(2), 148–151.

Srole, L. (1962). *Mental health in the metropolis: The Midtown Manhattan Study.* New York, NY: McGraw-Hill.

Stegenga, J. (2011). Is meta-analysis the platinum standard? *Studies in History and Philosophy of Biological and Biomedical Sciences, 42,* 497–507.

Stigler, S. (1992). A historical view of statistical concepts in psychology and educational research. *American Journal of Education, 101*(1), 60–70.

Stouffer, S. A., Lumsdaine, A. A., Lumsdaine, M. H., Williams, R. M., Jr., Smith, M. B., Janis, I. L., . . . Cottrell, L. S., Jr. (1949). *The American soldier: Combat and its aftermath, Vol. II.* Princeton, NJ: Princeton University Press.

Stouffer, S., Suchman, E., Devinney, L., Star, S., & Williams, R., Jr. (1949). *The American soldier: Adjustment during Army life, Vol. I.* Princeton, NJ: Princeton University Press.

Streptomycin in Tuberculosis Trials Committee. (1948). Streptomycin treatment of pulmonary tuberculosis. A medical research council investigation. *British Medical Journal, 2*(4582), 769–782.

Susser, M. (1985). Epidemiology in the United States after World War II: The evolution of technique. *Epidemiology Review, 7,* 147–177.

Susser, M., & Watson, W. (1962). *Sociology in medicine.* Oxford, UK: Oxford University Press.

Szklo, M., & Nieto, J. (2012). *Epidemiology* (3rd ed.). Burlington, MA: Jones and Bartlett.

Tashakkori, A., & Teddlie, C. (Eds.). (2003). *Handbook of mixed methods in social and behavioral research.* Thousand Oaks, CA. Sage.

Tashakkori, A., & Teddlie, C. (Eds.). (2010). *Handbook of mixed methods in social and behavioral research* (2nd ed.). Thousand Oaks, CA. Sage.

Teddlie, C., & Tashakkori, A. (2009). *Foundations of mixed methods research: Integrating quantitative and qualitative approaches in the social and behavioral sciences.* Thousand Oaks, CA. Sage.

Temple, R. (1986). *The genius of China: 3,000 years of science, discovery, and invention.* New York, NY: Simon and Schuster.

Van De Belt, T., Engelen, L., Berben, S., & Schoonhoven, L. (2010). Definition of Health 2.0 and Medicine 2.0: A systematic review. *Journal of Medical Internet Research, 12*(2), e18.

van der Vaart, R., Drossaert, C., de Heus, M., Taal, E., & van de Laar, M. (2013). Measuring actual eHealth literacy among patients with rheumatic diseases: A qualitative analysis of problems encountered using Health 1.0 and Health 2.0 applications. *Journal of Medical Internet Research, 15*(2), e27.

Wholey, J., Hatry, H., & Newcomer, K. (2010). *Handbook of practical program evaluation* (3rd ed.). San Francisco, CA: Jossey-Bass.

The world fact book. (2013). Retrieved from https://www.cia.gov/library/publications/the-world-factbook

World Health Organization. (2013). *The top ten causes of death. Fact sheet #310.* Retrieved from http://www.who.int/mediacentre/factsheets/fs310/en/

Wynder, E., & Graham, E. (1950). Tobacco smoking as a possible etiologic factor in bronchogenic carcinoma: A study of 684 proved cases. *Journal of the American Medical Association, 143,* 329–336.

Zuehike, E. (2011). *The demographic and health surveys at 25 years and beyond.* Washington, DC: Population Reference Bureau.

NOTES

1. Although the modern RCT became part of contemporary public health practice in the first half of the 20th century, its conceptual roots date back to the 11th century, when Persian physician and philosopher Avicenna completed *The Canon of Medicine* in 1025. In this series of medical texts he wrote a precise guide for practical experimentation in the process of discovering and proving the effectiveness of medical drugs and substances.

2. Note that the history of censuses extends back to some of the earliest civilizations—such as Babylon and Rome—where they were used primarily for tax collection purposes. The first U.S. census was conducted in 1790.

3. The HIV prevention landscape is rapidly changing. Male circumcision has proven effective in reducing HIV transmission (Auvert et al., 2005; Bailey et al., 2007; Gray et al. 2007). Pre-exposure prophylaxis has also been shown to be effective among certain populations (Baeten et al., 2012; Grant et al., 2010), leading the FDA to approve the antiretroviral drug Truvada for HIV prevention. A vaginal microbicide gel has shown promise during a "proof-of-concept" trial showing efficacy (Abdool Karim et al., 2010) and a confirmatory trial is underway at the time of writing. Several HIV vaccines are also undergoing clinical trials, with more candidates in the pipeline.

4. Other terms used to describe a similar concept include: eHealth, Health 2.0, and Medicine 2.0.

5. A caveat here is that although cause of mortality is an informative measure, it does not take into account the health of those who survive and the burden of disease they face. WHO now routinely measures the disability-adjusted life year (DALY), a time-based measure that combines years of life lost due to premature mortality and years of life lost due to time lived in states of less than full health.

PART I

Planning and Preparing for Research

2

Designing Research

Heidi W. Reynolds and Greg Guest

Many of this book's chapters, particularly those in Part II, discuss research design. But these discussions occur in the context of a particular type of research or method. In contrast, the contents in this chapter cover broader aspects of research planning and present basic research design principles that cut across all types of research. This chapter is therefore designed to give readers foundational knowledge for the pages that follow.

Scientific research is the systematic and organized gathering of information about a specific topic. Systematization of process across the design, data collection, and analysis phases of a study is what distinguishes scientific research from other forms of inquiry. Organization of and attention to procedures—both internal and external to a study—also characterize research. Though the degree of systematicity varies by the study design, all types of research share certain basic principles and elements of design.

Viewed broadly, designing and planning research is a lot like planning a wedding. You need to think about

- your event well in advance of its occurrence,
- which and how many people to invite (sampling and sample sizes),
- how to invite them (recruitment),
- what activities will be included (method selection),
- costs and budget parameters,

- the location of the event (site selection),
- potential obstacles/problems (will Uncle Fred get drunk and table dance?), and
- how much time your event will take.

Other parallels include

- the larger the event is, the more difficult to plan and the more expensive it is;
- the more planners involved, the more expertise is included, but the longer it will take to reach consensus and plan (individual personalities are a key variable in this!);
- no matter how much planning you do, you can't anticipate or control exactly how the event will play out (refer back to Uncle Fred); and
- the fewer events and activities, the more control you have over the details; conversely, less control with more events and activities.

Research design is also—or at least should be—a highly iterative process. Going back to our wedding analogy, imagine the following (not uncommon) scenario. You and your fiancé have spent hours and hours planning your special day. Your dream wedding is set in motion. But after careful scrutiny of the projected costs, you realize that you can't afford it all, so you decide to cut costs by, say, inviting fewer guests and/or cutting back on food. Changes in either of these will, in turn, have consequences for you and your wedding guests. Or perhaps an even more stressful scenario occurs. Your future mother-in-law (in research the analogues might be funders, Institutional Review Boards, local stakeholders, research partners, or all four!) demands changing or removing one or more of the carefully thought out elements and/or adding an activity. These demands will often happen late in the planning process. Wanting to please your spouse's mother, you scramble to make the "suggested" changes and incorporate them into a revised wedding plan. These changes will have a snowball effect on other event parameters (often the budget), which will subsequently need to be adjusted. Welcome to the world of research design.

The basic principle that the wedding analogy is intended to convey is that research design is a complicated, iterative, and often frustrating process. To help readers with this complex process, we outline a series of high-level steps in the design process. The sections that follow describe in more detail each of these steps. Table 2.6 at the end of this chapter outlines this process in more detail and presents options and considerations for each decision point discussed.

FIND YOUR FOCUS

Identify the Research Problem

The research problem, at least as we definite it here, refers to the broad theoretical or real-world problem that motivates a researcher to initiate the research design process in the first place. It is the driving force behind a study. Depending on which textbook you

Basic Steps in the Design Process (often revised at every step)

Find your focus

- Identify the research problem
- Specify research objectives
- Transform objectives into research questions and hypotheses

Narrow your focus

- Decide on the type of research study and design(s)
- Clarify units of observation and units of analysis
- Determine sample and recruitment procedures
- Operationalize study measures

Define data collection and management procedures

- Decide on the mechanics of data collection
- Develop data entry, storage, and transmission standards

Consider external logistics

- Consider research scope, time, and resources
- Consider research site context

Document the research plan

- Develop a protocol
- Draft an analysis plan
- Plan for communicating results

read, the research problem might also be referred to as the goal, aim, or purpose of a study. Theoretically, research problems can emerge from anywhere, but in reality they usually come from one or more of the following, nonmutually exclusive sources:

- *A funder.* This can come in the form of a personally communicated request, but much more commonly it is expressed through a formal funding announcement such as a request for proposals or applications (RFP, RFA).

- *The literature.* A literature review may reveal a gap in knowledge about a particular topic and/or may inspire a researcher to develop and evaluate a new theory.
- *A real-world problem.* The fundamental purpose of public health is to improve the well-being of communities and populations. Surveillance data, or personal experience with a particularly vulnerable population, can bring to light a public health problem and prompt a researcher (or funder) to seek a "solution."

When put into writing, a research problem is typically communicated in one or two sentences near the beginning of a research study description. It often begins something like "The aim/goal/purpose of this study is to . . ." and then continues with a brief description of the study's desired outcome. Note that research problems can vary immensely in scope and detail. A general rule to remember: The smaller the scope of the research problem, and the more detailed its description, the easier it is to operationalize and execute.

Regardless of how focused and detailed a research problem is, a few sentences simply cannot provide enough information to begin the design process. A research problem first must be transformed into one or more research objectives.

Specify Research Objectives

A research problem is a brief statement of the purpose and overall goal of a research study. In a very few cases, it is detailed and simple enough to guide development of a research plan. In the vast majority of cases, though, a research problem must be deconstructed and made more explicit. Research objectives should conceptually fall under the scope of the research problem and simultaneously describe in more detail what the study intends to accomplish. They are actionable and provide a bridge between the larger research problem and the more detailed and refined research question(s) and/or hypotheses, which we describe later. A good way to think about and describe a research objective is to begin with the preposition *to* and follow it with a verb. These are some of the more commonly used verbs in this regard:

Identify

Explore

Describe

Explain

Compare

Assess

Evaluate

Measure

Predict

Test

Note that the choice of verb is important, since it conveys what type of general approach the research design will take. Looking at the verbs above from left to right, an underlying pattern of increasing structure in design is observable. *Exploring* a topic requires less structure than, say, *evaluating* or *testing* something. The verbs on the left side above imply a more descriptive-type study. As they move to the right they become increasingly relational and then explanatory.

Be mindful of infusing meaning-laden words into an objective. Words like *cause, relationship,* and *difference*, among other words, can substantially change the meaning of an objective even if the initial verb is constant. Consider the following four objectives:

- To identify the sanitation issues in community X.
- To identify the cause of sanitation issues in community X.
- To identify the different sanitation issues between communities X and Y.
- To identify the relationship between sanitation issues and dysentery in community X.

The first objective lends itself to an exploratory qualitative study. The second objective requires looking deeper and designing a causal study. The third objective requires a comparative design. And objective four is correlative in nature. All of these warrant very different types of studies.

The take-home point is that objectives must be carefully thought out and written in a precise and explicit manner. Figuring out how to phrase your research objectives is the first step in honing in on what you want to actually accomplish with your research. Moreover, most proposals and protocols require explicitly delineated objectives. The conceptual relationship between a research problem, objectives, and research questions/hypotheses (discussed next) is depicted in Figure 2.1.

Progressing from the research problem to explicit study objectives is probably one of the most critical steps in the design process. The total number and specificity of the objectives shape the scope and nature of the study. But developing objectives is not just a scientific enterprise, it is also a political and economic one. Different audiences for your research will have different expectations regarding its design and associated outcomes. Some audiences, for example, require more precision and/or rigor than others. Logistical factors also place a relatively firm boundary around study parameters. Budget and time are two of the stronger constraints, but other factors, such as the local political context (see Chapter 4) and access to the study population and data sources, can significantly affect the shape of a study.

Transform Objectives Into Research Questions and Hypotheses

Once the objectives have been specified, the next step is to operationalize them and transform the *to* statements into research questions and/or hypotheses. Research questions and hypotheses more precisely describe what the research findings will inform.

Figure 2.1 Conceptual Relationship Between Research Problem, Objectives, and Research Questions/Hypotheses

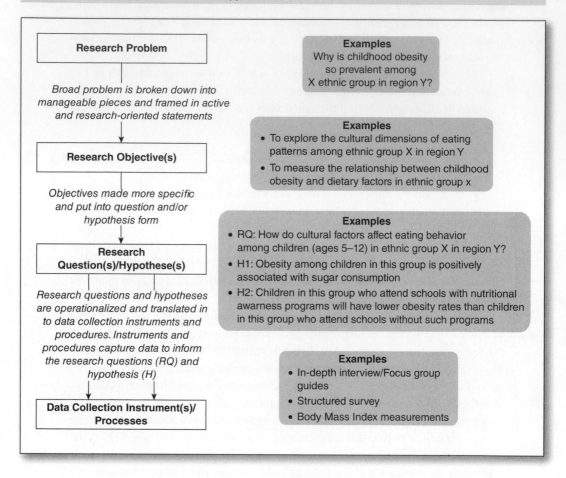

Types of Research Questions

Part of the research question development process is deciding how you will approach the topic and what you want to be able to say with the data you collect and analyze. There are three general types of research questions (Gilson, 2012; Robson, 2011; Shi, 2008). The first type, **descriptive or exploratory**, seeks to understand a particular phenomenon or problem when little is known about it or there is a need to understand it in a new context, for example, to *explore* the characteristics, motivations, and medical history of women who delay childbearing until an advanced age. The second type, **relational**, seeks to understand the relationship between two concepts or measures. Relational questions investigate associations rather than causal relationships, for example, what is the *relationship* between women's access to family planning services and delayed childbearing? **Causal** questions seek to understand whether one variable causes changes in the outcome variable of interest, for example, does use of a particular contraceptive device cause women to have trouble conceiving when they decide they are ready? Relational and causal questions are more often used to understand the effect of a health service or intervention on key outcomes, but they might also be used to understand the factors associated with certain behaviors—like the influence of social support on the use of health care services by people who use illegal drugs—in order to inform interventions.

Descriptive (aka exploratory) research questions seek to answer questions about a phenomenon. How many or how much are affected or implicated? Who is involved? Where does the phenomenon occur? For example, infant male circumcision is not routinely practiced in East Africa, so Young and colleagues (2012) interviewed parents in hospitals in a province in Kenya. They talked with parents who did and did not accept the procedure in order to understand more about their decision-making processes related to the procedure and whether they experienced any barriers or facilitators to uptake (Young et al., 2012).

Relational and causal (aka explanatory) research questions are evaluative in nature and seek to understand whether changes in one factor, such as the implementation of or improvement to a program, results in changes in behaviors, knowledge, and health outcomes (Gilson, 2012). Relational and causal research questions can also be formulated to understand why and how changes occurred. Understanding the mechanisms that resulted in change (not just whether the change occurred, yes or no) can help make recommendations for future research and program and policy implementation. For example, a 1989 study by Bongaarts and colleagues was one of the studies that helped uncover a strong population-level association between the presence of male circumcision and lower HIV prevalence in African contexts (Bongaarts, Reining, Way, & Conant, 1989). They noted that in areas and among cultures where circumcision was rare, HIV prevalence was higher. Among areas where male circumcision was common, HIV prevalence was lower. This study is relational because the research cannot demonstrate whether the lack of male circumcision caused lower HIV prevalence. These relational studies were, however, critical in the development of hypotheses which led to clinical trials of male circumcision. The subsequent randomized control trials eventually demonstrated at the individual level that male circumcision can reduce the risk of acquiring HIV prevalence by up to 53%–60% (Bailey et al., 2007; R. H. Gray et al., 2007).

Whichever the type, a good research question is clearly articulated, focused, answerable, and measureable (Gilson, 2012). In other words, it should be clear what concepts are to be measured, the relationships of those concepts, and it should be possible to answer the questions with data that can be feasibly collected. We need to be pragmatic and balance the scope and size of the study against available resources and the utility of the answers provided by the research (Robson, 2011). Above all, a good research question should yield results that are useful to inform policy, programs, or theory or serves to move along the field of inquiry. Therefore, when formulating research questions, it is important to be able to articulate what the research results will add to the existing knowledge base, to whom it will be useful, and how the results will be useful (Gilson, 2012).

For exploratory research, research questions are typically stated in the form of an actual question. Most research questions, though, can be translated into hypotheses that contain a statement about a direction of influence of cause and effect. In other words, a hypothesis restates the research question in a way that describes the expected relationship between two or more variables (Fisher & Foreit, 2002). For example:

- Variable A is associated with variable B
  - ___ Areas with higher levels of male circumcision are associated with lower levels of HIV.
- A change in variable A will result in an increase or decrease in variable B
  - ___ Adult male circumcision will result in decreased risk of HIV acquisition for men.

The hypothesis describes the relationship between the independent variable (e.g., male circumcision) and dependent variables (HIV). It also implies directionality (male circumcision influences HIV acquisition, not the reverse). The independent variable is often an intervention or program in public health research, such as the introduction of electronic medical records. But the independent variable can also be some other factor, such as education level, that is hypothesized to be associated with or cause a change in the dependent variable. The dependent variable is the outcome that is influenced, often health behaviors or health status, for example.

A note about different terminology: Different disciplines may use different words for independent or dependent variables. For example, independent variables may also be called exposure variables or predictor variables. Dependent variables may be called outcomes or response variables.

Literature Reviews

As mentioned above, developing research questions and hypotheses requires specificity and precision. This, in turn, requires a certain degree of insight about where the knowledge gaps and/or applied needs are. A literature review will help you understand what is already known about your research topic. Literature reviews serve many purposes, detailed in Table 2.1. The most rigorous type of literature is that which is peer reviewed—those books and manuscripts that went through a process of independent review by scholars with relevant expertise in the field of study. While support for study ideas will be viewed more credibly if backed up by the peer-reviewed literature, often good information—and possibly more recent and timely information—exists in the "grey literature." That is information that exists in conference presentations, reports, or working papers from various organizations, usually on their websites. The decision to include grey literature may be strengthened if the intervention being reviewed is complex, has a complex outcome, or lacks outcomes measures; is underrepresented in the peer-reviewed literature; lacks quality evidence in the peer-reviewed literature; or takes place in a context that is important to implementation (Benzies, Premji, Hayden, & Serrett, 2006).

Table 2.1   Uses for Literature Reviews

Within a given field of inquiry, literature reviews can help you:	*For a particular project or study, a literature review can help you:*
• understand areas for future research • identify patterns within existing studies • reveal potentially conflicting findings • define measures or identify variations in measures • reveal what research methods, questionnaires, instruments, scales, and conceptual models have been applied previously (Robson, 2011)	• specify and refine your research question • develop a strong rationale for the need for the research • support your study design, instruments, and measures

Systematic reviews are different from literature reviews in that they are, as you might imagine, more systematic. They still cover the literature and summarize what is known, but typically systematic reviews are an end rather than a means, resulting in a comprehensive understanding of what is known about the effectiveness of health interventions. Typically, the process involves several partners, the results reflect precisely what is and is not known about interventions, and results are used to inform policy or clinical decisions (Institute of Medicine, 2011). The Institute of Medicine has produced very specific standards for systematic reviews.[1]

Resources for conducting literature reviews include library databases, electronic databases (e.g., Pubmed, CINAHL, PsycINFO, SSCI, AgeInfo, CareData, Social Services Abstracts, Popline, EMBASE), and search engines such as Google Scholar. A more complete list is available at the end of this chapter (see Search Engines and Databases for Conducting Literature Reviews). Take the time to learn how to effectively use keywords in your search; how to narrow your search using parentheses and *or, and,* or *not* statements; and truncation or other "advanced" features. The more thorough your literature search is, the more important it becomes to document your search strategy by documenting the combination of key words you have used and your strategy for eliminating and retaining articles to review.

As you may know, bibliographic citation management software is widely available now, and there are a number of both paid and free packages to choose from (e.g., Endnote, Procite). Programs may be hosted on your own personal computer or may be web-based or hosted by a central server. They are tools that can help store and organize and create reference lists of the materials you have gathered. They can also help you create formatted bibliographies or references lists and according to the style you need. They also serve as search engines within the databases you have created or have access to.

Using Theory and Conceptual Models to Inform/Refine Research Questions

Theory, research, and practice are all linked. Research provides evidence that informs how to organize and target interventions to improve care and ultimately health outcomes. Theory drives research priorities and how research is carried out. Theory is "a set of interrelated concepts, definitions, and propositions that presents a systematic view of events or situations by specifying relationship among variables in order to explain and predict the events or situations" (Glanz, Lewis, & Rimer 1997, p. 21). Theories help researchers know *who* to target as the subject of research, *what* the researcher needs to know before developing the research or the program of study, and *how* to shape interventions of study so that they have a greater likelihood of having a positive effect on outcomes of interest. The Appendix at the end of this book provides a description of the main theories and models used in public health research and practice.

Conceptual models are used to summarize existing knowledge about the relationships between variables of interest and to illustrate the research question using concept boxes and arrows. A conceptual model is "a diagram of proposed causal linkages among a set of concepts believed to be related to a particular public health problem" (Earp & Ennett, 1991, p. 164). A *concept* is an abstract idea or phenomenon that can be observed or measured. *Variables* are the operational definitions of the concepts (Glanz et al., 1997). At the center, a conceptual model contains the independent variable (or cause or intervention) that leads to an outcome (or dependent variable; Figure 2.2). Conceptual models are typically read from left to right, but other formulations exist. The model allows for mediating variables (an intervening explanatory variable in between the independent and outcome variable), antecedent variables, and modifying variables (variables that affect the direction or strength of the relationship between the independent and outcome variables). In Figure 2.2 we use a light example of proposal and marriage to illustrate the relationship of some of these variables.

Figure 2.2 Conceptual Model of Marriage Proposal Leading to Marriage

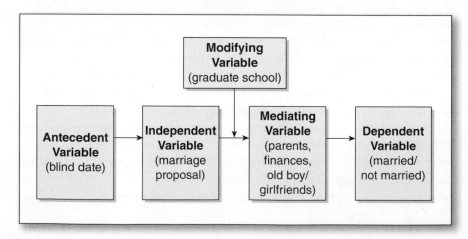

Although not shown in Figure 2.2, confounding variables are commonly included in conceptual models. They are factors that act to influence both the independent variable and the outcome or dependent variable. For example, while use of antenatal care is typically associated with better maternal and infant outcomes, pregnancy complications might be a confounding variable in the relationship between use of antenatal care and pregnancy outcome (Figure 2.3). A woman who experiences complication in a pregnancy might be more likely to use more antenatal care, and those pregnancy complications may also result in poorer pregnancy outcomes.

Figure 2.3   Example of a Variable Confounding the Relationship Between the Independent and Dependent Variable

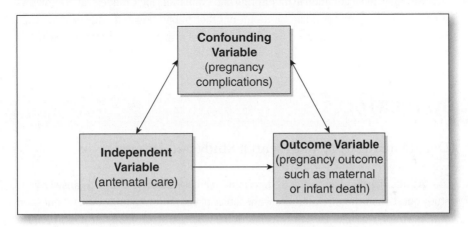

A research conceptual model does not tell the researcher how to intervene, but rather how the intervention is expected to influence the outcomes of interest and the other factors that influence the effectiveness of the intervention. For research purposes, the concepts are translated into variables and are operationally defined so that they can be measured. Researchers typically include in the conceptual model only those variables that they can measure, though sometimes researchers include variables they know to influence the other variables but that they are not measuring. However, conceptual models are meant to be parsimonious. Table 2.2 provides examples in order to demonstrate the increasing specificity from concepts to variables and measures.

Table 2.2   Examples of Concept, Variable, and Measure

Concept	Variable	Measure
Use of maternal health care services	Seek antenatal care	Attended antenatal care with a trained provider four or more times during pregnancy (Y/N)
Economic strengthening	Social cash transfer intervention	Ultra poor household with orphans and vulnerable children receives US$20 per month (Y/N)

Conceptual models also help during data analysis because they describe the hierarchical relationships between factors. For example, poverty is often associated with poor health, but poverty is not the cause of poor health per se. Poverty acts through variables such as malnutrition to affect health outcomes like diarrhea in children. In multivariable and multivariate analyses (like those using linear and logistic regression models), researchers typically want to assess the effect of the independent variable (in this case malnutrition) on the outcome (diarrhea) taking into account the other factors (poverty). The analyst will want to understand the effect of malnutrition without taking into account other variables as well as adjusting for other variables. Thus, she or he may have three models, one with malnutrition alone, one with poverty alone, and one with both malnutrition and poverty (looking at the effects on diarrhea).

Although most common in monitoring and evaluation, logic models (also known as program impact pathways) can be useful in other public research endeavors as well. Logic models are linear, left-to-right models that describe program inputs and activities expected to influence outputs, outcomes, and impact.

NARROW YOUR FOCUS

Decide on the Type of Research Study and Design(s)

At this stage you are ready to determine the best research design to answer your study question. As noted earlier, the word choice of your research objective and question starts to imply a design. The key is to determine which study design is the most effective way to answer your research question.

Basic Types of Research Studies

As stated above, there are different types of research questions: descriptive, relational, and causal. These types of research questions translate into either exploratory or explanatory research. **Exploratory** research seeks to understand new or complex phenomena and to generate hypotheses, particularly when little is known about a topic. Once more information is known about a situation or context, descriptive research is used to describe phenomena and characteristics of people and their contexts. **Explanatory** research is carried out to try to understand the factors causing or associated with knowledge, behavior, health, or other variables and the relationship between various factors and the outcomes (Robson, 2011). Explanatory research is interested in the relationships (i.e., causal or associative) between variables (Gilson, 2012).

Descriptive Studies

The type of research question will inform the study design, and descriptive questions usually translate into simpler study designs. Descriptive studies are observational, do not attempt to assign causality, and are good for problem identification. They are good at answering who, what, why, when, where, and so what (Grimes & Schulz, 2002).

Descriptive studies are conducted to investigate a population's health service needs, experiences, or behaviors in order to inform interventions. When descriptive studies gather information about experiences with health services or a particular intervention, they may actually be considered a posttest-only design, which is described in the context of study designs below. Types of descriptive studies include the following:

- *Case studies:* A comprehensive focus on a single phenomenon (Yin, 1999). Qualitative and quantitative data can be used, and the researcher can rely on multiple types of data collection. Examples include studies of a financial system in a hospital, the political structure of a community, or policies of a managed care system. The methods used to select cases can vary widely; a case may be selected because it is thought to be a critical case, extreme case, revelatory case, model case, or modal case.

- *Cross-sectional studies:* In a cross-sectional study, data are collected at one point in time. A variety of quantitative and qualitative methods can be employed with a sample of units (e.g., people, hospitals) to gather data about a particular health service or policy or to gain understanding about a particular phenomenon, measure, or context. Descriptive surveys aim to describe pictures of a situation or problem or program (Veney & Kaluzny, 1998). Other data may be used in cross-sectional descriptive studies, including structured or semistructured interviews, reviews of documents, or observations.

- *Trend design:* In a trend design, two or more cross-sectional studies are conducted over time. Data, often quantitative, are compiled to demonstrate how variables of interest change over time. An important data source for trend analyses in the health services is routine program information (Veney & Kaluzny, 1998). Information about number of clients served, client characteristics such as sex and age, diagnostic classification, and so on provide information about patterns of use of a particular program. Other trend data can come from state, national, or international statistics agencies tracking disease and injury prevalence and use of services.

- *Panel design:* A panel design is similar to a trend design in that data are collected at two or more points over time, but in a panel design data are collected from the same people or cases.

- *Case-control and cohort studies* (either retrospective or prospective): These are two other types of descriptive observational studies and are commonly used in epidemiology to understand disease etiology, incidence, prevalence, causes, and risk factors (Mann, 2003). You can find more information about cohort and case-control studies in Chapter 7.

Relational and Causal Studies

Relational and causal studies are used to understand a relationship between independent and dependent variables. In the case of causal or explanatory studies, there is also an attempt to demonstrate a causal relationship. Interventions range from true experimental to quasi-experimental and nonexperimental designs (Table 2.3). The main feature of **true experimental designs** is that randomization is used to assign units into intervention (or experimental) and control groups. The unit of randomization can be at the level of the individuals or it can be at higher levels, such as a hospital or facility, or geographic unit such as a district. Randomization is a technique that can deal with most of the threats to internal validity (see below), particularly selection. In other words, it helps increase our confidence that the participants in each intervention and the control group are similar in characteristics that might otherwise act to independently influence the outcome of interest.

True experiments, while having many positive attributes as a study design, also have some drawbacks. For one, true experiments do not do well with explaining complex social issues; when outcomes of true experiments are unexpected, researchers often face difficulties in explaining the reasons for those results (Robson, 2011). Some interventions, particularly in health services or psychosocial areas, are complex or operate through complex pathways of influence that may be difficult to randomize or assign adequate control groups. Another problem can arise when true experiments rely on volunteers for participating in studies. The simple act of volunteering may mean that the participants are more motivated or interested in the study and therefore may react to the intervention differently from the rest of the population. This difference may cause problems when the intervention is made available to the general population but does not have the same effects as under experimental conditions (see Chapter 16 for a discussion of efficacy versus effectiveness randomized controlled trials).

Quasi-experimental designs again involve an intervention group and a comparison group, but control groups are determined by means other than randomization. Quasi-experimental designs are suitable for environments where it is not feasible to randomize. In the nonequivalent control group design, the individual is not usually the primary sampling unit. Usually the groups are made up of units such as hospitals or facilities, or geographic units such as districts. A nonequivalent control group design has pre- and posttest measures for both the intervention and comparison groups; the main difference is that there is no randomization into groups. Researchers have other techniques they can use to try to make the intervention and comparison groups as similar as possible. They can rely on *matching*, whereby researchers try to make key characteristics as similar as possible between intervention and comparison groups. For example, in a situation where the groups are health facilities, researchers might try to match on characteristics such as number of beds, number of doctors or medical staff, rural/urban location, catchment area size, services offered, and so on. Also, multivariable and multivariate analysis methods can be used to try to control for differences between intervention and comparison groups. The main risk in both of these methods is that the researcher cannot control for or identify all factors that may result in differences between intervention and comparison groups (that is, researchers can never rule out selection bias).

Time series designs can often offer convincing evidence of changes due to interventions. In a time series design, the comparison group is actually repeated measures that occur prior to an intervention. Time series designs are useful when the boundaries of interventions, such as mass media campaigns, are difficult to define, determine, or contain. Thus, control or comparison groups are not feasible. The more measures that are taken before and after the intervention the better. These measures can be plotted on a graph for visual interpretation of effect, but researchers can also use analytic methods to test for statistical differences. A main limitation of time series designs is that some measures might naturally change over time. For example, more and more adolescents will naturally initiate sexual activity over time. A related model is a regression-discontinuity design. In this model, intervention and comparison groups are determined based on defining a criterion cutoff value, with one group falling above the value and the other falling below.

Nonexperimental designs are more appropriate for collecting descriptive information about a program or for problem diagnosis (Fisher & Foreit, 2002). In a posttest-only design, measures are taken with in an intervention group only after the intervention has occurred. Thus, this design is good for investigating demand for the intervention; characteristics of people participating in the intervention; understanding provider perspectives, knowledge, or skills implementing the intervention; or clients' satisfaction with the intervention.

Pre- and posttest study designs have no comparison group, but measures are made before and after the intervention. While researchers cannot make statements about the levels of change that are attributed to an intervention, pre- and posttest designs can be useful for piloting new interventions in order to get a sense of the potential for effectiveness before engaging in a more rigorous design.

A static group comparison has postintervention-only measures, but in both intervention and comparison groups. Because assignment into groups is not randomized and there is no baseline measure by which to compare changes over time, a researcher must seriously consider the added value of collecting data in the comparison group. It may be sufficient to stick with a posttest-only design and save costs associated with the additional data collection in the comparison group, if the research cannot ensure adequate matching or statistical analysis to justify the inclusion of the comparison group.

Table 2.3   Summary of Types of Study Designs for Research and Evaluation

Type of Design	Study Design	Random Assignment	Intervention Group	Control or Comparison Group	Measures Occur Before Intervention	Measures Occur After Intervention
Experimental	Pretest-posttest control group design	Yes	Yes	Yes	Yes	Yes
	Posttest-only control group design	Yes	Yes	Yes	No	Yes
Quasi-experimental	Nonequivalent control group	No	Yes	Yes	Yes	Yes
	Time series design	No	Yes	Yes (historical control)	Yes	Yes
Nonexperimental	Posttest-only design	No	Yes	No	No	Yes
	Pretest-posttest design	No	Yes	No	Yes	Yes
	Static-group comparison	No	Yes	Yes	No	Yes

Variations on Common Study Designs

Thus far we have described basic study designs, but there are a number of other designs that build on these. For example, it is possible to have participants assigned to two different intervention groups (A and B) and compare that to a control group, or to have participants assigned to an intervention group (A) and an enhanced intervention group. Whether you want to compare A and B to the control group or (A vs. C) and (B vs. C) and (A vs. B) depends on the research question. Similarly, it is possible that you might want to compare one intervention group to two control groups. The more complex your design, the larger the sample size required.

In some cases, you might investigate whether two factors interact to increase their effect on the outcome. This **factorial design** results in a number of combinations including (A vs. C), (B vs. C), and (A*B vs. C). Economic components could be added here to understand more about the value of the additional component. For example, if providers are trained in a particular technique in the classroom setting, a researcher may be interested in whether the addition of web-based training enhances the providers' skills. The study design would compare the effect of training only with training plus web component. An excellent example of randomized control trial with a factorial design compared the effects of different supplementation during pregnancy to prevent neural tube defects (MRC Vitamin Study Research Group, 1991). Women were assigned to one of four groups: folic acid only (A), folic acid and other vitamins (B), no vitamins or folic acid (C), or other vitamins but no folic acid (D). The design allowed the researchers to understand that folic acid had a 72% protective effect against neural tube defects while there was no significant protective effect provided by the other vitamins.

In a **parametric** or **dose-response analysis**, researchers are interested in the effect of different levels of exposure to an intervention. The concept comes from clinical studies of whether increasing (or decreasing) drug doses results in corresponding improvements in health.

A **stepped-wedge design** is increasing in popularity recently as an alternative to randomized control trials. Stepped-wedge designs can be useful when it is not feasible to exclude groups in order to create control or comparison groups, or if is not feasible to delay program implementation in order to get baseline measures. In a stepped-wedge design, groups are randomly selected to receive the intervention in phases. The advantage of this design is that it allows for all groups to eventually receive the intervention, but in a phased process that is usually compatible with program implementation. In some cases it may also allow for dose responses analyses to see whether increased exposure to the intervention is associated with changes in study outcomes.

Structure and Method/Design Selection

The degree of structure in a research project overall, and in the data collection processes more specifically, will help define both your method selection and the type of findings you will generate. In an ideal world, the overall process of scientific inquiry follows a funnel pattern, starting off with broader and more general types of questioning and moving to more specific and structured types of inquiry as more about a topic is learned. In this context, "research process" can refer to a single study with multiple components or the larger, collective body of multiple scientific studies pertaining to a particular topic (which can take place over years, decades, or even centuries).

In the earliest stages of the research process, the focus is likely to be exploratory and the selection of data collection methods and development of instruments will reflect this. Not surprisingly, the early stages in the overall research process are when qualitative, and less structured, forms of inquiry are often employed. Using less structured forms of inquiry in the incipient stages of research improves inquiry validity (that is, ensures that researchers are asking the right questions and in the right way). On the other end of the spectrum, rigorous hypothesis testing, such as in randomized controlled trials, requires a substantial amount of structure (Figure 2.4).

Figure 2.4 Structure and Implications for Research Design

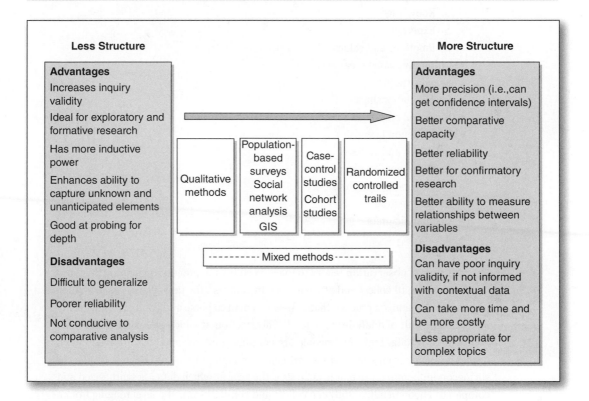

Looking at Figure 2.4, you'll notice that structure and the flexibility and inductive process that characterize lack of structure each come with advantages and disadvantages. More flexible, less structured forms of inquiry can help enhance inquiry validity, identify locally relevant issues, and contribute to a deeper understanding of a given research topic. They are not, however, well suited to comparative analyses. They are even less useful for directly testing hypotheses. As a researcher, you will need to decide where your specific study context fits on the structure continuum.

Clarify Units of Observation and Units of Analysis

After a literature review, you will know where additional research is needed, and research questions(s) will begin to crystalize. Conceptualizing and specifying what you want to collect data from and/or about—the unit of observation—is another step in the research question development process. It is important to clarify this in the early stages of designing your research. Below is a list of the more common domains of observation in public health research. Note that many studies include two or more of these, often in a relational framework:

- Human behavior
- Human psychological aspects
  - o Attitudes/opinions
  - o Perceptions
  - o Knowledge
  - o Experiences
  - o Emotions and values
- Culturally shared meanings
- Social structures
- Social relationships
- Biological outcomes
- Socioeconomic metrics
- Processes and systems
- Environmental context
- Disease incidence/prevalence
- Disease vectors
- Geographic units
- Events

The **unit of observation** relates to the data collection process by defining the types of data you plan to collect and at what level. In contrast, the unit of analysis in a study pertains to the analytic process; that is, how you plan to parse and compare data during analysis. The **unit of analysis** is the level of abstraction at which you will look for variability in your data. Individual people are common units of analysis in public health research, as are groups defined by particular demographics, such as race, gender, or socioeconomic status. The unit of analysis is the level at which data are synthesized and compared. Theoretically, a study can collect and compare data at a level ranging from a specific isolated behavior (episode) to a country and its attributes. Some commonly employed units of observation in health research include the following:

- Country or other large geographic region
- City/town/village
- Neighborhoods, districts, or areas within a city/town/village
- Institution (e.g., company, hospital, NGO)
- Household

- Dyad (e.g., a married couple, patient/doctor)
- Individual
- Event

Note that the unit of observation and unit of analysis are often, but not always, the same thing. For example, a study may collect data from and about individuals (unit of observation) in a community, but aggregate those data during analysis and compare data among two or more communities (unit of analysis). Or biological data may be the unit of observation, but more than likely the unit of analysis in this case will be individuals. A cardinal rule in research design is to make sure that your unit of observation is at the same, or preferably more granular, level of abstraction as your unit of analysis. Once collected, data can always be aggregated. They can never be disaggregated.

Determine Sample and Recruitment Procedures

Public health researchers must decide how to select their study samples and how many items to include in their sample. A *sample* is a subset of a population of people, health facilities, households, geographic units, events, and so on. Chapter 17 covers the conceptual and practical aspects of sampling and recruitment. It is important to note here, however, that sampling is a critical component of research design. Sampling procedures determine how much a researcher can extrapolate and generalize (or not) beyond a study sample. A study that has high external validity (or generalizability) provides greater insight into how the behavior, knowledge, an intervention, disease pathways, or incidence observed in one study would apply (or not) in other geographic areas, with different participants, or when made available to a larger segment of the population from which the original study participants were drawn (that is, scale up).

Operationalize Study Measures

Earlier in this chapter we discussed how studies consist of *concepts* to be measured by *variables*. At this point in the study design you will need to operationalize those variables for measurement. This means making more precise how you will measure the variable. In social research, verbal or self-report are the most common kinds of measurement (Singleton, Straits, & Straits, 1993). For example, questions are asked of respondents about their background characteristics such as levels of education, their knowledge and attitudes, and certain health behaviors. These measures can also be combined to make composite measures, scales, or indexes (more information about scale development and validation is in Chapter 13). Measures may also be obtained through observation or through review of existing records or documentation. Chapter 11 has more information about observing client-provider interactions, for example, to study quality of health care. Other observed measures may include medical assessment of weight, height, blood pressure, blood or urine samples, and such. Existing records or documents may include health records, public or private documents, and written or video communications (Singleton et al., 1993).

The operationalization of measures is highly dependent on what you have defined as the research question and hypothesis. There are pragmatic considerations as well about what is feasible. Questionnaires have to be of reasonable length so as to not overburden the respondent, and all measures and procedures have to be ethically and technically feasible. See Table 2.2 above for examples of concepts, variables, and measures. Operationalizing your study measures will help you determine the data you need to obtain those measures. Broad data categories include primary data, or data collected by you for your study, and secondary data, which are existing sources of data (see Chapter 9). Data can be obtained from self-reports, observation, or biological sources.

The tool that will measure your variable is called an **instrument**. This can be a survey, device, checklist, procedure, or any other measurement tool. Prior to conducting the research, ensure that your instrument is reliable (measures are reproducible at different times or by different observers) and valid (data measure what they are actually supposed to measure). This is typically done through a process of pretesting (or pilot testing) the instrument. Then, in order to ensure proper use of the instrument, researchers train any data collection or study staff who will use the instrument. Additional information about survey design and implementation is in Chapter 12.

Validity

Within the research methods literature, there is big V validity and little v validity. The former refers to the concept as a whole, while the latter refers to specific subtypes of validity. As the term *validity* is commonly used in research vernacular across multiple disciplines, the definitions associated with it vary by field. Below are a few definitions of the general concept of validity (big V):

- "An account is valid or true if it represents accurately those features of the phenomena, that it is intended to describe, explain or theorize" (Hammersley, 1992, p. 69)
- "The accuracy and trustworthiness of instruments, data and findings in research" (Bernard, 2013, p. 45)
- "The degree to which a test measures what it is intended to measure" (Social Science Dictionary, 2008)
- "Validity can be considered as the extent to which a measurement, test, or study measures what it purports to measure" (Kirch, 2008, p. 1440)
- "The degree to which data in a research study are accurate and credible" (D. E. Gray, 2009, p. 582)
- "The validity of a measure is the extent to which it actually assesses what it purports to measure" (Shi, 2008, p. 464)

The definitions represented (and typically those not represented here as well) encompass a cross-cutting theme: the notion that we are actually assessing what we are intending to assess.

The subtypes of validity most commonly discussed are face validity, content validity, construct validity, criterion validity, external validity, and internal validity (although one can find many more types of validity described throughout the literature; see Bernard, 2013; Maxwell, 1992). We provide a brief definition of several subtypes in Table 2.4.

Table 2.4   Subtypes of Validity

Type of Validity	Definition
Face	The indicator for a concept (e.g., question, scale) intuitively makes sense; determined by consensus among researchers
Content	The degree to which an instrument has the appropriate breadth and depth of content for measuring a complex construct or concept
Construct	The degree to which a measure relates to other variables as expected within a system of theoretical relationships
Criterion (predictive) validity	The degree to which a measure relates to some external criterion that is known to be valid
External	The degree to which study findings are relevant to other populations and contexts (i.e., generalizability)
Internal	The degree to which one can be certain that changes in the dependent variable were actually caused by the experimental treatment

Threats to Validity

There are a number of threats to validity that can undermine the confidence that researchers or others have in a study's findings. At the most fundamental level, threats to internal validity apply to all research designs. Internal validity relates to whether the study's design and data collection methods accurately capture and address what the objectives seek to achieve. External review of the study design, by a diverse audience, can minimize problems associated with validity at this level, as can prestudy formative inquiry. Pretesting study instruments among the target population is another critical activity in this regard.

Several commonly encountered threats to internal validity affect causal studies, including the following (Campbell & Stanley, 1963; Singleton et al., 1993):

• *History:* Events external to the independent variable of interest that happen in the participants' environment during the course of the study and exert an influence on the outcome. The Haiti earthquake and election violence in Kenya, both of which displaced thousands of people, disrupted access to antiretroviral treatment for those who are HIV positive (Oser, Ojikutu, Odek, Ogunlayi, & Bakualufu Ntumba, 2012).

• *Maturation:* Psychological or physical events that occur over time to study participants as part of natural processes regardless of study influences. Changes in height, weight, or intellectual development occurring naturally may influence study outcomes of interest independent of the variable of interest.

- *Testing or observation effect:* The act of being observed may result in a participant intentionally or unintentionally changing their behavior because they know they are being observed. Participating in surveys or questionnaires can have an independent influence on those scores across repeated measures. Some tasks, like taking tests, get easier with practice.

- *Inconsistent instrumentation or measurement:* Changes to the measurement instrument result in changes in scores independent from the main variable of interest. For example, an observer assigning scores will get better at scoring over time, or alternatively, the observer gets bored and pays less attention. It may also happen that a measurement instrument such as a scale or blood pressure machine is poorly calibrated or an interview question is poorly written.

- *Statistical regression or regression to the mean:* This refers to the tendency for outlying scores, behaviors, or measures to move closer to the mean. This can influence studies of people with extreme characteristics, such as low scores on a test.

- *Selection:* Differences in the characteristics of individuals composing the intervention and control groups, present prior to any intervention, might affect observed outcomes. Interventions are often targeted to areas or populations with greatest need for the intervention or service, so there may be challenges to identifying an adequate control group.

- *Attrition:* Most studies experience some loss-to-follow-up—some participants willingly drop out over time, they cannot be located for additional data collection efforts, or they die. The threat to internal validity comes in when there are differences in the characteristics of people who drop out over time between the intervention and control groups.

Those are some of the traditional threats to internal validity. Another problem that can occur is ambiguity about the causal direction (Robson, 2011), meaning that for some research questions/findings, it is difficult to determine which variable is independent and which is dependent (the outcome). For example, does use of contraceptive methods increase women's educational attainment, or does more education increase contraceptive use? Differential treatment effects can also be a problem (Robson, 2011). This can happen when a person assigned to an intervention or drug treatment does not receive the full intervention or take the whole drug dose. Conversely, participants in a control group may have access to the intervention or treatment. This is sometimes called *contamination* or *diffusion* and is more likely to happen when interventions are not based at the individual level but are applied at higher levels such as a health facility or within a close-knit community.

The concept of external validity is concerned with what happens after the study and the degree to which study findings are relevant to other populations and contexts. *Generalizability* is another term used to describe the degree to which studies of effective interventions will be able to be replicated in other populations. External validity can be established by ensuring that the population participating in the study is representative of the population as a whole that will eventually benefit from the intervention (Gertler, Martinez, Premand, Rawlings, & Vermeersch, 2011). Random selection of participants for a study enhances representativeness.

DEFINE DATA COLLECTION AND MANAGEMENT PROCEDURES

Decide on the Mechanics of Data Collection

Once your study design and data collection methods have been determined, you can turn your attention to the physical means of data collection. Will someone from the research team collect data from/about individuals directly (as in clinician- or interviewer-administered instruments)? If not, what will be your data sources, and how will you define what is included and excluded? If so, how will data be recorded? Paper and pencil is the traditional method and still commonly used. Data collectors, however, are increasingly taking advantage of digital data capture devices, such as PDAs, iPods, and iPads (Figures 2.5a–b), or other devices such as digital imagery or videos. One of the advantages of using digital methods of data collection is that data are usually entered directly into a database, avoiding an extra data entry step. One of the disadvantages is that setting up the data collection system often requires a lot of up-front programming. Electronic devices also need to be charged, necessitating reliable power sources in the field. And electronic devices can also simply fail.

Another option is to collect data remotely and/or without direct contact with a study participant. Examples of remote techniques include telephone (including text messages), mail, or the Internet. Audio computer-assisted self-interviews (ACASI) is a commonly used remote data collection technique (Figure 2.5c). ACASI involves computer-administered questions that participants read and hear. Participants are automatically led through the survey based on how they respond. A purported advantage of remote techniques such as ACASI is that they enhance the accuracy of self-reported data, at least in contexts where the topic is sensitive in nature (e.g., criminal behavior, condom use). Remote data collection techniques, however, can lead to more missing data items, since a data collector is not there to ensure completion of the instrument. Also, remote techniques are generally not well suited to complex and conceptually difficult questions, where a data collector may need to be present to explain questions. The In Focus section on mobile data collection strategies, at the end of Chapter 21, provides more information on mobile and digital data collection methods.

If you will be collecting primary data from study participants, be mindful of the characteristics and skills of the person/people collecting data. Sex, race, ethnicity,

Figure 2.5a Screenshot of PDA-Administered Survey (courtesy of FHI 360)

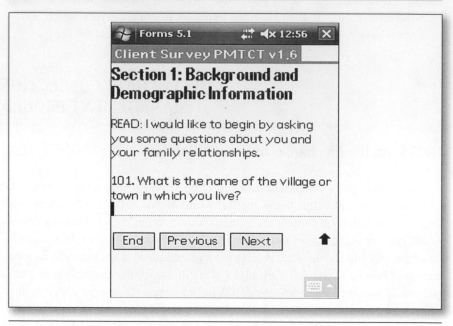

Source: Courtesy of FHI 360.

Figure 2.5b Screenshot of iPod-Administered Survey (courtesy of FHI 360)

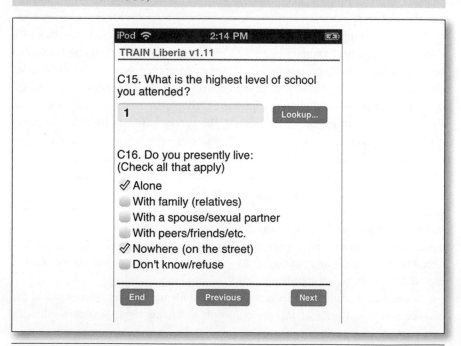

Source: Courtesy of FHI 360.

Figure 2.5c   Audio Computer-Assisted Self-Interview (ACASI)

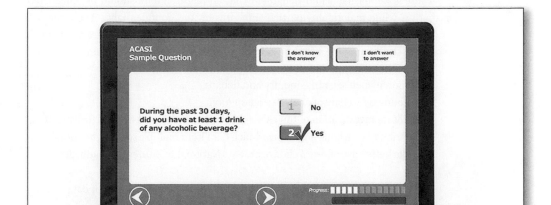

Source: Tufts University's ACASI System: http://acasi.tufts.edu.

language, age, and education level may all factor in to how well data collectors are able to elicit information from study participants. Depending on the data collection method, the collector may need to have special skills such as qualitative interviewing experience or experience drawing biological samples.

Develop Data Entry, Storage, and Transmission Standards

Data entry requires you or research team members to have skills using the data entry software and in entering data, verifying data, and cleaning data. This applies to all types of data, whether focus group transcripts, survey data, or biological samples. Consider how you will identify and follow up on skipped questions, illogical or illegible responses, or ambiguous data.

Data storage is another important concern. How will questionnaires, biological samples, or electronic data be stored? How will you securely transfer data? How and when will questionnaires and data be disposed of after the study is finished and all papers are written? Developing and distributing a written record of standard operating procedures—a project procedures manual—goes a long way toward establishing and maintaining the integrity of the research design, protecting human subjects, and ultimately successfully executing a study.

Data Sharing

There is increasing acknowledgment that all research data should be considered for sharing, while maintaining participants' privacy and confidentiality. There may be more demand for access to large databases and population-based studies than small, descriptive studies, but the scientific community notes that accessible data will

- reinforce open scientific inquiry and debate,
- encourage diversity of analysis and opinion,
- facilitate investigation of topics not within the scope of the initial investigators,
- contribute to creating data sets in which data from multiple sources are combined,
- make better use of research investment (National Institutes of Health, 2003).

Prior to conducting studies with multiple partners, the negotiation of data sharing agreements and third-party data-sharing plans can avoid many problems and disagreements about who "owns" the data. Data-sharing agreements define roles and responsibilities with research partnerships, clarify who maintains the data and study documentation, and outlines arrangements for handling third-party requests for data (from people not directly involved in the study who want to use the data for secondary analysis).

CONSIDER EXTERNAL LOGISTICS

Research Scope, Time, and Resources

Every researcher wants to design and execute the "perfect" study. Clients and funders want this too. The challenge for researchers is that clients and funders typically want the perfect research study done quickly and cheaply. Figure 2.6 is a simple, yet useful graphic to conceptualize the balance of research scope with time and resources. Increasing one element almost always means that you will have to adjust at least one other element. Otherwise, quality is sacrificed.

Study timelines, therefore, require careful calculation and realistic schedules. Resources—financial, human, and material—must be identified. Scope is reflected in your research objectives and is the most ambiguous of the three elements. The larger the scope, the more time and resources (labor and cost) it will require to execute.

If funders and/or clients expect too much for too little, you must educate them on the effects such demands will have on the quality of the end product. Provide them with outcome scenarios based on different decision routes. Easier said than done, but still easier than explaining, *post facto*, why your data are substandard, why the project is behind schedule, or why you went over budget.

Consider Research Site Context

Understanding the physical, political, and cultural context of a research site is critical to successful implementation and completion of a research study. Key stakeholders need

Figure 2.6   Balancing Time, Resources, and Scope

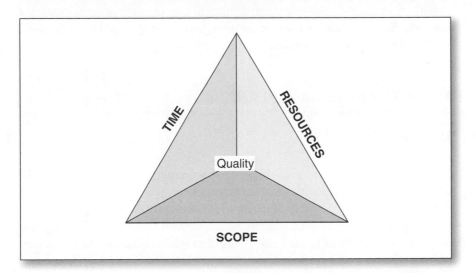

to be engaged, at least at some level, prior to study design and implementation. For example, one of our students was conducting a participant observation exercise in a department store for a research methods course. The student had been carrying out his assignment for no more than a few minutes before being told to leave by the store's manager. Informing the manager of what he wanted to do and why *before* engaging in the activity would have likely resulted in a different outcome. Needless to say, for real research studies the stakes are much higher and the political context much more complicated. Chapter 4 provides examples of the importance of community engagement.

Community-based participatory research (CBPR) is a specific approach that engages stakeholders in the research process, increases understanding of the research site, and is gaining attention as an approach that has the potential to bridge the gap between research and practice (Wallerstein & Duran, 2010). Researchers work with communities as an equitable partner throughout the research process, including deciding on how to use the research results to improve programs and intervention. The approach typically relies on multiple methods, both qualitative and quantitative, and primary and secondary data sources (Minkler et al., n.d.). CBPR can help increase external validity so that research findings are more easily translated into other settings. The approach has also been documented to affect policy and lead to programs that are more sustainable and equitable (Minkler et al., n.d.; Wallerstein & Duran, 2010). For more information on CBPR, refer to the In Focus section at the end of Chapter 4.

Understanding the physical context of where the study will take place is also essential. A personal visit to a field site can help you make determinations about appropriateness or fit for study objectives. Guest was designing procedures to select a sample from among female vendors (presumably at higher risk for HIV) in one of East Africa's largest markets. The only information available was the estimated size of the market and the knowledge that vendors could be located in various types of stalls, or be ambulatory, moving from one location to another. He designed an elaborate sampling plan that included several steps and strategies—cluster, systematic, and simple random sampling.

During a prestudy site visit, Guest and his local collaborator met with the market administrator, who informed them that he had a complete list of all the market vendors and would be willing to share this with them. Within a 10-minute conversation, the sampling plan went from a complex combination of strategies to a simple random sample based on the comprehensive list of vendors.

DOCUMENT THE RESEARCH PLAN

Develop a Protocol

A research protocol is a formal document that describes the procedures that make up a research study. The length and complexity of a protocol varies with the size and nature of a given study. A protocol for a clinical trial, involving an investigational drug, for example, will be much more complicated and detailed than a protocol for a small, qualitative study involving minimal risk. Though the extensiveness of protocols will vary, many contain the following sections:

Rationale for the Study

General Design of the Study

Objectives of the Research

Outcome Variables (for causal, predictive, and associative studies)

Description of the Target Population(s)

Participant Eligibility Criteria

Sampling Procedures and Sample Size Justification

Recruitment Procedures

Data Management Plan/Procedures

Analysis Plan Summary

Procedure for Protecting Research Participants (if applicable)

Plans for Communicating Results

A protocol is important for several reasons. First, protocol development requires a researcher to think about and write down all of the research procedures and how they relate to one another. This is an excellent exercise for tightening up a research design. A second reason is that a protocol provides a written record of study procedures that is distributed among study team members (and others). Having a central document for everyone to reference helps ensure (though by no means guarantees) consistent application of study procedures. If staff turnover on a project is expected to be high, particularly among key personnel, the importance of a protocol in this regard is amplified. Finally, in most cases, researchers are required to write and submit a protocol for others to review. External reviewers most often include research ethics committees (see Chapter 3), funders of the research, and key stakeholders (government officials, community leaders, community advisory boards, and so on). Prior to external review, protocols should go through internal scientific peer review to increase the quality of the proposed study.

Draft an Analysis Plan

A data analysis plan should be developed during the study protocol process and prior to study implementation in order to ensure that the anticipated data will, in fact, be able to answer your study questions. An analysis plan includes many of the same details as a study protocol (sample sizes, sampling strategy, unit of analysis) and describes the specific analyses planned to assess the relationship between the main independent and dependent variables. It can also include table shells, for proposed presentation of statistical results, and proposed statistical analyses and statistical tests. For quantitative studies, the analysis plan will include the type of univariate, bivariate, and multivariable and multivariate analysis methods that will be used, including statistical tests. Procedures for developing scales or combining key variables are also described. For qualitative studies, describe the general procedures for reviewing transcripts, identifying and coding themes, and interpreting the data. For more clinical studies, describe plans for monitoring participant safety (including involving data and safety monitoring board), for excluding or discontinuing participants, and/or early stoppage rules. Table 2.5 outlines some of the major components in an analysis plan.

Plan for Communicating Results

Communicating your study results goes beyond just writing up a paper or a report and sending it out into the world. Planning for dissemination starts during study

Table 2.5   Items to Consider Including in an Analysis Plan

- Specify how many separate analyses will be conducted and the timeline for each.
- For each separate analysis specify the following:
  - which research question(s) it will inform and how
  - precisely which data will be used
  - independent and key dependent variables (if applicable)
  - analytic or statistical technique(s) to be employed
  - how data from different data collection methods will be integrated
  - any assumptions that are embodied in the analysis

development. In order to communicate your results effectively, you need to think about the audience(s) for the findings even before you begin the study. In other words, who will be most interested in your study results. If your study is commissioned, then the primary user of your results will be the person, people, or group that commissioned the study. Primary users may include a donor or funder, a program director or staff, or a government agency. Secondary users include other people or groups who are interested in your study results, such as community groups, other similar programs and researchers, and program planners, for example.

Further, it is important to communicate your results in a style and format that will be accessible to different audiences. Academic audiences may be interested in a comprehensive report or peer-reviewed publication. But the people most likely to use your results—policymakers, program planners, and so on—may not have the research method background to understand a detailed explanation of your methods and assumptions. Moreover, they are likely very busy and under pressure to digest a lot of information at one time. Having an executive summary or short statement about the study findings and their resulting policy and program implications may increase the likelihood that a busy health director reads and understands your main findings. Equally important to how you present the findings is what you say about the findings. Clear statements, bullet points, summary boxes, graphics, illustrations, and pictures appeal to the busy reader. Other nonwritten media like oral and poster presentations, webcasts, video, and other electronic and social media can help get your message across. One way to ensure that your key messages are conveyed is to reinforce the message via different mechanisms. Perhaps you release the report, make a presentation, then meet individually with key stakeholders. Disseminating and applying research findings are covered in more detail in Chapters 22 and 23.

SUMMARY

In this chapter we covered the basic principles of research design, with the exception of sampling, which is covered in Chapter 17. We presented questions for consideration and suggestions to help provide guidance in making decisions about developing research questions and choosing a research design and data collection methods. To help organize this abundance of information, we've condensed and summarized most of the key decision points in research design in Table 2.6. We have written the steps in a general chronological order following the sequence in which they are often considered during research design. But research design is a messy, iterative process and often involves considering multiple factors simultaneously while constantly adjusting and revising components (note the last step!). Despite our best efforts, these are not exhaustive lists of options. The options are also not mutually exclusive. Any one study can embody, for example, multiple objectives, populations, sampling strategies, data collection methods, and so on (see, for example, Chapter 19 on mixed methods). And these elements can be combined in countless ways. Table 2.6 is intended as an organizational and planning tool, not as a fixed procedural map to a successful research design.

Table 2.6 Research Design Steps and Options/Considerations

Step	Options/considerations
Find a research problem	Funder-driven, literature, real-world problem
Create study objective(s)	To identify, explore, describe, explain, compare, assess, evaluate, measure, predict, test, etc.
Specify research questions/hypotheses	Descriptive/exploratory, relational, causal Research questions vs. hypotheses Nondirectional vs. directional hypotheses Literature review and/or conceptual models should inform these

Choose basic research design	Descriptive
	    Case study
	    Cross-sectional
	    Trend analysis
	    Case-control
	    Cohort
	
	Relational
	    Quasi-experimental
	    Experimental
	• Mono-method vs. mixed methods
	• Specify independent and dependent variables

Select domains of observation and units of analysis (for *each* objective)	Domains of observation
	• Human behavior
	• Human psychological aspects
	   o Attitudes/opinions
	   o Perceptions
	   o Knowledge
	   o Experiences
	   o Emotions and values
	• Culturally shared meanings
	• Social structures
	• Social relationships
	• Biological outcomes
	• Socioeconomic metrics
	• Processes and systems
	• Environmental context
	• Disease incidence/prevalence

(Continued)

Table 2.6 (Continued)

Step	Options/considerations
	• Disease vectors • Geographic units • Events Units of Analysis • Country or other large geographic region • City/town/village • Neighborhoods, districts, or areas within a city/town/village • Institution • Household • Dyad • Individual • Event

Establish sampling and recruiting procedures (for *each* population and data collection method)
 	
  Define the study population(s) and geographic parameters
 	
  Determine sampling flexibility
 	
  Determine sampling strategy(ies)
 	
  Determine/estimate sample size(s)
 	
  Determine recruitment method(s)
	• Number of sites
	• Study population(s) and eligibility criteria
	• Inductive vs. a priori
	• Census
	• Purposive (choose type; see Table 2.1)
	• Quota
	• Convenience
	• Simple random
	• Systematic
	• Other
	
	Media-based
	• Posters/flyers
	• Newspaper/magazine
	• Radio/TV
	• Internet
	
	Investigator initiated
	• Door-to-door
	• Facility-based
	• Intercept
	• Email
	• Phone
	• Mail
	
	Socially based
	• Chain referral
	• External referral
	
	Panel/list-based
	• National panel
	• Facility/affiliation based panel

Step	*Options/considerations*
Operationalize study measures; determine structure and data collection method (for *each* objective)	Specify variables and variable measures. Define operational measures for instruments. • Primary vs. secondary data • Self-reports • Observation • Biological indicators See Figure 2.2.
Identify potential threats to validity	General validity • Not enough contextual information • Untested instruments Internal validity • History • Maturation • Observation effect • Poor measurement • Regression to the mean • Selection • Attrition
Data collection and management	Form of administration • Interviewer/clinician vs. participant Data capture method • Paper and pencil • Computer (ACASI) • Internet • PDA, iPad, etc. • Mail • Phone • Text message (cell) Data sharing
Ethical considerations	See Chapter 3
External logistics	Scope, time, and resources Site context • Nature of study population • Local and international politics • Infrastructure and accessibility
Document the research plan	Protocol Analysis plan
Review, revise, and repeat	Include collaborators (client, funder, research partners, stakeholders, etc.) in review process

ADDITIONAL RESOURCES

Books

Bordens, K., & Barrington Abbott, B. (2010). *Research design and methods: A process approach* (8th ed.). New York, NY: McGraw-Hill.

Garrard, J. (2010). *Health sciences literature review made easy: The matrix method* (3rd ed.). Sudbury, MA: Jones and Bartlett.

Hulley, S. B., Cummings, S. R., Browner, W. S., Grady, D. G., & Newman, T. B. (2007). *Designing clinical research* (3rd ed.). Philadelphia, PA: Lippincott Williams & Wilkins.

Jacobsen, K. (2011). *Introduction to health research methods.* Sudbury, MA: Jones and Bartlett.

Mitchell, M., & Jolley, J. (2012). *Research design explained* (8th ed.). Belmont, CA: Wadsworth Cengage Learning.

Polgar. S., & Thomas, S. (2008). *Introduction to research in the health sciences* (5th ed.). New York, NY: Churchill Livingstone.

Search Engines and Databases for Conducting Literature Reviews

- **Popline**—reproductive health literature database. www.popline.org

- **PubMed**—primary component is MEDLINE, which is the U.S. National Library of Medicine's database of journal articles in life sciences and biomedicine in particular. www.ncbi.nlm.nih.gov/pubmed

- **EMBASE**—source for international biomedical literature; includes MEDLINE records often used for pharmaceutical literature related to drugs and devices. www.embase.com

- **CINAHL** (Cumulative Index to Nursing and Allied Health Literature)—includes literature about nursing, allied health, biomedicine, and heath care. www.ebscohost.com/academic/the-cinahl-database

- **AMED**—alternative medicines database from the British Library that contains journal in three subject areas: allied medical professions, including physiotherapy, occupational therapy, rehabilitation, speech and language therapy, and podiatry; complementary medicine; and palliative care. www.ebscohost.com/academic/amed

- **National Center for Health Statistics**—U.S. data from birth and death records, medical records, interview surveys, and through direct physical exams and laboratory testing. www.hsrmethods.org/DataSources/National%20Center%20for%20Health%20Statistics.aspx

- **Web of Science**—includes access to six citation databases with thousands of journals, including open access journals, and conference proceedings from many disciplines such as agriculture, biological sciences, engineering, medical and life sciences, physical and chemical sciences, anthropology, law, library sciences, architecture, and humanities. http://thomsonreuters.com/web-of-science

- **PsycINFO**—database of peer-reviewed journals, books, and dissertations in behavioral sciences and mental health. www.apa.org/pubs/databases/psycinfo/index.aspx

- **EconLit**—American Economic Association electronic bibliography. www.aeaweb.org/econlit

- **ClinicalTrials**.gov—database of trials sponsored by National Institutes of Health, other federal agencies, and private industry. http://clinicaltrials.gov

REFERENCES

Bailey, R. C., Moses, S., Parker, C. B., Agot, K., Maclean, I., Krieger, J. N., . . . Ndinya-Achola, J. O. (2007). Male circumcision for HIV prevention in young men in Kisumu, Kenya: A randomised controlled trial. *Lancet, 369*(9562), 643–656.

Benzies, K. M., Premji, S., Hayden, A. K., & Serrett, K. (2006). State-of-the-evidence reviews: Advantages and challenges of including grey literature. *Worldviews on Evidence-Based Nursing, 3*(2), 55–61.

Bernard, H. (2013). *Social research methods: Qualitative and quantitative approaches* (2nd ed.). Thousand Oaks, CA: Sage.

Bongaarts, J., Reining, P., Way, P., & Conant, F. (1989). The relationship between male circumcision and HIV infection in African populations. *AIDS, 3,* 373–377.

Campbell, D. T., & Stanley, J. C. (1963). *Experimental and quasi-experimental designs for research.* Boston, MA: Houghton Mifflin.

Earp, J. A., & Ennett, S. T. (1991). Conceptual models for health education research and practice. *Health Education Research, 6*(2), 163–171,

Fisher, A. A., & Foreit, J. R. (2002). *Designing HIV/AIDS intervention studies: An operations research handbook.* Washington, DC: Population Council.

Gertler, P. J., Martinez, S., Premand, P., Rawlings, L. B., & Vermeersch, C. M. J. (2011). *Impact evaluation in practice.* Washington, DC: World Bank.

Gilson, L. (Ed.). (2012). *Health policy and systems research. A methodology reader.* Geneva, Switzerland: World Health Organization.

Glanz, K., Lewis, F. M., & Rimer, B. K. (1997). Linking theory, research, and practice. In K. Glanz, F. M. Lewis, & B. K. Rimer (Eds.), *Health behavior and health education: Theory, research, and practice* (2nd ed., pp. 19–35). San Francisco, CA: Jossey-Bass.

Gray, D. E. (2009). *Doing research in the real world* (2nd ed.). Thousand Oaks, CA: Sage.

Gray, R. H., Kigozi, G., Serwadda, D., Makumbi, F., Watya, S., Nalugoda, F., . . . Wawer, M. J. (2007). Male circumcision for HIV prevention in men in Rakai, Uganda: A randomised trial. *Lancet, 369*(9562), 657–666.

Grimes, D. A., & Schulz, K. F. (2002). Descriptive studies: What they can and cannot do. *Lancet, 359*(9301), 145–149.

Hammersley, M. (1992). *What's wrong with ethnography?* New York, NY: Routledge.

Institute of Medicine. (2011). Finding what works in health care: Standards for systematic reviews. *Report Brief.* Retrieved from http://www.iom.edu/~/media/Files/Report%20Files/2011/Finding-What-Works-in-Health-Care-Standards-for-Systematic-Reviews/Standards%20for%20Systematic%20Review%202010%20Report%20Brief.pdf

Kirch, W. (2008). Validity. In W. Kirch (Ed.), *Encyclopedia of public health* (pp. 1440). New York, NY: Springer.

Mann, C. J. (2003). Observational research methods. Research design II: Cohort, cross sectional, and case-control studies. *Emergency Medicine Journal, 20,* 54–60.

Maxwell, J. (1992). Understanding and validity in qualitative research. *Harvard Educational Review, 62,* 279–300.

Minkler, M., Vásquez, V. B., Chang, C., Miller, J., Rubin, V., & Blackwell, A. G., . . . Bell, J. (n.d.). *Promoting health public policy through community-based participatory research: Ten case studies.* Oakland, CA: Policylink. Retrieved from http://www.policylink.org/atf/cf/%7B97C6D565-BB43-406D-A6D5-ECA3BBF35AF0%7D/CBPR_PromotingHealthyPublicPolicy_final.pdf

MRC Vitamin Study Research Group. (1991). Prevention of neural tube defects: Results of the medical research council vitamin study. *Lancet, 338*(8760), 131–137.

National Institutes of Health. (2003). *NIH data sharing policy and implementation guidance.* Retrieved from http://grants.nih.gov/grants/policy/data_sharing/data_sharing_guidance .htm

Oser, R., Ojikutu, B., Odek, W., Ogunlayi, M., & Bakualufu Ntumba, J. (2012). *HIV treatment in complex emergencies.* Arlington, VA: USAID, AIDS Support and Technical Assistance Resources Project. Retrieved from http://www.aidstar-one.com/sites/default/files/ AIDSTAR-One_Report_HIVTreatment_EmergencyPlanning.pdf

Robson, C. (2011). *Real world research* (3rd ed.). West Sussex, UK: Wiley.

Shi, L. (2008). *Health services research methods* (2nd ed.). Clifton Park, NY: Delmar Learning.

Singleton, R. A., Straits, B. C., & Straits, M. M. (1993). *Approaches to social research* (2nd ed.). New York, NY: Oxford University Press.

Social Science Dictionary. (2008). *Validity.* Retrieved from http://www.socialsciencedictionary .com/validity

Veney, J. E., & Kaluzny, A. D. (1998). *Evaluation and decision making for health services* (3rd ed.). Chicago, IL: Health Administration Press.

Wallerstein, N., & Duran, B. (2010). Community-based participatory research contributions to intervention research: The intersection of science and practice to improve health equity. *American Journal of Public Health, 100*(Suppl. 1), S40–S46.

Yin, R. K. (1999). Enhancing the quality of case studies in health services research. *Health Services Research, 34*(5 pt. 2), 1209–1224.

Young, M. R., Odoyo-June, E., Nordstrom, S. K., Irwin, T. E., Ongong'a, D. O., Ochomo, B., . . . Bailey, R. C. (2012). Factors associated with uptake of infant male circumcision for HIV prevention in Western Kenya. *Pediatrics,* 130, e175–e182.

NOTE

1. http://www.iom.edu/Reports/2011/Finding-What-Works-in-Health-Care-Standards-for-Systematic-Reviews/Standards.aspx.

3

Research Ethics and Working With Institutional Review Boards

Amy Corneli and David Borasky

As evidenced by the previous two chapters, there are myriad methods and research designs in use in public health research. One constant among them is the need for consideration of research ethics. All students, post-docs, and new and established scientists have the ethical obligation to adhere to recognized ethical standards when conducting human subject research. While a thorough discussion of the ethical issues researchers must consider is beyond the scope of this chapter, we provide an overview of the key ethical issues to consider during the development of your research, during its implementation, and after the research has concluded. We also provide detailed, practical guidance on how to describe the protections of human subjects in a research protocol and what to expect when a protocol is formally reviewed by an ethics review committee (commonly known as an Institutional Review Board, or IRB). Suggested readings for a fuller review of research ethics are listed at the end of this chapter in the Additional Resources section. We start with a brief history and overview of the ethics guidelines and regulations for research with human subjects. We primarily focus on the guidelines and regulations for the ethical conduct of research in the United States; a link to the *International Compilation of Human Research Standards*, a document which describes the ethical regulations and guidelines for over 100 countries, can be found in the Additional Resources section.

ETHICS GUIDELINES AND REGULATIONS

Chapter 1 briefly mentioned some of the ethics guidelines and regulations that serve as the foundation for the ethical conduct of human subject research. In this section, we provide additional information on four key ethics guidelines: the Nuremburg Code, the Declaration of Helsinki, *The Belmont Report,* and the Council for International Organizations of Medical Sciences' *International Ethical Guidelines for Biomedical Research Involving Human Subjects.* We also highlight information from the U.S. Code of Federal Regulations.

Nuremburg Code

The Nuremburg Code was the first of several ethics guidance documents on human subjects research. It was a product of the Nuremburg Trials held following

---

WHAT ARE ETHICS STANDARDS, GUIDELINES, AND REGULATIONS?

Human subject research is governed by overlapping **ethics standards**, **guidelines**, **regulations**, and **institutional policies**, and it is important to understand how they interrelate and apply to your research.

- **Ethics standards** are the guiding principles that should govern the design and conduct of the research. They are generally considered universal and are reflected across all guidelines, regulations, and policies.
- **Guidelines** can be issued by international bodies, such as the UNAIDS (www.unaids.org/en/media/unaids/contentassets/documents/unaidspublication/2012/jc1399_ethical_considerations_en.pdf) or more focused groups like the HIV Prevention Trials Network (http://hptn.org/web%20documents/EWG/HPTNEthicsGuidanceV10Jun2009.pdf). Guidelines do not carry the weight of law and are therefore not enforceable. However, they are often considered to represent best practices.
- **Regulations**, which are typically developed at the national level, set the rules for implementing the ethical standards. Unlike guidelines, regulations can be enforced by regulatory authorities. Regulations identify specific requirements for conducting the research and for the documentation of compliance, and they impose penalties for noncompliance.
- **Institutional policies** are developed by organizations that conduct research to define at the institutional level how all relevant standards, guidelines, and regulations will be incorporated in the research implemented by the organization.

World War II for the prosecution of Nazi war crimes, including experiments conducted by Nazi physician-researchers on prisoners in concentration camps. Accordingly, the 1949 Nuremburg Code focuses on the rights of research participants. The first of 10 guidance points in the code states that "the voluntary consent of the human subject is absolutely essential," and another guidance point states that participants should be able to freely stop their participation at any time. Other key ethical aspects of human subjects research are also described, including the obligation to reduce the risks to study participants and that only "scientifically qualified persons" should conduct research. At the time, the Nuremburg Code was viewed as a punitive measure against German war criminals and not as a document for the larger world of medical researchers. However, it remains a cornerstone document in the world of contemporary research ethics. To read the entire Nuremburg Code, visit www.hhs.gov/ohrp/archive/nurcode.html.

Declaration of Helsinki

The World Medical Assembly (WMA) initially adopted the Declaration of Helsinki in 1964, and several revisions have occurred over the years, with the last revision published in 2013. As described in the declaration, guidance is primarily directed toward physicians and focuses on the ethical principles for medical research involving human subjects, particularly when data collected are identifiable. However, the WMA encourages all researchers conducting human subjects medical research to follow their guidelines. The declaration is divided into multiple sections. It begins with general principles and then provides more detailed guidance on informed consent, privacy and confidentiality, and post-trial provisions, for example. To read the entire Declaration of Helsinki, visit www.wma.net/en/20activities/10ethics/10helsinki.

The Belmont Report

The U.S. National Commission for the Protection of Human Subjects of Biomedical and Behavioral Research was created in 1974 following exposure in the popular press of the "Tuskegee Study of Untreated Syphilis in the Negro Male"—known infamously as the Tuskegee study. The Tuskegee study was conducted from 1932 to 1972 in Alabama by researchers from the U.S. Public Health Service. The purpose was to study the natural progression of syphilis in African American men. The study began before treatment for syphilis was available, yet when a treatment was discovered, it was not provided to participants. The study continued for decades without informing participants of the purpose of the research, providing treatment, or providing accurate information to obtain meaningful participant consent (Centers for Disease Control and Prevention [CDC], 2012). In response, the Commission was charged with identifying the ethical principles that should be followed during the conduct of biomedical and behavioral research. Three basic ethical principles were identified and described in the commission's 1978 *Belmont Report: Ethical Principles and Guidelines for the Protection of Human Subjects of Research*. The meaning of the principles and how each can be applied in research are described below, as detailed in the report:

Respect for persons—The ethical principle of respect for persons is explained by two overall ideas: (1) "individuals should be treated as autonomous agents," meaning that individuals have the self-determination and capacity to make decisions for themselves, and (2) "persons with diminished autonomy are entitled to protection," meaning that special protections should be given to those individuals who are not capable of self-determination, such as individuals with certain illnesses or mental disabilities or individuals who are incarcerated. Informed consent is the main application of the ethical principle respect for persons.

Beneficence—The ethical principle of beneficence is also explained by two overall ideas: (1) "minimize possible risks" and (2) "maximize possible benefits." Beneficence is primarily applied in research through a careful review of the risk/benefit ratio to determine that the potential benefits justify the risks. Not only are the risks and benefits to the study participant considered when evaluating the risk/benefit ratio, the risks and benefits to the study participants' community and society in general may also be included. In some ethical constructs an additional principle of nonmaleficence is included. Nonmaleficence suggests an elimination of risks or the concept of "do no harm." However, the elimination of all risks is not considered possible, and strict adherence to nonmaleficence would make it impossible to expose research subjects to even the smallest risk of harm, regardless of the benefits.

Justice—The main premise of the ethical principle of justice is "who ought to receive the benefits of research and bear its burdens?" In practice, the ethical principle of justice is applied by the fair selection of the study population, where the potential benefits and risks of research are distributed equally or fairly among study populations. Justice also means "avoiding exploitation of research participants and their communities" (MacQueen & Sugarman, 2003, p. 41).

To read the entire *Belmont Report*, visit www.hhs.gov/ohrp/policy/belmont .html.

The Council for International Organizations of Medical Sciences Guidelines

CIOMS, in collaboration with the World Health Organization, issued the *International Ethical Guidelines for Biomedical Research Involving Human Subjects* in 1982. The CIOMS guidelines, as they are commonly called, were last revised in 2002. They were developed to provide an international perspective on research ethics, following concerns about the applicability of the Declaration of Helsinki to developed countries and the need for guidelines that addressed issues unique to the developing world. The guidelines focus on applying universal ethical principles while respecting cultural values:

An issue, mainly for those countries and perhaps less pertinent now than in the past, has been the extent to which ethical principles are considered universal or as culturally relative—the universalist versus the pluralist view. The challenge to international research ethics is to apply universal ethical principles to biomedical research in a multicultural world with a multiplicity of health-care systems and considerable variation in standards of health care. The Guidelines take the position that research involving human subjects must not violate any universally applicable ethical standards, but acknowledge that, in superficial aspects, the application of the ethical principles, e.g., in relation to individual autonomy and informed consent, needs to take account of cultural values, while respecting absolutely the ethical standards. (CIOMS, 2002, p. 11)

Like the Declaration of Helsinki, the CIOMS guidelines are not regulations and therefore cannot be enforced. To read all 21 of the CIOMS guidelines visit www.cioms .ch/publications/layout_guide2002.pdf.

Although the documents described above have been critiqued over the years and are contradictory at times (Vanderpool, 2001), they still serve today as the foundation for guidance on the ethical conduct of research with human subjects.

U.S. Code of Federal Regulations

For U.S. government–funded human subjects research in medicine and health, researchers are obligated to follow the U.S. Code of Federal Regulations, Title 45, Part 46 issued by the U.S. Department of Health and Human Services (DHHS, 2009). The regulations, commonly referred to as 45 CFR 46, are divided into four subparts:

- *Subpart A: Basic HHS Policy for Protection of Human Research Subjects.* Subpart A includes information such as what is in the purview of the policy; the requirements of institutions and IRBs, including membership, functions and operations, and review; and the requirements and documentation of informed consent. Subpart A is also referred to as "The Common Rule" and is followed by 17 other U.S. departments and agencies such as the Department of Education and the Environmental Protection Agency.
- Subparts B through D describe additional protections for study populations who are considered vulnerable:
  - Subpart B: Additional Protections for Pregnant Women, Human Fetuses, and Neonates Involved in Research
  - Subpart C: Additional Protections Pertaining to Biomedical and Behavioral Research Involving Prisoners as Subjects
  - Subpart D: Additional Protections for Children Involved as Subjects in Research
- *Subpart E: Registration of Institutional Review Boards.* This section was added in 2009 and includes information on IRB registration.

While these regulations apply only to U.S. government–funded research, institutions and IRBs typically apply them to all human subjects research, regardless of the funding source. To read the full text of 45 CFR 46, visit www.hhs.gov/ohrp/humansub-jects/guidance/45cfr46.html.

Take a moment to read these guidelines and regulations and become familiar with them. Refer to them as you develop your research idea into a protocol, and consider how they can be applied in your research. The next section provides guidance on how to do this.

PLANNING YOUR RESEARCH

Often in research protocols, the section that describes human subjects protections is located *after* a description of the research objectives, study design, and methods, sometimes appearing as an afterthought. Yet ethical considerations are intertwined with decisions about objectives, design, and methods when developing a research idea into a scientifically rigorous and ethically sound study. Research planning usually begins with discussions around a budding research question or hypothesis, potential study populations, and a geographical setting(s) in which to conduct the research. Use these initial discussions to consider the ethical implications of the various research possibilities (Sieber, 2000).

What Ethical Issues Should Be Considered When Developing a Research Idea Into a Research Protocol?

Listed below are several guidance points on integrating ethics issues into research planning and design discussions:

Study Population

Study populations are typically chosen because the research topic of interest affects them in some way (e.g., a community has a high prevalence of a particular illness or practices a specific health behavior). When discussing a potential study population from an ethical perspective, consider the following two questions:

1. *Are they chosen equitably?* The equitable selection of a study population is related to the ethical principle of justice. A population should not be selected for mere convenience or for studies where the expected benefits of the research would extend only to individuals in another population.

2. *Are they considered a vulnerable population that might require additional protections?* Populations are considered vulnerable when there are circumstances that limit an individual's ability to make informed decisions about participating in research. Some populations, such as prisoners, pregnant women, and children are considered vulnerable populations in the U.S. regulations, and special protections apply to these populations. Their involvement in research must be justified in order to satisfy the ethical principle of justice. If you intend to conduct research with one of these populations, refer to the U.S. Code of Federal Regulations (DHHS, 2009) and consult with your IRB for specific guidance to follow.

Potential Risks to Participants

Another ethical consideration is risk to participants. Risk is the possibility that a study participant will experience harm while participating in the research. Risks are generally grouped into four categories (Levine, 1988):

- *Physical* risks are typically "pain, suffering, or physical injury" (Prentice & Gordon, 2001, p. L-4) and can also include discomforts such as minor pain or bruising from having blood drawn. While physical risks can occur in any type of research, they most often occur in biomedical research (Prentice & Gordon, 2001).
- *Psychological* harms include the "participant's negative perception of self, emotional suffering (e.g., anxiety or shame), or aberrations in thought or behavior" (National Bioethics Advisory Committee [NBAC], 2001a, p. 71). Distress and anger are also psychological harms that could occur from sharing information with study staff that is sensitive or embarrassing to the participant (NBAC, 2001a), such as during a survey on sexual behaviors.
- *Social* risks include harms "to a person in the context of his or her social interactions with others" (Prentice & Gordon, 2001, p. L-5). The amount of potential risk or harm that could occur is associated with the sensitivity of the research objectives and data collected, and particularly to the participants' perspective on others knowing about their study participation or learning their responses to study questions or procedures (Prentice & Gordon, 2001).
- *Economic* risks occur when a participant incurs a financial cost as a result of participation in the research (Weijer, 2001). For example, loss of employment is a potential economic risk if confidentiality is breached in research on employee-employer relationships (Prentice & Gordon, 2001).

Following the ethical principle of beneficence, the role of a researcher is to minimize the risks to participants as much as possible while maximizing the benefits of research participation. When designing your research, consider each type of risk and whether there is potential for it to affect participants in your study. Consideration should also be given to whether your study may pose any of these risks to individuals related to the participants or to society (Levine, 1988), that is, people in the community where the research is conducted, as mentioned earlier. Include in your protocol a description of each potential risk to study participants and society and the specific procedures you will take to minimize the risks, to the extent possible. The IRB will evaluate whether the risks of your research are reasonable in relation to the anticipated benefits.

Potential Benefits to Participants

Benefits are items or activities participants receive as part of their participation in research that are not directly related to the overall research objective. For example, the objective of a particular biomedical HIV prevention clinical trial is to evaluate whether an oral antiretroviral drug taken daily can reduce the risk of

HIV-negative individuals acquiring HIV and is safe. As benefits of study participation, participants receive contraceptives and care and treatment for common illnesses free of charge. These activities are considered benefits as they can provide a health benefit to the participant, but the activities are not related to the overall objective of the clinical trial.

Some participants may find personal fulfillment in completing study procedures because of the opportunity to contribute to the advancement of science or to share information about themselves with others. These can be indirect benefits of research, particularly of social or behavioral research, although it is not guaranteed that every participant will find study participation beneficial in these ways. Incentives for participation, such as payment for time and inconvenience, are typically not considered "benefits" from a research ethics perspective, and therefore are not listed as such in the protocol or informed consent materials.

Privacy and Confidentiality

Privacy and *confidentiality* are two terms that are often interpreted to be synonymous, but they have different (yet connected) meanings. Privacy means the "control over the extent, timing, and circumstances of sharing oneself (physically, behaviorally, or intellectually) with others" (DHHS, 1993). Confidentiality means "the treatment of information that an individual has disclosed in a relationship of trust and with the expectation that it will not be divulged to others without permission in ways that are inconsistent with the understanding of the original disclosure" (DHHS, 1993). Privacy most often comes into play during the recruitment and data collection phases of research; it is incumbent upon the researcher to ensure that participants are selected for and approached about research discreetly and that participants have a safe and respectful place to share their study data (whether an interview or a blood sample). Confidentiality more often relates to the data management side of things, from the time the data are collected to final analysis and reporting, making sure that the participant's identity and information are kept within the research team, as specified in the protocol and agreed upon during informed consent. Both concepts are related to the ethical principles of respect for persons and of beneficence, and they are of particular importance in research where the primary risk to participants is a breach of confidentiality or lack of privacy.

When writing a research protocol, you'll need to consider and provide explicit strategies for how you will protect participants' privacy and keep the information they give you confidential to the extent possible. For example, a researcher wanted to conduct in-depth interviews with HIV-negative women on how they reduce their risk of acquiring HIV. During protocol development, the researcher considered strategies to maintain participants' privacy and described in the protocol that the interviews would be conducted in a private room. In addition, the researcher noted that a sign would be placed on the door reading "interview in progress" to ensure that no one entered the room during an interview. These strategies limited others from seeing the participant during the interview *or* hearing what she was saying, thereby reducing the potential for any harm if others observed the individual's interview. Another privacy consideration is the location of the interviews. In our example, the interviews were initially planned to be conducted at a facility that also provides care and treatment to individuals with HIV, as this would be convenient for the study staff. However, these interviews were planned with HIV-negative women in a geographic location where stigmatization toward people with HIV still occurs. After consideration, researchers were concerned that participants could be perceived to have HIV—and subsequently stigmatized—if seen entering this facility for the interview. The researchers therefore identified another location in the community that was not affiliated with HIV services where they could conduct the interviews. Privacy is also related to how potential participants are identified, contacted, and invited to enroll in research by research staff. For example, research staff should recruit participants in a way that does not identify them as having certain characteristics, especially if those characteristics would cause any potential harm if known to others.

Once participants enroll in your study and data are collected, several procedures must be implemented to reduce the possibility of a breach of confidentiality. Procedures typically used to maintain confidentiality are listed in the text box that follows. Although implementation of these procedures is good standard practice, according to the U.S. Code of Federal Regulations (DHHS, 2009), procedures to protect confidentiality are needed only for identifiable data—those data that clearly link individuals to the information collected about or provided by them. See information provided in the Additional Resources section at the end of the chapter for more detail on the type of information that is considered identifiable.

A third term that is often conflated with privacy and confidentiality is *anonymity*. Whereas privacy and confidentiality are related to the ways in which identity and information are protected, anonymity occurs when data or information has been completely de-identified and no linking code is retained that would enable re-identification. This is often possible only in research where data are collected from participants at only one time point (and therefore a list linking the participant's name to their study identification number is not needed) and when broad demographic information is collected, such as age and education. Data that were originally considered identifiable can become unidentifiable if identifiers, such as the list linking the participant name and study identification number, are destroyed and potentially identifiable demographics are removed from the data set.

Procedures to protect participants' privacy and keep their information confidential should be described in the study consent form (see below), to allow potential participants to make an informed decision on whether those procedures are acceptable to them based on the information being requested in the research. Potential participants should also be made aware of the potential consequences that could occur with a breach of confidentiality (CIOMS, 2002) or if their privacy is not maintained. The informed consent form should also describe that these protections cannot be fully guaranteed, as unforeseen circumstances may occur where privacy is compromised and data are viewed by others. In situations where there are limits

PROCEDURES TO REDUCE BREACHES IN CONFIDENTIALITY

- Never include the participant's name or other identifiable information (such as an address, telephone number, or birthdate) on any data collection form, such as a survey or interview notes.
- Use a participant identification number on all data collection forms and other documents including participant data.
- Collect participant names and other identifiable information only if needed for participant follow-up or if data are to be collected at multiple time points. Participant names may not need to be collected and documented for a one-time interview.
- Collect only identifiers that are needed for participant follow-up, to adequately describe the study population, or to answer the research questions.
- Store all hard copies of data in locked file cabinets and in a location where only a few members of the research team have access.
- Keep signed informed consent forms in a locked file cabinet separate from those containing participant data.
- Password-protect each electronic file containing participant data, such as interview transcripts.
- Only store data on password-protected computers. If data are to be stored on a shared network drive, limit access to that drive to research staff.
- Limit storing data on laptops or thumb drives that can easily be stolen or lost.
- If conducting interviews that are audio-recorded:
  - Store audiotapes under lock and key when not in use (i.e., being transcribed), and destroy after analysis is over or the associated manuscript is published.
  - Transfer digital files from the digital recorder to a password-protected computer and delete from the digital recorder (before deleting, consider making a back-up of the data in a secure location).
- Destroy all identifiers as soon as is feasibly possible.

to confidentiality, such as with the mandatory reporting requirements related to communicable diseases or the disclosure of activity such as child abuse, these limits should be described in the informed consent process and forms.

The steps described in this section reduce the potential for an invasion of participants' privacy and confidentiality breaches. Research participants may also feel more comfortable with the researcher and be more willing to share information in the study, knowing that their information will be protected to the extent possible.

CERTIFICATES OF CONFIDENTIALITY

If you know from the design phase that your research will address a topic that is highly sensitive, involves illegal behavior, or could be the source of future legal proceedings *and* you will be collecting and keeping identifiable information, you might consider (and your IRB may recommend) a Certificate of Confidentiality.

Certificates of Confidentiality are issued by the National Institutes of Health to protect identifiable research information from forced disclosure. They allow the investigator and others who have access to research records to refuse to disclose identifying information on research participants in any civil, criminal, administrative, legislative, or other proceeding, whether at the federal, state, or local level. By protecting researchers and institutions from being compelled to disclose information that would identify research subjects, Certificates of Confidentiality help achieve the research objectives and promote participation in studies by helping to ensure confidentiality and privacy to participants. Certificates of Confidentiality do not, however, override mandatory reporting requirements for issues like child abuse, imminent threats to safety, or public health reporting of communicable diseases, and these limitations of protection must be addressed in the consent form.

Certificates are recommended for many types of research, including the following:

- research on HIV, AIDS, and other STDs
- studies that collect information on sexual attitudes, preferences, or practices
- studies on the use of alcohol, drugs, or other addictive products
- studies that collect information on illegal conduct
- studies that gather information that if released could be damaging to a participant's financial standing, employability, or reputation in the community
- research involving information that might lead to social stigmatization or discrimination if it were disclosed
- research on participants' psychological well-being or mental health
- genetic studies, including those that collect and store biological samples for future use
- research on behavioral interventions and epidemiologic studies

If you believe your research may benefit from a Certificate of Confidentiality, check with your local IRB to determine whether and how to request one.

Source: NIH (2013); Guest, Namey, Mitchell 2013, pp. 335–336.

Informed Consent

As evident in the ethics guidelines and regulations overview, informed consent is a fundamental aspect of human subjects research. According to the Belmont Report, individuals can only give their informed consent if three elements are present: information, comprehension, and voluntariness.

Information

Information means that a sufficient amount of detail about the research must be disclosed to the potential participant during the informed consent process, allowing the individual to make an informed decision on whether she or he would like to participate. The basic elements of informed consent, as defined by 45 CFR 46.116(a), include the type of information that must be provided to potential participants in U.S.-funded research (see text box that follows). For some types of research, other elements of informed consent should be included, and these are described in detail in 45 CFR 46.116(b).

The CIOMS guidelines describe 26 types of information that should be provided to individuals during the informed consent process. The guidelines extend beyond the elements described in 45 CRF 46.116(a) and include information such as a description of posttrial access to proven interventions and the requirement to disseminate research findings to study participants. Importantly, the CIOMS (2002) guidelines also state that information must be provided "in the language or another form of communication that the individual can understand" (p. 37). The National Bioethics Advisory Commission (NBAC; 2001a) also places emphasis on how information is disclosed, and recommends that information "must be adapted to the potential participant's capacities and characteristics" (p. 97). It also recommends that "researchers should develop culturally appropriate ways to disclose information" (NBAC, 2001b, p. 40) so that the consent process is respectful of both the individual's decision on whether to participate in research *and* the cultural aspects that define that sense of individual, for example, seeking permission from community leaders for the research to be conducted in their community. To identify meaningful and culturally appropriate consent form language, researchers often conduct formative research with the study population and their communities and consult with community advisory boards (Corneli et al., 2006). Many IRBs also require that informed consent forms be written at a basic reading level.

BASIC ELEMENTS OF INFORMED CONSENT AS DEFINED IN 45 CFR 46.116(A)

1. A statement that the study involves research, an explanation of the purposes of the research and the expected duration of the subject's participation, a description of the procedures to be followed, and identification of any procedures which are experimental

2. A description of any reasonably foreseeable risks or discomforts to the subject

3. A description of any benefits to the subject or to others which may reasonably be expected from the research

4. A disclosure of appropriate alternative procedures or courses of treatment, if any, that might be advantageous to the subject

5. A statement describing the extent, if any, to which confidentiality of records identifying the subject will be maintained

6. For research involving more than minimal risk, an explanation as to whether any compensation and an explanation as to whether any medical treatments are available if injury occurs and, if so, what they consist of or where further information may be obtained

7. An explanation of whom to contact for answers to pertinent questions about the research and research subjects' rights, and whom to contact in the event of a research-related injury to the subject

8. A statement that participation is voluntary, refusal to participate will involve no penalty or loss of benefits to which the subject is otherwise entitled, and the subject may discontinue participation at any time without penalty or loss of benefits to which the subject is otherwise entitled

Source: U.S. Department of Health and Human Services (DHHS). (2009). 45 Code of Federal Regulations 46. Federal Register.

Comprehension

Disclosing information in meaningful ways is likely to enhance potential participants' understanding of the information, which is the second condition of informed consent outlined by the Belmont Report: comprehension. Under this condition, for individuals to give consent that is truly informed, they must sufficiently understand the information disclosed to them during the informed consent process. The Belmont Report states that "investigators are responsible for ascertaining that the subject has comprehended the information" (section c1). Similar statements are found in the CIOMS guidelines and the Declaration of Helsinki. The Belmont Report and the CIOMS guidelines also state that quizzes or tests can be used to assess comprehension. Yet determining what is sufficient understanding and how it can be measured is complicated. Currently, no shared definition of sufficient understanding exists, nor does agreement on how much information participants must understand to participate in research (e.g., only some key elements, all elements). Several studies have evaluated methods to improve the disclosure of consent information, but no method has shown consistent improvement across studies (Cohn & Larson, 2007; Flory & Emanuel, 2004). Several studies have also evaluated methods to measure comprehension of informed consent (Joffe, Cook, Cleary, Clark, & Weeks, 2001), although no standard method is currently used across studies. Nonetheless, informed consent comprehension quizzes or tests are increasingly being used in research as part of the informed consent process (Chaisson, Kass, Chengeta, Mathebula, & Samandari, 2011), particularly among research involving more than minimal risk.

Voluntariness

The third condition of informed consent outlined by the Belmont Report is voluntariness. As described in the report, informed consent is only valid if it is given voluntarily and obtained in "conditions free of coercion and undue influence" (section C2).

In practice, NBAC and others (NBAC, 2001b; Woodsong & Karim, 2005) emphasize that informed consent should be "a process and not merely a form to be signed in a routine manner" (NBAC, 2001a, p. 98). NBAC (2001a) describes how this process should work:

> From an ethics perspective, the informed consent process is the critical communication link between the prospective participant and the investigator, beginning with the initial approach of the investigator to the participant (e.g., via a flyer, brochure, or any advertisement regarding the research study) and continuing until the end of the project. It should be an active process of sharing information by both partners, throughout which the participant at any time is able to freely decide whether to withdraw or continue participating in the research. (p. 100)

Some researchers believe that too much attention is given to information disclosure and less to the other two conditions of informed consent, in part due to how the basic elements of informed consent are described in 45 CFR 46.116(a). NBAC (2001a) summarizes Vanderpool's (2001) concern on this issue:

> Although the regulations pertaining to informed consent (45 CFR 46.116; 21 CFR 50.20) begin with a paragraph from the Belmont Report related to the "three elements" of consent—information, comprehension, and voluntariness—the actual procedures emphasize disclosure requirements, and in so doing may distort the understanding of the ethical principle of respect for persons. Especially in the context of requirements that informed consent be documented using signed, written forms, this exclusive emphasis on information leads investigators and IRBs to equate informed consent with the information provided in a consent form and to focus mostly on disclosure to participants. Thus, these regulations fail to emphasize the informed consent *process* and to attend to the importance of comprehension and voluntariness. (pp. 98–99)

Such emphasis on information disclosure may impact consent form length. Consent forms have continued to lengthen over time, and lengthy consent forms have been shown to limit understanding of research (Beardsley, Jefford, & Mileshkin, 2007). In general, research on informed consent has shown that study participants often do not fully understand the information disclosed during the informed consent process (Sugarman et al., 1999).

In certain circumstances, written documentation of informed consent may be waived. As described in 45 CFR 46.117(c), this may occur when (1) the signed informed consent form is the "only record linking the subject and the research" and "the principal risk would be potential harm resulting from a breach of confidentiality," and (2) the research is of minimal risk and "involves no procedures for which written consent is normally required outside of the research context."

The procedures described above involve obtaining informed consent from legal, competent adults. Other procedures must be followed if your study participants include minors or individuals who are not competent to provide their individual informed consent. For research involving minors,[1] informed assent should be obtained, meaning that the minor agrees to participate in the research. And in most cases, parental permission must also be obtained, meaning that a parent or legal guardian gives her or his permission for the minor to participate. It is the IRB's responsibility to determine when minors are capable of providing assent, taking into account the age, maturity, and psychological state of the minors involved. For some types of research, such as research with neglected or abused children, IRBs can waive the requirement of parental permission provided that an alternative mechanism for protecting the children has been identified. In research with adults who are not capable of providing their informed consent, a legally authorized representative can give informed consent on the behalf of the individual. The determination of who may serve as a legally authorized representative for research purposes is determined by state law in the jurisdiction where the research will be implemented.

When writing consent forms for your research, check that all basic elements of informed consent as described in 45 CFR 46.116(a) are included unless formally waived by the IRB. Within the structure of the basic elements, keep consent forms short and write them at a basic reading level. (See the text box below for a sample form used to obtain oral informed consent.) Information should also be included in your protocol on how you plan to obtain informed consent (e.g., who administers the consent form; how is it administered—is it read aloud or does the participant read it; location of discussion); how or if you will assess participant comprehension of the information disclosed during the informed consent process; and what procedures will be used to obtain a *voluntary* informed consent, free from coercion and undue influence.

Participant Inducement

Inducements are often used in research to create interest and encourage individuals to participate or to remain in the research. Inducements can be monetary, such as giving participants $100 if they enroll in the research and another $100 if they complete all research-related activities. Other monetary inducements include reimbursing participants for costs incurred from participating in the research, such as transportation costs, or compensating participants for their time. Inducements can also be of nonmonetary value, such as access to health care. The ethics of some of these practices are still disputed, and determining what is ethically appropriate and inappropriate can be difficult. Yet without inducements, potential participants

---

ORAL INFORMED CONSENT FORM

INTERVIEWS AND FOCUS GROUPS WITH [POPULATION] IN DURHAM, NC

The [Name of] Project

Background/Purpose

The **[Name of] Project** is a X-year research study taking place in Durham, North Carolina. One goal of this study is to learn more about [Topic 1]. The other goal of this study is to collect information on how [Population] in Durham view and use health care.

We will use what we learn in this study to develop guidelines for [Topic 1]. We will also use what we learn to provide information on how [Population] decide when to seek medical care. The [Funder Name] is funding this study. This study is conducted by [Research Institution], a nonprofit organization based in Durham, North Carolina.

We will invite about 385 [Population] living in the city of Durham, North Carolina, to take part in this study.

You are being invited to take part in a one-on-one interview or focus group discussion because you are [Population plus specific eligibility requirements].

These interviews and focus groups are considered research and we must ask for your permission to take part. This consent form tells you what will happen during this study so you can decide whether you would like to take part.

Procedures

If you agree to take part in this study, you will be randomly chosen to participate in either a one-on-one interview or a focus group discussion. 1 in 11 people who agree to take part will be contacted to participate in a one-on-one interview. The other 10 will be contacted to schedule a time for the focus group.

The topics we will ask you about are the same in both the interviews and focus groups. We will be asking you for your experiences and opinions with health care and doctors in the Durham community. Some of the questions will ask you to reflect on your own experiences and others will ask you to comment on the Durham community more generally.

If you are chosen for a one-on-one interview, the interviewer will contact you to set up a time for the interview. If you are chosen for a focus group, you will be invited to join a group of about 8 [Population]. The recruiter will work with you to find the group that best fits your schedule. Some people may not be able to attend any of the offered group times and will not be enrolled. Interviews and focus groups will last up to 2 hours.

Both interviews and focus group discussions will be held in a private area. We will record the interviews and focus groups with a digital voice recorder so that we can make an exact written record of what was said. After this research project is finished, the digital recording will be permanently destroyed. If you do not want to be recorded, you can choose not to take part in the research. Before the interview or focus group, we will ask you questions about yourself, like your age, education, and health.

Risks and/or Discomforts

The risks of taking part in the research are small, if any. Some questions could make you feel uncomfortable or embarrassed. If this happens, you may refuse to answer any question and you may stop taking part at any time. In the focus groups, we will ask everyone in the group to respect each other and not to talk with others about who said what during the discussion. However, we cannot promise that people will not share what has been discussed with others, so please consider this before answering the questions.

Benefits

There are no direct benefits for taking part in this research, though findings from this study will help improve [Topic 1]. The information we learn about [Population's] views and use of health care in the Durham community will also [describe output].

Voluntary Participation

Your participation in the research is voluntary. You do not have to take part and you are free to leave the study at any time.

Confidentiality

We will keep the information you tell us and your name and contact information confidential, to the extent possible. We will destroy the digital voice recording once the research is completed. We will not write your name in our notes or in any report or publication about this research. We will do our best

(Continued)

(Continued)

to keep this information from being seen by others. Our notes will be kept in a locked cabinet except when they are being used by members of the research team for research purposes. The recorded file will be stored on computers that are protected by a password and on back-up disks kept in the locked file cabinet.

Compensation

You will receive [$XX] for participating in this study. We will also provide a voucher for parking at the study site, if applicable.

Questions

If you have any questions about this research, you may contact the study leader, [PI Name], at [Institution]. Tel: [XXX-XXX-XXXX], email: xxxx@xxx.xxx.

Your Rights as a Participant

This research has been reviewed and approved by [name of IRB] in Durham, North Carolina. This committee reviews research studies so that they help protect participants. If you have any questions about how are you being treated by the study or your rights as a research participant you may contact [name of IRB, plus contact information].

Do you have any questions?

Please note that by agreeing to participate in this study, you are agreeing to be randomized to either a one-on-one interview or a focus group discussion.

Do you agree to participate in this study?   _____Yes   _____No

Verification of Consent

The above document that explains the benefits, risks, and procedures of the research study named [Study Name] was read and explained to the individual and he/she agrees to take part.

_____
Written name and surname of the person who obtained consent

_____   _____
Signature of the person who   Date (mm/dd/yy)
obtained consent

may not have interest or the financial means to participate in research, and some may feel that they are exploited (Scott-Jones, 2000), particularly if participating in research with few benefits. For these reasons, give careful consideration to the incentives and/or payments provided to participants in your study. We have referenced several articles in the Additional Resources section for readers with an interest in this area, but here we briefly summarize the main points.

The core ethical concern with inducements is that they must not be excessive or reach the point where they become an *undue inducement*. This means that the perceived worth of the incentive prevents potential participants from carefully considering the risks and benefits of the research (Scott-Jones, 2000) and may lead them to enroll in research against their better judgment, as described by CIOMS (2002):

> Subjects may be reimbursed for lost earnings, travel costs and other expenses incurred in taking part in a study; they may also receive free medical services. Subjects, particularly those who receive no direct benefit from research, may also be paid or otherwise compensated for inconvenience and time spent. The payments should not be so large, however, or the medical services so extensive, as to induce prospective subjects to consent to participate in the research against their better judgment ("undue inducement"). All payments, reimbursements and medical services provided to research subjects must have been approved by an ethical review committee. (p. 45)

While no formula exists for identifying ethically appropriate inducements, consider the following factors when deciding on the inducements to provide in your study: the local context, national guidelines, the study design, the extent of participant involvement, cultural norms, and participant vulnerabilities, if any (Grady, 2005). It is important to point out that inducements should not be considered a benefit of research participation, as noted earlier. Otherwise, researchers could offer higher payments to counterbalance the risks of the research. In your protocol, you must provide sufficient description of the inducements and how they were determined, so the reviewing IRB can make the final decision about whether your proposed inducements are ethically appropriate.

In summary, we suggest visiting your institution's Office of Research (or similar) website in the early stages of developing your research idea. Many institutions provide guidance on ethics-related issues to consider when developing your protocol and describe the detailed information on human subjects protections they expect in research protocols. Many also provide informed consent templates and other template language that can be used in your protocol.

Once your research protocol is finalized, it must be reviewed and approved by an ethics review committee, sometimes called an Ethics Committee, a Research Ethics Board, or an IRB. In this chapter, we refer to an ethics review committee as an IRB.

INSTITUTIONAL REVIEW BOARDS

What Is an Institutional Review Board?

An IRB is an ethics review committee "responsible for safeguarding the rights, safety, and well-being of the research subjects" (CIOMS, 2002, p. 25). According to the U.S. Code of Federal Regulations (DHHS, 2009), an IRB must consist of at least five committee members of various expertise related to the types of research typically reviewed by the IRB. Also, one member must have no affiliation with the institution, at least one member must primarily focus on scientific issues, and at least one member must primarily focus on nonscientific issues (45 CFR 46.107). Among public health IRBs, committee members are generally public health researchers and others affiliated with public health. Most academic research institutions have their own IRB(s), and researchers from that institution, including all students, must submit their proposed research to the IRB for review and approval before any research activities with participants can begin. If your institution does not have an internal IRB, check with your academic department to learn if there is an established partnership with a nearby IRB that can review your proposed research.

IRBs review and approve *research* with *human subjects*. Both of these qualifiers require further explanation in the context of public health research. According to the U.S. Code of Federal Regulations (DHHS, 2009), research is "a systematic investigation, including research development, testing and evaluation, designed to develop or contribute to generalizable knowledge" (45 CFR 46.102(d)). In some situations, it is difficult to discern if an activity should be considered research or nonresearch. A good example is evaluation of an intervention. Whether that evaluation is considered research or nonresearch depends on the purpose of the activity (CDC, 2010) and how you intend to use the data collected from the evaluation. Ultimately, in most cases, it is best to check with your institution's IRB about any proposed activity that involves the collection of data, as it is the responsibility of the IRB to determine if your activity should be classified as research or nonresearch. For readers who are interested in learning more about research and nonresearch determination, please see suggested guidance from the CDC (2010).

The second qualifier above—human subjects—is defined by the U.S. Code of Federal Regulations (DHHS, 2009) as "a living individual about whom an investigator (whether professional or student) conducting research obtains 1) data through intervention or interaction with the individual, or 2) identifiable private information" (45 CFR 46.102(f)). The first category above—collecting data directly from an individual as part of the research—is easier to interpret than the second category. If, as part of your research, you interact (e.g., communicate in some way) or intervene (e.g., deliver a health program, draw blood) directly with an individual for the purposes of documenting information about an individual, then it is considered research with human subjects (Office of Human Research Projections [OHRP], 2008). The second part of the definition, concerning private information, may need more explanation. Information is considered *private* when the person who originally provided the information did so without any intention for it to become public. Information contained in medical records is an example; patients provide information to doctors with the understanding that the information will remain private. Information that is considered *identifiable* can be linked to a specific individual either directly or through coded means such as participant identification numbers (OHRP, 2008).

Determinations about what constitutes research with human subjects should be of particular interest to readers conducting secondary data analysis, as described in Chapter 9. Researchers conducting secondary analysis will not interact or intervene directly with study participants. However, if the researcher of the *original* research can link the data used in the second analysis to the study participant who provided that information, IRB approval will likely be needed. If identifiers are not linked with the data, IRB review may also be needed, but the study will likely be exempt from ongoing review. Again, it is always best to check with your institution's IRB for specific guidance.

What Documents Must Be Submitted to the IRB?

In general, IRBs require submission and review of the protocol, informed consent materials, study questionnaires, recruitment scripts, and any materials provided to the participant. Most IRBs also require that you submit a separate application that summarizes your protocol. Other documentation may be requested depending on the type of proposed research. Most IRBs give specific details on how to submit a research protocol for review and list the accompanying materials to be submitted. Several IRBs have or are in the process of transitioning to an online submission process. While the required information to submit is typically the same as with a paper submission, an online submission is environmentally friendly and facilitates storage, communication about, and documentation of IRB records.

What Happens After I Submit My Protocol to the IRB?

When an IRB first receives a protocol, a determination is made on how the protocol should be reviewed. There are typically three levels of IRB review:

1. *Exempt from ongoing review:* Research that poses very little risk to participants may qualify to be exempt from ongoing review. This means that you do not have to subsequently submit your protocol for annual review. The U.S. Code of Federal Regulations (DHHS, 2009) describes specific categories of research that IRBs may deem to be exempt from ongoing review (in 45CFR 46.101(b)(1)-(6)), such as observation of people in public places if information gathered is not identifiable (i.e., will not identify the people who were observed).

2. *Expedited review:* An expedited review means that a designated member or members of the IRB, rather than the full board, review the protocol. The designated member or members can approve, approve with required changes, or disapprove the research. The OHRP (1998) has issued guidance that IRBs can use to determine the types of research that qualify for an expedited review. Such research involves no more than minimal risk and can include both biomedical and behavioral research, depending on the procedures and populations involved.

For example, most research involving interviews, surveys, and focus group discussions with nonvulnerable populations qualifies for expedited review.

3. *Full board:* A full board review means that the IRB determined that a protocol should be reviewed and discussed by all members (or a quorum) of the committee at a scheduled meeting. At the end of the discussion, the members of the IRB vote on whether the protocol should be approved, approved with required changes, not approved, or tabled until the next meeting (e.g., in situations where the IRB requests more information from the investigator). Depending on the IRB's review, protocols that are not approved may be resubmitted to the IRB at a later date after all concerns have been addressed.

Protocols assigned to a full board review typically describe research that poses more than minimal risk to participants, such as a clinical trial of an investigative drug, and/or includes vulnerable populations, such as children or pregnant women.

Note: As described above in the What Is an Institutional Review Board? section, it may be difficult to discern in some situations whether a proposed data collection activity is considered research that requires prospective IRB review and approval. It is best to check with your institution's IRB about any proposed activity that involves the collection of data, as it is the responsibility of the IRB to determine if your activity should be classified as research or nonresearch.

Will More Than One IRB Need to Review My Research?

In some situations, more than one IRB must review and approve a proposed research study. This occurs in situations where researchers from different institutions collaborate on a protocol. The IRBs from each investigator's institution must review and approve the research, unless an agreement is made among the institutions' IRBs where one IRB defers review to another. Review from multiple IRBs may also be needed in situations where the sponsor of the research (i.e., the institution of the researcher who received the funding) is located in a different country than where the research will take place. According to the CIOMS (2002) guidelines, research should be reviewed by an ethics review committee associated with the sponsoring institution and in the country where the research is to be conducted. In situations where multiple IRBs must review a research study, any changes required by one IRB must be approved by the other IRB, and all IRBs must approve the research before it can be implemented. In short, final IRB approvals must be unanimous.

Does the IRB Need to Review Approved Research on an Ongoing Basis?

All research, except for the small number of very low-risk studies determined by the IRB to be exempt from ongoing review, must be reviewed on an ongoing basis—at least once per year—by an IRB, according to the U.S. Code of Federal Regulations. There are many reasons to be in regular contact with your IRB during the course of your research, as described below.

Continuing Review

All nonexempt IRB-approved protocols must be reapproved by the IRB after a certain period of time. The IRB stipulates the renewal date in their approval letter, which is typically one year from the initial approval date. Researchers must submit the required renewal materials well in advance of the renewal date to allow the IRB time to review the materials, ask the researcher and have answered any questions they may have, and provide a renewal approval before the initial approval period has expired.

Check with your institution's IRB about the specific information and materials that must be submitted for renewal. Items typically include the protocol, informed consent forms, and a progress report detailing things like the number of participants enrolled to date, the number of participants who withdrew from the research, any new significant findings from related research that may impact the current research, a description of any changes since the last review, any changes in the risk/benefit ratio, and any protocol deviations, adverse events, or social harms.

If the IRB approval renewal is not obtained by the expiration date of the prior approval, all study activities must be halted, except those that are necessary to ensure the safety of participants, until the approval is renewed.

Amendments

Often after a research study begins, unanticipated changes are needed. Before any changes can be implemented in an approved protocol, an amendment to the protocol that describes all proposed changes must be submitted, reviewed, and approved by the IRB. When an amendment is submitted to the IRB, researchers should describe the proposed change(s), the rationale for the proposed change, and any impact the change has on the potential risk of harm toward participants. Any proposed change to an approved consent form must also be reviewed and approved by the IRB.

Amendments to studies that were approved through expedited review are typically processed in the same manner. Major amendments to protocols that were reviewed during a full board meeting will most likely be reviewed during a full board meeting.

Social Harms

Social harms are related to the social risks described earlier in the chapter. When a social harm occurs, the situation, the context surrounding the situation, and how the investigators addressed the situation are typically reported to the IRB(s).

Unanticipated Problems and Adverse Events

Unanticipated problems involving risks to subjects or others and adverse events can happen in any type of research, though they are more likely to occur in biomedical research than in social and behavioral research. If an individual is harmed while participating in your study, regardless of whether it is associated with your study or not, it must be reported to the IRB(s) in a timely manner. For more information on definitions of unanticipated problems and adverse events and related information, refer to *Guidance on Reviewing and Reporting Unanticipated Problems Involving Risk to Subjects or Others and Adverse Events*, listed in the Additional Resources section.

Protocol Deviations

Once a research protocol is approved by the IRB(s), the research team is expected to follow the procedures described in the protocol. If the investigator determines a different approach should be used for any aspect of the research, an amendment describing the new approach must be submitted and approved before it is implemented. A protocol deviation is when an investigator or study staff member makes a change in the approved research after IRB approval is obtained, does something that is not described in the protocol, or varies an approved procedure in some way from what is described in the protocol. When this occurs, the investigator must inform the IRB that a protocol deviation has occurred. IRBs typically want to be told this information as soon as possible after it occurs, and they will request information about the deviation such as the date of the violation, a description of what occurred, the reason for the protocol violation, and the corrective action that was taken so the circumstance does not happen again. At times investigators may need to deviate from an approved protocol to protect the safety of the participants or others. When this occurs, the deviation must still be reported to the IRB(s). Examples of protocol deviations include a breach in confidentiality, missing or incomplete informed consent, and enrolling subjects who do not meet the study's inclusion/exclusion criteria.

End of Data Collection

After all data have been collected, some IRBs will allow the research to be classified as closed, which means that continuing IRB review will no longer be necessary. This primarily occurs when all contact with the participants has ended and the data can no longer be linked to any individual participant. Other IRBs, however, prefer to provide continuing review until all data have been analyzed and published.

Ethics Training

Most institutions and a growing number of sponsors require that all individuals involved in the design and conduct of research receive basic instruction in research ethics prior to the initiation of research. This is done to ensure a common understanding of the ethical issues involved when implementing human subjects research. Researchers should note in their protocols that staff will receive such training. A popular ethics training courses is the Collaborative Institutional Training Initiative (CITI; www.citiprogram.org).

The Health Insurance Portability and Accountability Act (HIPAA)

In addition to the human subjects regulations discussed above, HIPAA requirements may also apply to your research. HIPAA is a U.S. federal law aimed at protecting health information by establishing standards for the use and disclosure of individually identifiable health information (known as Protected Health Information, or PHI) that is created or received by a health care entity. HIPAA took effect in April 2003 with new procedures for collecting and sharing patient information used in research. Under HIPAA, researchers who wish to use PHI for research purposes must obtain a signed authorization from each individual or obtain a waiver of authorization. Institutions are required to establish a Privacy Board to review and approve requests for waivers of authorization for use and disclosure of PHI for research purposes. At many institutions, the IRB serves as the Privacy Board, in part so researchers are not obliged to apply to two separate committees.

THE GLOBAL RESEARCH LANDSCAPE

The last several decades have seen a dramatic increase in the amount of research being conducted internationally, particularly in countries with limited resources. This has led to increased concerns about the exploitation of the people in these settings who are invited to participate in research, even when the research has clear local public health goals such as preventing HIV infection or developing a vaccine to protect against malaria. At the root of these concerns is the suggestion that many of the people who would be likely candidates for research participation are vulnerable to undue influence to participate because of low literacy, poverty, and/or limited access to basic health care—or that the communities who participate in the research will not benefit from the results. The ethical principle of justice demands that the populations who bear the burdens of the research should also stand to receive any benefits of the research. In the global context this has fueled debate about posttrial access to effective interventions and therapies. Sponsors of research may be reasonably expected to commit to making the effective intervention or therapy that was tested in that setting locally available after the trial.

Researchers working internationally must be aware of these realities and be prepared to address them when developing the study plan. Managing these issues may require a different approach to recruitment and informed consent, as well as assisting those who do enroll in the study with their non-study-related health care issues. Identifying and collaborating with a local research partner and community stakeholders can be very effective strategies for appropriately incorporating local ethical and cultural issues, particularly when working in an unfamiliar country.

Local Ethics Review

The growth in international research has been paralleled by the development of local capacity for ethics review. While many low-resource countries may currently lack a robust research ethics infrastructure, such as well-developed regulations, mature IRBs, and effective enforcement mechanisms, they may still have capacity for ethics review. Certainly local IRBs are in an excellent position to review research and determine if it is compatible with the local context and culture, particularly in the areas of recruitment and informed consent (Gilman & Garcia, 2004). For example, when a local IRB reviews a research proposal, it determines whether the local laws have been considered, such as the age of majority, what constitutes legal documentation of consent (signature), and who can give permission for children and others with diminished consent capacity to participate in research. Many local IRBs also request that researchers describe in their protocol steps that they and others (e.g., advocates, drug companies) will take to promote access to any product proven effective by the research among those individuals who participated in the research and their communities, as mentioned above.

Practical Issues When Working With Local IRBs

The growth and maturation of in-country or local IRBs has produced an expectation that research be reviewed by an IRB in the country where the research is being conducted, in addition to any reviews that are required in the country of the research sponsor or lead investigator (CIOMS, 2002). When working with the local IRB, take the following factors into account:

- In many places, limited resources mean that local IRBs have backlogs of several months in the queue of protocols or documentation they have to review. This should be factored in to your research timeline.
- As in the United States, many local IRBs will have specific guidelines for submission and application processes that must be strictly adhered to. Failure to follow the local requirements may mean that your application is rejected without being reviewed, and the revised application sent back to the end of the queue.
- Both the local IRB and the sponsor country IRB may require the submission of translations (along with verifications such as back-translations) that must be addressed prior to approval.
- Finally, when the research is funded by the U.S. Department of Health and Human Services, including the National Institutes of Health and CDC, the collaborating institution in the host country will be required to obtain a Federalwide Assurance (FWA) from the OHRP and to register the local IRB as part of that process. The OHRP website has all of the information required to obtain an FWA, and the application can be submitted electronically (www.hhs.gov/ohrp/assurances/assurances/index.html). Assurances are typically issued within 30 days of receipt of the application by OHRP. The OHRP website also includes a database of institutions that have FWAs as well as registered IRBs that can be searched by country. The International Activities office within OHRP is also a useful resource. When working with U.S. government sponsors other than the Department of Health and Human Services, check with the sponsor to determine if an assurance is required.

CURRENT ISSUES AND FUTURE DIRECTIONS

Bioethics

The field of bioethics continues to evolve alongside advances in human subjects research, medicine, and public health. New ethical considerations will emerge in the literature with the development of new research approaches, such as the novel approach to HIV prevention using conditional cash transfers to decrease HIV risk (e.g., paying participants money as an incentive to remain HIV negative) and suggested guidance for ethical review by London, Borasky, Bhan, and the Ethics Working Group of the HIV Prevention Trials Network (2012; e.g., whether the cash transfer is a benefit of the research and considerations for evaluating the risk/benefit ratio). Advances in genomics research which rely on pooled data from biobanks or large data repositories (necessary for population-level research in genetic disorders) also raise new questions about privacy and confidentiality, since DNA samples are by their nature identifiable (Rothstein, 2005). At the same time, longstanding ethical issues, such as the quality of informed consent, will continue to occupy the attention of ethicists and researchers who conduct empirical research on research ethics (Flory & Emanuel, 2004; Sugarman et al., 1999).

Research Using the Internet

Researchers can now use the online environment to recruit, collect data, and interact with research subjects and their avatars directly. The use of the Internet as a research tool raises several new scientific, ethical, and regulatory challenges. Researchers who want to utilize the Internet for their studies must take these challenges into account when planning and implementing research. While the anonymity that the World Wide Web provides may make some individuals more likely to participate, it can also lead to the collection of inaccurate data. In addition, it may be impossible to completely verify that individuals who participate online are who they claim to be. In most Internet-based research it is also impossible to obtain legal documentation of informed consent, and as a result the IRB may be asked to grant a waiver of documentation of consent. The evolving social media environment has also presented challenges to maintaining privacy and confidentiality. Finally, data collected online—and especially sensitive data—requires sufficient data security measures to help protect the confidentiality of the data and the privacy of subjects. Research teams should consider adding personnel with Internet technology security expertise to their study teams to help manage these issues.

CONCLUSION

Ethical considerations reach across all stages of public health research, from development and implementation of the study design to providing posttrial access to interventions proven effective. The ethical guidelines and regulations reviewed here serve as a starting point for best practices, though issues pertaining to ethics are not often straightforward or served by template language. IRBs, local partners, and community stakeholder advisory mechanisms are key resources for making determinations about ethical issues. Chapter 4 provides suggestions for developing stakeholder relationships to facilitate these and other elements of public health research.

ADDITIONAL RESOURCES

Ethics guidelines and regulations in countries other than the United States: U.S. Department of Health and Human Services. (2012). *International compilation of human research standards.* Retrieved from http://www.hhs.gov/ohrp/international/intlcompilation/intlcompilation.html

Ethics regulatory and guidance development timeline: Israel, M., & Hay, I. (2006). Codes and principles. In *Research ethics for social scientists* (pp. 23–39). London, UK: Sage.

Concerns with current regulations on human subject research: Emanuel, E. J., Wood, A., Fleischman, A., Bowen, A., Getz, K. A., Grady, C., . . . Sugarman, J. (2004). Oversight of human participants research: Identifying problems to evaluate reform proposals. *Annals of Internal Medicine, 141,* 282–291.

Information that is considered identifiable in research: Jones, E. (2009*). HIPAA "protected health information": What does PHI include?* Retrieved from http://www.hipaa.com/2009/09/hipaa-protected-health-information-what-does-phi-include

Privacy and confidentiality: Folkman, S. (2000). Privacy and confidentiality. In B. D. Sales & S. Folkman (Eds.), *Ethics in research with human subjects* (pp. 13–26). Washington, DC: American Psychological Association.

Inducements and compensation:

- Dickert, N., & Grady, C. (1999). What's the price of a research subject? Approaches to payment for research participation. *New England Journal of Medicine, 341,* 198–203.
- Emanuel, E. J., Currie, X. E., Herman, A., & Project Phidisa. (2005). Undue inducement in clinical research in developing countries: Is it a worry? *Lancet, 366,* 336–340.
- Macklin, R. (1981). On paying money to research subjects: "Due" and "undue" inducements. *IRB, 5,* 1–6.

Informed consent:

- Beauchamp, T. (2011). Informed consent: Its history, meaning, and present challenges. *Cambridge Quarterly of Healthcare Ethics, 20,* 515–523.

- Faden, R., & Beauchamp, T. (1986). *A history and theory of informed consent.* New York, NY: Oxford University Press.
- Nelson, R. M., Beauchamp, T., Miller, V. A., Reynolds, W., Ittenbach, R. F., & Luce, M. F. (2011). The concept of voluntary consent. *American Journal of Bioethics, 11,* 6–16.

Global Health:

- Lavery, J. V., Grady, C., Wahl, E. R., & Emanuel, E. J. (2007). *Ethical issues in international biomedical research: A casebook.* New York, NY: Oxford University Press.
- Nuffield Council. (2005). *The ethics of research related to healthcare in developing countries: A follow-up discussion paper.* Retrieved from http://www.nuffield bioethics.org/research-developing-countries

Information on unanticipated problems and adverse events: U.S. Department of Health and Human Services. (2007). *Guidance on reviewing and reporting unanticipated problems involving risk to subjects or others and adverse events.* http://www.hhs.gov/ohrp/policy/advevntguid.html

The latest in the field of bioethics:
- Organizations related to bioethics:
  - PRIM&R. http://www.primr.org
  - American Society for Bioethics and Humanities. http://www.asbh.org
- Bioethics-related journals:
  - *IRB: Ethics and Human Research.* http://www.thehastingscenter.org/Publications/IRB/Default.aspx
  - *Journal of Medical Ethics.* http://jme.bmj.com
  - *American Journal of Bioethics.* http://www.bioethics.net/journals
  - *Journal of Empirical Research on Human Research Ethics.* http://ucpressjournals.com/journal.php?j=jer

REFERENCES

Beardsley, E., Jefford, M., & Mileshkin L. (2007). Longer consent forms for clinical trials compromise patient understanding: So why are they lengthening? *Journal of Clinical Oncology, 25,* 13–44.

Centers for Disease Control and Prevention. (2010). *Distinguishing public health research and public health nonresearch.* Retrieved from http://www.cdc.gov/od/science/integrity/docs/cdc-policy-distinguishing-public-health-research-nonresearch.pdf

Centers for Disease Control and Prevention. (2011). *U.S. Public Health Service syphilis study at Tuskegee.* Retrieved from http://www.cdc.gov/tuskegee/timeline.htm

Chaisson, L. H., Kass, N. E., Chengeta, B., Mathebula, U., & Samandari, T. (2011). Repeated assessments of informed consent comprehension among HIV-infected participants of a three-year clinical trial in Botswana. *PLoS One, 6,* e22696.

Cohn, E., & Larson E. (2007). Improving participant comprehension in the informed consent process. *Journal of Nursing Scholarship, 39,* 273–280.

Corneli, A. L., Bentley, M. E., Sorenson, J. R., Henderson, G. E., van der Horst, C., Moses, A., . . . Jamieson, D. J. (2006). Using formative research to develop a context-specific approach to informed consent for clinical trials. *Journal of Empirical Research on Human Research Ethics, 1,* 45–60.

Council for International Organizations of Medical Sciences. (2002). *International ethical guidelines for biomedical research involving human subjects.* Geneva, Switzerland: CIOMS. Retrieved from http://www.cioms.ch/publications/layout_guide2002.pdf

Flory, J., & Emanuel, E. (2004). Interventions to improve research participants' understanding in informed consent for research: A systematic review. *Journal of the American Medical Association, 292,* 593–601.

Gilman, R. H., & Garcia, H. H. (2004). Ethics review procedures for research in developing countries: A basic presumption of guilt. *Canadian Medical Association Journal, 171,* 248–249.

Grady, C. (2005). Payment of clinical research subjects. *Journal of Clinical Investigation, 115,* 1681–1687.

Joffe, S., Cook, E. F., Cleary, P. D., Clark, J. W., & Weeks, J. C. (2001). Quality of informed consent: A new measure of understanding among research subjects. *Journal of the National Cancer Institute, 93,* 139–147.

Levine, R. J. (1988). *Ethics and regulation of clinical research* (2nd ed.). New Haven, CT: Yale University Press.

London, A. J., Borasky, D. A., Bhan, A., & Ethics Working Group of the HIV Prevention Trials Network. (2012). Improving ethical review of research involving incentives for health promotion. *PLoS Med, 9,* e1001193.

MacQueen, K. M., & Sugarman, J. (2003). *HIV Prevention Trials Network: Ethics guidance for research.* Retrieved from http://www.hptn.org/Web%20Documents/EWG/HPTNEthics GuidanceFINAL15April2003.pdf

National Bioethics Advisory Committee. (2001a). Assessing risks and potential benefits and evaluating vulnerability. In *Ethical and Policy Issues in Research Involving Human Participants* (Vol. 1, pp. 69–96). Bethesda, MD: Author.

National Bioethics Advisory Committee. (2001b). Voluntary informed consent. In *Ethical and Policy Issues in International Research: Clinical Trials in Developing Countries* (Vol. 1, pp. 35–53). Bethesda, MD: Author.

National Commission for the Protection of Human Subjects of Biomedical and Behavioral Research. (1978). *The Belmont Report: Ethical principles and guidelines for the protection of human subjects of research.* Washington, DC: U.S. Government Printing Office. Retrieved from http://www.hhs.gov/ohrp/policy/belmont.html

National Institutes of Health. (2013). *Certificates of confidentiality kiosk.* Retrieved from http://grants.nih.gov/grants/policy/coc/

Office of Human Research Projections. (1998). *Categories of research that may be reviewed by the Institutional Review Board (IRB) through an expedited review procedures.* Retrieved from http://www.hhs.gov/ohrp/policy/expedited98.html

Office of Human Research Projections. (2008). *Guidance on research involving coded private information or biological specimens.* Retrieved from http://www.hhs.gov/ohrp/policy/cdebiol.html

Prentice, E. D., & Gordon, B. G. (2001). Institutional Review Board assessment of risks and benefits associated with research. In *Ethical and Policy Issues in Research Involving Human Subject* (Vol. 2, pp. L1–L16). Bethesda, MD: National Bioethics Advisory Commission.

Rothstein, M. A. (2005). Expanding the ethical analysis of biobanks. *Journal of Law, Medicine & Ethics, 33,* 89–101.

Scott-Jones, D. (2000). Recruitment of research participants. In B. D. Sales & S. Folkman (Eds.), *Ethics in research with human subjects* (pp. 27–34). Washington, DC: American Psychological Association.

Sieber, J. E. (2000). Planning research: Basic ethical decision-making. In B. D. Sales & S. Folkman (Eds.), *Ethics in research with human subjects* (pp. 13–26). Washington, DC: American Psychological Association.

Sugarman, J., McCrory, D. C., Powell, D., Krasny, A., Adams, B., Ball, E., & Cassell, C. (1999). Empirical research on informed consent. An annotated bibliography. *Hastings Center Report, 29*, S1–42.

U.S. Department of Health and Human Services. (1993). *Institutional Review Board guidebook glossary.* Retrieved from http://www.hhs.gov/ohrp/archive/irb/irb_glossary.htm

U.S. Department of Health and Human Services. (2009). 45 Code of Federal Regulations 46. *Federal Register.*

Vanderpool, H. Y. (2001). Unfulfilled promise: How the Belmont Report can amend the Code of Federal Regulations Title 45 Part 46—Protection of Human Subjects. In *Ethical and Policy Issues in Research Involving Human Subject* (Vol. 2, pp. O1–O20). Bethesda, MD: National Bioethics Advisory Commission.

Weijer, C. (2001). The ethical analysis of risks and potential benefits in human subjects research: History, theory, and implications for U.S. regulation. In *Ethical and Policy Issues in Research Involving Human Subject* (Vol. 2, pp. P1–P29). Bethesda, MD: National Bioethics Advisory Commission.

Woodsong, C., & Karim, Q. A. (2005). A model designed to enhance informed consent: Experiences from the HIV prevention trials network. *American Journal of Public Health, 95*, 412–419.

World Medical Association. (2008). *Declaration of Helsinki: Ethical principles for medical research involving human subjects.* As amended by the 59th WMA General Assembly, Seoul, Korea. Retrieved from www.wma.net/en/30publications/10policies/b3

NOTE

1. In the U.S., minors are persons who have not attained the legal age for consent to treatments or procedures involved in the research, under the applicable law of the jurisdiction in which the research will be conducted. The age of majority should be confirmed in national laws when working outside of the U.S. The definition of minors, however, can vary among countries.

4

Community Engagement in Public Health Research

Dázon Dixon Diallo and Paula M. Frew

In 2006 the National Institutes of Health (NIH) began emphasizing translational research, or research focusing on the translation of scientific discoveries into practical applications to improve human health. Community engagement (CE) and community-engaged research (CEnR) have become increasingly viewed as the keystone to translational science (Michener et al., 2012), as funders, researchers, and policymakers have recognized that the elimination of persistent health inequities requires the engagement of multiple perspectives, resources, and skills (Schulz et al. 2011). Indeed, The Centers for Disease Control and Prevention's (CDC) Ten Essential Services for Public Health include two community engagement–related functions:

- Inform, educate, and empower people about health issues;
- Mobilize community partnerships and actions to identify and solve health problems. (CDC, 2012)

A community-engaged research approach can enable researchers to strengthen the links between research and practice and enhance translational results because, although research programs and policy are "defined at regional and national levels," the "community is, literally, where prevention and intervention take place" (MacQueen et al., 2001, p. 1929). In recent years, for example, community engagement and mobilization have been essential to programs addressing smoking cessation, obesity, cancer, heart disease, and other health concerns (Ahmed & Palermo, 2010; Minkler & Wallerstein, 2008).

The purpose of this chapter is to describe the role of community engagement in public research and to offer guidance and conceptual frameworks on how to cultivate community involvement in public health research. While community engagement is essential to all types of public health research and issues, we draw on our extensive experience in engaging diverse communities, primarily among ethnic and racial minorities in urban southern U.S. cities, in HIV prevention and treatment research. HIV provides an effective lens through which to view community engagement for two key reasons: (1) since the beginning of the epidemic, community involvement has played a central role in prevention and treatment efforts, and (2) historically, the research agenda for HIV/AIDS has been driven by a dynamic partnership between affected and scientific communities. We provide several examples of how community engagement has successfully (and sometimes unsuccessfully) been used in this particular field to illustrate how it may be applied to other public health issues as well.

DEFINITIONS AND CONSTRUCTS IN COMMUNITY ENGAGEMENT (CE)

The concept of community engagement arose from participatory action research traditions (Crotty, 2003; MacQueen et al., 2001; Miller & Shinn, 2005), which focus on building public trust in research through consultation, dialogue, and collaboration with communities, particularly among minority and marginalized populations (Smith et al., 2007).

Community engagement has been characterized as addressing health issues from an ecological perspective for the promotion of "learning and empowerment, equalizing power among participants, integrating knowledge and change for the mutual benefit of all partners, and ultimately disseminating findings and knowledge gained to all partners" (Israel, Schulz, Parker, & Becker 1998; Schulz, Krieger, & Galea, 2002). Although no one unified definition of CE exists in the public health sphere, the definitions extant in the literature tend to share three common themes: collaboration, communication, and respect.

KEY DEFINITIONS

Community is defined as "a group of people with diverse characteristics who are linked by social ties, share common perspectives, and engage in joint action in geographical locations or settings" (MacQueen et al., 2001). MacQueen et al. (2001) further characterize community by five essential core elements:

1. Joint action (cohesion and identity)

2. Locus (sense of place)

3. Sharing (common interests and perspectives)

4. Social ties (the community foundation)

5. Diversity (heterogeneous social complexity)

Community engagement is "the process of working collaboratively with and through groups of people affiliated by geographic proximity, special interest, or similar situations to address issues affecting the well-being of those people." In public health this process typically "involves partnerships and coalitions that help mobilize resources and influence systems, change relationships among partners, and serve as catalysts for changing policies, programs, and practices" (CDC, 1997, p. 9; see also Fawcett et al., 1995).

Community-engaged research is an approach to conducting scientific inquiry that follows the process and principles of community engagement.

Participatory action research is a collaborative approach to conducting research that aims to bridge science and clinical practice. The key characteristic of this approach—collaboration between consumers and researchers—often increases the relevance of research while maintaining the standards of scientific rigor (White, Suchowierska, & Campbell, 2004).

Community-based participatory research (CBPR) is "a collaborative approach to research that equitably involves all partners in the research process and recognizes the unique strengths that each brings. CBPR begins with a research topic of importance to the community and has the aim of combining knowledge with action and achieving social change to improve health outcomes and eliminate health disparities" (Kellogg Health Scholars Program, 2003–2013; see In Focus at the end of this chapter).

Another key concept in community engagement is the degree to which a community is involved in a research endeavor, which can be viewed along a continuum. Table 4.1 compares three general research approaches, with respect to level of engagement with the community, across all phases of the research process. Note that the table is for heuristic purposes only. In reality, most projects will involve a variety of techniques that blur the boundaries between the approaches presented. At the most involved, or engaged, end of the continuum is community-based participatory research (CBPR), which has been in existence for some years (Fleischman, 2007; Green, George, Daniel, Frankish, & Herbert, 1995; Schulz et al., 2002). Collaboration with target groups using CBPR methods has been shown to be effective in overcoming issues of mistrust and suspicion of research (Hatch, Moss, Saran, Presley-Cantrell, & Mallory, 1993). Moreover, community involvement in health promotion initiatives has been shown to enhance dissemination and utilization of research findings (Bracht, 2001; Leung, Yen, & Minkler, 2004).

Table 4.1 Comparison of Traditional, Community-Engaged, and Community-Based Participatory Research

	Type of Research		
	Traditional	*Community-Engaged*	*Community-Based Participatory*
Research objective	Based on epidemiologic data and funding priorities	Community input in identifying locally relevant issues	Full participation of community in identifying issues of greatest importance
Study design	Design based entirely on scientific rigor and feasibility	Researchers work with community to ensure study design is culturally acceptable	Community intimately involved with study design
Recruitment and retention	Based on scientific issues and "best guesses" regarding how to best reach community members	Researchers consult with community representatives on recruitment and retention strategies	Community representatives provide guidance on recruitment and retention strategies and aid in recruitment
Instrument design	Instruments adopted/ adapted from other studies and tested chiefly with psychometric analytic methods	Instruments adopted from other studies and tested/adapted to fit local populations	Instruments developed with community input and tested in similar populations
Data collection	Conducted by academic researchers or individuals with no connection to the community	Community members involved in some aspects of data collection	Conducted by members of the community, to the extent possible based on available skill sets; focus on capacity building
Analysis and interpretation	Academic researchers own the data, conduct analysis, and interpret the findings	Academic researchers share results of analysis with community members for comments and interpretation	Data are shared; community members and academic researchers work together to interpret results
Dissemination	Results published in peer-reviewed academic journals	Results disseminated in community venues as well	Community members assist academic researchers to disseminate data

Source: Adapted from: Mary Anne McDonald, "Practicing Community-Engaged Research." On-line module, Duke Center for Community Engaged Research.

COMMUNITY ENGAGEMENT IN PUBLIC HEALTH RESEARCH

Regardless of the research approach taken, some level of community engagement is likely necessary for public health projects, as humans are social beings located within geographic and social communities that influence ideas and behaviors. Indeed, many of the public health theories covered in the Appendix explicitly or implicitly recognize the effects of social and environmental factors on health. As Morgan and Lifshay (2006) summarize:

> The public health issues of the 21st century include chronic diseases (such as cancer, obesity and diabetes), gun violence, and homelessness, as well as communicable disease and maternal and child health. These problems affect low-income and minority populations disproportionately and are influenced by the physical, social and economic environments in which people live. To address these complex health issues effectively, modern [public health practitioners] must broaden their approaches and use a spectrum of strategies to build community capacity and promote community health. To carry out these functions and address the public health disparities of today, local health departments [and public health practitioners] must expand their ability to engage communities. (p. 1)

CE and HIV Prevention Research

Similar to other health disparities, the HIV epidemic has demonstrated that engagement of the most affected communities is a successful approach to effective interventions, though defining community involvement and implementing it successfully often present numerous challenges. Community involvement in HIV research (as with other types of public health research) raises a spectrum of social and ethical questions, especially when the concerned communities include people who are disadvantaged because of ethnicity, income, gender, class, or sexuality (Strauss, 1999).

The evolution of community engagement in HIV and AIDS research and programming is a well-documented process as described in recent historical texts and films about activist movements to advance the AIDS research agenda in the United States and globally (Killen, Harrington, & Fauci, 2012). Groups of people living with HIV/AIDS and their allies demonstrated against and protested the lack of inclusion of the affected communities in all stages of research design and implementation. For example, we acknowledge the radically effective and pioneering activism of the AIDS Coalition to Unleash Power (ACTUP) and the Treatment Action Group (TAG) of the USA and Treatment Action Campaign of South Africa. These activists have brought increased attention to the need for community engagement and recognition that inclusion and transparency are ethical responsibilities. In 2007, the Joint United Nations Programme on HIV/AIDS (UNAIDS) copublished with the

World Health Organization (WHO) a sentinel document, *Ethical Considerations in HIV Biomedical Prevention Trials*, which noted:

> To ensure the ethical and scientific quality of proposed research, its relevance to the affected community, and its acceptance by the affected community, community representatives should be involved in an early and sustained manner in the design, development, implementation and distribution of results. (p. 2)

Beyond these ethical imperatives, experience has shown that failing to involve communities in HIV clinical research can threaten the viability of the trials (West et al., 2008), potentially wasting scarce public health resources.

Lessons Learned From the Failure to Engage Community

In July 2004, a drug called tenofovir disoproxil fumarate (TDF), an antiretroviral used to treat AIDS, was being tested as a pre-exposure prophylaxis—something that could be taken daily by uninfected persons to prevent HIV acquisition. Clinical trials were planned in four countries among female sex workers as well as two sites in the United States among other populations at higher risk for HIV acquisition. The multi-country trial was funded by the U.S. National Institutes of Health and the Bill and Melinda Gates Foundation. The trials were implemented by Family Health International in Ghana, Nigeria, and Cameroon, and (expected to be) in Cambodia by the University of California, San Francisco and University of New South Wales.

Prior to implementation at the Cambodian site, increasing pressure from activist groups and affiliated nongovernmental organizations (NGOs) persuaded the Cambodian Prime Minister to halt the initiation of the trial (Cohen, 2004). Although the research team assigned to Cambodia attempted to bring sex workers into a community advisory group for the study, the efforts failed because of strong community mistrust (Page-Shafer et al., 2005). On the surface, it appeared that the research team followed WHO (2002) guidelines on community participation to ensure adequate informed consent, study material translation, and advisement on recruitment and retention practices (Page-Shafer et al., 2005), yet the community felt patronized. In particular, community representatives expressed concern that the participants felt a lack of power in the situation. They also perceived a lack of sensitivity from the research team to engage in dialogue with the community about their needs and concerns prior to study implementation (Page-Shafer et al., 2005). The Cambodian government eventually intervened and the clinical trial never got underway.

The Cambodian TDF study experience highlights important distinctions with respect to community engagement, community involvement, and community consultation. They are not synonymous terms. In Cambodia, the effort failed in part because of inadequate formative research in the community prior to study implementation. The perception among potential participants was that the needs, desires, and concerns of the community were not important considerations. Provisions for "community consultation" in the development of the study protocol, recruitment and retention methods, and other research team concerns were therefore rebuffed. With a growing demand on behalf of communities to have more control in the development and conduct of research, the nuanced nature of the community's involvement has become an important issue of concern (Dickert & Sugarman, 2005; Green & Mercer, 2001; Swartz & Kagee, 2006). Thus, building on the definitions presented earlier, *community engagement* is also an umbrella term for an encompassing endeavor which includes behavioral research, community input and advisement, and empowerment and advocacy.

A FRAMEWORK FOR THE COMMUNITY ENGAGEMENT PROCESS

Guiding Values and Principles

The NIH Director's Council of Public Representatives (COPR) is a federal advisory committee comprising members of the public who consult with the NIH on issues related to public participation in NIH activities. In 2010, COPR developed a framework that includes a set of values linked with strategies and expected outcomes for CE (Table 4.2).

Table 4.2   Core Principles and Strategies for Community Engagement in Research

Core Principles of Community Engagement	Core Strategies to Effect Community Engagement
1. Definition and scope of community engagement in research	1. Define community and identify partners.
2. Strong community-academic partnerships	2. Learn the etiquette of community engagement.
3. Equitable power and responsibility	3. Build a sustainable network of CEnR researchers.
4. Capacity building	4. Recognize the need to develop new methodologies.
5. Effective dissemination of plans	5. Improve translation and dissemination plans.

Source: Michener L, Cook J, Ahmed SM, Yonas MA, Coyne-Beasley T, Aguilar-Gaxiola S. Aligning the goals of community-engaged research: why and how academic health centers can successfully engage with communities to improve health. Acad Med. 2012 Mar;87(3):285–91.

Building on these values, we recognize that, beyond the generally accepted definition of community, it is important that specific individuals, organizations, and institutions in a community are identified and included as partners in the research. Communities are complex systems in which individual memberships may reflect multiple interests and represent a diverse set of demographics, including race, gender, age, and sexual orientation. Michener and colleagues (2012) provide a guide for academic health centers, discussing the types and layers of prospective community partners with whom to engage and collaborate. Among these groups are neighborhood organizations and leaders, faith-based organizations, community-based health practitioners, and governmental agencies. Political support for public health initiatives invariably begins with community engagement. And funding and support at the local, state, and national levels is influenced by what are perceived to be the needs of the community (CTSA, 2011).

For many underserved and historically abused communities, the benefits of medical or public health research may be unclear. Likewise, the possible benefits of collaborating with researchers may not be recognized or believed by community members. Thus, before a CEnR agenda can be built, the community must first learn the principles of community engagement. It is, therefore, incumbent upon researchers to understand themselves and be able to cogently explain the underlying rationale behind planned research, collaborative principles, and the importance of community involvement in the research process (Ahmed & Palermo, 2010). Researchers should also study the background and history of the community to be engaged. This enables researchers to highlight and explain the potential benefits of teaming up with researchers *to the community and its members.*

This concept of teamwork includes capacity building as well. Consider subcontracts to and from partners in the community. Long-term, committed partnerships between communities and local researchers require building a training pipeline that sparks interest in research in precollege students, makes community engagement a required competency for doctoral and medical students as well as residents and post-doctoral fellows, and rewards researchers for community-engaged projects that lead to improved outcomes. This can be done at a number of levels. For example, in the academic health center setting, schools can provide training for all university students and researchers through required coursework, self-paced modules, and certification (CTSA, 2011).

Enacting Community Engagement

As we can see from the principles and strategies that guide CE, strong value is placed on collaboration, partnerships, and sustainability. So how do we enact these values or principles? Community engagement can be conceptualized as having three general phases, depicted in Figure 4.1.

An Example of Successful Community-Academic Partnership

In 2009, SisterLove—a reproductive justice organization for women in Atlanta—expanded their scope and capacity to be a reliable and long-term community-based

Figure 4.1   Phases of Community Engagement

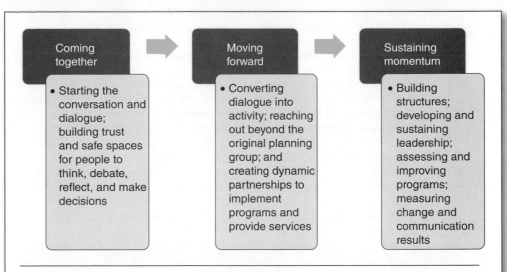

Source: Minnesota Department of Health (n.d.).

These broad phases can be broken down into smaller components. The updated version of the guidelines for CE mentioned earlier (CTSA, 2011), for example, provide an excellent summary of the basic steps required for successful community engagement. Rather than paraphrasing them, we have reproduced excerpts of them here. You can find the full text of the most recent version at www.atsdr.cdc.gov/communityengagement.

Before Starting a Community Engagement Effort . . .

1. Be clear about the purposes or goals of the engagement effort and the populations and/or communities you want to engage.

   Those wishing to engage the community need to be able to communicate to that community why its participation is worthwhile. Of course, simply being able to articulate that involvement is worthwhile does not guarantee participation. Those implementing the effort should be prepared for a variety of responses from the community. There may be many barriers to engagement, and appropriate compensation should be provided to participants. The processes for involvement and participation must be appropriate for meeting the overall goals and objectives of the engagement.

2. Become knowledgeable about the community's culture, economic conditions, social networks, political and power structures, norms and values, demographic trends, history, and experience with efforts by outside groups to engage the community in various programs. Learn about the community's perceptions of those initiating the engagement activities.

(Continued)

(Continued)

It is important to learn as much about the community as possible, through both qualitative and quantitative methods, and from as many sources as feasible. Many of the organizing concepts, models, and frameworks presented in the Appendix of this volume support this principle. Social ecological theories, for example, emphasize the need to understand the larger physical and social/cultural environment and its interaction with individual health behaviors. An understanding of how the community perceives the benefits and costs of participating will facilitate decision making and consensus building and will translate into improved program planning, design, policy development, organization, and advocacy. The concept of stages of diffusion of innovation highlights the need to assess the community's readiness to adopt new strategies. Understanding the community will help leaders in the engagement effort map community assets, develop a picture of how business is done, and identify the individuals and groups whose support is necessary, including which individuals or groups must be approached and involved in the initial stages of engagement.

For Engagement to Occur, It Is Necessary to . . .

3. Go to the community, establish relationships, build trust, work with the formal and informal leadership, and seek commitment from community organizations and leaders to create processes for mobilizing the community.

   Engagement is based on community support. The literature on community participation and organization illuminates this principle and suggests that positive change is more likely to occur when community members are an integral part of a program's development and implementation. All partners must be actively respected from the start. For example, meeting with key community leaders and groups in their surroundings helps to build trust for a true partnership. Such meetings provide the organizers of engagement activities with more information about the community, its concerns, and the factors that will facilitate or constrain participation. In addition, community members need to see and experience "real" benefits for the extra time, effort, and involvement they are asked to give. Once a successful rapport is established, meetings and exchanges with community members can build into an ongoing and substantive partnership.

4. Remember and accept that collective self-determination is the responsibility and right of all people in a community. No external entity should assume it can bestow on a community the power to act in its own self-interest.

   Just because an institution or organization introduces itself into the community does not mean that it automatically becomes of the community. An organization is of the community when it is controlled by individuals or groups who are members of the community. This concept of self-determination is central to the concept of community empowerment. The dynamic can be quite complex, however, because communities themselves may have factions that contend for power and influence. More broadly, it should be recognized that internal and external forces may be at play in any engagement effort. As addressed in Principle 6, a diversity of ideas may be encountered and negotiated throughout the engagement process.

5. Partnering with the community is necessary to create change and improve health.

   Organizing concepts, models, and frameworks such as social ecology, community participation, and community organization speak to the relationship between community partnerships and positive change. Indeed, community-based participatory research and current approaches to translational research explicitly recognize that community engagement significantly enhances the potential for research to lead to improved health by improving participation in the research, its implementation, and dissemination of its findings. Community engagement based on improving health takes place in the context of and must respond to economic, social, and political trends that affect health and health disparities. Furthermore, equitable community partnerships and transparent discussions of power are more likely to lead to desired outcomes (see Principle 4). The individuals and groups involved in a partnership must identify opportunities for co-learning and feel that they each have something meaningful to contribute to the pursuit of improved health, while at the same time seeing something to gain.

6. All aspects of community engagement must recognize and respect the diversity of the community. Awareness of the various cultures of a community and other factors affecting diversity must be paramount in planning, designing, and implementing approaches to engaging a community.

   Diversity may be related to economic, educational, employment, or health status as well as differences in culture, language, race, ethnicity, age, gender, mobility, literacy, or personal interests. These elements of diversity may affect individuals' and communities' access to health care delivery, their health status, and their response to community engagement efforts. For example, the processes, strategies, and techniques used to engage the community must be respectful of and complement cultural traditions. The systems perspective suggests attention to another element of community diversity: the diversity of roles that different people and organizations play in the functioning of a community. Engaging these diverse populations will require the use of multiple engagement strategies.

7. Community engagement can be sustained only by identifying and mobilizing community assets and strengths and by developing the community's capacity and resources to make decisions and take action.

   Community assets include the interests, skills, and experiences of individuals and local organizations as well as the networks of relationships that connect them. Individual and institutional resources such as facilities, materials, skills, and economic power all can be mobilized for community health decision making and action. In brief, community members and institutions should be viewed as resources to bring about change and take action. The discussion of community participation earlier highlighted the need to offer an exchange of resources to ensure community participation. Of course, depending on the "trigger" for the engagement process (e.g., a funded mandate vs. a more grassroots effort), resources are likely to be quite varied.

   (Continued)

(Continued)

8. Organizations that wish to engage a community as well as individuals seeking to effect change must be prepared to release control of actions or interventions to the community and be flexible enough to meet its changing needs.

   Engaging the community is ultimately about facilitating community-driven action . . . Community action should include the many elements of a community that are needed for the action to be sustained while still creating a manageable process. Community engagement will create changes in relationships and in the way institutions and individuals demonstrate their capacity and strength to act on specific issues. In environments characterized by dynamism and constant change, coalitions, networks, and new alliances are likely to emerge. Efforts made to engage communities will affect the nature of public and private programs, policies, and resource allocation. Those implementing efforts to engage a community must be prepared to anticipate and respond to these changes.

9. Community collaboration requires long-term commitment by the engaging organization and its partners.

   Community engagement sometimes occurs around a specific, time-limited initiative. More commonly, however, community participation and mobilization need nurturing over the long term. Moreover, long-term partnerships have the greatest capacity for making a difference in the health of the population. Not surprisingly, building trust and helping communities develop the capacity and infrastructure for successful community action takes time. Before individuals and organizations can gain influence and become players and partners in decision making and action steps taken by communities relative to their health, they may need additional resources, knowledge, and skills. For example, partners might need long-term technical assistance and training related to the organizational and technical knowledge necessary to address issues of concern. The probability of sustained engagement and effective programming increases when community participants are active partners in the process.

Source: Adapted from CTSA (2011).

participatory research partner addressing the sexual health needs of women of color. For more than a decade, SisterLove has participated as a research partner with research teams at Emory University. The SisterLove-Emory research partnerships have resulted in clinical and behavioral studies in HIV prevention, including, but not limited to, HIV vaccines, microbicides, treatment modalities, research literacy, and qualitative assessments of community readiness to engage in trials. The SisterLove-Emory team has a long track record of recruiting women living with HIV and those vulnerable to infection into clinical research studies. For example, among AIDS Clinical Trial Group sites in the United States, the Emory clinical trials unit has benefitted from SisterLove's promotion of participation in HIV clinical research; the site is consistently ranked among the top sites enrolling women and minorities. The history of this relationship allowed for SisterLove's inclusion in the Emory site implementation of the HIV Prevention Trials Network's (HPTN) 064 HIV SeroIncidence Study in Women, also known as ISIS. The ISIS study was a multisite, prospective observational clinical trial designed to estimate incidence rates of HIV infection among women at risk for HIV acquisition in the United States and to determine the feasibility of enrolling and following at-risk women (Eshleman et al., 2012; Hodder et al., 2013).

SisterLove collaborated as a CBPR partner in the ISIS study and supported the study in the following ways:

- Engaging in robust community participation at all stages of development and implementation
- Serving as community representatives on the local protocol team
- Providing community consultation to the national HPTN 064/ISIS research team
- Maintaining an active presence at community events and in day-to-day activities
- Identifying key stakeholders (civic leadership, NGO leadership, etc.)
- Providing community contacts/advocates
- Supporting ongoing community feedback through the local Emory Hope Clinic Community Advisory Board and the HPTN Community Working Group (Vermund et al., 2010)

In appreciation for the successful participation of SisterLove as a key CBPR partner, the Emory research team wrote,

> This work has led to increased minority participation in local research. Through identification of multilevel factors influencing HIV clinical trials participation, and subsequent development and implementation of a culturally tailored intervention to address participation barriers, we have realized significant increases in women and minorities study enrollment. (Woodruff Health Sciences Center, 2012; see box on Hope in Our Soul program)

The future work of this dynamic CBPR relationship will include the implementation of a new clinical trial in which the CBPR model proposed will require more integration of behavioral and clinical research. The model by Lau and colleagues (2011) offers a useful conceptual framework for this approach (Figure 4.2).

Figure 4.2 Conceptual Model for Integrated Behavioral-Clinical Research

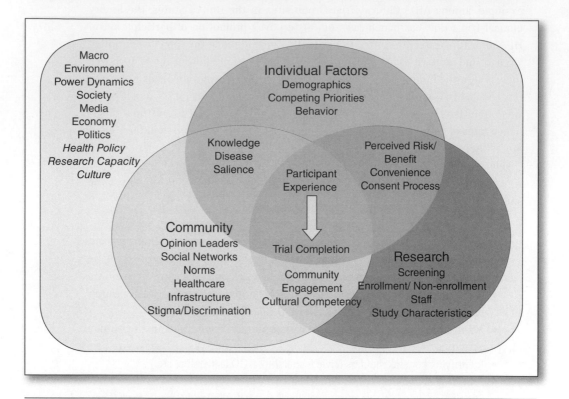

Source: Lau et al. (2011).

CASE STUDY: WHY THERE IS "HOPE IN OUR SOUL"

Given the disparities in HIV/AIDS rates between Blacks and Whites, several faith-based interventions have been developed to address key issues in HIV prevention, to both eliminate health-related disparities and promote healthy sexual behavior (Moss, Gallaread, Siller, & Klausner, 2004; Zahner & Corrado, 2004). Our previous studies highlighted the need to work with faith-based institutions to develop and implement "culture-centered" HIV biomedical prevention research programs in churches to effectively address HIV/AIDS and related health disparities issues (Dutta-Bergman, 2005; Frew et al., 2008). The Black church serves many roles in the community, including but not limited to a bank, a political organization, a party space, a spiritual base, and the center of the community (Pattillo-McCoy, 1998), providing potential to serve as the center for health promotion activities specifically targeting African Americans (Kotecki, 2002). Yet there has been hesitation within the Black church to address issues pertaining to HIV/AIDS for fear of condoning behaviors that are associated with HIV transmission (Griffin, 2006; Harris, 2010). Nonmutually monogamous sexual behavior and homosexual orientation were considered deviant by the Black church. Therefore, Black churches often criticized and condemned these practices, along with premarital sex and alcohol and drug use (Harris, 2010; Higginbotham, 1993). As the face of HIV/AIDS began to change, the Black church's stance on sexuality did not alter. African Americans were increasingly becoming infected with HIV/AIDS and some felt as if the response of the Black church was to ignore the problem (Douglas & Hopson, 2001; Harris, 2010).

Thus, we developed and implemented the Hope in Our Soul and, more recently, Dose of Hope programs with members of the Black church and our Atlanta HIV Biomedical Prevention Research Community Collaborative members. These programs address several barriers to clinical research participation, including trust in the medical community, myths and stigmas related to clinical research, time commitments, and lack of knowledge about clinical trials. Our focus has been to encourage of church leaders and congregants to learn about health disparities affecting the community and the landscape of clinical research issues including ethics in the post-Tuskegee era, to empower discussion about research protections and approaches to address health disparities, and to facilitate message dissemination to others in social networks. In particular, the curricula and related communication strategies encourage message dissemination from the pulpit. We also aimed to increase the proportion of racial and ethnic minorities enrolled in biomedical research studies.

The programs have been successfully implemented with several churches throughout Atlanta. We utilized CBPR approaches in designing the intervention and employed best practice strategies including building trust with the community, hiring community members as lead staff, and delivering cultural competency training to increase the knowledge and skills necessary to work with this special group (Brach & Fraser, 2000).

Formative findings from the Hope in Our Soul program indicate that it reached a wide range of participants in terms of employment, sexual orientation, educational attainment, and household income. Participants indicated greater interest in HIV vaccine research participation; the influences of positive research attitudes (OR = .362, p = .033), the influences of friends and family ("subjective norms"; OR = .211, p = .025), and attention to those persuasive forces ("motivation to comply") were of considerable importance (OR = 3.981, p = .017) in achieving our aims. Thus, we

(Continued)

(Continued)

learned that it was critical not only to cultivate positive attitudes toward research through inclusion of church leaders, including health and wellness ministry staff, but also to continue to engage family, friends, and social networks in the program.

Figure 4.3   Hope in Our Soul CE Conceptual Model

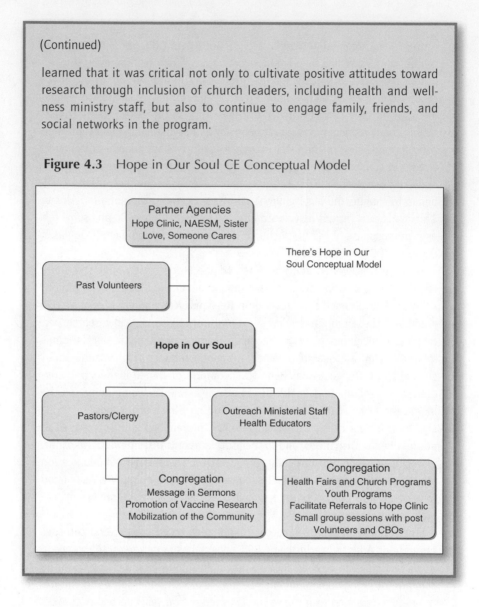

COMMUNITY ENGAGEMENT IN THE GLOBAL CONTEXT

The idea of community engagement as an ethical requirement for research involving human participants, particularly marginalized populations, has made its way into international research ethics guidelines and reports from a variety of organizations around the world (Tindana et al., 2011). Increased efforts by international advocacy groups such as the Global Campaign for Microbicides, AIDS Vaccine Advocacy Coalition, the International Council of AIDS Service Organizations, and others outside of the field of HIV prevention have contributed to the growing body of community stakeholders who are research literate and have the capacity to engage meaningfully with ongoing HIV prevention research trials. The recent development of international guidelines and reports for community engagement practice have provided a collection of standards and expectations (CTSA, 2011; International Council of AIDS Service Organizations, 2007) that could lead to the development of more empirical data regarding the role that community and stakeholder engagement has in collaborative clinical research—data that are currently lacking (Tindana et al., 2011). There is still debate, for example, about how the effectiveness of CE should be conceptualized and measured (Tindana et al., 2011). In their seminal article "Grand Challenges in Global Health: Community Engagement in Research in Developing Countries," Tindana and colleagues (2007) capture stories of two well-documented examples of CE in practice, especially in international collaborative research, presented below.

The CAPRISA Model

The Centre for the AIDS Program of Research in South Africa (CAPRISA) is an AIDS research institute based in Durban, South Africa. CAPRISA has a community program in Vulindlela, about 60 kilometers from Durban. The purpose of the CAPRISA Community Program is to support and facilitate community involvement and informed participation in all CAPRISA projects, starting at protocol development through to data collection. CAPRISA undertakes a host of measureable strategies, including the innovative community research support groups (CRSGs), which are specific bodies aimed at preparing community stakeholders for participation in CAPRISA research projects. Research results are fed back to the community at monthly CRSG meetings in plenary form, and additional focus group discussions are arranged to capture particular issues.

CAPRISA has been in the process of empirically measuring the impact of the many CE initiatives for participant recruitment, retention, and positive feedback. According to the report, prior to CAPRISA, in Vulindlela, the local community had little knowledge of HIV research, and discussion of HIV/AIDS at traditional community gatherings was considered taboo. Open discussion of HIV/AIDS is now common at traditional gatherings, and posters raising awareness of the pandemic are a regular feature. Many community members credit CAPRISA engagement efforts with sensitizing the community to the HIV/AIDS pandemic; helping to reduce the stigma attached to the disease; and enabling relevant, world-class HIV/AIDS research in the region, including the groundbreaking proof of concept ARV-based microbicide trial results of CAPRISA 004 (Abdool Karim et al., 2010; Sokal et al., 2013).

The Navrongo Model

In a northern district of Ghana, the Navrongo Health Research Center initiated a community-based research project to develop, test, and evaluate approaches to rural health service delivery using a combination of strategies. The key stakeholders in this project were community leaders—traditionally known as chiefs—district health authorities, development partners, and researchers. The Center embarked on a series of consultations with the chiefs and residents of the district, who contributed to the design of the project, known as the Navrongo Experiment. This model of following cultural tradition and protocol has been incorporated into a policy known as the Ghana Community-Based Health Planning and Services Initiative. Unique features of the Navrongo model include processes for

- going into the community to meet with community leaders before initiating a research activity;
- gathering chiefs, elders, opinion leaders, and community members, along with researchers, to deliberate on a proposed research agenda; and
- consolidating and communicating community views and concerns.

A publication called *What Works, What Fails* shares the experiences of the Navrongo Experiment. It notes that while community participation is important, translating the concept into practical terms at the local level can be difficult. Significant institutional, economic, social, health, and environmental concerns of community members must be addressed if efforts are to succeed (Navrongo Health Research Centre, 2001).

As these stories model the successes and challenges related to engaging community and stakeholders, it is clear that as community education becomes more widely expected as a feature of ethical international collaborative research, it will become important to identify good community engagement practices and be able to describe in detail how they contribute to community engagement effectiveness (Tindana et al., 2011).

EMERGING TRENDS AND FUTURE DIRECTIONS

Historically, community engagement in HIV and AIDS research began with demands from community activists and has evolved into a comprehensive and integrated component of clinical, behavioral, and social science research. Beginning with the establishment of Community Advisory Boards, which have become a standard of practice in HIV research, the scope of community engagement has expanded to include many defined forms of meaningful involvement with affected communities. Emerging trends in the interest of addressing both communities' and researchers' concerns for ethical clinical and nonclinical research properly include community engagement at every stage of the trial or study, community-based participatory research, campus and community partnerships for research, and community advisory boards and institutional review boards.

Additionally, the burgeoning integration of behavioral and social science with biomedical/clinical research will require that the meaningful integration of affected communities and stakeholders is ensured. This integration is a clear indication of the need to further increase the role, support, and resources for community-based participatory and action research. Increased participation requires a broader and more effective approach to introducing or improving research literacy in communities. CBPR is inclusive of the involvement of individuals as well as community organizations and civil society. Community-based organizations and NGOs need support to increase capacity to design and implement research with institutional and academic partners. (See In Focus on CBPR at the end of this chapter.)

Community engagement in biomedical and public health research is also a proven sustainable pathway to educating and recruiting hard-to-reach, underserved, and historically excluded populations from clinical trials and other nonclinical research. The increased influence of stakeholder and community involvement can have measurable impact in the fields of translation and implementation science, subsequently building the capacity of communities to become critical partners to help identify, strategize, and solve community-level health challenges where they live, work, play, and pray.

There is a significant body of research that justifies, and defends well, the need for community engagement in research, and particularly in HIV trials, but little is published on the measureable impacts of direct involvement of affected communities and stakeholders or on the experience of community engagement in practice (Marsh, Kamuya, Rowa, Gikonyo, & Molyneux, 2008). Establishing and building on an evidence base, documenting the impact of CE on research outcomes, and reporting the utilization of findings, would benefit researchers, public health practitioners, and communities alike.

ADDITIONAL RESOURCES

Aguilar-Gaxiola, S., McCloskey, D. J., & Michener, L. (2012). *Researchers and their communities: The challenge of meaningful community engagement.* Bethesda, MD: National Institutes of Health, National Center for Research Resources. Retrieved from https://www.dtmi.duke.edu/about-us/organization/duke-center-for-community-research/Resources/TheChallengeMeaningful CommunityEngagement-monograph6_30.pdf

Institute of Medicine. (2011). *Exploring challenges, progress and new models for engaging the public in the clinical research enterprise.* Washington, DC: National Academies Press.

Joint United Nations Programme on HIV/AIDS. (2011). *Good participatory practice: Guidelines for biomedical HIV prevention trials.* Geneva, Switzerland: Author.

Leykum, L. K., Pugh, J. A., Lanham, H. J., Harmon, J., & McDaniel, R. R. (2009). Implementation research design: Integrating participatory action research into randomized controlled trials—A debate. *Implementation Science, 4*(69). Retrieved from http://www.implementation-science.com

Mallery, C., Ganachari, D., Fernandez, J., Smeeding, L., Robinson, S., Moon, M., . . . Siegel, J. (2012). *Innovative methods in stakeholder engagement: An environmental scan.* Rockville, MD: Agency for Healthcare Research and Quality. Retrieved from http://www.effectivehealthcare.ahrq .gov/tasks/sites/ehc/assets/File/CF_Innovation-in-Stakeholder-Engagement_Literature Review.pdf

REFERENCES

Abdool Karim, Q., Abdool Karim, S., Frohlich J., Grobler, A., Baxter, C., Mansoor, L., . . . Taylor, D. (2010). Effectiveness and safety of tenofovir gel, an antiretroviral microbicide, for the prevention of HIV infection in women. *Science, 329,* 1168–1174.

Ahmed, S. M., & Palermo, A. G. (2010). Community engagement in research: Frame-works for education and peer review. *American Journal of Public Health, 100,* 1380–1387.

Brach, C., & Fraser, I. (2000). Can cultural competency reduce racial and ethnic health disparities? A review and conceptual model [Review]. *Medical Care Research and Review, 57*(Suppl 1), 181–217.

Bracht, N. (2001). Community partnership strategies in health campaigns. In R. E. Rice & C. K. Atkin (Eds.), *Public communication campaigns* (3rd ed., pp. 323–342). Thousand Oaks, CA: Sage.

Centers for Disease Control and Prevention. (1997). *Principles of community engagement.* Atlanta, GA: Author.

Centers for Disease Control and Prevention. (2012). Estimated HIV incidence in the United States, 2007–2010. *HIV Surveillance Supplemental Report, 17*(4). Retrieved from http://www.cdc.gov/hiv/topics/surveillance/resources/reports/#supplemental

Cohen, J. (2004). AIDS research: Cambodian leader throws novel prevention trial into limbo. *Science, 305,* 1092.

Crotty, M. (2003). *The Foundations of Social Research: Meaning and Perspectives in the Research Process.* London: Sage.

CTSA Community Engagement Key Function Committee Task Force on the Principles of Community Engagement. (2011). *Principles of community engagement* (2nd ed.). Washington, DC: U.S. Department of Health and Human Services. Retrieved from http://www.atsdr.cdc.gov/communityengagement

Dickert, N., & Sugarman, J. (2005). Ethical goals of community consultation in research. *American Journal of Public Health, 95,* 1123–1128.

Douglas, K. B., & Hopson, R. E. (2001). Understanding the Black church: Dynamics of change. *Journal of Religious Thought, 56*(2), 95–13.

Dutta-Bergman, M. J. (2005). Theory and practice in health communication campaigns: A critical interrogation. *Health Communication, 18*(2), 103–122.

Eshleman, S. H., Hughes, J. P., Laeyendecker, O., Wang, J., Brookmeyer, R., Johnson-Lewis, L., . . . Hodder, S. (2012). Use of a multi-faceted approach to analyze HIV incidence in a cohort study of women in the United States: HIV Prevention Trials Network 064 Study. *Journal of Infectious Diseases, 207,* 223–231.

Fawcett, S. B., Paine-Andrews, A., Harris, K. J., Francisco, V. T., Richter, K. P., Lewis, R. K., . . . Schmid, T. L. (1995). *Evaluating community efforts to prevent cardiovascular diseases.* Atlanta, GA: Centers for Disease Control and Prevention, National Center for Chronic Disease Prevention and Health Promotion.

Fleischman, A. R. (2007). Community engagement in urban health research. *Journal of Urban Health, 84,* 469–471..

Frew, P. M., del Rio, C., Clifton, S., Archibald, M., Hormes, J., & Mulligan, M. J. (2008). Factors influencing HIV vaccine community engagement in the urban South. *Journal of Community Health, 33,* 259–269.

Green, L. W., George, M. A., Daniel, M., Frankish, C. J., & Herbert, C. J. (1995). *Study of participatory research in health promotion.* Vancouver: University of British Columbia, Royal Society of Canada.

Green, L. W., & Mercer, S. L. (2001). Can public health researchers and agencies reconcile the push from funding bodies and the pull from communities? *American Journal of Public Health, 91,* 1926–1929.

Griffin, H. (2006). *Their own received them not: African American lesbians and gays in the Black church.* Cleveland, OH: Pilgrim.

Harris, A. (2010). Sex, stigma, and the Holy Ghost: The Black church and the construction of AIDS in New York City. *Journal of African American Studies, 14,* 21–43.

Hatch, J., Moss, N., Saran, A., Presley-Cantrell, L., & Mallory, C. (1993). Community research: Partnerships in Black communities. *American Journal of Preventive Medicine, 16*(3), 27–31.

Higginbotham, E. (1993). *Righteous discontent: The women's movement in the Black Baptist Church, 1880–1920.* Cambridge, MA: Harvard University Press.

Hodder, S. L., Justman, J., Hughes, J. P., Wang, J., Haley, D. F., Adimora, A. A., . . . Women's HIVSeroIncidence Study Team. (2013). HIV acquisition among women from selected areas of the United States: A cohort study. *Annals of Internal Medicine, 158*(1), 10–18.

International Council of AIDS Service Organizations. (2007). *Community involvement in HIV vaccine research:* Making it work. Toronto, Ontario, Canada: Author.

Israel, B. A., Schulz, A. J., Parker, E. A., & Becker, A. B. (1998). Review of community-based research: Assessing partnership approaches to improve public health. *Annual Review of Public Health, 19*, 173–202.

Joint United Nations Programme on HIV/AIDS. (2011). *Good participatory practice: Guidelines for biomedical HIV research trials.* Geneva, Switzerland: Author.

Joint United Nations Programme on HIV/AIDS & World Health Organization. (2007). *Ethical considerations in HIV biomedical prevention trials.* Geneva, Switzerland: UNAIDS.

Kellogg Health Scholars Program. (2003–2013). *Community track.* Retrieved from http://www.kellogghealthscholars.org/about/community.cfm

Killen, J., Harrington, M., & Fauci, A. S. (2012). MSM, AIDS research activism, and HAART. *Lancet, 380*, 314–316.

Kotecki, C. N. (2002). Developing a health promotion program for faith-based communities. *Journal of Holistic Nursing Practice, 16*(3), 61–69.

Lau, C. Y., Swann, E. M., Singh, S., Kafaar, Z., Meissner, H. I., & Stansbury, J. P. (2011). Conceptual framework for behavior and social science in HIV vaccine clinical research. *Vaccine, 29*, 7794–7800.

Leung, M. W., Yen, I. H., & Minkler, M. (2004). Community-based participatory research: A promising approach for increasing epidemiology's relevance in the 21st century. *International Journal of Epidemiology, 33*, 499–506.

MacQueen, K. M., McLellan, E., Metzger, D., Kegeles, S., Strauss, R. P., Scotti, R., . . . Trotter, R. T. (2001). What is community? An evidence-based definition for participatory public health. *American Journal of Public Health, 91*, 1929–1937.

Marsh, V., Kamuya, D., Rowa, Y., Gikonyo, C., & Molyneux, S. (2008). Beginning community engagement at a busy biomedical research programme: Experiences from the KEMRI CGMRC-Wellcome Trust Research Programme, Kilifi, Kenya. *Social Science & Medicine, 67*, 721–733.

Michener, L., Cook, J., Ahmed, S. M., Yonas, M. A., Coyne-Beasley, T., & Aguilar-Gaxiola, S. (2012). Aligning the goals of community-engaged research: Why and how academic health centers can successfully engage with communities to improve health. *Academic Medicine, 87*, 285–291.

Miller, R. L., & Shinn, M. (2005). Learning from communities: Overcoming difficulties in dissemination of prevention and promotion efforts. *American Journal of Community Psychology, 35*(3/4), 169–183.

Minkler, M., & Wallerstein, N. (2008). The growing support for CBPR. In M. Minkler & N. Wallerstein (Eds.), *Community-based participatory research for health: From process to outcomes* (2nd ed., p. 544). San Francisco, CA: Jossey-Bass.

Minnesota Department of Health. (n.d.). *Community engagement.* Retrieved from http://www.health.state.mn.us/strategies/engagement.pdf

Morgan, M. A., & Lifshay, J. (2006). *Community engagement in public health.* Martinez, CA: Contra Costa Department of Health Services, Public Health Division. Retrieved from http://barhii.org/resources/downloads/community_engagement.pdf

Moss, N. J., Gallaread, A., Siller, J., & Klausner, J. D. (2004). "Street medicine": Collaborating with a faith-based organization to screen at-risk youths for sexually transmitted diseases. *American Journal of Public Health, 94*, 1081–1084.

Navrongo Health Research Centre. (2001). *What works, what fails.* Retrieved from http://pdf.usaid.gov/pdf_docs/Pnact200.pdf

Page-Shafer, K., Saphonn, V., Sun, L. P., Vun, M. C., Cooper, D. A., & Kaldor, J. M. (2005). HIV prevention research in a resource-limited setting: The experience of planning a trial in Cambodia. *Lancet, 366*, 1499–1503.

Pattillo-McCoy, M. (1998). Church culture as a strategy of action in the Black community. *American Sociological Review, 63*, 767–784.

Schulz, A. J. Israel, B. A., Coombe, C. M., Gaines, C., Reyes, A. G., Rowe, A., . . . Weir, S. (2011). A community-based participatory planning process and multilevel intervention design: Toward eliminating cardiovascular health inequities. *Health Promotion Practice, 12,* 900–911.

Schulz, A. J., Krieger, J., & Galea, S. (2002). Addressing social determinants of health: Community-based participatory approaches to research and practice. *Health Education and Behavior, 29,* 287–295.

Smith, Y. R., Johnson, A. M., Newman, L. A., Greene, A., Johnson, T. R. B., & Rogers, J. L. (2007). Perceptions of clinical research participation among African American women. *Journal of Women's Health, 16,* 423–505.

Sokal, D. C., Karim, Q. A., Sibeko, S., Yende-Zuma, N., Mansoor, L. E., Baxter, C., . . . Karim, S. S. (2013). Safety of tenofovir gel, a vaginal microbicide, in South African women: Results of the CAPRISA 004 Trial. *Antiviretroviral Therapy, 18,* 301–310.

Strauss, R. P. (1999). Community advisory board–investigator relationships in community-based HIV/AIDS research. In N. M. P. King, G. E. Henderson, & J. Stein (Eds.), Beyond regulations: Ethics in human subjects research (pp. 94–101). Chapel Hill: University of North Carolina Press.

Swartz, L., & Kagee, A. (2006). Community participation in AIDS vaccine trials: Empowerment or science? *Social Science & Medicine, 63,* 1143–1146.

Tindana, P. O., Rozmovits, L., Boulanger, R. F., Bandewar, S. V., Aborigo, R. A., Hodgson, A. V., . . . Lavery, J. V. (2011). Aligning community engagement with traditional authority structures in global health research: A case study from northern Ghana. *American Journal of Public Health, 101,* 1857–1867.

Tindana, P. O., Singh, J. A., Tracy, C. S., Upshur, R. E. G., Daar, A. S., Singer, P. A., . . . Lavery, J. V. (2007). Grand challenges in global health: Community engagement in research in developing countries. *PLoS Medicine, 4*(9), e273.

University of Southern California, Office for the Protection of Research Subjects. (2013). *Frequently asked questions about community-engaged research.* Retrieved from http://oprs.usc.edu/files/2013/01/Frequently_Asked_Questions_about_Community-Engaged_Research.pdf

Vermund, S. H., Hodder, S. L., Justman, J. E., Koblin, B. A., Mastro, T. D., Mayer, K. H., . . . El Sadr, W. M. (2010). Addressing research priorities for prevention of HIV infection in the United States. *Clinical Infectious Disease, 50,* S1490S155.

West, S. G., Duan, N., Pequegnat, W., Gaist, P., Des Jarlais, D. C., Holtgrave, D., . . . Mullen, P. D. (2008). Alternatives to the randomized controlled trial. *American Journal of Public Health, 98,* 1359–1366.

White, G. W., Suchowierska, M., & Campbell, M. (2004). Developing and systematically implementing participatory action research. *Archives of Physical Medicine and Rehabilitation, 85*(Supplement 2), S3–S12.

World Health Organization. (2002). *Community participation in local health and sustainable development: Approaches and techniques.* Geneva, Switzerland: Author.

Woodruff Health Sciences Center. (2012). *HIV rates for black women in parts of U.S., including Atlanta, much higher than previously estimated.* Retrieved from http://news.emory.edu/stories/2012/03/hiv_rates_for_black_women_higher_than_estimated/index.html

Zahner, S. J., & Corrado, S. M. (2004). Local health department partnerships with faith-based organizations. *Journal of Public Health Management Practice, 10,* 258–265.

IN FOCUS

Community-Based Participatory Research
Karen Hacker and Greg Guest

The preceding chapter illustrates the importance of directly engaging with communities during the research process. Community-engaged research exists on a continuum ranging from simply doing research in a community setting to doing research that fully engages community partners. Community-based participatory research (CBPR) represents the latter end of this spectrum. It encourages full participation of community partners in every aspect of the research process. The equitable aspects of the partnership and the participatory nature of the work distinguish CBPR from traditional research approaches.

A CBPR approach is particularly useful for addressing emergent problems and conducting formative research, and as a strategy to engage hard-to-reach populations. Conversely, CBPR is less appropriate for highly controlled study designs, as its participatory nature requires flexibility of process. Israel, Eng, Schulz, and Parker (2005) outline core principles of CBPR (IF Table 1). For a more detailed description, we refer readers to Hacker (2013), the source from which this section was adapted, as well as Wallerstein and Duran (2006).

IF Table 1   Core Principles of CBPR

Community as a unit of identity	Understanding and identifying "the community" for the purposes of CBPR projects is an important first step in the CBPR process. Communities are made up of people linked by social ties who share common perspectives or interests and may also share a geographic location (MacQueen et al., 2001).
Builds on strengths and resources within the community	In CBPR, the community, as represented by its members, is a participant in the process and brings a variety of skill sets that are different than but equally as valuable as academic skills. Corburn (2005) refers to this knowledge as *street knowledge*. The strengths of a given community can be brought to bear to implement solutions once identified. This offers the potential for sustainable change.

(Continued)

(Continued)

Collaborative and equitable partnership across all phases of research	CBPR hinges on the researcher-community partnerships that are formed (Christopher, Watts, McCormick, & Young, 2008). These partnerships are built on mutual respect and trust. Researchers should recognize the inherent inequities that exist between community members and investigators and try to address them via transparency, communication, shared decision making, and appropriate allocation of resources.
Co-learning and capacity building among all partners	One of the outcomes of a CBPR approach is the co-learning that takes place by both community members and researchers. As the investigator learns of the community realities and the meaning of interactions from community members, so too the community members gain competencies in data use, critical thinking, and evaluation.
Balance between knowledge generation and intervention for the benefit of all partners	CBPR is nested in real-world issues and the need for action. Balancing the demands of community action with the needs of research can be challenging. Pacing may differ, analytic methods may clash, and dissemination efforts may conflict. When the CBPR process works best, it can satisfy both needs. Expectations should, therefore, be discussed up front and frequently throughout the process.
Focus on the local relevance, and social determinants of public health problems	The problems explored in CBPR studies are generally of great relevance to the communities involved. As such, CBPR necessarily will involve social determinants as important factors to be considered and explored.
Cyclical and iterative process	CBPR is often perceived as a cyclical process involving numerous phases from question development to data collection and analysis. As with the quality-improvement cycles used in health care improvement and business (Plan Do Study Act), the process often opens the door to new and emerging questions, which in turn requires an investigative process.
Inclusion of all partners in the dissemination of results	Dissemination of findings in CBPR needs to benefit all parties. Yet it often means different things to researchers than it does to community partners, and it may require different formats and venues. In

	addition, the time sequencing may be different. There is usually a more rapid demand for results at the community level than in academic realms. Thus, negotiating types of dissemination and what can be disseminated when is an important element in CBPR work.
Long-term and sustainable process	To fully engage in CBPR, the researcher needs to consider the time involved for specific projects but also to nurture relationships outside of shorter-term projects. In order to establish the trust needed to fully engage in CBPR, a long-term commitment will likely extend beyond the specific project to other worthy projects that partners feel are appropriate. The long-term nature of CBPR needs to be considered up front, as part of the research planning process.

Source: Adapted from Israel et al. (2005).

Steps in the CBPR Process

Step 1: Defining the Community

Community can be defined by geography, by condition, or by other common concerns/characteristics. If you want to work with immigrants, think through the groups that might represent this population and contact them. If you want to work with a geographic community, consider the organizations or institutions that serve the community.

Step 2: Engaging the Community and Assessing Its Needs

After determining your target community, the engagement process can begin. Examine available data on the community. Census data are an excellent source when thinking about geographic populations. Contact the local health department to see what data they might share. Local newspapers are also helpful in learning about local politics and issues. Educate yourself about a community before you engage its members.

To build on the available data, contact leaders of active community groups such as schools, community-based organizations, advocacy groups, religious groups, and service agencies. Meet with stakeholders and find out what they perceive as the challenges in their community. Visit programs. Meet, and informally interview, their staff. These early introductions serve to establish rapport and trust for all future interactions.

A needs assessment is a critical step in developing a CBPR agenda, particularly if the researcher is unfamiliar with the community. The data that a researcher obtains in this engagement process are instrumental for community mapping; that is, they contribute to developing an in-depth understanding of the community's social and political structure, its resources, and the issues that concern its community. Identifying social networks, the local social/political landscape, and existing infrastructure fosters understanding of how things get done, what opportunities there are for change, and who can help sustain change in the future.

COMMUNITY ADVISORY BOARDS

Community advisory boards (CABs) are a fundamental component of community-based participatory research. Their members are representatives of the local community who advise and negotiate with researchers about research activities in their community. CABs help to ensure that research processes and outcomes benefit the community, that community members are part of the analysis and interpretation of data, and have input into the dissemination of results. Some CABs are temporarily created for a particular research project, but many have a more permanent place in the community and may be affiliated with specific community or research institutions. Responsibilities of a CAB vary by context. For a specific project a CAB's role is negotiated between its members and researchers. Much like an IRB (see Chapter 3), the CAB plays a role in protecting the well-being of the community with respect to research activity. However, it is important to note that CABs are not the same as IRBs. They do not have the formal regulatory responsibilities, nor the breadth of coverage, that IRBs possess.

Step 3: Refine the Research Question

Community members are very helpful in identifying the topic of interest but may not have the skills to operationalize the research question. Work with community partners to help refine the research questions. Sharing your knowledge of the literature and the existing evidence base will help in this process. Part of your role is to educate the community about what is already known about the subject from a research perspective, just as the community will educate you about the subject from their perspective.

Step 4: Design and Methods

Once researchers and community members agree on the research question(s), the investigator and community members should work together to determine the most appropriate research strategy. While the investigator is likely to know more about the possible methods for investigation, the community partners know which methods are feasible from a political and logistical standpoint.

Step 5: Roles and Responsibilities

Roles and responsibilities for research conduct, and their budgetary implications, should be delineated in partnership with the community representatives. Transparent communication and establishing a memorandum of agreement (MOA) are useful in this regard. Items typically found in a MOA include the following:

- Description of partners (who are the parties entering into the agreement)
- Dates (beginning and end of project)
- Roles and responsibilities (who will actually do what; what each party agrees to do)
- Scope of work
- Timeline
- Deliverables (what is expected of each partner and by what date)
- Budget (how much, billing procedures)
- Publication rights and authorship
- Use of names of partners
- Data ownership (who owns data and how they can be used)

Step 6: Conduct Research

Successful implementation of the research is largely dependent on how well roles and procedures are defined early on, and on staff training. The involvement of community members in data collection builds research capacity within the community. During the research process, it is important to review progress regularly at community meetings, to deal with unexpected challenges, and to ensure the work gets done according to the protocol.

Step 7: Analysis and Interpretation

Roles in analysis often depend on expertise, time, and interest. For example, analyzing quantitative data using statistical methods is often left to the research team, who has the required technical expertise. However, there may be community members who want to learn more, which presents an ideal opportunity to build local research capacity.

It is also important to recognize and address issues of data ownership. Data ownership should be negotiated up front, as data are the property not only of the researcher but also of the community partners (in some cases a third party, such as a funder, may own the data). Negotiating up front about how data will be used, shared, and stored will mitigate future problems. MOAs can facilitate this process.

Step 8: Dissemination

As a researcher, you are likely to be interested in peer-reviewed journals, while community partners are much more likely to want immediate dissemination so that they can act on the results. Agendas can conflict, and the two dissemination strategies may have different timelines. Open and transparent communication about the dissemination process is, therefore, essential. Collaborative dissemination is cumbersome, but diverse perspectives enrich the final products, make them more relevant to the community, and enhance the likelihood of sustainable outcomes.

Additional Resources

Blumenthal, D., DiClemente R., Braithwaite, R., & Smith, S. (Eds.). (2013). *Community-based participatory health research: Issues, methods, and translation to practice* (2nd ed.). New York, NY: Springer.

Israel, B., Eng, E., Schulz, A., & Parker, E. (Eds.). (2012). *Methods in community-based participatory research for health* (2nd ed.). San Francisco, CA: Jossey-Bass.

Jason, L., & Glenwick, D. (Eds.). (2012). *Methodological approaches to community-based research.* Washington, DC: American Psychological Association.

Minkler, M., & Wallerstein, N. (Eds.). (2008). *Community-based participatory research for health: From process to outcomes* (2nd ed.). San Francisco, CA: Jossey-Bass.

Note

1. This In Focus section is adapted from *Community-Based Participatory Research* (Hacker, 2013). Readers are encouraged to refer to the original source for more detail.

References

Christopher, S., Watts, V., McCormick, A. K., & Young, S. (2008). Building and maintaining trust in a community-based participatory research partnership. *American Journal of Public Health, 98,* 1398–1406.

Corburn, J. (2005). *Street science: Community knowledge and environmental health justice.* Cambridge, MA: MIT Press.

Hacker, K. (2013). *Community-based participatory research.* Thousand Oaks, CA: Sage.

Israel, B., Eng, E., Schulz, A., & Parker, E. (2005). Introduction to methods in community-based participatory research for health. In B. Israel, E. Eng, A. Schulz, & E. Parker (Eds.), *Methods in community-based participatory research for health* (pp. 2–26). San Francisco, CA: Jossey-Bass.

MacQueen, K., McLellan, E., Metzger, D., Kegeles, S., Strauss, R., Scotti, R., . . . Trotter, R. (2001). What is community? An evidence-based definition for participatory public health. *American Journal of Public Health, 91,* 1929–1938.

Wallerstein, N. B., & Duran, B. (2006). Using community-based participatory research to address health disparities. *Health Promotion Practice, 7,* 312–323.

PART II

Traditional Epidemiologic Methods and Designs

5

Public Health Surveillance and Research

From Data to Action

Donna F. Stroup, Stephen B. Thacker[1], and C. Kay Smith

Public health surveillance, from the French *veiller sur*, meaning *to watch over*, is defined as

> the ongoing, systematic collection, analysis, and interpretation of health-related data with the *a priori* purpose of preventing or controlling disease or injury and identifying unusual events of public health importance, followed by the dissemination and use of such information for public health action. (Lee & Thacker, 2011, p. 637)

Surveillance can involve data collection mandated by state and local law, with the intent of prioritizing the needs of society over those of the individual, in order for public health practitioners to proceed without delay to identify and control health risks (Snider & Stroup, 1997). Given its primary function as a tool for monitoring public health, surveillance itself is not a research activity (Council for International Organizations of Medical Sciences, 2009), but as you will see in this and other chapters throughout this book, data arising from public health surveillance activities present multiple opportunities for public health research using a variety of methods.

A BRIEF HISTORY

This core public health function of monitoring health status to identify and solve community health problems began with infectious conditions (see Table 5.1). However, decline in incidence of certain infectious conditions, continuing challenges posed by HIV infection and AIDS, tuberculosis (TB), and malaria, and the "spread" of heart disease, stroke, cancer, diabetes, and mental illness to low-resource countries has led to development of surveillance for a broad spectrum of health conditions (Table 5.2).

Table 5.1 Selected Events in the History of Public Health Surveillance

1662	John Graunt analyzes reports of births and deaths (London).
1680s	Johann Peter Franc performs numerical analyses of mortality data (Germany).
1741	In the United States, tavern keepers are required to report contagious diseases (Rhode Island).
1766	Police take responsibility for community health (Germany).
1788	Leaders of the French Revolution declare the health of the people is the responsibility of the state.
1839	England and Wales initiate mortality reporting.
1849	Sir Edwin Chadwick documents the link between poverty and disease (England).
1859	Lemuel Shattuck develops nomenclature for diseases and causes of death, establishes collection of health data by age, sex, occupation, socioeconomic status, and location (Massachusetts).
1878	The U.S. Congress passes the National Quarantine Act*; this mandate results in the first issue of *The Bulletin of the Public Health*.
1888	Mandatory reporting of 11 communicable diseases is instituted and recorded on death certificates (Italy).
1893	List of causes of death is published by the International Statistical Institute.
	In the U.S., Michigan becomes the first state to require reporting of infectious diseases.

1911	The United Kingdom institutes use of surveillance data from the National Health Insurance program.
1918	50 U.S. cities perform morbidity surveillance for pneumonia and influenza.
1935	The first national health survey is conducted in the United States.
1943	Denmark creates the first registry (for cancer); in the United Kingdom, first sickness survey is conducted.
1955	Active surveillance begins for poliomyelitis in the U.S.
1961	The *Morbidity and Mortality Weekly Report* is moved to the Communicable Disease Center.
1963	Alexander D. Langmuir defines the modern concept of surveillance to include analysis, dissemination, and link to public health action.
1965	The Epidemiological Surveillance Unit in the Division of Communicable Diseases is established at the World Health Organization (WHO) headquarters, Geneva, Switzerland.
1966	WHO's *Communicable Disease Surveillance Reports* begins publication.
1967	The General Practitioner's Sentinel Systems is developed (United Kingdom, Netherlands).
	Global smallpox surveillance begins.
1968	WHO applies communicable disease surveillance to diseases (rather than individuals with disease) and extends surveillance to noninfectious conditions.
1981	Acquired immunodeficiency syndrome surveillance is initiated in the U.S.
1988	All U.S. states begin reporting notifiable diseases electronically to the Centers for Disease Control.
1995	New York City's first syndromic surveillance systems are established to detect outbreaks of waterborne illness.
2001	After the World Trade Center and anthrax attacks, use of syndromic surveillance systems is enhanced with emergency departments, over-the-counter and prescription pharmacy sales, and worker absenteeism.

*Required the Surgeon General of the U.S. Marine-Hospital Service to collect reports on the sanitary condition of vessels departing for the United States and to give notice of these vessels to federal and state officers through weekly abstracts.

Table 5.2 Selected Health Events for Public Health Surveillance

- Mortality
- Communicable diseases
- Noncommunicable diseases
- Birth defects
- Abortions and pregnancy outcomes
- Environmental hazards
- Environmental air and water quality
- Injuries
- Behavioral risk factors
- Health practices
- Animal reservoirs and vector distribution
- Vaccine/drug usage and reactions
- Growth, development, and nutrition
- Occupational safety
- Animal health
- Nosocomial infections
- Mental illness

APPLICATIONS TO PUBLIC HEALTH RESEARCH

Across the areas of public health listed in Table 5.2, surveillance offers the necessary foundation for public health policy, practice, and research by providing both longitudinal and real-time data on which education, programs, and decisions can be based. For example, surveillance data have been crucial in identifying health disparities related to education (Jemal et al., 2008), differential access to health care and treatment (Smedley, Stith, & Nelson, 2003), and social context (Thorpe, Brandon, & LaVeist, 2008) as well as in the incidence of particular diseases, like cancer (see Table 5.3).

Table 5.3 Overall Cancer Incidence and Death Rates per 1,000,000 in the Population, United States, 2000–2004[a]

	All sites	
Racial/ethnic group	Incidence	Death
All	470.1	192.7
African American/Black	504.1	238.8
Asian/Pacific Islander	314.9	115.5
Hispanic/Latino	356.0	129.1
American Indian/Alaska Native	297.6	160.4
White	477.5	190.7

[a]Age-adjusted to 2000 U.S. standard million population.

Source: Centers for Disease Control and Prevention (2013b).

In this chapter, we review the relevance of public health surveillance to public health research by discussing types of research questions that can be answered using surveillance data. We present examples from a range of health conditions and countries, along with selected examples of global research and surveillance activities, and provide practical guidance in using data from surveillance systems for research.

THE CONTRIBUTION OF PUBLIC HEALTH SURVEILLANCE TO RESEARCH

Implementation of randomized controlled trials (ideal for confirmatory research studies) is difficult for public health. Practical and ethical difficulties arise in defining the intervention, implementing random allocation methods, measuring outcomes controlled adequately for confounders, and defining adequate theoretical frameworks (Rychetnik, Frommer, Hawe, & Shiell, 2002; see also Chapter 1). Thus, in public health, researchers turn to data from *secondary sources* for baseline measures (Chapter 9). Secondary sources, in turn, are typically based on data from health surveys that measure health indicators, often at repeated intervals, on a sample from a population (see Chapter 12). Such surveys can be distinguished from those used in surveillance in that they often collect information for wider use (i.e., without a specific surveillance purpose in mind), while surveillance systems that use routine, repeated surveys as their data collection tool ensure that data are analyzed, interpreted, and disseminated *for specific public health action* (Kalsbeek, 2004). A surveillance system concerned with sexual violence, for example, might use data from police records, death certificates, hospitals, and community surveys. Research into concepts and methods for measuring social class and other aspects of socioeconomic position (e.g., income, poverty, deprivation, wealth, education) have informed guidelines for collecting these data in surveillance systems (Krieger, Williams, & Moss, 1997).

The most useful surveillance systems for research have the following characteristics:

- *Established*: Ongoing rather than one-time, and the data have been analyzed so that data collection problems are caught and remedied; data collection methodology is consistent over time
- *Sensitive*: Capture a high proportion of the incidents within a population
- *Specific*: Capture a low proportion of nonincidents (false positives)
- *Generalizable*: Cover a large, easily described general population (e.g., "all women residents of Tunisia") rather than cases in a client database or in only one local institution
- *Informative*: Include enough pertinent data to be of interest (e.g., "crisis call received by police" might not include sufficient information)
- *Available*: Easy to obtain (e.g., website, routine reports)

Many discussions of surveillance have been organized around its uses, listed in Table 5.4 (Thacker, 2010). Below, we present examples from among these uses to illustrate the types of public health research questions that can be addressed using surveillance data.

Table 5.4 Uses of Public Health Surveillance

- ○ Quantitative estimates of magnitude of health problem
- ○ Portrayal of the history of disease
- ○ Generation and testing of hypotheses
- ○ Detection of epidemics
- ○ Documentation of the distribution and spread of a health event
- ○ Facilitation of epidemiologic and laboratory research
- ○ Evaluation of control and prevention measures
- ○ Monitoring of changes in infectious agents
- ○ Monitoring of isolation activities
- ○ Detection of changes in health practice
- ○ Planning of public health actions and use of resources
- ○ Appropriation and allocation of prevention and care resources

Source: Thacker (2010).

Documenting the Magnitude of the Problem

Finding evidence to demonstrate the severity or spread of a particular health problem is a basic step for public health research. For example, body mass index (BMI) is a simple index of weight-for-height used to classify overweight and obesity among adults, defined as excessive fat accumulation that affects health. According to the World Health Organization (WHO), a BMI ≥ 25 is overweight and a BMI ≥ 30 is obesity. Global surveillance data reveal that in 2008, approximately 1.5 billion adults ages ≥ 20 years were overweight, more than 1/10 of the adult population. The numbers are important in relation to the health sequelae of living with a high BMI: 2.8 million adults die each year from being overweight or obese, more than from being underweight (WHO, 2013a). Additionally, such chronic conditions as diabetes, ischemic heart disease, and certain cancers are attributable to overweight and obesity, resulting in high morbidity and mortality. Research designs employing longitudinal analysis of BMI trends can use these public health surveillance data to document changes in and health-related outcomes of overweight and obesity, as a first step toward addressing these health concerns.

Revealing the History of a Disease

Research into the history of a disease (progression in incidence over time) also uses surveillance data. For example, after establishment of the Malaria Control in War Areas Program in 1942 (now the Centers for Disease Control and Prevention), malaria rates decreased until the early 1950s, when infected military personnel returned from Korea. A downward trend continued until the mid-1960s, when malaria increased among veterans of the Vietnam War (Figure 5.1). Research using these surveillance data helped to identify factors that contribute to mortality among U.S. travelers to malarial zones (Greenberg & Lobel, 1990).

Figure 5.1   Malaria Rates by Year, United States, 1930–2010

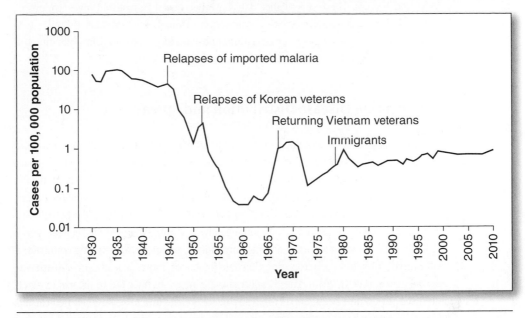

Source: Adapted from Centers for Disease Control and Prevention (2009).

Generating and Testing Research Hypotheses

Surveillance data can also provide solid source material for generating and testing hypotheses as part of the public health research process. For instance, in 2010, Nigerian public health officials observed higher-than-expected numbers of childhood illnesses and deaths in rural northwestern Nigeria, the majority among children under 5 years of age. Although symptoms seemed consistent with malaria, ill children failed to respond to malaria treatment. Because residents of all four villages were involved with gold ore-processing activities, heavy metals were hypothesized to be a potential illness source. To further assess this hypothesis, data from serosurveys, environmental sampling, international surveillance for mortality, and blood lead levels were analyzed longitudinally, and public health officials demonstrated that childhood deaths in these villages were caused by acute lead poisoning. This research, which began with hunches based on surveillance data of child mortality, led to measures to stop the exposure (Dooyema et al., 2012).

Detecting Epidemics

Epidemic detection and prevention—one of the hallmarks of surveillance—offers multiple opportunities for research. Worldwide, foodborne diseases, and more especially diarrheal diseases, are often a cause of morbidity and mortality. In countries with high socioeconomic status, surveillance for foodborne disease is a fundamental component of food safety systems. The U.S. Foodborne Diseases Active Surveillance Network (FoodNet) conducts laboratory-based surveillance for *Campylobacter, Cryptosporidium, Cyclospora, Listeria, Salmonella,* Shiga toxin-producing *Escherichia coli* O157 and non-O157, *Shigella, Vibrio,* and *Yersinia.* These surveillance data have been used in research investigations of outbreaks of disease associated with consumption of unpasteurized dairy products (see Chapter 6 for more on outbreak investigation) and have also been used in evaluating the effectiveness of legislation in disease prevention (Langer et al., 2012).

Documenting Disease Distribution and Spread

Surveillance data have helped track the spread of cancers across the globe, spurring new research as surveillance findings are reported. In part a result of the world's aging population and in part related to the increasing prevalence of smoking in economically developing countries, approximately 12.7 million cancer cases and 7.6 million cancer deaths are estimated to have occurred during 2008 (WHO, 2010). Of these, 56% of the cases and 64% of the deaths occurred in the economically developing world. Breast cancer is now the leading cause of cancer death among women in economically developing countries, a shift from the previous decade, during which the most common cause of cancer death was cervical cancer (WHO, 2010). These cancer surveillance data have led to diverse research initiatives: review and evaluation of tobacco control policies and programs, biomedical and behavioral research on vaccination (for viral agents associated with liver and cervical cancers), early detection and treatment, and evaluation of the effectiveness of campaigns promoting physical activity and healthier diet (Jemal et al., 2011).

Epidemiologic and Laboratory Research

For approximately 60 years, the WHO Global Influenza Surveillance Network has worked to reduce the threat posed by influenza. During 2009, the network responded to an H1N1 pandemic. This surveillance activity has led to basic and applied epidemiologic and laboratory research to build the evidence base for improved influenza prevention, diagnosis, and treatment. For example, research into antiviral susceptibility monitoring and gene sequencing has led to increased laboratory capacity (Stöhr, 2003). This was further demonstrated when laboratory research into the emerging influenza strain (H7N9) in China in early 2013 revealed that the new strain is resistant to the antiviral treatment that had been effective against previous influenza strains (Hirschler, 2013).

Evaluation Research

In the current public health environment, evidence—often in the form of health outcomes—dominates decision making at all levels. As mentioned in some of the previous examples, surveillance data are commonly used in evaluation research because they provide consistent, longitudinal data for a general population. In South Africa, for instance, surveillance data were used to assess efforts to prevent mother-to-child (MTC) HIV transmission (Goga et al., 2011). In 2002, South Africa began a national prevention program to prevent MTC HIV transmission through comprehensive antenatal HIV testing and provision of antiretroviral prophylaxis or treatment for mothers and infants. Nine years later, South Africa's MTC HIV transmission rate had declined from an estimated 25% to < 4% at 4–8 weeks after birth. This dramatic reduction was a measure of the success of the MTC prevention program; however, related research has revealed that voluntary counseling and testing for HIV are underused, and more applied social and behavioral research is needed to improve knowledge about how couples in sub-Saharan Africa deal with the risks for HIV infection (Painter, 2001).

Surveillance data were also used to evaluate the effectiveness of isolation activities for Ebola in Africa (Figure 5.2). Research analyzing mortality data by onset time enabled the implementation of case isolation in a timely manner and revealed differences in the epidemiology of the virus in rural and urban settings. The surveillance data revealed that during epidemics in rural settings, multiple introductions of the virus into the human population occurred through contact with wildlife, but in urban settings, a single introduction of the virus in the community was responsible for the epidemic. The investigators concluded that "active surveillance is key to containing outbreaks of Ebola and Marburg viruses" (Allaranga et al., 2010, p. 37).

Figure 5.2 Ebola Surveillance, Kikwit, Zaire; Distribution of Cases by Date of Onset of Symptoms and by Professional Status, 1995

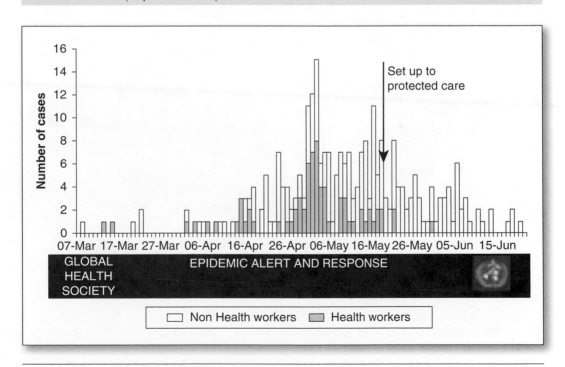

Source: Allaranga, Y., Kone, M. L., Formenty, P.,Libama, F., Boumandouki, P., Woodfill, C. J., Sow, I., Duale, S., Alemu,W.,& Yada, A. (2010). Lessons learned during active epidemiological surveillance of Ebola and Marburg viral hemorrhagic fever epidemics in Africa. *East African Journal of Public Health, 7,* 32–36.

Research on Changes in Infectious Agents

Reduction in TB incidence has been challenged by the emergence of multidrug-resistant (MDR) and extensively drug-resistant (XDR) forms of the bacteria. Data from the Global Drug Resistance Surveillance Project indicate that changes are occurring in this infectious agent (Figure 5.3; WHO, 2007). These data serve as the basis for a multitude of research questions, for epidemiologists, laboratory scientists, and social scientists alike. How and where are MDR and XDR forms of TB spreading most quickly? What are the genetic foundations of changes in the bacteria? What are the most effective TB infection prevention interventions, and how can we best communicate or implement them? Each requires different research methodology, but all begin with trends identified or hypotheses generated through review of surveillance data.

Figure 5.3   Global Surveillance for Drug-Resistant Tuberculosis

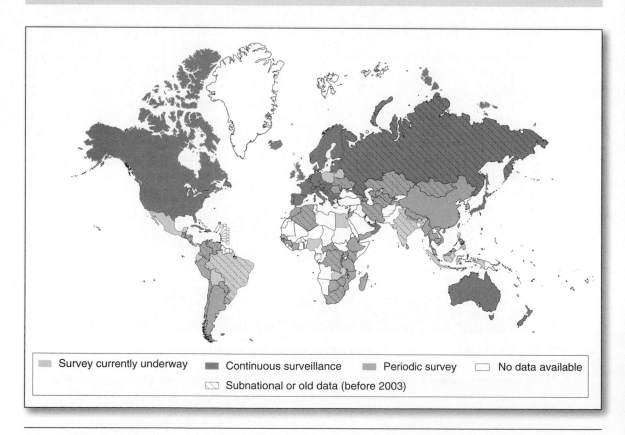

Survey currently underway   Continuous surveillance   Periodic survey   No data available

Subnational or old data (before 2003)

Source: WHO (2007).

Health Practice Research

Surveillance can aid in determining when changes in health practices warrant research activities. Health practices include protective behaviors, like going for a mammogram or using a seat belt, or risk behaviors, like having unprotected sex or smoking cigarettes. Where documenting these types of practices by using surveillance is possible, the data can indicate the effects on health. For example, two communities in Tanzania experienced extremely high malaria transmission during the 1990s. By 2001–2003, after high usage rates (75% of all age groups) of noninsecticide-treated bed nets, a 4.2-fold reduction in malaria transmission was observed (Russell et al., 2010). Because data were readily available regarding high bed net usage among that population, malaria control programs were able to transition easily to insecticide-treated bed nets for even greater protection against the disease vector.

Policy Research

Research using surveillance data can also be used to develop policy strategy, draft legislation, evaluate proposed legislation, or monitor program progress. For example, we know that folic acid use before pregnancy confers a decreased risk for neural tube defects; however, 20%–50% of pregnancies are unplanned (Burris & Werler, 2011). The research question was whether medical providers should recommend folic acid or folic acid–containing multivitamins for their nonpregnant female patients of childbearing age. To address the question, researchers used a cross-sectional study design and surveillance data from CDC's National Ambulatory Medical Care Survey and National Hospital Ambulatory Medical Care Survey. The research revealed that provider-ordered folic acid/multivitamins were most common for women ages 30–34 years, but were differentially offered to women who receive Medicaid and whose race/ethnicity was other than White, Black, or Hispanic. The researchers concluded that while preventive care visits are an important venue for counseling regarding the benefits of folic acid for women of childbearing age, they appear to be underused for certain women (Burris & Werler, 2011). These findings could then be used to suggest a policy for health practitioners to follow with women of childbearing age.

In another example, we see how global surveillance for polio had direct utility for resource allocation. The majority of countries in Europe and North America effectively eliminated endemic transmission of wild poliovirus within a few years after introduction of *inactivated poliovirus vaccine* (IPV) in 1955. Striking results from well-organized national vaccination days in Central America resulted in the 1985 regional polio eradication initiative in the Americas. Surveillance data–based research regarding the effectiveness of these initiatives prompted the World Health Assembly to adopt a resolution in 1988 to eradicate polio worldwide by 2000, by allocating resources to reduce the disease burden in low-resource countries through assistance provided by WHO, the United Nations International Children's Emergency Fund, Rotary International, and CDC (Cochi & Kew, 2008). Policy research can also address collaboration among government agencies like these, which is necessary to translate findings from surveillance and monitoring into responses to urgent threats (Mitka, 2010).

PRACTICAL GUIDANCE FOR PUBLIC HEALTH SURVEILLANCE

The previous examples demonstrate how effective public health research depends on high-quality surveillance systems and the data they produce. In this section, we discuss the pieces and types of surveillance systems, how to work with data from an existing system, and how to evaluate the quality of data generated, so that you might employ surveillance data in your own projects.

Getting to Know a Surveillance System

To effectively use a surveillance system for research purposes, you will need a working understanding of the specifics of the system. Any effectual surveillance system should have a clear statement of purpose and use. Determine which health events are under surveillance and when and how these events are tracked, and then proceed to identify the data sources and type of surveillance reporting used.

Data Source

Case definition. The utility of surveillance data for research is dependent on aspects of the case definition. Case definitions include four components: clinical information about the disease (e.g., fever, diarrhea, intestinal cramps), characteristics about the persons who are affected (e.g., age and sex of ill persons), information about the location or place where the exposure occurred (e.g., meal eaten at the company picnic), and specification of time during which the illness onset occurred and the length of time the symptoms lasted (e.g., diarrhea within 24–48 hours after eating potato salad at the picnic and lasting for 3 days). An example can be seen in the worldwide outbreak of severe acute respiratory syndrome (SARS) in mainland China, Hong Kong, Taiwan, Singapore, Vietnam, Canada, and eventually 32 countries or regions. The first case with typical symptoms of SARS emerged in Guangdong Province, China, with the onset date of November 16, 2002. Subsequently, a case definition for "atypical infectious pneumonia," later termed SARS, was developed and modified during the course of the SARS epidemic (Table 5.5).

System Types

In a *passive surveillance* system, data are collected from all potential providers but without solicitation from individual providers (London School of Hygiene and Tropical Medicine, 2009). Consequently, system developers are dependent on data providers (usually physicians, laboratories, and other health care providers) for reporting, and the data provided are usually minimal. Sometimes the providers are required by law to produce the information, as in the Notifiable Diseases Surveillance System in the United States (Doyle, Glynn, & Groseclose, 2002) or for quarantinable diseases globally (Baker & Fidler, 2006). In contrast, *active surveillance* involves searching for cases, often with staff contacting providers directly. Use of data from passive surveillance systems for research is influenced by consideration of completeness and data quality.

Table 5.5   Case Definition for SARS in China, 2002–2003*

	First period	*Second period*	*Third period*
Date	November 16, 2002–April 20, 2003	April 20–May 1, 2003	After May 1, 2003
Probable case	[2 + 3 + 4 +5] or [1.1 + 2 + 3 + 4]	[1.2 + 2 + 3 + 4] or [1.1 + 2 + 4] or [1.2 + 2 + 4 + 5]	[1.2 + 2 + 3 + 4] or [1.1 + 2 + 4] or [1.2 + 2 + 4 + 5]
Suspected case	[2 + 3 + 4] or [1 + 2 + 3]	[2 + 3 + 4] or [1.1 + 2 + 3] or [1.2 + 2 + 4]	[2 + 3 + 4] or [1.1 + 2 + 3] or [1.2 + 2 + 4]
Under medical observation	N/A	[1.2 + 2 + 3]	[1.2 + 2 + 3]
Confirmed case	N/A	N/A	Based on laboratory findings for SARS-CoV probable SARS case and with positive on one or more of 6.1, 6.2, or 6.3

Source: Adapted from Feng et al. (2009).

CoV = coronavirus; N/A = not applicable; SARS = severe acute respiratory syndrome.

* The numbers in the table cells correspond to the criteria listed below. For example, to be classified as a probable case occurring during the first period, criteria 2, 3, 4, and 5 or 1.1, 2, 3, and 4 had to have been met.

1. Epidemiological history
    1.1 Having close contact with a patient or being a member of an infected cluster, or having infected other persons.
    1.2 Having visited or resided in a city or area where SARS cases were reported with secondary transmission during 2 weeks before onset of symptoms.

2. Symptoms and signs of febrile respiratory illness (i.e., fever $\geq 38°C$, cough, difficulty with breathing, shortness of breath).

3. White blood cell count in peripheral blood is not increased, some decreased (leukocyte count $\leq 10.0 \times 10^9/L$).

4. Radiograph of chest with abnormalities (evidence of infiltrates consistent with pneumonia or respiratory distress syndrome on chest radiograph).

5. Antibiotic treatment is ineffective (within 72 hours).

6. A person with positive laboratory findings for SARS-CoV based on one or more of the following diagnostic criteria:
    6.1 Polymerase chain reaction (PCR) positive; at least two different clinical specimens (e.g., nasopharyngeal, stool) or the same clinical specimen collected on two or more occasions during the course of the illness.
    6.2 Seroconversion by enzyme-linked immunosorbent assay or indirect fluorescent antibody (negative antibody test on acute serum followed by positive antibody test on convalescent phase serum tested in parallel or fourfold or greater increase in antibody titer between acute and convalescent phase sera tested in parallel).
    6.3 Virus isolation (isolation in cell culture of SARS).

Sentinel surveillance relies on agreement from a sample of reporting sources to report all or a sample of conditions. Reporting sources tend to have an interest in the condition under surveillance; therefore, data might not be widely generalizable and might not provide specificity about etiology. However, these can give earlier information at lower cost. In a context of low resources, inadequate health facilities, superstitions that discourage reporting, suppression of reporting, and inadequate diagnostic techniques, a Japanese nongovernmental organization developed a sentinel surveillance system for selected infectious diseases, involving a network of experts and managers (Figure 5.4). Data from the system enabled time-series research in acute flaccid paralysis and prevalence of HIV, syphilis, hepatitis B, and hepatitis C (Arita et al., 2004). Research on the usefulness of sentinel surveillance during the 2009 influenza pandemic supported the vaccination of groups at high risk (Donaldson et al., 2009).

Syndromic surveillance has been defined as "an investigational approach where health department staff, assisted by automated data acquisition and generation of statistical alerts, monitor disease indicators in real-time or near real-time to detect outbreaks of disease earlier than would otherwise be possible with traditional surveillance" (CDC, 2004, p. 2). These systems rely on near real-time automated data collection and analysis from multiple information sources, including general practitioners,

Figure 5.4 Alumni for Global Disease Surveillance Network, 2003

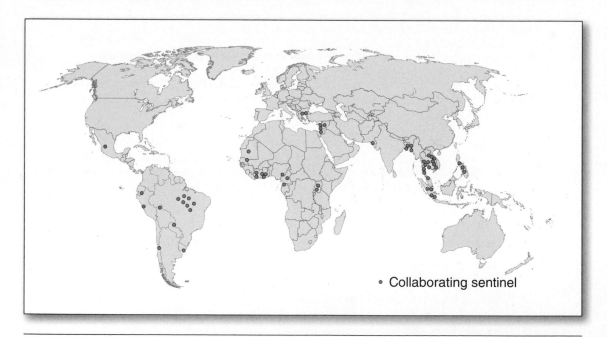

• Collaborating sentinel

Source: Reprinted from *The Lancet,* Vol. 4, Arita, I., Nakane, M., Kojima, K., Yoshihara, N., Nakano, T., & El-Gohary, A. (2004). Role of a sentinel surveillance system in the context of global surveillance of infectious diseases, 171–177. Copyright 2004, with permission from Elsevier.

emergency departments, pharmacy sales, telephone helplines, Internet queries, and veterinary clinics (Soler et al., 2011). Data can be used to monitor spread and impact, or absence of impact, of known or unknown events on the basis of signs and symptoms (Soler et al., 2011). Syndromic surveillance has proven utility for research in cardiovascular morbidity (Mathes, Ito, & Matte, 2011) and for influenza-like illness (Chan, Tamblyn, Charland, & Buckeridge, 2011), but has limitations for hospital infections (Carnevale et al., 2011).

Using Data From a Surveillance System

Legal and Ethical Concerns

Although increasing availability of surveillance data offers multiple opportunities for public health research, the end of the 20th century brought concerns highlighting ethics (Levine, 1996). Data sharing is generally accepted as important for full data utility (Quigg, Hughes, & Bellis, 2012); however, any use of public health surveillance data for research requires a consideration of any laws or ethical imperatives affecting the data collection (Neslund, Goodman, Hodge, & Middaugh, 2010). Even when data are collected under authority of some law, these laws might vary from one location to another, and ensuring data security and confidentiality is imperative. Surveillance data might be personal or stigmatizing, associated with identifiers, and allow direct or indirect identification of individuals. Model legislation developed in the 1990s includes specific actions to ensure confidentiality of public health data (Lawlor & Stone, 2001). When surveillance data are used to generate or test research hypotheses, research ethics, including institutional review board regulations, must be considered (Gitau-Mburu, 2008), including whether ethical principles of informed consent might apply to surveillance and potentially limit data collection and use (see Chapter 3 for more on research ethics).

Analysis

As with any analysis, the statistical analysis plan for research using surveillance data should be specific. For the majority of conditions, an analysis of crude numbers of cases and rates precedes a description of the group in which the condition occurs (person), where the condition occurs (place), and over what period (time). For instance, a plot of cases of influenza across time or by selected personal characteristics should precede a more technical analysis of trends or multivariable modeling. Analytic strategies for working with surveillance data range from simple to complex (see Chapter 19), particularly as new tools and increased computer capacity become available (Table 5.6). Scholarship is also available to guide your choice of analytic methods when using surveillance data for specific purposes, such as the following:

- detecting departures from expected patterns (Stroup, Williamson, Herndon, & Karon, 1989)
- detecting clusters of health events (Lawson & Kleinman, 2005)

- modeling trends (Box, Jenkins, & Reinsel, 2008; Holford, 2004)
- modeling spatial-temporal patterns (Devine, 2003; Waller, 2004)
- linking exposures and hazards to health outcomes (Mather et al., 2004)
- modeling incubation period (Brookmeyer, 2004; Hallett et al., 2008)
- incorporating geographic information systems (Tsui, Wong, Jiang, & Lin, 2011; Wertheim, Horby, & Woodall, 2012)

Table 5.6 Types of Surveillance Systems and Associated Analysis Types and Methods

Data collection design	Analysis purpose[a]	Statistical methods	Examples from literature
Case surveillance	Case counts/ rates (D)	Rates, standardized rates	Number of cases of poliomyelitis by country; age standardized rates of violent deaths by country
	Trend (I)	Time series, regression analysis, Poisson regression	Trends in HIV among MSM, UNAIDS regions
Syndromic surveillance	Geographic clustering (I,O)	Mapping and GIS, comparison observed-to-expected, cluster methods (e.g., scan statistic)	
	Temporal clustering (I,O)		
Behavioral surveillance	Prevalence of behaviors (D)	Weighted analysis related to survey design	
	Trends in behaviors (I)	Rates, linear or logistic analysis, polynomial regression	
Clinical outcomes	Rates (D)		
	Associated factors (I)	Survival analysis	

Source: Adapted from Sullivan, McKenna, Waller, Williamson, and Lee (2010).

D = descriptive; GIS = geographic information system; I = inferential; MSM = men who have sex with men; O = other; UNAIDS = Joint United Nations Programme on HIV/AIDS.

[a] Commission decision of July 12, 2003, amending Decision 2000/96/EC as regards the operation of dedicated surveillance networks.

Regardless of system design and analysis strategy, some general guidance about analysis of surveillance data applies. First, as is true of any secondary data set (see Chapter 9), taking the time to get to know the data before undertaking the analysis will save you time later. You might want to know whether certain sources or study periods are known for poor-quality reporting, whether some cases might be delayed because of diagnosis or resource constraints, or whether the surveillance system might be affected by increased public or political awareness of the condition.

Second, review your statistical analysis plan (developed in research planning) and begin with the simplest of analyses. Compare your planned analyses against the purpose of the system: Do your research questions match that purpose?

Third, assess whether more sophisticated analyses of the data are possible. Often, data quality will preclude complex analytic techniques. Moreover, your purpose might not require additional analyses.

Fourth, if more sophisticated statistical analyses are warranted, ensure that the data can support them. Verify any assumptions used within in the system, and tailor your analysis to take these into account. For example, if a weighted design was used for data collection, your analysis should reflect the use of sampling weights.

Fifth, surveillance data should be analyzed and interpreted at the level closest to the source generating the data. Local events might go unnoticed in a national data analysis.

Finally, plan how to disseminate results of your analysis to partners, collaborators, and those who are included in the surveillance system. Dissemination is critical to ongoing data quality and system utility.

Interpretation and Dissemination

After analysis is complete, your job is to interpret the results for the intended audience. Traditionally, surveillance results have been disseminated through written reports (e.g., *WHO Bulletin*, CDC's *Morbidity and Mortality Weekly Report*, peer-reviewed publications). In dissemination of research results from surveillance, consider extending authorship status to the data providers; in some cases, this might be a condition of data sharing. Even if not required, data acquisition and provision is a commonly accepted criterion for authorship, and at the least, research reports should be shared with surveillance providers for review and comment.

Beyond data providers, other audiences should be considered in your dissemination plans. Suppose, for example, that you have completed an analysis of behavioral surveillance data on sexual health risk among adolescents in South Africa. Your data demonstrate an increase in the number of persons ages 13–17 years who report engaging in sexual activity, not using a condom at each sexual encounter, and having insufficient knowledge of HIV prevention facts. Think about how you would interpret these results for three different audiences: (a) parents in the community, (b) physicians in this area, and (c) students in the local secondary school. This exercise might bring you to certain realizations. First, the details of statistical analyses previously discussed are of no interest (probably) to any of these audiences. (However, if you publish in a peer-reviewed journal to give validation to your findings, these will be of interest.) Second, the focus of the dissemination must be tailored to each audience. Public health research on the topic of surveillance dissemination has looked at communication, behavior, and informatics (Dixon, 2008). This research has revealed that effectiveness of dissemination campaigns is enhanced when combined with prevention strategies (e.g., education, enforcement of existing laws).

GLOBAL PUBLIC HEALTH RESEARCH AND SURVEILLANCE

Global Guidelines

We know that microorganisms do not respect political borders, nor do noncommunicable diseases for that matter. WHO's International Health Regulations (IHR) evolved from efforts to respond to the threat of the international spread of epidemics. Until 2005, IHR focused primarily on quarantinable diseases—cholera, plague, and yellow fever—as well as sanitary measures for seaports and airports. Revised in 2005, the new IHR acknowledges that antibiotic resistance might constitute "a public health emergency of international concern" and also includes events that might originate deliberately or that might involve chemical, radiologic, or infectious disease agents (Plotkin, Hardiman, González-Martin, & Rodier, 2007).

WHO develops guidelines for surveillance by member countries for a wide range of conditions for data comparability. For example, for chronic diseases, the WHO STEPwise approach to surveillance is a standardized method for collecting, analyzing, and disseminating data to facilitate monitoring within-country trends and comparisons across countries. The approach, recommending collection of a limited amount of useful information regularly, is being implemented for risk factor surveillance and for stroke (WHO, 2013c). Similar guidelines have been developed for malaria, cholera, meningococcal meningitis, influenza, HIV, foodborne infections, tuberculosis, polio, tropical diseases, child health and nutrition, school-based health, injury, and immunization (WHO, 2013b). For global surveillance of dengue fever and dengue hemorrhagic fever, WHO created DengueNet in partnership with WHO regional and country offices, ministries of health, WHO collaborating centers, and laboratories (WHO, 2003–2007).

Use of these guidelines for surveillance contributes to public health research by ensuring that data from different countries can be compared. For example, data from DengueNet has been used to develop global research priorities for

- diagnostics (methods for early specific detection of antibody, antigen, and RNA),
- treatment (antivirals and antimediators),
- pathogenesis (mechanism of immune enhancement, neutralization escape, T-cell responses, viral virulence determinants by serotype/genotype, molecular basis of viral interference, and mediators of plasma leakage/altered hemostasis),
- dengue vaccines,
- vector control (vector biology and modeling of dengue transmission), and
- evaluation (including cost-effectiveness) of novel mosquito control methods.

One analysis of the status of surveillance activities in WHO member countries and neighboring regions reported that, although territorial systems of surveillance are weak, threat of cross-border spread of infectious disease (particularly avian influenza) has lowered political barriers to international data collection (McKee & Atun, 2006). Indeed, recent SARS outbreaks and the influenza A (H1N1) pandemic provide evidence of the benefits of global surveillance (Castillo-Salgado, 2010).

Examples of Surveillance and Research in a Global Context

We present two examples of global surveillance development to demonstrate the importance of public health surveillance to research.

Western Europe

In many European countries, diseases of public health significance are selected for surveillance at the national level, although regional adaptations are possible. Although control measures are primarily country responsibilities, European Union (EU) data are beneficial for general trends and monitoring of EU regulations. In 1998, the European Parliament and European Council established a network for surveillance and control of communicable diseases in all EU countries (27 member states as of January 2007; *Decision No 2119/98/EC*, 1998), leading to an Early Warning and Response System for prevention and control of communicable diseases in Europe. The list of reportable conditions includes 44 diseases and two additional health concerns (antimicrobial resistance and nosocomial infections; *Commission Decision,* 1999). To coordinate the surveillance, 17 dedicated surveillance networks have been established (Ammon & de Valk, 2007).

These networks have been useful in responses to problems that cross country borders, particularly in outbreak investigation (see Chapter 6). In 2001, consumption of contaminated chocolate from Germany resulted in an outbreak of *Salmonella* serotype Oranienburg in Germany, Austria, Belgium, Denmark, Finland, the Netherlands, and Sweden. Data sharing through this network resulted in prompt action so that the chocolate was removed from shelves in Canada before cases occurred there (Werber et al., 2005). Utility of this system depends on standardization of variables collected, frequent evaluation of data quality, development of data format and transfer protocol that is compatible, rapid and useful feedback (including easy access to the entire database), and standard operating procedures and memoranda of understanding to ensure collaboration.

Asia

India is the second-most populous country in the world, with more than 1.2 billion people. Before 1997, poliomyelitis surveillance in India involved passive reporting. Widespread transmission of wild poliovirus types 1 and 3 persisted throughout the country, while type 2 was reported in only two provinces (Banerjee et al., 2000).

In 1999, the number of vaccination rounds was increased. In 2005, monovalent OPV1 and later monovalent OPV3 were introduced, and in 2007, the number of vaccination rounds in endemic areas was increased to a round every month. Still, polio incidence increased. Research based on these surveillance data indicated that the vaccine failure was attributable to multiple factors (Paul, 2009):

- environmental (inadequate sanitation)
- high birth rate, increasing number of susceptible people
- infrastructure (lack of health workers and facilities)
- social factors (religious groups electing not to vaccinate)
- vaccine failure (in vaccine or in host)

Further research led to the recommendation to switch to monovalent vaccine (Grassly et al., 2006). Support from the Global Polio Eradication Initiative (www.polio-eradication.org/Research.aspx) enabled research on

- evaluation and development of bivalent OPV,
- evaluation and implementation of the short-interval additional dose strategy,
- social mobilization strategies,
- vaccine efficacy,
- seroconversion, and
- mathematical modeling and to determine areas at risk for outbreaks after reinfection.

As a result of these surveillance and research activities, WHO has officially added India to the list of countries considered to have interrupted the transmission of polio. India has not had a case of polio since January 13, 2011, and no recent environmental samples have identified wild poliovirus ("India: Country Marks Year Without Polio," 2012).

CHALLENGES TO RESEARCH USING SURVEILLANCE DATA

Bioterrorism and Disaster Preparedness

In 1999, the United States developed guidance for the most serious threats of bioterrorism (CDC, n.d.) as measured by high mortality, major public health impact or social disruption, ease of agent dissemination, and medical treatment difficultly. The laws for reportable diseases include requirements to report unusual cases of disease or suspicious clusters. However, because legal authority for public health reporting rests with states, health departments must develop data-sharing protocols with other states and agencies (e.g., with agencies involved with law enforcement because of variation in state laws).

A major challenge to using surveillance for research is that initial symptoms might be nonspecific. During anthrax bioterrorism events of 2001, a physician treated a case of cutaneous anthrax for weeks before reporting it to health authorities (Bresnitz & Ziskin, 2004). Thus, health departments have a responsibility to train physicians and remove any barriers to reporting.

A second challenge is that cases might appear outside the clinician's office (e.g., at laboratories, in medical examiners' or coroners' offices). Nontraditional sources of information are needed (e.g., pharmacy sales, data from poison control centers, environmental monitoring, information from veterinary laboratories, data from law enforcement). Further, syndromic surveillance, discussed earlier, can contribute to bioterrorism preparedness (Stoto, 2008), although its utility is controversial (Reingold, 2003). The challenges of bioterrorism apply to surveillance in the context of natural or other types of human-made disasters as well. Surveillance-based research during and after any disaster can help strengthen public health and relief agency preparedness, but only if those surveillance data are reliable.

Electronic Developments

The Internet offers unprecedented opportunities for public health research, streamlining data entry and reporting and facilitating data access. In the United States, widespread use of computers to facilitate infectious disease surveillance activities began in 1988, when all states and U.S. territories began to use the National Electronic Telecommunication System for Surveillance, now the National Electronic Disease Surveillance System. A study reported that nearly all of a random sample of state health departments' Internet sites during 2005–2006 reported at least simple counts of selected reportable conditions; however, fewer than half of the sites reported recent antibiotic susceptibility data or information regarding a recent outbreak (M'ikanatha, Rohn, Welliver, McAdams, & Julian, 2007).

In addition to data entry and transmission, computer technologies offer opportunities for data access and analysis for research. The American Recovery and Reinvestment Act and the Health Information Technology for Economic and Clinical Health Act (both enacted in 2009) have given prominence to electronic health records and electronic medical records and offer opportunities for surveillance and research, particularly data mining (Hristidis, Varadarajan, Biondich, & Weiner, 2010). Full utility of these data for adding to knowledge and improving population health will depend on commitment to data sharing for research (Walport & Brest, 2011). A health information exchange (HIE) can facilitate secure access, use, and control of health information (American Health Information Management Association, 2012), though the establishment and implementation of these exchanges are still ongoing.

Another new development that affects surveillance is cloud technology. This mode of storing and working on data remotely enables software functions to move from the individual's local hardware to a central server that operates from a remote location (Pareek & Gautam, 2011) and can result in lower costs and greater transparency. BioSense, a U.S. surveillance initiative mandated in the Public Health Security and Bioterrorism Preparedness and Response Act of 2002 (CDC, 2013a) is a nationwide syndromic surveillance system for early detection and assessment of potential bioterrorism-related illness. It uses multiple sources (food supply, environmental data, and public health surveillance) and cloud technology to remove the need to manage physical storage.

Concerns have been raised about data security when using cloud and other electronic technology. Privacy laws for protection of patient confidentiality are complex and can be different for electronic records (Klein, 2011). An international standard (Myler & Broadbent, 2006) addresses data security and states that all stored information should have a designated owner whose responsibility it is to control access and protect confidentiality. Properly protected, the electronic availability of surveillance data offers new opportunities for research (see Table 5.7).

Table 5.7 Selected Public Health Surveillance Data Available for Research

System	Description	Data access	Research application
HIV/AIDS public use data set	Counts of AIDS cases reported during 1981–2002, by demographics; location; case-definition; month/year, and quarter-year of diagnosis, report, and death (if applicable); and HIV exposure group (risk factors for AIDS)	http://wonder.cdc.gov/AIDSPublic.html	AIDS and older Americans at the end of the twentieth century (Mack & Ory, 2003)
Cancer Incidence: Surveillance, Epidemiology, and End Results (SEER) registries	Cancer incidence data with associated population data; geographic areas available are county and SEER registry	http://seer.cancer.gov/index.html	Trends in racial and age disparities in definitive local therapy of early-stage breast cancer (Freedman, He, Winer, & Keating, 2009)
Global tobacco use prevalence	Prevalence of tobacco use throughout the world	www.who.int/gho/database/en	Patterns of global tobacco use in young people and implications for future chronic disease burden in adults (Warren, Jones, Erickson, & Asma, 2006)
Global obesity and overweight	BMI ≥ 25, by country	http://apps.who.int/ghodata	Overweight and obesity worldwide now estimated to involve 1.7 billion people (Deitel, 2003)

As public health takes advantage of electronic technology, it must not miss the groups of people who lack computer access or who rely on mobile technology. For example, in a 2006 Pew study, only 5.8% of Hispanic households reported having searched for health information online, compared with 79.7% of White non-Hispanic respondents (Rice, 2006). In addition, Blacks and Hispanics are more likely than Whites to have smartphones, but many government sites still do not perform well on mobile devices (Yelton, 2012).

Behavioral Surveillance

The role of behaviors in health and health care are well documented within public health, for both chronic and infectious conditions. Long recognized as important in HIV and AIDS surveillance, data regarding behaviors also are crucial in addressing health problems related to tobacco use, diet, and physical activity. In the United States, the Behavioral Risk Factor Surveillance System (BRFSS) is a system of health surveys designed to collect standard state-specific data on health risk behaviors, clinical preventive health practices, and health care access associated with leading causes of morbidity and mortality in the United States (Iachan et al., 2001). This system provides a unique source of risk behavior data for states, but also is useful for measuring progress toward national objectives. Other countries have translated parts of the questionnaire and adopted the methodology (Chen, Chiou, & Chen, 2008; see also Chapter 9 for more on the BRFSS).

Despite this system's success, it faces multiple challenges (Mokdad, 2009) that are shared by other telephone surveys. Nonresponse and reluctance to complete interviews affect data quality. More than 100 million telephone numbers have been listed on the National Do Not Call Registry since it began in 2003. Another challenge is presented by the number and nonrepresentative nature of mobile-phone-only households (Blumberg & Luke, 2008), while increasing diversity of the population requires that interviewers be trained in multiple languages. Collection of physical measurements would assist in validating self-reported data (e.g., height, weight). Survey staff are conducting studies to assess these challenges and are researching mixed-mode survey designs.

The Role of Surveillance in Research
Addressing Health Disparities

Public health surveillance systems provide the data that both monitor progress toward eliminating health disparities and enable identification of populations where disparities remain a serious challenge. The National Institutes of Health (NIH) Request for Applications for Research Centers of Excellence supported by NIH's National Center for Minority Health and Health Disparities highlights the critical role of surveillance systems in a published definition of *disparities* (PL 106-525):

Differences in the incidence, prevalence, morbidity, mortality, and burden of diseases and other adverse health conditions that exist among specific population groups. The specific population groups are African Americans, American Indians, Alaska Natives, Asian Americans, Hispanic Americans, Native Hawaiians, Pacific Islanders, subpopulations of all of the above, and medically underserved populations (i.e., socio-economically disadvantaged individuals in rural and urban areas).

The definition has been extended to include persons living with disabilities and those stigmatized because of sexual orientation.

Research into surveillance methods as they pertain to disparities should help practitioners design more effective systems, which in turn should enable public health programs to improve and provide more effective services to those whose health is compromised by their position in society. Improving the health of these populations might have a positive impact on other communities and on the social and political will to eliminate such disparities.

ADDITIONAL RESOURCES

Brookmeyer, R., & Stroup, D. F. (Eds.). (2004). *Monitoring the health of populations: Statistical principles and methods for public health surveillance.* New York, NY: Oxford University Press.

Chen, H., Zeng, D., & Yan, P. (2010). *Infectious disease informatics: Syndromic surveillance for public health and bio-defense.* New York, NY: Springer.

Gregg, M. B. (Ed.). (2008). *Field epidemiology* (3rd ed.). New York, NY: Oxford University Press.

Institute of Medicine & National Research Council. (2010). *BioWatch and public health surveillance: Evaluating systems for the early detection of biological threat.* Washington, DC: National Academies Press.

Lee, L. M., Teutsch, S. M., Thacker, S. B., & St. Louis, M. E. (Eds.). (2010). *Principles and practice of public health surveillance* (3rd ed.). New York, NY: Oxford University Press.

Stroup, D. F., & Teutsch, S. M. (Eds.). (1998). *Statistics in public health: Quantitative approaches to public health problems.* New York, NY: Oxford University Press.

Tango, T. (2010). *Statistical methods for disease clustering.* New York, NY: Springer.

Journals

Bulletin of the World Health Organization

Morbidity and Mortality Weekly Report (Centers for Disease Control and Prevention)

Western Pacific Surveillance and Response Journal

REFERENCES

Allaranga, Y., Kone, M. L., Formenty, P., Libama, F., Boumandouki, P., Woodfill, C. J., . . . Yada, A. (2010). Lessons learned during active epidemiological surveillance of Ebola and Marburg viral hemorrhagic fever epidemics in Africa. *East African Journal of Public Health, 7,* 32–36.

American Health Information Management Association. (2012). *What is health information?* Retrieved from http://www.ahima.org/careers/healthinfo?tabid=what

Ammon, A., & de Valk, H. (2007). Supranational surveillance in the European Union. In N. M. M'ikanatha, R. Lynfield, C. A. Van Beneden, & H. de Valk (Eds.), *Infectious disease surveillance* (pp. 69–78). Malden, MA: Blackwell.

Arita, I., Nakane, M., Kojima, K., Yoshihara, N., Nakano, T., & El-Gohary, A. (2004). Role of a sentinel surveillance system in the context of global surveillance of infectious diseases. *Lancet Infectious Diseases, 4,* 171–177.

Baker, M. G., & Fidler, D. P. (2006). Global public health surveillance under new international health regulations. *Emerging Infectious Diseases, 12,* 1058–1065.

Banerjee, K., Hlady, W. G., Andrus, J. K., Sarkar, S., Fitzsimmons, J., & Abeykoon, P. (2000). Poliomyelitis surveillance: The model used in India for polio eradication. *Bulletin of the World Health Organization, 78,* 321–329. Retrieved from http://www.scielosp.org/scielo.php?script=sci_serial&pid=0042-9686&lng=en&nrm=iso

Blumberg, S. J., & Luke, J. V. (2008). *Wireless substitution: Early release of estimates from the National Health Interview Survey, July–December 2007.* Retrieved from http://www.cdc.gov/nchs/data/nhis/earlyrelease/wireless200805.htm

Box, G. E. P., Jenkins, G. H., & Reinsel, G. C. (2008). *Time series analysis: Forecasting and control* (4th ed.). New York, NY: Wiley.

Bresnitz, E. A., & Ziskin, L. S. (2004). An epidemiologist's view of bioterrorism. *New Jersey Medicine, 101*(Suppl), 26–31.

Brookmeyer, R. (2004). Temporal factors in epidemics: The role of the incubation period. In R. Brookmeyer & D. F. Stroup (Eds.), *Monitoring the health of populations: Statistical principles and methods for public health surveillance.* New York, NY: Oxford University Press.

Burris, H. H., & Werler, M. M. (2011). U.S. provider reported folic acid or multivitamin ordering for non-pregnant women of childbearing age: NAMCS and NHAMCS, 2005–2006. *Maternal and Child Health Journal, 15,* 352–359.

Carnevale, R. J., Talbot, T. R., Schaffner, W., Bloch, K. C., Daniels, T. L., & Miller, R. A. (2011). Evaluating the utility of syndromic surveillance algorithms for screening to detect potentially clonal hospital infection outbreaks. *Journal of the American Medical Informatics Association, 18,* 466–472.

Castillo-Salgado, C. (2010). Trends and directions of global public health surveillance. *Epidemiologic Reviews, 32,* 93–109.

Centers for Disease Control and Prevention. (2004). Framework for evaluating public health surveillance systems for early detection of outbreaks: Recommendations from the CDC working group. *MMWR Recommendations and Reports, 53*(RR-5), 1–11.

Centers for Disease Control and Prevention. (2009). Summary of notifiable diseases—United States. *MMWR Summary of Notifiable Diseases, 58.*

Centers for Disease Control and Prevention. (2013a). *BioSense program.* Retrieved from http://www.cdc.gov/biosense

Centers for Disease Control and Prevention. (2013b). United States cancer statistics. Retrieved from http://wonder.cdc.gov/cancer.HTML

Centers for Disease Control and Prevention. (n.d.). *Emergency preparedness and response: Bioterrorism agents/diseases.* Retrieved from http://www.bt.cdc.gov/agent/agentlist.asp

Chan, E. H., Tamblyn, R., Charland, K. M., & Buckeridge, D. L. (2011). Outpatient physician billing data for age and setting specific syndromic surveillance of influenza-like illness. *Journal of Biomedical Informatics, 44,* 221–228.

Chen, Y. H., Chiou, H. Y., & Chen, P. L. (2008). The development of a Chinese version of the tobacco use subscale of the behavioral risk factor surveillance system (BRFSS). *Preventive Medicine, 46,* 591–595.

Cochi, S. L., & Kew, O. (2008). Polio today: Are we on the verge of global eradication? *Journal of the American Medical Association, 300,* 839–841.

Commission Decision of 22 December 1999 (2000/57/EC) on the early warning and response system for the prevention and control of communicable diseases under Decision 2119/98/EC of the European Parliament and of the Council. (1999). Retrieved from http://eur-lex.europa.eu/LexUriServ/LexUriServ.do?uri=CELEX:32000D0057:EN:NOT

Council for International Organizations of Medical Sciences. (2009). *International guidelines for ethical review of epidemiological studies.* Geneva, Switzerland: World Health Organization.

Decision No 2119/98/EC of the European Parliament and of the Council of 24 September 1998 setting up a network for the epidemiological surveillance and control of communicable diseases in the Community. (1998). Retrieved from http://eur-lex.europa.eu/LexUriServ/LexUriServ.do?uri=CELEX:31998D2119:EN:NOT

Deitel, M. (2003). Overweight and obesity worldwide now estimated to involve 1.7 billion people. *Obesity Surgery, 13,* 329–330.

Devine, O. (2003). Exploring temporal and spatial patterns in public health surveillance data. In R. Brookmeyer & D. F. Stroup (Eds.), *Monitoring the health of populations: Statistical principles and methods for public health surveillance* (pp. 71–98). New York, NY: Oxford University Press.

Dixon, G. D. (2008). Information dissemination. In G. L. Fisher & N. A. Roget (Eds.), *Encyclopedia of substance abuse prevention, treatment, and recovery* (pp. 483-486). Thousand Oaks, CA: Sage.

Donaldson, L. J., Rutter, P. D., Ellis, B. M., Greaves, F. E., Mytton, O. T., Pebody, R. G., & Yardley, I. E. (2009). Mortality from pandemic A/H1N1 2009 influenza in England: Public health surveillance study. *British Medical Journal, 339,* 5213.

Dooyema, C. A., Neri, A., Lo, Y. C., Durant, J., Dargan, P. I., Swarthout, T, . . . Brown, M. J. (2012). Outbreak of fatal childhood lead poisoning related to artisanal gold mining in northwestern Nigeria, 2010. *Environmental Health Perspectives, 120,* 601–607.

Doyle, T. J., Glynn, M. K., & Groseclose, S. L. (2002). Completeness of notifiable infectious disease reporting in the United States: An analytical literature review. *American Journal of Epidemiology, 155,* 866–874.

Feng, D., De Vlas, S. J., Fang, L. Q., Han, X. N., Zhao, W. J., Sheng, S., . . . Cao, W. C. (2009). The SARS epidemic in mainland China: Bringing together all epidemiological data. *Tropical Medicine and International Health, 14*(Supp 1), 4–12.

Freedman, R. A., He, Y., Winer, E. P., & Keating, N. L. (2009). Trends in racial and age disparities in definitive local therapy of early-stage breast cancer. *Journal of Clinical Oncology, 27,* 713–719.

Gitau-Mburu, D. (2008). Should public health be exempt from ethical regulations? Intricacies of research versus activity. *East African Journal of Public Health, 5,* 160–162.

Goga, A., Dinh, T. H., Dlamini, N., Mosala, T., Lombard, C., Puren, A., . . . Jackson, D. (2011, July). *Impact of the national prevention of mother to child transmission (PMTCT) program on mother-to-child transmission of HIV (MTCT), South Africa, 2010.* Paper presented at the 6th International AIDS Society Conference, Rome, Italy. Retrieved from http://pag.ias2011.org/abstracts.aspx?aid=1176

Grassly, N. C., Fraser, C., Wenger, J., Deshpande, J. M., Sutter, R. W., Heymann, D. L., & Aylward, R. B. (2006). New strategies for the elimination of polio from India. *Science, 314,* 1150–1153.

Greenberg, A. E., & Lobel H. O. (1990). Mortality from *Plasmodium falciparum* malaria in travelers from the United States, 1959 to 1987. *Annals of Internal Medicine, 113,* 326–327.

Hallett, T. B., Zaba, B., Todd, J., Lopman, B., Mwita, W., Biraro, S., & Gregson, S. (2008). Estimating incidence from prevalence in generalised HIV epidemics: Methods and validation. *PloS Medicine, 5,* e80. Retrieved from http://www.plosmedicine.org

Hirschler, B. (2013, May 28). Drug resistance in new China bird flu raises concern. *Reuters.* Retrieved from http://www.reuters.com

Holford, T. R. (2004). Temporal factors in public health surveillance: Sorting out age, period, and cohort effects. In R. Brookmeyer & D. F. Stroup (Eds.), *Monitoring the health of populations: Statistical principles and methods for public health surveillance* (pp. 99–126). New York, NY: Oxford University Press.

Hristidis, V., Varadarajan, R. R., Biondich, P., & Weiner, M. (2010). Information discovery on electronic health records using authority flow techniques. *BioMed Central Medical Informatics and Decision Making, 10,* 64.

Iachan, R., Schulman, J., Powell-Griner, E., Nelson, D. E., Mariolis, P., & Stanwyck, C. (2001). Pooling state telephone survey health data for national estimates: The CDC Behavioral Risk Factor Surveillance System. In M. L. Cynamon & R. A. Kulka (Eds.), *Proceedings of the Seventh Conference on Health Survey Research Methods, Dallas, Texas* (pp. 221–226). Hyattsville, MD: U.S. Department of Health and Human Services, Centers for Disease Control and Prevention. Retrieved from http://www.cdc.gov/nchs/data/conf/conf07.pdf

India: Country marks year without polio. (2012). *Science, 335,* 268.

Jemal, A., Bray, F., Center, M. M., Ferlay, J., Ward, E., & Forman, D. (2011). Global cancer statistics. *CA: A Cancer Journal for Clinicians, 61,* 69–90.

Jemal, A., Thun, M. J., Ward, E. E., Henley, S. J., Cokkinides, V. E., & Murray, T. E. (2008). Mortality from leading causes by education and race in the United States, 2001. *American Journal of Preventive Medicine, 34,* 1–8.

Kalsbeek, W. D. (2004). The use of surveys in public health surveillance: Monitoring high risk populations. In R. Brookmeyer & D. F. Stroup (Eds.), *Monitoring the health of populations: Statistical principles and methods for public health surveillance* (pp. 37–70). New York, NY: Oxford University Press.

Klein, C. A. (2011). Cloudy confidentiality: Clinical and legal implications of cloud computing in health care. *Journal of the American Academy of Psychiatry Law, 39,* 571–578.

Krieger, N., Williams, D. R., & Moss, N. E. (1997). Measuring social class in U.S. public health research: Concepts, methodologies, and guidelines. *Annual Review of Public Health, 18,* 341–378.

Langer, A. J., Ayers, T., Grass, J., Lynch, M., Angulo, F. J., & Mahon, B. E. (2012). Nonpasteurized dairy products, disease outbreaks, and state laws—United States, 1993–2006. *Emerging Infectious Diseases, 18,* 385–391.

Lawlor, D. A., & Stone T. (2001). Public health and data protection: An inevitable collision or potential for a meeting of minds? *International Journal of Epidemiology, 30,* 1221–1225.

Lawson, A. B., & Kleinman, K. (Eds.). (2005). *Spatial and syndromic surveillance for public health.* New York, NY: Wiley.

Lee, L. M., & Thacker, S. B. (2011). Public health surveillance and knowing about health in the context of growing sources of health data. *American Journal of Preventive Medicine, 41,* 636–640.

Levine, R. J. (1996). International codes and guidelines for research ethics: A critical appraisal. In H. Y. Vanderpool (Ed.), *The ethics of research involving human subjects: Facing the 21st century.* Frederick, MD: University Publication Group.

London School of Hygiene and Tropical Medicine. (2009). Types of surveillance. In *Epidemiological Tools in Conflict-Affected Populations.* London, England: London School of Hygiene and Tropical Medicine. Retrieved from http://conflict.lshtm.ac.uk/page_75.htm

Mack, K. A., & Ory, M. G. (2003). AIDS and older Americans at the end of the twentieth century. *Journal of Acquired Immune Deficiency Syndromes, 33,* S68–S75.

Mather, F. J., White, L. E., Langlois, C., Shorter, C. F., Swalm, M., Shaffer, J. G., & Hartley, W. R. (2004). Statistical methods for linking health, exposure, and hazards. *Environmental Health Perspectives, 112,* 1440–1445.

Mathes, R. W., Ito, K., & Matte, T. (2011). Assessing syndromic surveillance of cardiovascular outcomes from emergency department chief complaint data in New York City. *PLoS One, 6*, e14677.

McKee, M., & Atun, R. (2006). Beyond borders: Public health surveillance. *Lancet, 367*, 1224–1226.

M'ikanatha, N. M., Rohn, D. D., Welliver, D. P., McAdams, T., & Julian, K. G. (2007). Use of the World Wide Web to enhance infectious disease surveillance. In N. M. M'ikanatha, R. Lynfield, C. A. Van Beneden, & H. de Valk (Eds.), *Infectious disease surveillance* (pp. 281–293). Malden, MA: Blackwell.

Mitka, M. (2010). Surveillance efforts lacking. *Journal of the American Medical Association, 303*, 499.

Mokdad, A. H. (2009). The Behavioral Risk Factor Surveillance System: Past, present, and future. *Annual Review of Public Health, 30*, 43–54.

Myler, E., & Broadbent, G. (2006, November–December). ISO 17799: Standard for security. *Information Management Journal*, pp. 43–52. Retrieved from http://www.arma.org/book-store/files/myler_broadbent.pdf

Neslund, V. S., Goodman, R. A., Hodge, J. G., & Middaugh, J. P. (2010). Legal considerations in public health surveillance in the United States. In L. M. Lee, S. M. Teutsch, S. B. Thacker, & M. E. St. Louis (Eds.), *Principles and practice of public health surveillance* (3rd ed., pp. 217–235). New York, NY: Oxford University Press.

Painter, T. M. (2001). Voluntary counseling and testing for couples: A high-leverage intervention for HIV/AIDS prevention in sub-Saharan Africa. *Social Science and Medicine, 53*, 1397–1411.

Pareek, R., & Gautam A. (2011). Cloud computing. *Journal of Global Research in Computer Science, 2.* Retrieved from http://www.jgrcs.info/index.php/jgrcs/index

Paul, Y. (2009). Oral polio vaccines and their role in polio eradication in India. *Expert Review of Vaccines, 8*, 35–41.

Plotkin, B. J., Hardiman, M., González-Martin, F., & Rodier, G. (2007). Infectious disease surveillance and the International Health Regulations. In N. M. M'ikanatha, R. Lynfield, C. A. Van Beneden, & H. de Valk (Eds.), *Infectious disease surveillance* (pp. 18–31). Malden, MA: Blackwell.

Public Law 106-525 (2000). Minority Health and Health Disparities Research and Education Act, 2498.

Quigg, Z., Hughes, K., & Bellis, M. A. (2012). Data sharing for prevention: A case study in the development of a comprehensive emergency department injury surveillance system and its use in preventing violence and alcohol-related harms. *Injury Prevention, 18*, 315–320.

Reingold, A. (2003). If syndromic surveillance is the answer, what is the question? *Biosecurity and Bioterrorism, 1*, 77–81.

Rice, R. E. (2006). Influences, usage, and outcomes of Internet health information searching: Multivariate results from the Pew surveys. *International Journal of Medical Informatics, 75*, 8–28.

Russell, T. L., Lwetoijera, D. W., Maliti, D., Chipwaza, B., Kihonda, J., Charlwood, J. D., . . . Killeen, G. F. (2010). Impact of promoting longer-lasting insecticide treatment of bed nets upon malaria transmission in a rural Tanzanian setting with pre-existing high coverage of untreated nets. *Malaria Journal, 9*, 187. Retrieved from http://www.malariajournal.com

Rychetnik, L., Frommer, M., Hawe, P., & Shiell, A. (2002). Criteria for evaluating evidence on public health interventions. *Journal of Epidemiology and Community Health, 56*, 119–127.

Smedley, B. D., Stith, A. Y., & Nelson, A. R. (Eds.). (2003). *Unequal treatment: Confronting racial and ethnic disparities in health care.* Washington, DC: National Academies Press.

Snider, D. E., Jr. & Stroup, D. F. (1997). Defining research when it comes to public health. *Public Health Reports, 112*, 29–32.

Soler, M. S., Fouillet, A., Viso, A. C., Josseran, L., Smith, G. E., Elliot, A. J., . . . Krafft, T. (2011). Assessment of syndromic surveillance in Europe: Triple S Project. *Lancet, 378,* 1833–1834.

Stöhr, K. (2003). The global agenda on influenza surveillance and control. *Vaccine, 21,* 1744–1748.

Stoto, M. A. (2008). Public health surveillance in the twenty-first century: Achieving population health goals while protecting individuals' privacy and confidentiality. *Georgetown Law Journal, 96,* 703–718.

Stroup, D. F., Williamson, G. D., Herndon, J. L., & Karon, J. M. (1989). Detection of aberrations in the occurrence of notifiable diseases surveillance data. *Statistics in Medicine, 8,* 323–329.

Sullivan, P. S., McKenna, M. T., Waller, L. A., Williamson, G. D., & Lee, L. M. (2010). Analyzing and interpreting public health surveillance data. In L. M. Lee, S. M. Teutsch, S. B. Thacker, & M. E. St. Louis (Eds.), *Principles and practice of public health surveillance* (3rd ed., pp. 88–145). New York, NY: Oxford University Press.

Thacker, S. B. (2010). Historical development. In L. M. Lee, S. M. Teutsch, S. B. Thacker, & M. E. St. Louis (Eds.), *Principles and practice of public health surveillance* (3rd ed., pp. 1–17). New York, NY: Oxford University Press.

Thorpe, R. J., Jr., Brandon, D. T., & LaVeist, T. A. (2008). Social context as an explanation for race disparities in hypertension: Findings from the Exploring Health Disparities in Integrated Communities (EHDIC) Study. *Social Science and Medicine, 67,* 1604–1611.

Tsui, K.-L., Wong, S. Y., Jiang, W., & Lin, C.-J. (2011). Recent research and developments in temporal and spatiotemporal surveillance for public health. *IEEE Transactions on Reliability, 60,* 49–58.

Waller, L. A. (2004). Detecting disease clustering in time or space. In R. Brookmeyer & D. F. Stroup (Eds.), *Monitoring the health of populations: Statistical principles and methods for public health surveillance* (pp. 167–202). New York, NY: Oxford University Press.

Walport, M., & Brest, P. (2011). Sharing research data to improve public health. *Lancet, 377,* 537–539.

Warren, C. W., Jones, N. R., Erickson, M. P., & Asma, S. (2006). Patterns of global tobacco use in young people and implications for future chronic disease burden in adults. *Lancet, 367,* 749–753.

Werber, D., Dreesman, J., Feil, F., van Treeck, U., Fell, G., Ethelberg, S., . . . Ammon, A. (2005). International outbreak of *Salmonella* Oranienburg due to German chocolate. *BMC Infectious Diseases, 5*(7). Retrieved from http://www.biomedcentral.com

Wertheim, H. F. L., Horby, P., & Woodall, J. P. (Eds.). (2012). *Atlas of human infectious diseases.* Chichester, UK: Wiley-Blackwell.

World Health Organization. (2003–2007). *About the Global Health Atlas.* Retrieved from http://apps.who.int/globalatlas/default.asp

World Health Organization. (2007). *Global MDR-TB and XDR-TB response plan 2007–2008.* Geneva, Switzerland: Author. Retrieved from http://www.who.int/tb/publications/2007/mdr_xdr_global_response_plan.pdf

World Health Organization, International Agency for Research on Cancer. (2010). *GLOBOCAN 2008.* Retrieved from http://globocan.iarc.fr/

World Health Organization. (2013a). *Overweight and obesity. Fact sheet 311.* Retrieved from http://www.who.int/mediacentre/factsheets/fs311/en/index.html

World Health Organization. (2013b). *Public health surveillance.* Retrieved from http://www.who.int/topics/public_health_surveillance/en/

World Health Organization. (2013c). *STEPwise approach to surveillance (STEPS).* Retrieved from http://www.who.int/chp/steps/en/

Yelton, A. (2012). Mobile websites. *Library Technology Reports, 48,* 9–21.

NOTE

1. In February 2013, a beacon of epidemiology and research was extinguished when Dr. Stephen B. Thacker died after a sudden diagnosis of Creutzfeldt-Jakob disease. His work reported here and numerous other imprints on public health are a legacy to public health research, improving the health of communities around the world.

6

Outbreak Investigation

Douglas H. Hamilton

As mentioned in the previous chapter, one of the uses of surveillance data is to help identify outbreaks of disease. In the fall of 1994, a Public Health Functions Steering Committee, comprising federal agencies and major national public health organizations, defined the 10 essential public health services and included, as Number 2, to "diagnose and investigate health problems and health hazards in the community" (Centers for Disease Control and Prevention [CDC], 2013). The committee mentioned outbreak investigation specifically as a way to diagnose and investigate health problems. **Outbreak investigation** involves recognizing a problem, collecting relevant information, analyzing likely risk factors, identifying and implementing appropriate control measures, evaluating the effectiveness of the control measures, and communicating the investigation results. This chapter describes the general steps that are undertaken in investigating an outbreak. These principles apply to the investigation of an acute infectious disease, but can also be applied to other kinds of outbreaks, including environmental, occupational, injury, or chronic disease problems.

OUTBREAK INVESTIGATION AS PUBLIC HEALTH RESEARCH AND PRACTICE

The most obvious reason for an outbreak investigation is to identify the source or mode of disease transmission so that control measures can be implemented to limit further spread of the disease. The information gathered in the investigation is important for evaluating the effectiveness of those control measures as well. Outbreak investigations offer other important opportunities for public health professionals in that they provide a natural experiment where investigators can evaluate the effect of an exposure or other risk factors that are impractical or unethical to conduct in a controlled experiment that uses humans or animals. For example, in 1991, endocrinologists in Massachusetts reported five cases of suspected hypervitaminosis D (an excess of vitamin D) to local health authorities. Investigation of this outbreak revealed that the affected persons had consumed milk from a specific local dairy that had been inadvertently overfortifying its milk with 30–35 times the recommended amounts of vitamin D. Investigators studied 243 exposed persons and were able to document the clinical effects of this type of exposure. Devising a clinical study to expose a similar group of persons to such excess levels of vitamin D would have been unreasonable (Scanlon, Blank, & Sinks, 1992).

Outbreaks also allow investigators to study the natural history of a given disease and sometimes the opportunity to characterize a new problem. Before the introduction of West Nile virus (WNV) into North America, studies in Africa, the Middle East, and Eastern Europe had characterized the clinical syndromes associated with WNV infections, but did not measure the extent of asymptomatic infection or mild illness. Serosurveys conducted during the 1999 outbreak of WNV among an immunologically naïve population in New York City revealed that, for every case of WNV meningoencephalitis, 30 additional probable cases of mild WNV fever and 140 persons with symptomless or mildly symptomatic infections were identified (Mostashari et al., 2001).

Other important reasons to investigate outbreaks include

- responding to political or public pressures to identify an outbreak cause (e.g., a foodborne outbreak after a community gathering and public concern that an intentional or negligent contamination of the food item had occurred),
- fulfilling statutory requirements for the health office to investigate outbreaks (e.g., an outbreak that involves a commercial establishment or product), and
- training health workers in disease investigation and control.

Figure 6.1 lists the key steps in an outbreak investigation and forms the outline for the remainder of this chapter. Keep in mind two key points about this list. First, it is not a rigid, sequential task list. When conducting an actual investigation, epidemiologists usually perform multiple steps simultaneously. For example, investigators often try to identify patients while they are verifying the diagnosis and trying to confirm that an epidemic is occurring. Because the primary role of public health workers is to protect the public's health, one of the last steps in the sequence—implement and evaluate control measures—should be undertaken as soon as practicable control measures are identified. The second crucial point is that this is simply one way of approaching outbreak investigations. Undoubtedly, other protocols are equally effective.

Figure 6.1   Guidelines for Epidemiologic Field Investigations

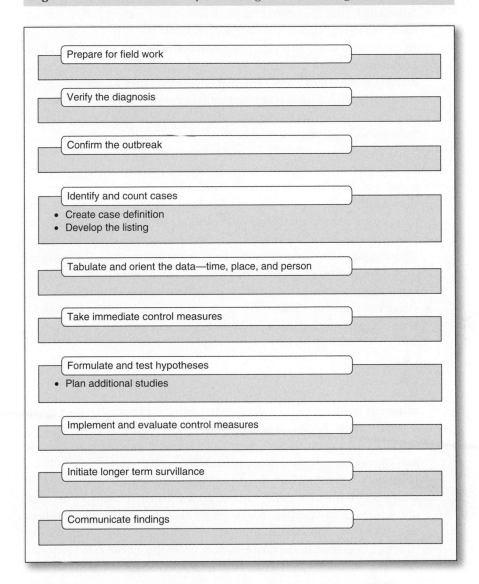

Prepare for field work

Verify the diagnosis

Confirm the outbreak

Identify and count cases
- Create case definition
- Develop the listing

Tabulate and orient the data—time, place, and person

Take immediate control measures

Formulate and test hypotheses
- Plan additional studies

Implement and evaluate control measures

Initiate longer term survillance

Communicate findings

CONDUCTING AN OUTBREAK INVESTIGATION

Prepare for Field Work

Depending on the setting in which investigators are working, they will have administrative and scientific tasks that must be completed before beginning the investigation.

Administrative

- **Jurisdiction.** Have you notified the persons with legal authority about the outbreak, and has the request for assistance come from the correct authorities? An astute clinician will often bring a potential problem to health authorities' attention but might not have the authority to initiate a public health investigation. For example, in the United States, "health" is under each state's jurisdiction. Federal authorities must not conduct an investigation unless they are invited by the state authorities, typically the state epidemiologist. Similar jurisdictional restrictions between local and state authorities also might apply within states.

- **Team composition.** Who will be on the investigation team, and who will be providing support from a distance (e.g., the central public health office)? Who is included in the chain of command for the team?

- **Resources.** What supplies (office or laboratory) will the team need? How will transportation be managed? How will the lines of communication between team members be managed? Will computer and Internet access be readily available? What lodging and meals for team members need to be prearranged? These items can be straightforward in a domestic investigation but considerably challenging in a resource-poor (rural or low-socioeconomic) environment.

- **Other.** What travel documents does each team member need? Does overtime for team members need to be preapproved?

Scientific

- **Background information on the suspected agent or mode of transmission.** To prepare for the investigation, team members gather information on likely agents and risk factors. Possible resources include the scientific literature, local or national subject-matter experts, records of similar past investigations, and reliable Internet sites (the CDC or research centers and universities).

- **Laboratory support and specimen handling.** What types of samples will the team most likely collect (environmental, clinical, other)? What types of collection equipment and specimen containers are needed? What are the conditions for sample shipping (room temperature, wet ice, dry ice)? How will the samples be shipped (commercial shipping firm, mail, courier)? Remember to involve the laboratory authorities early in an investigation, especially if you anticipate a substantial volume of samples.

- **Personal protection equipment.** What measures do you need to take for team members' safety? Consider such safety precautions as barrier protection (gloves, gown, and masks), respirators (have team members been fit-tested?), vaccinations, and prophylactic medications. These items might not be readily available in remote locations.

- **Current response.** What types of control measures have already been put into place? Medical treatments can change the clinical picture for individual patients just as community intervention measures can alter the disease profile in the community.

• **Local theories.** What do the local authorities think is causing the outbreak? This is a crucial question to ask the person requesting the investigation. Although investigators should maintain an open mind regarding all possible causes of the outbreak, the local authorities will have been working on the problem before calling for assistance. They likely will have considered and eliminated certain causes of the outbreak and can provide useful guidance to the team at the outset.

Verify the Diagnosis

As soon as possible, verify that the reports of disease or conditions causing the outbreak are accurate. The goal of this step is to rule out misdiagnosis, laboratory error, and pseudoepidemics. This can occur when either a real clustering of false infections or an artifactual clustering of real infections occurs. At the beginning of an investigation, if possible, the team should visit in person, interview, and even examine the patients. The team should review the medical records and, if indicated, obtain clinical specimens to confirm laboratory test results at a provincial or national reference laboratory to rule out laboratory error.

If clinical features are incompatible with laboratory results and the diagnosis cannot be verified, consider the possibility of a false infection. For example, false-positive diagnoses can result from contaminated antiseptic used to prepare skin for drawing blood cultures, use of nonsterile syringes to collect specimens for blood cultures, or environmental contamination of specimens during processing in the laboratory. For example, during an outbreak of neonatal sepsis among pediatric patients at two regional hospitals, investigators noted that the relatively mild illness reported among the patients was not typical of *Serratia* sepsis, which was also an unusual causative agent among this population. The investigation revealed that the blood collection tubes used by the two hospitals were contaminated with the outbreak strain of *Serratia* (Hoffman et al., 1976).

More recently, in a 2010–2011 outbreak of pertussis in New York, health officials identified 542 patients with laboratory-confirmed pertussis, but also noted that many of the patients did not have clinically compatible symptoms. They were able to demonstrate that certain pertussis vaccines contained considerable amounts of polymerase-chain reaction–detectable *Bordetella pertussis* DNA, and environmental sampling had identified the presence of this DNA in clinic environments. They postulated that inadvertent transfer of DNA from clinic environmental surfaces to clinical specimens resulted in contamination and led to false-positive results (Maxted et al., 2012).

Artifactual clustering of real infections can occur as a result of a change in the sensitivity of case finding, rather than an actual increase in disease incidence. To rule out artifactual clustering, consider the following questions:

• Has a new, more sensitive diagnostic test been introduced?
• Has the surveillance definition for the disease changed?

- Has a new practitioner entered the community who is either ordering more diagnostic tests or using different diagnostic criteria?
- Has public awareness about the disease led to more people seeking clinical evaluation?

> **Practical Point**: Try to obtain clinical specimens or other samples already isolated for possible additional testing and analysis at the outset of the investigation. Obtaining samples as soon as possible—before they have been discarded by a laboratory—is crucial. Samples can always be thrown away, but they cannot be retrieved after they have been discarded.

Confirm the Outbreak

After the team has verified the diagnosis, the next crucial step is confirming that an outbreak is occurring. From the perspective of an epidemiologist, the terms *outbreak* and *epidemic* are synonymous: "The occurrence in a community or region of cases of illness, specific health-related behavior, or other health-related events clearly in excess of normal expectancy. The community or region and the period in which the cases occur are specified precisely" (Last, 1995, p. 54).

The key elements of this definition are *time*, *place*, and *person*. Of note, the public's perception of these terms is often considerably different from the epidemiologist's. *Outbreak* is often regarded by the public as a smaller, highly localized increase in disease occurrence, whereas *epidemic* is interpreted as a much more serious, widespread, and likely threatening increase in disease. Public health workers should be aware of the potential impact of how they describe a problem to the public. The public reaction to the statement "We have an outbreak of *Salmonella* in our city" will likely be quite different than the reaction to "We have an epidemic of *Salmonella* in our city." Sometimes, however, health authorities might want to elicit a more vigorous public response; hence, we hear such phrases as "the epidemic of teenage pregnancy" or "the obesity epidemic."

Other terms that are used when describing an increase in disease but are not synonymous with *outbreak* include the following (Last, 1995):

- **Cluster:** An aggregation of unusual events in place or time that is perceived to be greater than expected. The focus of the majority of cluster investigations is to try to determine what the actual expected rate is.
- **Endemic:** The constant presence of a disease or infectious agent within a given geographic area or among a population group.
- **Hyperendemic:** A disease that is constantly present at high incidence or prevalence rates and that affects all age groups equally.
- **Pandemic:** An epidemic occurring worldwide or throughout a geographic region, crossing international boundaries, and usually affecting a substantial number of persons.

How much in excess of normal expectancy is required before an increased number of cases constitutes an outbreak? It depends. Multiple factors can be considered when making this decision, including the following:

- How prevalent is the disease among the population?
- How severe is the disease (e.g., does it result in death or serious disability)?
- How transmissible is the disease?
- Does this disease usually occur seasonally?
- Are specific populations at high risk (e.g., older persons, young children, immunocompromised persons)?

For certain conditions that rarely occur among a given population (e.g., rabies, plague, meningococcal meningitis), a single case might be considered more than expected. For conditions that are endemic in a community (e.g., salmonellosis, histoplasmosis), determining how many cases are more than expected might be much more difficult. For other conditions (e.g., seasonal influenza) that occur regularly in the community with relatively high numbers, health officials might calculate expected rates on the basis of a moving 5- to 10-year average to establish an epidemic threshold. For instance, by examining influenza rates in the United States for 1972–1985, researchers defined an epidemic as the number of observed cases increasing above the predetermined epidemic threshold that was set at 1.64 standard deviations higher than the predicted mean. During this period, 4 years occurred when the number of cases exceeded the epidemic threshold (Figure 6.2; Lui & Kendal, 1987).

During an outbreak response, investigators should count the number of cases and compare that with the predicted baseline number of cases for a defined time and place. So if you were asked to investigate an outbreak of surgical wound infections in a community hospital, your team would need to get an estimate of the number of such cases that normally occur. You could review the discharge records for the previous month or months. However, when using historical data to compare the magnitude of the current problem with the baseline, using rates is imperative. If the hospital had six surgical wound infections this month but the records reveal only two the month before and three each of the preceding months, is this an outbreak? Perhaps. What if the hospital had just opened up a new surgical suite and tripled the number of surgical cases performed? In that instance, the case rate this month might be the same as for previous months.

What if the team is asked to investigate an apparent increase in pediatric cases of severe respiratory syncytial virus (RSV) infections? Comparing the rates to the previous months might not be an accurate indication. RSV is a seasonal disease; therefore, the team should compare the rates in the facility for the same period the previous year or the year before that.

Calculating a baseline rate for a hospital outbreak is probably a best-case scenario. In community investigations, determining the baseline might be more difficult, and investigators might encounter problems that lack available data, have incomplete reporting or inefficient surveillance, or have absent or varying case definitions. For instance, in June 1981, investigators reported five cases of *Pneumocystis carinii* pneumonia (PCP) among young homosexual men in Los Angeles. This was an

Figure 6.2 Regional Pneumonia and Influenza-Associated Deaths Reported to the National Center for Health Statistics, 1975–1981

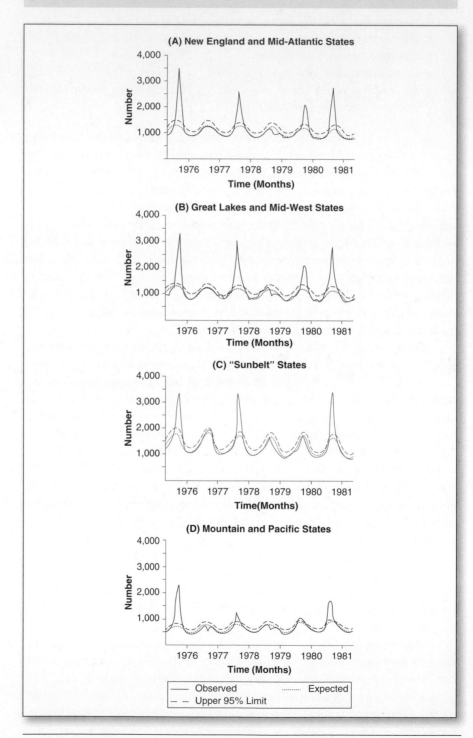

Source: Lui and Kendal (1987).

unusual group of patients because they did not fit the profile of PCP patients: persons who typically have a known severe immunodeficiency (CDC, 1981). Was this an epidemic? To answer this question, a large team of public health workers conducted active surveillance and reviewed available tumor registries and other medical information systems. They were able to gather the information illustrated in Figure 6.3 (CDC, 1982).

Figure 6.3   Incidence of Kaposi's Sarcoma (KS), *Pneumocystis carinii* Pneumonia (PCP), and Other Opportunistic Infections in the United States, 1979–1981

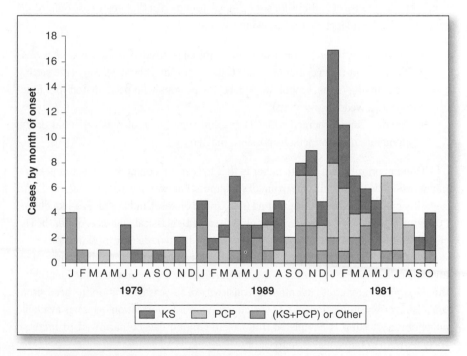

Source: CDC (1982).

Their data revealed a clear increase over the expected number of cases that began in 1980. This report documented the beginning of the HIV/AIDS epidemic in the United States. However, the effort to collect and analyze the data necessary to make this determination took 6 months. Establishing a baseline and verifying an epidemic can be a difficult and time-consuming process.

Identify and Count Cases

After confirming the existence of an outbreak, the next task is to identify as many cases as possible. The term that epidemiologists often use is *casting a broad net*. Investigators want to find as many cases as possible (sensitivity) without including noncases (specificity).

IMPORTANT TERMS

Sensitivity: the proportion of truly positive individuals that are identified as diseased by the test (true positive rate).

Specificity: the proportion of truly negative individuals who are identified as disease free by the test (true negative rate).

A critical element of case finding is establishing a clear, easily applied case definition. As with the case definitions for surveillance discussed in Chapter 5, case definitions for outbreaks should include the following elements:

- **Time:** specify when the disease occurred (often referred to as the *outbreak period*)
- **Place:** might be a geographic place (e.g., town, state, country), a specific setting (e.g., nursing home, school, workplace), or persons who participated in a function (e.g., wedding, meeting)
- **Person:** clinical characteristics (signs and symptoms) of those affected or the laboratory tests for persons possibly affected

One important point to remember is that for certain conditions, infected persons might present with an entire spectrum of symptoms. For example, patients infected with hepatitis might have no symptoms at all (subclinical disease), mild influenza-like illness, nondescript abdominal complaints, frank disease with classical jaundice, or death. The case definition might need to be designed to select different disease presentations.

A case definition is not necessarily static and can change during the course of an investigation. Initially, the working definition might be overly sensitive for identifying the maximum number of patients. The sensitivity of the case definition in these situations is inversely proportional to its specificity. As more information becomes available or laboratory testing is completed, the case definition can be narrowed to increase specificity. An example may help to clarify.

During an investigation of a Legionnaires' disease outbreak in Indiana, the team started their case finding with a highly sensitive case definition, as follows:

Case: Illness in a person who was in Bloomington, Indiana [**place**], during the 2 weeks before illness onset [**time**] and who presented with a fever of $\geq 39.2°C$, radiologic evidence of pneumonia, and no bacterial isolates of clinical significance [**person**].

As the investigation proceeded and more laboratory data became available, they narrowed their case definition by requiring laboratory data to differentiate a *confirmed case* from a *presumptive case*, as follows (Dondero et al., 1980):

Confirmed case: A case where paired sera demonstrate a fourfold or greater increase in indirect fluorescent antibody titer to ≥ 128.

Presumptive case: A case with only a single serum sample available that demonstrates a convalescent-phase indirect fluorescent antibody titer of ≥ 256.

The initial case definition was highly sensitive and would likely have caught the majority of the patients with Legionnaires' disease who had sought clinical care. However, the specificity of the definition was lower and, therefore, might also have identified patients with viral pneumonia or other bacterial agents that were not isolated by laboratory testing. The confirmed case diagnosis has the advantage of not including these noncases, but at a cost of greater time and expense required to obtain the laboratory tests and a smaller sample size for the data analysis.

Practical Point: In most instances, the case definition will be applied by various members of the team in the process of case finding. Therefore, the definition needs to be unambiguous. If the case definition is "illness in a person with pneumonia, fever, and diarrhea," what are the potential problems?

- **Pneumonia:** Is this patient-reported pneumonia, clinician-diagnosed, or by radiologic evidence?
- **Fever:** How high does a patient's temperature have to be? (Many patients will report having a fever, but when asked how high, they will report, "I felt hot.")
- **Diarrhea:** One person's diarrhea might be another person's regular bowel pattern.

Be sure that your case definition has clear parameters (e.g., illness in a person with clinician-diagnosed pneumonia, oral temperature > 100ºF, and three or more loose bowel movements within 24 hours). Clearly defining how the definition should be applied is integral to obtaining accurate data.

After the case definition is developed, it should be used in a systematic search of the affected location to find cases. Identifying all of the affected patients in an outbreak is unnecessary; gathering a sample of the affected population where the sample size provides enough data to make statistically valid inferences about exposure and disease is all that is necessary. However, using a systematic approach to finding affected patients is important to avoid introducing an ascertainment bias into your sample.

Take case-control investigations, for example. Case-patients and control subjects often have been identified by conducting random-digit-dialing of telephone exchanges that match the numbers of known case-patients. This works because the three-digit exchange number tends to be restricted to a specific geographic area. Historically, the concern about this technique has been the potential for missing persons without telephones. If this group is different from the persons with telephones (socioeconomic status, education, race/ethnicity, renters versus homeowners), the sample will not reflect the general population. More recently, the dramatic increase in the use of cell phones has affected the utility of using telephone numbers to match for geographic area. Concerns now include the potential for age bias, since cell phones might be disproportionately used by younger persons (Kempf & Remington, 2007).

Using multiple sources to identify patients during an investigation is therefore crucial, and the team should consider several possible sources:

- **Medical offices:** The obvious first place to find affected persons is in hospitals, clinics, or physicians' offices in the area. The advantage of this approach is that it is relatively convenient, the data quality is usually good, and you often have diagnostic data that are helpful in the investigation. The disadvantage is that only persons with more severe illness will seek medical attention, and the persons you identify will be the sicker among all affected persons.

- **Laboratories:** During an infectious disease outbreak, laboratories are possibly the most important place to start. The data are usually reliable and can provide confirmation of specific diagnoses. In addition, laboratories often serve multiple providers and might provide results for a wider geographic area than just one clinical facility. The disadvantage is the same as with medical facilities—only patients who have sought care will be represented.

- **Surveillance data:** Public health surveillance data might be a valuable way to identify cases. The biggest challenge is the likely time lag between occurrence of disease and reporting to the surveillance system. During rapidly evolving outbreaks, this can be a serious limitation.

- **Institutions:** Large employers or schools often have clinics or systems for tracking absences.

- **Targeted surveys:** Sometimes conducting a community survey is necessary to identify affected persons. These might be random-sample surveys based on an established sampling frame, cluster surveys, or convenience surveys. A key consideration is whether the sampling technique used generates a sample that is representative of the community.

- **Friends/contacts:** Case finding might involve asking patients to identify others who are also sick. The main disadvantage with this approach is the potential for overmatching case-patients with control subjects (i.e., finding controls who are too similar to case-patients than a control from the general population would be).

- **Local/tribal/community leaders:** In smaller communities, the local leaders can be a resource for identifying ill persons. This is especially important in communities with limited resources.

- **Media/press:** Using the media for identifying cases can be a double-edged sword. In some instances, identification of a potential source of an outbreak by the press can seriously bias the reporting of affected persons—ill persons who were not exposed to the publicized risk factor might fail to report their illness, or persons who are not ill might report simply because they were exposed. In other cases, press attention helps by raising public awareness and encouraging ill persons to contact health care providers for evaluation.

- **Social media:** Public health investigators have used this resource as a way to contact widely dispersed groups of possible patients quickly. During a recent investigation of respiratory illness among attendees at a conference, all 715 attendees from 30 countries were contacted through social media (Twitter, Facebook, SurveyMonkey, and relevant blogs). One major limitation of this resource is susceptibility to reporting bias (Reed et al., 2011).

- **Pharmacy records:** Local pharmacies can help identify persons who have purchased specific antibiotics or medications for symptoms (e.g., diarrhea, respiratory disease).
- **Novel data sources:** Investigators can use other resources as applicable, too (e.g., credit card receipts for patrons of a particular restaurant). Recently, a multistate outbreak of *Salmonella* was linked to contaminated pepper in a delicatessen meat product sold at a national warehouse club. The investigation team made extensive use of data collected from club membership cards linked to a database of every purchase made (CDC, 2010; see the case study at the end of this chapter).

When you are collecting case data, it is always helpful to construct a line list (Table 6.1). This is a simple way to record case information in a ledger, computer spreadsheet, or by another means. Each row in the line listing records the information for an individual patient; the columns include information on demographics (age, race, sex), contact information (address, telephone number), key times/dates (onset of symptoms, treatments, time of diagnoses, and so forth), and potential risk factors. Depending on the situation, other specific information might be included in the line listing (e.g., in a hospital-acquired infection: date of admission, wards, procedures, laboratory results, and staff caring for the patient).

With so much modern technology at our fingertips, we have a tendency to put all available information into a computer database or spreadsheet immediately. Although this is an important step for the eventual data analysis, early in the investigation a simple paper line listing is a quick and easy way to look for patterns.

Tabulate and Orient the Data—Time, Place, and Person

After the cases have been identified and the data collected, the next step is to tabulate and orient the data in terms of time, place, and person. Initial steps in this process typically include the following:

- **Time:** drawing an epidemic curve (i.e., graphing the number of cases across a time span)
- **Place:** drawing a spot map that indicates specific cases or case rates by location
- **Person:** thoroughly describing patients' characteristics

When investigators analyze the data to answer when, where, and who, they are describing the situation and the sample population. This process is often referred to as *descriptive epidemiology*.

This information is then analyzed and used to develop hypotheses to explain the cause, source, mode of spread, or other aspects of the outbreak (i.e., the how and why). Investigators usually will analyze the existing data or conduct additional studies to

Table 6.1 Example Line Listing of Hepatitis A Cases

ID	Date of Diagnosis	Town	Age (Years)	Sex	Hosp	Jaundice	Outbreak	IV Drugs	IgM Pos	Highest ALT*
01	01/05	B	74	M	Y	N	N	N	Y	232
02	01/06	J	29	M	N	Y	N	Y	Y	285
03	01/08	k	37	M	Y	Y	N	N	Y	3250
04	01/19	J	3	F	N	N	N	N	Y	1100
05	01/30	C	39	M	N	Y	N	N	Y	4146
06	02/02	D	23	M	Y	Y	N	Y	Y	1271
07	02/03	F	19	M	Y	Y	N	N	Y	300
08	02/05	I	44	M	N	Y	N	N	Y	766
09	02/19	G	28	M	Y	N	N	Y	Y	23
10	02/22	E	29	F	N	Y	Y	N	Y	543
11	02/23	A	21	F	Y	Y	Y	N	Y	1897
12	02/24	H	43	M	N	Y	Y	N	Y	1220
13	02/26	B	49	F	N	N	N	N	Y	644
14	02/26	H	42	F	N	N	Y	N	Y	2581
15	02/27	E	59	F	Y	Y	Y	N	Y	2892
16	02/27	E	18	M	Y	N	Y	N	Y	814
17	02/27	A	19	M	N	Y	Y	N	Y	2812
18	02/28	E	63	F	Y	Y	Y	N	Y	4218
19	02/28	E	61	F	Y	Y	Y	N	Y	3410
20	02/29	A	40	M	N	Y	Y	N	Y	4297

*ALT = Alanine aminotransferase

Source: CDC (2012, p. 2-2).

examine the association between disease status and exposure to potential risk factors. This process is referred to as *analytical epidemiology* (see the following descriptions).

Time

In an outbreak investigation, key events should be chronologically ordered to create a framework. The following aspects should be determined:

1. The time of onset of manifestations among patients and their contacts

2. The period of exposure to the causal agent or potential risk factors

3. Time when treatments were administered or control measures implemented; as noted previously, this can change the clinical picture for individual patients or the epidemic curve in a community when an effective control measure is implemented

4. Time of potentially related events or unusual circumstances that might relate to the outbreak: Did the persons who became ill recently attend a large gathering? Did a power outage occur that might have affected food storage? Did a storm lead to contamination of the water supply?

During an outbreak of coccidioidomycosis (a fungal lung infection, also known as San Joaquin fever) in 1994 in California, the majority of the patients and the highest attack rates were identified in Simi Valley. Investigators noted that the Northridge earthquake, magnitude 6.7, had occurred 7 days earlier. Because of the geography of Simi Valley, multiple landslides had occurred, generating large dust clouds. They postulated and eventually demonstrated that exposure to the dust clouds, which contained large amounts of fungal arthrospores, was a major risk factor for disease (Schneider et al., 1997).

An essential way to evaluate the time component of an outbreak is to use the data from the case finding to construct an epidemic curve, commonly called an *epicurve*. The epicurve is a simple histogram that plots the number of cases on the y-axis (the vertical axis) and the time of onset, or in certain instances the time of death, on the x-axis (the horizontal axis). Certain factors should be kept in mind when constructing an epicurve:

- Because time is continuous, each interval is contiguous; thus, no gaps exist between the different periods (this is a histogram, not a bar chart).
- Each patient is represented by a box of uniform size where the x-axis dimension is the time interval when the person became ill. Therefore, the area under the epicurve is proportional to the number of cases.
- The time interval on the x-axis is, by convention, one-quarter to one-third of the incubation period. If the interval is less than this value, it will stretch out the epicurve, and if it is considerably more, it will compress the epicurve. If the epicurve is distorted, making inferences about the transmission mode in the outbreak is difficult. For example, in an investigation of a *Salmonella* species outbreak where the incubation often is in a 12- to 16-hour range, the time interval on the epicurve should be 4 hours. However, with an investigation of an outbreak caused by an unknown agent where the incubation period has not been calculated, constructing an epicurve with the correct x-axis scale is difficult.

Epicurves

Examination of the shape of the epicurve is often helpful in determining the mode of transmission for a particular outbreak.

Point-source outbreaks

One of the most common presentations occurs with a single exposure of a susceptible population to the causative agent. This is referred to as a *point-source outbreak*. In point-source outbreaks, the epicurve typically indicates a single peak with a fairly steep leading edge and a more gradual downslope (Figure 6.4).

Figure 6.4   Cases of Gastrointestinal Illness by Time of Onset of Symptoms

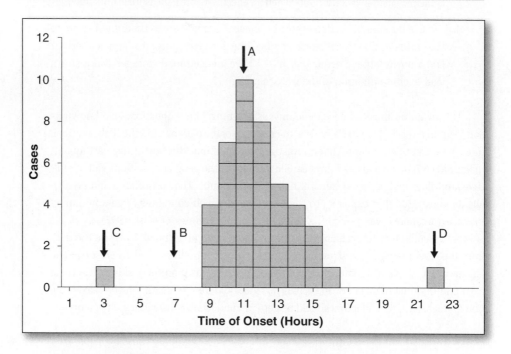

This type of epicurve can be extremely helpful during the early investigative stages. In this example, the median point of the curve is demonstrated by arrow A, the common exposure is indicated by arrow B, and the incubation period for the disease is the time interval between A and B. Also in this example, two cases fall outside of the general population of cases and are marked by arrows C and D. These latter two cases are commonly referred to as *outliers*. In an investigation where a point-source exposure is apparent, the agent causing the outbreak is known, but the common exposure is unknown; investigators can use the known incubation period and median of the epicurve to calculate the likely period of exposure (arrow B). They then focus their investigation on the period around point B. Alternatively, if a common exposure is known but the specific agent is unknown, the team can use the epicurve to estimate the incubation period for the causative agent. This information is highly useful in narrowing down potential causes.

Practical Point: The outliers in investigations often provide extremely useful information and should be examined carefully. In Figure 6.4, two cases are clearly outside of the general group of cases, one of them occurring before the common exposure. If this were a foodborne outbreak, what possible explanations might exist for these cases?

- This might represent errors in the data collection or coding.
- They might be random cases completely unrelated to the outbreak investigation.
- Case C might represent the person who prepared the contaminated food item.
- The person associated with Case D might have been exposed to a small innoculum (simply tasted someone else's food).
- The person associated with Case D might have eaten the contaminated food item after the common exposure (leftovers).
- Case D might be a secondary case (i.e., the person was exposed to an ill person rather than directly to the food source).

In July 1976, a severe respiratory disease broke out among persons who had attended the American Legion Convention held at a Philadelphia, Pennsylvania, hotel. The causative agent for this outbreak and the mode of transmission were unknown at the time. The epicurve for this outbreak (Figure 6.5; CDC, unpublished data, 1976) was highly indicative of a point-source outbreak. In this instance, the point source was the American Legion Convention. The team also recognized that the time spent in the lobby of the convention hotel was directly proportional to the risk for acquiring the disease (Fraser at al., 1977). The causative agent was subsequently identified as a novel gram-negative coccobacillus later named *Legionellae pneumophila* (Legionnaires' disease). This particular organism grows in stagnant water sources (e.g., cooling towers), and the investigation revealed that the main outflow for the hotel's cooling system was into the lobby.

One challenge that investigators faced during the 1976 outbreak was the unknown incubation for this newly discovered disease. Unsure of what interval to use for the x-axis, they drew multiple epicurves that resulted in differently shaped curves, based on how compressed or stretched the x-axis time intervals were drawn. The correct epicurve (Figure 6.5) indicated a point-source; however, other epicurves indicated other transmission modes, as described in the following section.

Propagated transmission outbreaks

In disease outbreaks where the infectious agent is transmitted *person to person*, the epicurve will typically demonstrate a biphasic pattern with two or more peaks (this is also referred to as *propagated transmission*). In the following hypothetical example

Figure 6.5 Legionnaires' Disease by Date of Onset, Philadelphia, Pennsylvania, July 1–August 18, 1976

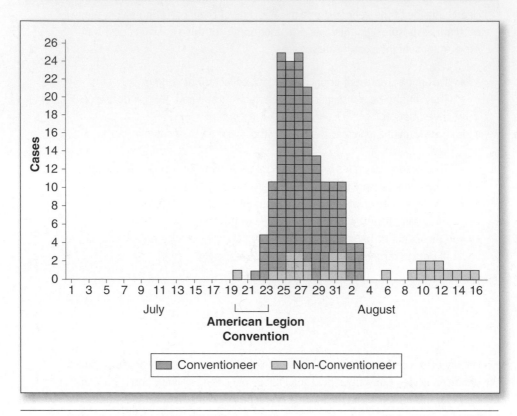

Source: CDC, unpublished data, 1976.

(Figure 6.6), a child infected with measles is introduced to a school where none of the children are immune (arrow A). The infected child acts as a point-source, and an initial group of cases (arrow B) with a curve similar to the point-source example described previously occurs (i.e., the time interval between the arrival of the infected child and the median of the first peak is equal to the disease incubation period). As these initial patients become ill, they infect other susceptible patients, and a wave of secondary cases occurs (arrow C). The time interval between the median of the primary and secondary case peaks is equal to the disease incubation period. Figure 6.6 depicts a textbook person-to-person transmission; in reality, the curve rarely looks this clean. Typically, the peaks indicate greater dispersion, and a clean and obvious delineation between the primary and secondary cases does not exist.

For example, from March 27 to May 5, 1995, seven suspected cases of viral hemorrhagic fever were identified in Kikwit, Zaire, a city of 400,000 people located approximately 200 kilometers east of the capital city, Kinshasa. All seven ill persons died (Figure 6.7). Additional suspect cases were identified. Serologic testing of specimens from Kikwit was consistent with Ebola-like virus infection. This was the beginning of a major Ebola outbreak. The epicurve prepared by the field teams (CDC, unpublished data,1995)

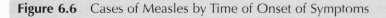

Figure 6.6   Cases of Measles by Time of Onset of Symptoms

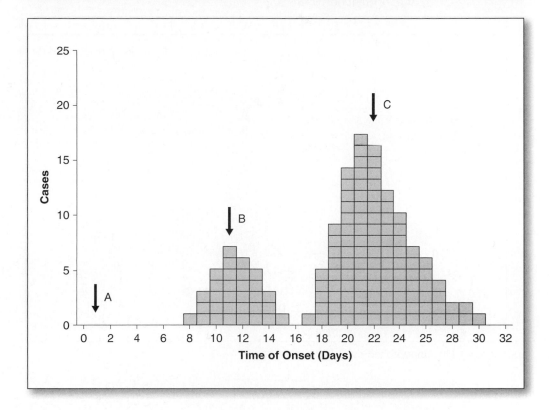

reveals a pattern typical for a person-to-person transmission mode, the mechanism usually observed in Ebola outbreaks where transmission is through direct contact with contaminated bodily fluids. This graph illustrates five fairly clear cycles of transmission where the incubation period appears to be 12–16 days. During this outbreak, a total of 315 cases with a 78% case-fatality rate occurred. Twenty-five percent of the cases occurred among health care workers (Breman, van der Groen, Peters, & Heymann, 1997). As the outbreak continued, the data curve tended to spread out, and the separation between the cycles was not as clean. This was likely caused by individual differences in susceptibility, size of inoculum, and time of infection.

Continuous source outbreak

The third type of transmission that can be demonstrated by an epicurve is displayed in Figure 6.8. This type of pattern has a sharp upslope similar to the point-source outbreak. However, instead of a more gradual decline, a plateau phase continues for multiple incubation periods before the outbreak ends. For example, if a break occurs in a community's sewage system, leading to contamination of the water supply, a sharp increase probably will occur in the number of cases (sharp upslope). If the break is not repaired and the contamination continues, the number of infections will continue and eventually reach a steady state (plateau phase). When the break is repaired, the cases will decline.

Figure 6.7 Suspected Viral Hemorrhagic Fever Deaths, Bandundu Province, Zaire, April–June 1995

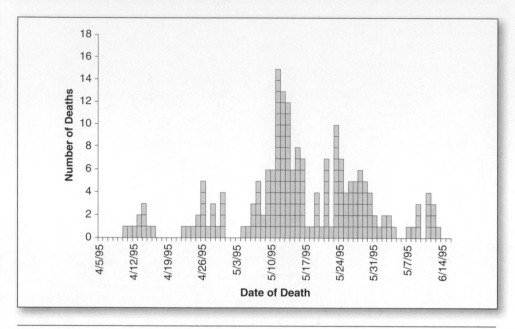

Source: CDC, unpublished data, 1995.

Figure 6.8 Distribution of Hepatitis A Cases by Month of Onset

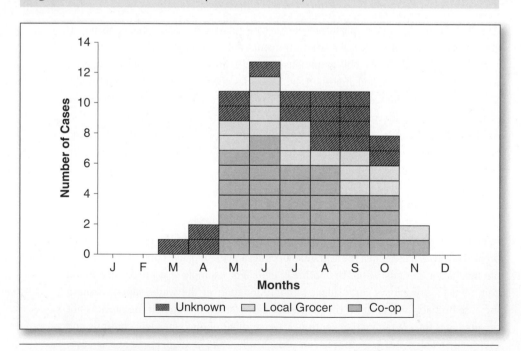

Source: CDC, unpublished data, 1981.

The example in Figure 6.8 is taken from a field investigation of hepatitis A in California (CDC, unpublished data, 1981). Person-to-person transmission is a common mechanism identified in hepatitis A outbreaks; however, in this instance, the team was able to rule this out as a likely mechanism. The epicurve revealed a potential continuous source outbreak, and the team was able to identify a specific brand of orange juice, sold at multiple locations, as the implicated item. A single lot of contaminated product had been sold as a frozen concentrate. Because consumers had bought the contaminated juice and stored it in their freezers until use, this served as a continuous source of infectious agent.

Place

The second of the three primary descriptive categories (time, place, and person) must be considered next. When orienting patient data to place, consider the following:

- **Residence:** Where do the affected persons live? What hotel rooms did they stay in? For hospitalized patients, what rooms were they in?
- **Occupation:** Where do they work? Where do they go to school?
- **Activity sites:** Where do they go for recreational activities? Where do they shop? What other leisure activities do they have? At a convention or meeting, what sessions did they attend?
- **Exposure sites:** Map their proximity to known exposure sites (e.g., near a water tower in a legionellosis outbreak).

One of the key tools of the epidemiologist for assessing place-based factors is the spot map. This is a way to map the location of the patients by using one or more of the variables described. Spot maps can be useful when drawn at different observation levels. For example, maps can be used to describe the location of cases within a building or other structure, at the neighborhood or city block level, or at the county or state level. Maps can be oriented toward residence or specific exposure sites (e.g., areas visited during a convention, meeting, or rooms in which known patients are hospitalized), or they can be oriented to include certain activity sites.

Figure 6.9 is based on one of the most iconic spot maps of all time—John Snow's investigation of the Broad Street pump mentioned in Chapter 1 (Snow, Frost, & Richardson, 1936). In 1854, the prevailing theory of infectious disease transmission was the miasma theory that disease was caused by bad air; the modern germ theory of disease had not been widely disseminated. On the basis of earlier work with cholera, Snow, a London anesthesiologist, believed that contaminated water might be the cholera transmission route. During the 1854 outbreak, Snow decided to map out the locations of where all the persons with cholera either lived or worked. Because of his suspicion that water played a key role, he mapped out the public water pumps in the affected areas and questioned patients about where they got their water supply. It became clear from his initial map that patients were clustered around the Broad Street pump. The map clearly indicated a much higher density of cases clustered around the Broad Street pump

(Pump A) than the other four pumps in the area (Figure 6.9). Outliers also supported his conclusion that the pump was a risk factor for cholera. The first outlier consisted of ill persons from outside of the immediate area who had traveled to get their water from the Broad Street pump because it was reputed to be of higher quality than other water sources. Second, Snow noted a two-block area just east of the pump where no cases had occurred. When he investigated, he discovered that this was a brewery that had a separate deep-well water supply. In addition, workers were allowed a daily ration of malt liquor! The legend is that Snow, on recognizing the danger posed by the pump, removed the pump handle and stopped the outbreak. In reality, he presented his findings to the local borough council, and they ordered the pump closed.

Figure 6.10 is an example of a spot map drawn for an outbreak known to be associated with a facility (CDC, unpublished data, 2007). This map illustrates the berthing space on a Navy ship where one patient had cavitary tuberculosis that had been misdiagnosed as atypical pneumonia. With this map, the investigators displayed the sleeping spaces of the index patient (the box with the x), the general air

Figure 6.9 Distribution of Cholera Cases and Implicated Water Well, Golden Square Area of London, August–September 1854

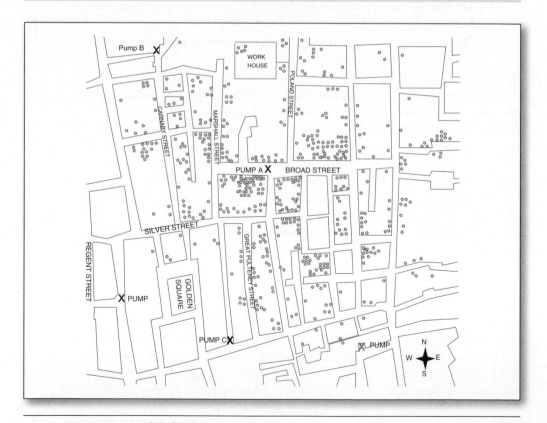

Source: Snow, Frost, and Richardson (1936).

Figure 6.10   Spot Map Showing the Berths of Persons Infected With Tuberculosis

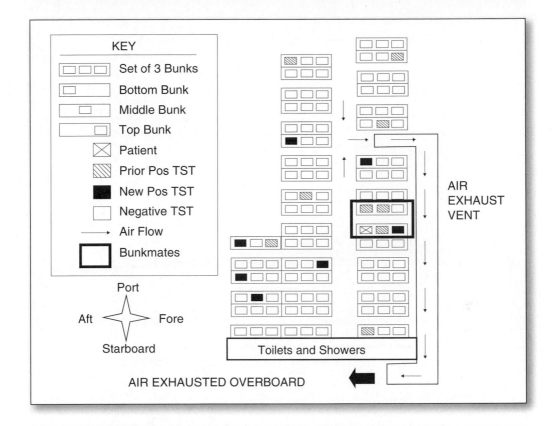

Source: CDC, unpublished data, 2007.

flow in the compartment, and persons with evidence of new tuberculosis infection (black boxes). This map helped prioritize the contact investigation and, because of the index patient's proximity to the main outflow vent, helped explain why so few cases occurred among the other sailors in the berthing compartment (CDC, 2007).

USING PLACE TO SOLVE AN ANTHRAX OUTBREAK

Perhaps one of the best examples of using place as a tool in solving an outbreak involved anthrax infections that occurred in the Russian town of Sverdlovsk in 1979 (Figure 6.11).

(Continued)

Figure 6.11 Onset of Illness by Week, Among Fatal Cases of Anthrax, Sverdlovsk, Russia, 1979

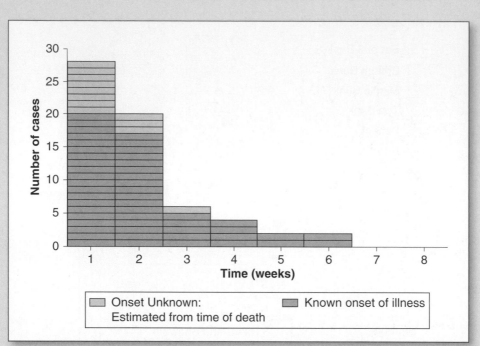

Source: Meselson et al. (1994).

Anthrax is a bacterial enzootic pathogen that has a stable spore stage, which is infectious for humans. As a result of these properties, this organism has been adapted for use as a biologic weapon. Anthrax infection among humans takes three forms. Cutaneous anthrax (95% of naturally occurring human cases) has a case-fatality rate of 5%–20%. Gastrointestinal anthrax caused by consumption of contaminated food products has a case-fatality rate of 25%–60%. Pulmonary anthrax, caused by inhalation of aerosolized spores, is estimated to have a case-fatality rate > 85% (Heymann, 2008; Mandell, Bennett, & Dolin, 2005).

During the 1979 Sverdlovsk outbreak, 96 human cases of anthrax infection were reported, with 64 deaths. At the time, Western authorities were suspicious that this was inhalational anthrax caused by a release from a military microbiologic facility that was believed to be a bioweapons production facility (Defense Intelligence Agency, 1986). Animal cases also occurred in the region, and the Soviet health authorities reported that the infected persons had contracted gastrointestinal anthrax when they obtained contaminated meat on the black market. In 1991, newly elected Russian Federation President Boris Yeltsin, who had been the head Communist Party official in Sverdlovsk in 1979, authorized a reinvestigation of the incident by a team of Western and Russian scientists. Despite attempts by the KGB (Committee for State Security) in 1979 to confiscate all of the data from the investigation, the team led by Harvard professor Matthew Meselson had access to patient records as well as clinical specimens (Meselson et al., 1994). The specimen analysis clearly indicated that the persons who died had suffered from inhalational, not gastrointestinal anthrax.

Anthrax has a usual incubation period of 1–7 days, but depending on the initial inoculum, this can extend to 60 days. The epicurve for this outbreak is highly indicative of a point-source transmission (sharp increase with more gradual decrease), which is consistent with an inadvertent release of an aerosol form of the bacteria. Investigators noted that the age distribution of the patients did not include children (the youngest patient was aged 24 years); therefore, they focused their investigation on where persons were during daylight hours (presumably, the adults were at work and the children at school). The team obtained a satellite photo of Sverdlovsk and mapped out the daytime locations for the patients (Figure 6.12).

Figure 6.12   Map of Sverdlovsk, Russia, Showing Location of Fatal Cases of Anthrax, 1979

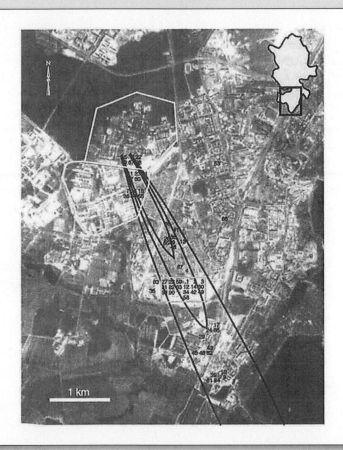

Source: Meselson et al. (1994).

In this photo, each of the cases is indicated by a case number. The shape at the top left of the map outlines the Microbiology and Virology Institute, which the investigators labeled Compound 19. The adjacent shape outlines Compound 32, another part of the military complex, and the rectangle below that outlines an open-air tile factory where many of the infected persons worked.

The locations of the cases were tightly clustered around a line extending from Compound 19 and projecting 330° to the southwest. During the same period that the human cases were occurring, anthrax cases among domestic animals were being reported in the villages surrounding Sverdlovsk 50 kilometers away. When the investigators mapped the location of the villages, they found that they also lay along the line oriented at 330° from Compound 19. These observations were highly indicative of a windborne plume of anthrax originating at Compound 19.

The investigators had an apparent point-source transmission with a known agent, a probable source of the organism, but an unknown period of exposure. By using the epi-curve and the incubation period for anthrax, they were able to calculate the median onset of disease and focus their investigation on April 2. The meteorologic data from an airport located 10 miles from the ceramics factory revealed that the predominant wind pattern in April was east to west. Approximately 2% of the time, the winds blew from the north along a southeasterly vector (330°); April 2 was one of those days.

In 1992, the Russian government admitted that Compound 19 had been part of an offensive biologic weapons program. The release occurred when air filters on the factory exhaust were not properly activated (Christopher, Cieslak, Pavlin, & Eitzen, 1997). Meselson et al. (1994) performed complex mathematical modeling based on the infectivity of anthrax spores, rates of infection among the exposed persons, and the case locations. They calculated that the upper limit for the amount of weaponized anthrax released in this outbreak was one gram.

Person

After identifying and counting cases and orienting the data in terms of time and place, thoroughly characterize the patients by collecting the following information:

- **Identifying information:** Name, address, telephone number, respondent (e.g., self, parent of child, spouse)
- **Demographic information:** Birthdate or age, sex, occupation, education, socioeconomic status
- **Clinical information:** Signs/symptoms, severity or outcome (hospitalization, death), time of onset, duration, documented medical care (name and telephone number in case contacting the provider is needed), preexisting medical conditions
- **Epidemiology:** Risk factor information (exposures and contacts), activities in which respondents might have participated, contacts with ill persons (are others ill in the family?), other factors shared in common among the other patients

The ultimate goal is to calculate and compare rates between groups on the basis of potential risk factors. For this reason, gathering denominator data is critically important for deriving rates for risk estimates. This crucial step is often overlooked. Unless groups being compared are identical in terms of size and composition, simple case counts cannot be compared.

Formulate and Test Hypotheses

After completing the descriptive epidemiologic study when the data have been analyzed in terms of time, place, and person, the next step is to use the results of this analysis to formulate and test hypotheses.

As noted previously, the primary reason for the investigation is to identify effective actions to control the outbreak and to prevent additional cases or a recurrence of the problem. Developing hypotheses that explain the outbreak by characterizing the type of exposure, the agent, source or reservoir, mode of transmission, or risk factors is therefore important.

At times, a hypothesis will be apparent from the descriptive analysis of the time, place, and person data. However, using other methods to develop a testable hypothesis might be necessary. Possible approaches include

- looking at previous outbreaks with similar agents or exposures,
- reviewing information obtained from case interviews,
- conducting open-ended questioning among patients or their contacts (hypothesis-generating interviews),
- reviewing anecdotes and impressions or ideas from local community members and leaders, and
- examining outliers (i.e., cases that did not occur during the expected time sequence for disease; early or late cases).

Testing the hypothesis can sometimes be accomplished with the descriptive data that already have been collected during the case finding. In the majority of cases, using comparison groups to evaluate the contribution of different risk factors is necessary. This frequently requires **planning additional studies** to collect the data needed to evaluate risk factors, and the two most commonly used study designs are the case-control study and the cohort study. Chapter 7 contains a detailed explanation of these study designs; here I provide a summary of the advantages and disadvantages of each design for outbreak investigation (Table 6.2).

Outbreak investigation teams typically start with a case-control study because it is usually faster, cheaper, and permits evaluation of multiple risk factors. After a specific risk factor has been identified, the team might conduct a cohort study to determine the specific risk associated with that exposure.

Implement and Evaluate Control Measures

As noted at the beginning of this chapter, public health officials should act as soon as they have a rational basis for implementing control measures. Public health

Table 6.2 Advantages and Disadvantages of Case-Control and Cohort Studies for Outbreak Investigation

	Advantages	Disadvantages
Case-control studies (use odds ratio as the measure of association)	• are quick and relatively inexpensive • require fewer study participants • permit evaluation of multiple exposures • are well suited for rare diseases	• are backward in that they begin with the disease and look back to the exposure (determining if the exposure preceded the disease might be problematic) • are unsuitable for rare exposures • cannot directly calculate the risk associated with a specific exposure because the number of control subjects is variable • are prone to bias in selecting the control subjects and prone to recall bias
Cohort studies (use risk ratio as the measure of association)	• have a logical temporal sequence (i.e., investigators start with the exposure and observe for occurrence of disease) • permit calculation of the risk associated with the exposure • allow evaluation of multiple outcomes from a single exposure (e.g., a study looking at smokers and nonsmokers enables evaluation of lung disease, cardiovascular, or cancer as potential outcomes) • are well suited to studies of rare exposures	• might require substantial numbers of subjects if the disease is rare • tend to be more challenging logistically (longer term, more participants, more expensive) • can be subject to bias if subjects drop out for specific reasons • might result in participants' behavior being influenced and the results being biased because the participants are being observed • are dependent on records being available (retrospective cohort studies)

authorities do not wait until the end of an investigation to implement control measures; instead, they implement them as soon as practicable. The big challenge for investigators is to determine when sufficient information is available on which to base a decision. Act too soon and unnecessary negative economic or social consequences might result for the persons affected by the control measure (e.g., closing a restaurant, causing loss of income). Act too slowly and additional persons might become ill who would have been spared. Unfortunately, no hard and fast rules exist on exactly when to implement control measures; each situation is unique.

Common control measures available to public health authorities include the following examples:

- **Eliminating or treating the source**: Recalling an implicated product, removing an infected food handler from work and providing medical treatment, or eliminating insect breeding sites
- **Cohorting patients**: A common approach in hospitals, child care, and other institutional settings
- **Preventing further exposures**: Washing hands and covering coughs during an influenza outbreak, safe food preparation practices, educational efforts to change knowledge and behaviors to limit HIV transmission
- **Protecting populations at risk**: Vaccination or chemoprophylaxis for persons at risk

Finally, evaluating the effect of control measures and adjusting the public health response accordingly is crucial. This might involve initiating **longer term surveillance** to monitor the ongoing effectiveness of control measures and to provide early warning of disease recurrence.

Communicate Findings

The final, critical step in any investigation (and one that is often omitted) is to prepare a written record of the investigation and outcomes. Writing the report

- provides a way for the team to formally convey recommendations to the requesting authority,
- might be an institutional requirement (i.e., the institution supporting the investigation will probably require a formal report for the official record),
- records the activities and methods for future reference (if the same type of problem occurs again, future investigators will be aided by seeing how a previous investigation was conducted),
- ensures rapid dissemination or notification to others regarding a serious problem having immediate implications (e.g., communicable diseases, a contaminated commercial product),
- shares experience with others if especially interesting, and
- provides communication skill training.

Different formats might be used for the team's report, including a preliminary written report to the requesting authority, a final written report, publication in a public health bulletin (i.e., a state health department newsletter or a national-level epidemiology bulletin), an article for a peer-reviewed journal, or as an abstract and presentation at a professional meeting.

OUTBREAK INVESTIGATION: A CASE STUDY

The following investigation, conducted by local, state, and federal health authorities in 2009, demonstrates many of the steps in an outbreak investigation (CDC, 2010).

Background

In 1996, public health authorities established a laboratory-based surveillance system called PulseNet. Participating public health laboratories from across the country perform standardized molecular subtyping of enteric pathogens by using DNA fingerprinting with a technique called *pulsed-field gel electrophoresis*. The resulting fingerprints are sent electronically to a database maintained at CDC. Computer algorithms are used to determine if a statistically significant increase is occurring in any given bacterial subtype. By looking at data from across the entire country, the PulseNet system frequently is able to identify clusters that might not be apparent to a single state or local health department laboratory.

Recognition of the Outbreak

During August–September 2009, the PulseNet system detected a multistate cluster of *Salmonella enteritidis* serotype Montevideo cultures from 13 states that had identical DNA fingerprints, indicating a possible common source. The observed number of reports approximated the expected baseline of two to three reports per week, and the PulseNet system continued to monitor this common pattern. In November, the number of reported infections with the outbreak strain had increased to 15–20 samples per week, and CDC initiated a multistate investigation. By November 30, CDC had identified 127 cases in 30 states (Figure 6.13; CDC, unpublished data, 2010).

At this point in the investigation, the team had already completed certain basic steps. They had first verified the diagnosis; because PulseNet is a laboratory-based surveillance system, this step was fairly simple. Next, they confirmed the epidemic by comparing the number of cases of a single strain of *Salmonella* Montevideo reported to the national system to the historical rate of reports for this organism. Finally, the samples reported to the PulseNet system were instrumental in the first phase of identifying and counting cases.

The investigators then began a case-control study to try to identify the risk factors for infection. The team created the following case definition: a laboratory-confirmed infection with the outbreak strain of *Salmonella* Montevideo in a person with diarrhea onset, or if that date was not available, isolation date on or after July 1, 2009. (Note that this definition includes the elements of time, place, and person—although it does not define *diarrhea*.)

The investigators identified a total of 272 cases (Figure 6.14). The epicurve is not indicative of a point-source or person-to-person transmission mechanism but is more consistent with an ongoing source of infection.

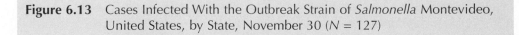

Figure 6.13   Cases Infected With the Outbreak Strain of *Salmonella* Montevideo, United States, by State, November 30 (*N* = 127)

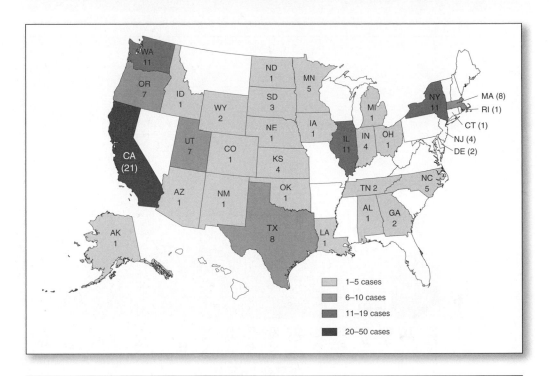

Source: CDC, unpublished data, 2010.

After gathering the basic descriptive data for this outbreak, the investigators began the process of hypothesis generating to try to identify potential risk factors for infection. They used different strategies.

- **"Shotgun questionnaire":** A long, standardized questionnaire that asked about > 300 possible exposures, including foods, beverages, and animal contact
- **Open-ended telephone interviews:** Less structured and focused on asking about travel, food consumption, and exposure to restaurants and grocery stores during the 7 days preceding illness
- **In-depth interviews:** Conducted in homes and included inventory of pantries and refrigerators

The open-ended questioning of one group of ill persons indicated that 58% reported having eaten salami, 75% reported having eaten delicatessen meats, and 55% reported having shopped at a national warehouse club store. Because the club store tracks purchases by all members, health officials in Washington were able to compile a complete record of all purchases made by seven ill persons. After

Figure 6.14 Number of Infections ($N = 272$) With the Outbreak Strain of *Salmonella* Montevideo, by Week of Isolation Date, United States, 2009–2010

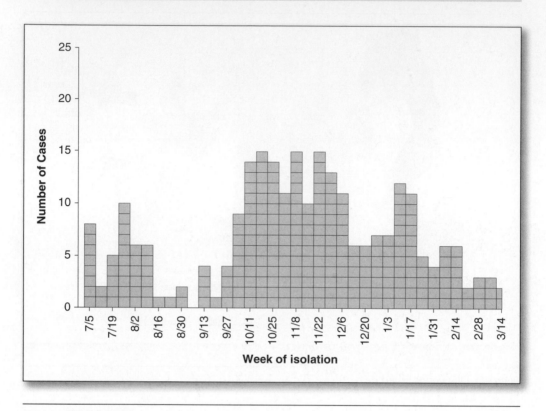

Source: CDC (2010).

reviewing over 750 pages of shopping records, the team identified a brand of delicatessen meat (Company A) that had been purchased by five of the seven patients before they became ill. By comparing shopping records for patients in other states, they were able to identify 19 persons who had purchased the Company A product an average of 4 days before onset of illness.

After identifying a possible source of the infection, the investigators set up a case-control study where the control subjects were matched to the case-patients by neighborhood by using a reverse telephone directory system. Exposures evaluated in this study included the Company A delicatessen meats as well as other food items reported in the hypothesis-generating questionnaires. This study revealed that case-patients were four to eight times more likely to have eaten any Italian-style delicatessen meat.

The outbreak strain of *Salmonella* Montevideo was isolated from eight samples of Company A delicatessen meat collected from case-patient households and from retail stores. Two of these samples were taken from intact, sealed products obtained from retail stores. At this point, the team had formulated and tested a hypothesis, and on the basis of the initial results, they had conducted additional studies to further support their findings.

Working in collaboration with the Food and Drug Administration, the team implemented the following three control measures:

- Multiple consumer health advisories were issued by CDC, the Food and Drug Administration, the U.S. Department of Agriculture, and state and local health departments.
- Company A voluntarily recalled 1.3 million pounds of Italian sausage products.
- Additional recalls of 132,000 pounds of deli meat products were issued.

Further investigation at the Company A plant did not reveal any obvious lapses in food preparation protocols that might explain the massive contamination. The meat products were cooked at temperatures adequate to kill any *Salmonella*. However, after cooking, the meat was rolled in spices to apply a red and black pepper coating. Samples of pepper from Company A were also determined to contain the outbreak strain of *Salmonella* Montevideo. Contaminated lots of pepper were traced back to two separate spice companies, and these tracebacks resulted in an additional recall of >100,000 pounds of pepper. Ongoing surveillance for the outbreak strain of *Salmonella* Montevideo was maintained by PulseNet.

Conclusion

This investigation illustrates the key steps in an outbreak investigation, as outlined in Figure 6.1. Of note, after the team identified a likely vehicle (the delicatessen meat), they implemented well-designed control measures to protect the public's health. However, they also planned additional studies during the traceback to confirm the specific source of the contamination. Armed with the additional information that the pepper was implicated as the source of contamination for the meat products, they implemented additional control measures.

CURRENT ISSUES AND FUTURE DIRECTIONS

The way outbreaks are identified and investigated will continue to evolve in response to changes in technology and informatics. We have already seen a dramatic increase in the number of disease outbreaks that are first identified through clusters of case-reports picked up by increasingly sophisticated surveillance systems (e.g., PulseNet). However, with increasing sensitivity of those systems, the new challenge is to sort through the growing number of detected clusters to identify the significant public health events. As information technology improves, public health will likely have access to more timely data through the expanding use of electronic health records (EHRs). Large medical systems like the Veterans Administration are already developing the capability for real-time detection of outbreaks through monitoring of their EHR system.

Information technology also increases the tools that investigators can use to gather data. The case study described previously demonstrates the use of computerized shopping records to identify exposures reliably. Monitoring the frequency of specific inquiries to online search sites is being developed as a technique for monitoring infectious disease spread like the flu (www.google.org/flutrends/us/#US). The Internet is also being used with increasing frequency not just to get information out to consumers, but to gather information from them. Administering outbreak questionnaires electronically can dramatically improve the response time and efficiency of an investigation and lead to more rapid identification of control measures. This methodology has potential limitations, though, the most obvious being data security and privacy concerns.

Finally, changes in the technology available to teams in the field will affect the way investigations are conducted. Small handheld devices make data collection easier and faster, and they reduce errors when data from different field teams are consolidated. These devices can also aid in the interview process through the use of memory aids like photos or maps. Improvements in GPS technology have made mapping by field teams much easier and more accurate, thus improving the element of "place" in many investigations.

ADDITIONAL RESOURCES

Centers for Disease Control and Prevention. (2006). *Principles of epidemiology in public health practice* (3rd ed.). Atlanta, GA: US Department of Health and Human Services, CDC. http://www.cdc.gov/osels/scientific_edu/SS1978/SS1978.pdf

Dworkin, M. (Ed.) (2011). *Cases in field epidemiology: A global perspective.* Sudbury, MA: Jones and Bartlett Learning.

Gregg, M. (Ed.). (2008). *Field epidemiology* (3rd ed.). New York, NY: Oxford University Press.

Pendergrast, M. (2010). *Inside the outbreaks: The elite medical detectives of the Epidemic Intelligence Service.* New York, NY: Houghton Mifflin Harcourt.

REFERENCES

Breman, J. G., van der Groen, G., Peters, C. J., & Heymann, D. L. (1997). International Colloquium on Ebola Virus Research: Summary report. *Journal of Infectious Diseases, 176,* 1058–1063.

Centers for Disease Control. (1981). Pneumocystis pneumonia—Los Angeles. *Morbidity and Mortality Weekly Report, 30,* 250–252.

Centers for Disease Control. (1982). Epidemiologic aspects of the current outbreak of Kaposi's sarcoma and opportunistic infections. *New England Journal of Medicine, 306*, 248–252.

Centers for Disease Control. (2012). *Principles of epidemiology in public health practice: An introduction to applied epidemiology and biostatistics* (3rd ed.). Atlanta, GA: U.S. Department of Health and Human Services.

Centers for Disease Control and Prevention. (2007). Brief report: Latent tuberculosis infection among sailors and civilians aboard *U.S.S. Ronald Reagan*—United States, January–July 2006. *Morbidity and Mortality Weekly Report, 55*, 1381–1382.

Centers for Disease Control and Prevention. (2010). *Salmonella* Montevideo infections associated with salami products made with contaminated imported black and red pepper—United States, July 2009–April 2010. *Morbidity and Mortality Weekly Report, 59*, 1647–1650.

Centers for Disease Control and Prevention. (2013). *The public health system and the 10 essential public health services*. Retrieved from http://www.cdc.gov/nphpsp/essentialservices.html

Christopher, G. W., Cieslak, T. J., Pavlin, J. A., & Eitzen, E. M., Jr. (1997). Biological warfare: A historical perspective. *Journal of the American Medical Association, 278*, 412–417.

Defense Intelligence Agency. (1986). *Soviet biological warfare threat* (Document no. DST-1610F-057-86). Washington, DC: U.S. Department of Defense. Retrieved from http://www.gwu.edu/~nsarchiv/NSAEBB/NSAEBB61/Sverd26.pdf

Dondero, T. J., Jr., Rendtorff, R. C., Mallison, G. F., Weeks, R. M., Levy, J. S., Wong, E. W., & Schaffner W. (1980). An outbreak of Legionnaires' disease associated with a contaminated air-conditioning cooling tower. *New England Journal of Medicine, 302*, 365–370.

Fraser, D. W., Tsai, T. R., Orenstein, W., Parkin, W. E., Beecham, H. J., Sharrar, R. G., . . . Brachman, P. S. (1977). Legionnaires' disease: Description of an epidemic of pneumonia. *New England Journal of Medicine, 297*, 1189–1197.

Heymann, D. L. (Ed.). (2008). *Control of communicable diseases manual* (19th ed.). Washington, DC: American Public Health Association.

Hoffman, P. C., Arnow, P. M., Goldmann, D. A., Parrott, P. L., Stamm, W. E., & McGowan, J. E., Jr. (1976). False-positive blood cultures association with nonsterile blood collection tubes. *Journal of the American Medical Association, 236*, 2073–2075.

Kempf, A. M., & Remington, P. L. (2007). New challenges for telephone survey research in the twenty-first century. *Annual Review of Public Health, 28*, 113–126.

Last, J. M. (Ed.). (1995). *A dictionary of epidemiology* (3rd ed.). Oxford, England: Oxford University Press.

Lui, K. J., & Kendal, A. P. (1987). Impact of influenza epidemics on mortality in the United States from October 1972 to May 1985. *American Journal of Public Health, 77*, 712–716.

Mandell, G. L., Bennett, J. E., & Dolin, R. (2005). *Principles and practice of infectious disease* (6th ed., Vol. 2). Philadelphia, PA: Elsevier, Churchill, Livingstone.

Maxted, A. M., Grant, D., Schulte, C., Rausch-Phung, E., Blog, D., Newman, A., & Martin, S. (2012, April). *Factors associated with false-positive polymerase chain reaction results during a pertussis outbreak—Jefferson County, New York, 2010–2011*. Paper presented at the 61st Annual Epidemic Intelligence Service Conference, Atlanta, GA. Retrieved from http://www.cdc.gov/EIS/downloads/2012.EIS.Conference.pdf

Meselson, M., Guillemin, J., Hugh-Jones, M., Langmuir, A., Popova, I., Shelokov, A., & Yampolskaya, O. (1994). The Sverdlovsk anthrax outbreak of 1979. *Science, 266*, 1202–1208.

Mostashari, F., Bunning, M. L., Kitsutani, P. T., Singer, D. A., Nash, D., Cooper, M. J., . . . Campbell, G. L. (2001). Epidemic West Nile encephalitis, New York, 1999: Results of a household-based seroepidemiological survey. *Lancet, 358*, 261–264.

Reed, C., Fleming-Dutra, K., Terashita, D., Kozak, N., Marquez, P., Garrison, L., . . . Masola, L. (2011, April). *Role of social media in investigating an outbreak: The good, the bad, and the ugly—Los Angeles, February 2011.* Paper presented at the 60th Annual Epidemic Intelligence Service Conference, Atlanta, GA.

Scanlon, K. S., Blank, S., & Sinks, T. (1992, April). *Health effects among persons exposed to excess vitamin D.* Presented at the 41st Annual Epidemic Intelligence Service Conference, Atlanta, GA.

Schneider, E., Hajjeh, R. A., Spiegel, R. A., Jibson, R. W., Harp, E. L., Marshall, G. A., . . . Werner, S. B. (1997). A coccidioidomycosis outbreak following the Northridge, Calif, earthquake. *Journal of the American Medical Association, 277,* 904–908.

Snow, J., Frost, W. H., & Richardson, B. W. (1936). *Snow on cholera.* London, England: Humphrey Milford, Oxford University Press.

7

Cohort and
Case-Control Studies[1]

Lee Warner and Deborah Dee

Despite their scientific rigor, experimental designs, namely randomized controlled trials (RCTs), in which investigators fully control the exposure assignment of study participants in controlled research settings (see Chapter 8), are not always an option for evaluating clinical, behavioral, or structural interventions. Feasibility issues, financial constraints, or ethical concerns regarding the assignment of participants to potentially harmful exposures often preclude the conduct of randomized trials (Deeks et al., 2003; Gregg, 2008; Victora, Habicht, & Bryce, 2004). In these situations, observational studies have yielded critical information benefitting public health. An **observational study**—often a cohort or case-control design—allows investigators to monitor the experiences of study participants, but with no control over exposure assignment. Brief definitions of cohort and case-control studies are provided in Chapter 1, and the relative advantages and disadvantages of each method outlined in Chapter 6. Here, we discuss each of these two study designs in more depth, starting with a history of their use in the context of public health. We then cover key terms, discuss methodological considerations associated with each design, and provide guidance on how to plan and implement both types of studies.

A BRIEF HISTORY

Several landmark cohort and case-control studies conducted during the 20th century greatly advanced the rigor of these designs. They range from studies published in the

1950s and 1960s that demonstrated the now well-established epidemiologic link between cigarette smoking and lung cancer (Doll & Hill, 1954, 1956) to a 1970s study that implicated diethylstilbestrol (DES), a drug given to women early in pregnancy to prevent miscarriage, as the primary cause of a rare vaginal cancer diagnosed among their daughters (Herbst, Ulfelder, & Poskanzer, 1971). Subsequent similarly designed studies have documented a host of reproductive-related problems among DES-exposed daughters and sons (Hoover et al., 2011).

The utility of cohort and case-control study designs was first noted nearly a century earlier, however, during John Snow's search for the cause of severe outbreaks of cholera that affected the Soho area of London in both 1849 and 1854 (Snow, 1855/1965). As described in Chapters 1 and 6, Snow had long theorized that cholera was attributable to ingestion of contaminated water (but was unsure of the vector). Upon discovering that the London households most severely affected by the cholera outbreak were served by only two water supply companies (one of which Snow had suspected to have contaminated water), Snow traveled door to door to gather data and record the identity of the supplier for each household. He ultimately determined through novel statistical and mapping techniques that residents of houses that had been provided contaminated water by the Southwark and Vauxhall Company had a mortality rate from cholera (315 deaths per 10,000 households) that was nearly 10 times higher than those supplied water by the competing Lambeth Company (37 deaths per 10,000 households). Moreover, through interviews with relatives of the deceased, Snow traced many of the cases to a single nearby water pump at the corner of Cambridge Street and Broad Street that was supplied water by the Southwark and Vauxhall Company—this is the infamous Broad Street pump whose handle was eventually removed to further stem the outbreak.

As well described by others (Friis & Sellers, 2004; Hennekens & Buring, 1987; Rothman, 2002), the elegance of what has come to be known as Snow's "natural experiment" was best summarized by Snow himself in his 1855 work, *On the Mode of Communication of Cholera:*

In the subdistricts enumerated . . . as being supplied by both Companies, the mixing of the supply is of the most intimate kind. The pipes of each company go down all the streets, and into nearly all the courts and alleys. A few houses are supplied by one Company and a few by the other, according to the decision of the owner or occupier at that time when the Water Companies were in active competition. In many cases a single house has a supply different from that on either side. Each company supplies both rich and poor, both large houses and small; there is no difference either in the condition or occupation of the persons receiving the water of the different Companies. Now it must be evident that, if the diminution of cholera, in the districts partly supplied with improved water, depended on this supply, the houses receiving it would be the houses enjoying the whole benefit of the diminutions of the malady, whilst the houses supplied by the water from Battersea Fields would suffer the same mortality as they would if the improved supply did not exist at all. . . . As there is no difference whatever, either in the houses or the people receiving the supply of the two Water Companies, or in any of the physical conditions with which they are surrounded, It is obvious that no experiment could have been devised which would more thoroughly test the effect of water supply on the progress of cholera than this, which circumstances placed ready made before the observer.

The experiment too, was on the grandest scale. No fewer than three hundred thousand people of both sexes, of every age and occupation, and of every rank and station, from gentlefolks down to the very poor, were divided into two groups without their choice, and, in most cases, without their knowledge; one group being supplied with water containing the sewage of London, and, amongst it, whatever might have come from the cholera patients, the other group having water quite free from such impurity.

To turn this grand experiment to account, all that was required was to learn the supply of water to each individual house where a fatal attack of cholera might occur. (Snow, 1855/1965, p. 75)

With this "natural experiment," Snow recognized the opportunity to observe that the study population, conditions, and setting present in London at the time offered a unique opportunity to undertake a cohort study to test his scientific hypothesis regarding the cause of cholera. The link between polluted drinking water and cholera could not have been evaluated with an experimental design, even today, as it would have been impractical and unethical to randomize one-half of the households in London to a highly suspected contaminated water source and the other half to a suspected clean drinking source during an outbreak.

In cases where randomized experiments are not feasible, as was the case with the cholera epidemic in London, scientists must rely on carefully executed observational study designs to advance public health. This chapter provides a general overview of the two most rigorous observational study designs: cohort and case-control studies. Within this context, we outline appropriate use of these study designs, discuss how to minimize key biases in these designs, and review the impact that these study designs have had on public health. We refer readers elsewhere for discussion of other commonly conducted observational study designs, including cross-sectional studies (i.e., surveys; see Chapter 12) and ecologic studies, both of which are less resource-intensive but also less rigorous approaches (Friis & Sellers, 2004; Kelsey, Whitemore, Evans, & Thompson, 1996; Rothman, 2002; Rothman, Greenland, & Lash, 2008).

KEY CONCEPTS AND DEFINITIONS

Cohort Studies

Cohort studies are investigations of one or more specified groups of people (i.e., the cohort) who are free of, but at risk for, disease; share some common characteristic or experience; and are followed over a defined period of time to assess development of disease or, alternately, another health outcome. Cohorts are defined based on the presence or absence of exposure to a suspected risk factor. In a cohort study, investigators select one group of individuals who possess the exposure of interest (hereafter referred to as the *exposed*) and another group who do not have the exposure (the *unexposed*) and proceed to follow both groups to compare the incidence (occurrence) of disease over some interval among people who were free of disease at the beginning of the interval. Cohort studies are also commonly referred to as follow-up or longitudinal studies.

Types of Cohort Studies

There are two primary types of cohort studies, prospective and retrospective, and one less common type, ambidirectional, all of which are defined based on the time at which follow-up begins (Figure 7.1). In prospective cohort studies, exposed and unexposed groups are identified and followed in real time for ascertainment of disease. In retrospective cohort studies, the exposed and unexposed groups are identified after both exposure and disease have already occurred (what is often referred to as *historical time*). Investigators are generally certain that exposure has preceded disease (e.g., from review of existing medical records), minimizing potential concerns about temporality. Ambidirectional studies employ a hybrid cohort design in which elements of both prospective and retrospective study designs are incorporated. Here, the exposed and unexposed groups are identified based on exposures that have occurred in the past, yet follow-up is both retrospective (such as for a short-term outcome that would have occurred relatively soon after exposure [Outcome/Disease 1 in Figure 7.1]) and prospective (such as for a longer term outcome that may occur years or decades after exposure [Outcome/Disease 2 in Figure 7.1]).

Figure 7.1 Prospective, Retrospective, and Ambidirectional Cohort Study Designs With Respect to the Time Follow-up Begins

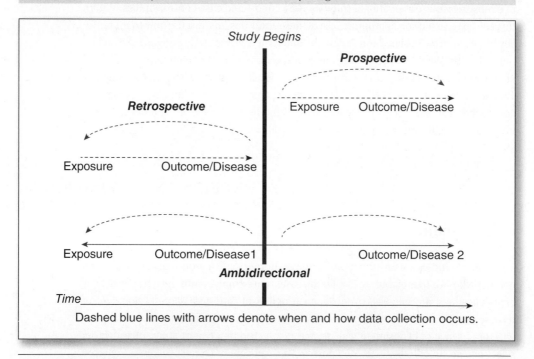

Source: Adapted from Chumney and Simpson (2006, p. 38); Grimes and Schulz (2002b, p. 341).

Selecting Cohorts

Cohorts based on exposure status

Cohorts can be selected in different ways, depending on the specific research questions being addressed. For instance, a cohort may be selected based on *exposure status* (i.e., whether or not individuals were exposed to a suspected risk factor). A classic example of this type of cohort selection occurred after World War II, when the United States and Japan collaborated to investigate the effects of ionizing radiation (the exposure) from atomic bombs on the development of leukemia (the disease) among survivors (Rothman et al., 2008). Investigators have continued to follow survivors to the present day to assess the effects of various levels of radiation exposure on the risk of leukemia incidence. In these investigations, a cohort study was the ideal design to explore the effects of radiation on health; it would have been unethical to conduct a randomized trial in which some individuals would be assigned to radiation exposure.

Related examples of the value and applicability of cohort studies include investigations of the health outcomes and potential dose-response effects of radiation among individuals exposed to radiation for medical reasons (e.g., diagnostic procedures, cancer treatment) or workers with occupational exposure to radiation. Findings from such cohort studies have contributed greatly toward improving the understanding of the health effects of radiation.

Cohorts selected based on a shared characteristic

Cohorts may also be selected through identification of some shared characteristic, such as place of residence or age. A classic example of this type of cohort identification is the Framingham Heart Study of cardiovascular disease, a prospective cohort study, in which individuals who lived in Framingham, Massachusetts (a shared characteristic), were eligible to participate if they were between the ages of 30 and 62 years (a *birth cohort*, another shared characteristic) and free of cardiovascular disease at the outset. The original cohort included over 5,000 men and women who were randomly selected from those who were eligible to participate, and who were followed from 1948 until 2005. Notably, the Framingham Study was also the first major cardiovascular study to recruit female participants, and it helped greatly improve knowledge about the incidence of coronary heart disease in women and the risk factors that are unique to women.

Examples of Investigations Using a Cohort Study Design

As detailed in Chapter 6, cohort study designs are a commonly used approach for investigating outbreaks associated with food exposures. For instance, investigators wanting to identify the source of an outbreak of gastroenteritis aboard a cruise ship often first obtain a list of people who were aboard the ship, collect detailed information about their food exposures and the timing of onset for any illnesses that occurred during the cruise, and then calculate the incidence of illness among those who did and did not eat each food item (also known as the *attack rate*). By comparing the attack rates, investigators can determine the food(s) associated with the highest risk of illness. This example uses a retrospective cohort design and is ideally suited for situations in which there is a well-defined population (here, the manifest of passengers on the cruise ship). In addition to outbreak investigations, retrospective cohort studies are also useful for conducting occupational epidemiologic investigations exploring the associations of job-related exposures and disease (e.g., asbestos exposure among those employed in mines, shipyards, construction, automobile repair shops, etc.; and risk of developing mesothelioma). Retrospective cohort studies are most practical and applicable when exposed and non-exposed groups can be clearly defined and located for data collection throughout the study. In cases where disease or illness has occurred, but the population giving rise to the cases is not well defined, a case-control study design is the better approach (Gregg, 2008).

Case-Control Studies

Case-control studies are investigations of whether exposure history differs between a group of individuals with a particular disease or health outcome (hereafter referred to as the *cases*) and a comparison group of individuals without disease (the *controls*). A case-control study differs fundamentally from a cohort study, in that a case-control study is initiated based on disease status (the presence or absence of a disease), whereas a cohort study begins based on exposure status (the presence or absence of an exposure). Of note, disease status has already occurred at the outset of both case-control and retrospective cohort studies; however, an important distinction is that case-control studies always first identify diseased and nondiseased individuals and then assess exposure status. Conversely, in retrospective cohort studies, both exposure and disease status are known from the outset, as is the temporality between exposure and disease.

Once individuals are classified as cases or controls, the investigator looks backward in time at the exposure histories of both groups. Exposure histories can be obtained from a variety of sources, such as medical records, employment records, laboratory results, or city or historical records (e.g., real estate or tax records). Histories can also be obtained through interviews and discussions with the individual or, for deceased individuals, with proxies such as family members, friends, or coworkers. Once exposure histories have been recorded, the investigator compares the prevalence of exposure among cases with that of controls. If exposure is associated with disease, the proportion of cases that was exposed differs from the proportion of controls that was exposed.

Selecting Cases and Controls

Source population

Prior to selection of cases and controls, the source population must be properly defined. The source population represents the population that gave rise to the cases; it is based on the eligibility criteria used to determine which individuals are considered to be cases. For example, the source population may come from the medical facility where the cases sought treatment (e.g., hospital, clinic). In this example, the source population would be composed of all individuals who theoretically would solicit care at that medical facility and be noted as having the disease of interest if they truly had it (Rothman et al., 2008). Carefully defined source populations are essential to ensuring appropriate, unbiased selection of cases and controls for a case-control study.

Identification of cases

Case-control studies often involve investigations of rare diseases or conditions, so it is often most practical to search for cases where they are most likely to be located, such as in medical care facilities where cases may have sought care or through population-based registries. Birth defect and cancer registries are two examples of registries that have been used to identify cases (Gordis, 2009; Gregg, 2008; Rothman et al., 2008). Registries tend to be reliable sources of information that enable investigators to identify cases quickly and inexpensively.

In the United States, the Centers for Disease Control and Prevention (CDC) administers the National Program of Cancer Registries (NPCR; www.cdc.gov/cancer/npcr), which was established in 1992 and collects data on the occurrence of cancer; the type, extent, and location of the cancer; and the type of initial treatment. As of 2013, NPCR supports central cancer registries in 45 states, the District of Columbia, Puerto Rico, and the U.S. Pacific Island Jurisdictions, with resulting data representing 96% of the U.S. population. The National Cancer Institute's Surveillance, Epidemiology, and End Results (SEER; http://seer.cancer.gov) Program includes nine population-based cancer registries and includes cancer cases that were diagnosed from 1973 to today (Kelsey et al., 1996). SEER is a key data source for epidemiologists studying various cancers and was designed to provide representation of different geographic regions and racial/ethnic groups in the United States (Kelsey et al., 1996). Together, NPCR and SEER collect cancer-related data for the entire U.S. population.

In studies of diseases where such registries do not exist, a researcher may turn to medical records for case finding. Most commonly, researchers using medical records identify cases by selecting all incident cases who obtained care at any of a number of a number of facilities, such as hospitals or clinics within a specified geographic region over a defined time period. Due to feasibility or cost constraints, researchers may be limited to including only one source (e.g., one hospital) in a study; however, where possible, use of multiple sources is preferable. With cases selected from only a single source, caution is warranted, as any results observed could be attributable to characteristics unique to that source (e.g., air quality or infection control practices at the source hospital), as opposed to specific exposures of the cases, thereby potentially affecting study validity and generalizability.

Another consideration in case selection is whether to use incident (newly diagnosed) or prevalent (new or previously diagnosed) cases. Investigators interested in disease etiology generally prefer to study incident cases, which can more easily distinguish temporality for exposures that occurred before disease onset versus afterward. In addition, use of incident cases prevents investigators from mistakenly attributing a risk factor as being associated with disease development, when it actually was associated with survival among those who developed disease. The primary disadvantage to using incident cases, however, entails the additional time needed to accrue a sufficient number of new diagnoses for study; with prevalent cases, a larger pool of individuals exists from which to identify cases because both new and previously diagnosed cases are included (assuming a disease is not rapidly fatal). Nevertheless, when using incident cases, some diseased individuals may have been missed or excluded, such as those who were too ill to participate or who died before being diagnosed.

Identification of controls

Proper selection of controls is critical to ensuring study validity and is the most challenging aspect for investigators conducting case-control studies. The primary aim of a case-control study is to determine the exposure-disease relationship by comparing the prevalence of exposure between cases and controls. As a result, control groups must be sampled independently of their exposure status and should reflect the prevalence of exposure in the underlying source population. If, for example, controls are selected from only the subset of nondiseased individuals who were not exposed to a suspected risk factor (i.e., ignoring those with exposure), the comparison of the percentage of cases versus controls that were exposed becomes distorted, thus introducing bias into the study.

As with cases, there are many potential sources from which to select controls. Controls may be chosen from populations of nonhospitalized persons who share similar residential characteristics as the cases, or from persons hospitalized for a health condition different from that under study. In addition to communities and hospitals as sources, controls may be identified through insurance company or school rosters, or from neighborhoods where the cases resided. Another means of identifying controls is through random digit dialing (RDD), whereby households are sampled based on a random selection of telephone numbers, with the goal of closely replicating the source population that gave rise to the cases (Gordis, 2009; Kelsey et al., 1996; Rothman et al., 2008). Typically, RDD-generated controls are matched to cases by some criterion, such as area code, to reflect similar geographic and environmental exposure profiles as the cases; however, advancements in telephone technology (e.g., introduction of cell phones) may make the RDD model less productive and reliable over time (Lee et al., 2011; Link, Mokdad, Stackhouse, & Flowers, 2006).

A concept in case-control designs that is sometimes hard to grasp is that, for some diseases and conditions, an individual actually can serve as both a control and a case within the same study (Kelsey et al., 1996; Rothman et al., 2008). For example, an individual chosen as a control who remains disease-free for the first 3 months of a study before developing the disease of interest in the 4th month would theoretically be eligible to serve as a control for 3 months and a case from month 4 until study completion. One way to conceptualize control selection is to remember that controls should be chosen in an unbiased way from among those individuals who would have been included as cases had they developed the disease being studied (Miettinen, 1985).

Nested Case-Control Studies

A "nested" study is one that is conducted within the context of other studies; in essence, case-control studies are nested studies because they are nested within the source population that gave rise to the cases (Rothman et al., 2008). Nested case-control studies are typically conducted within an existing cohort study. With the nested design, a cohort study is first initiated to identify disease-free exposed and non-exposed populations. As individuals develop disease, a case-control study is separately initiated to assess more in-depth exposure histories of cases and controls. Nesting the case-control study within an existing cohort study offers the advantage of being able to maximize use of baseline data that were collected in the cohort study (e.g., blood and serum samples, laboratory test results); more important, this design minimizes potential problems with temporality through use of information about exposure history that was collected before disease onset, which is thus less susceptible to recall bias (Gordis, 2009; Kelsey et al., 1996; Rothman et al., 2008).

Limitations of Observational Designs

Any epidemiologic study design is subject to bias, which may cause investigators to incorrectly conclude there is an association between exposure and outcome when one

EXAMPLE OF NESTED CASE-CONTROL STUDY DESIGN

Human papillomavirus (HPV) is common among young women, and certain types of HPV, especially types 16 and 18, are associated with cervical cancer. To investigate whether the amount of viral load of HPV 16 predicted development of cervical cancer, a nested case-control study was undertaken among women who were part of a cohort that participated in a cytological screening program begun in Sweden in 1967 (Josefsson et al., 2000). Biological specimens (cytological smears) had been collected from the cohort of women and stored; information was entered into a database beginning in 1969.

Researchers identified all women from the cohort who had at least one smear, whose first smear was considered normal, were younger than age 50 when they entered the cohort, and were available for phone interviews starting in 1996. Researchers then identified all incident cases of cervical carcinoma in situ by linking study-cohort data with Sweden's National Cancer Registry data from 1969 to 1995. For each case, researchers randomly selected five controls who were matched by date of first registered smear (within 90 days) and birth year. Controls were considered eligible if they had no history of in-situ or invasive cervical carcinoma or hysterectomy before the date of the case's diagnosis.

The prevalence of HPV 16 was higher among smears from cases (42%) than controls (7%), as was the amount of HPV 16 DNA. The odds of developing cervical carcinoma in situ for women with the highest amount of viral DNA were almost 70-fold higher than for women negative for HPV 16, allowing investigators to conclude that high amounts of HPV 16 DNA can predict the risk of developing cervical cancer long before any tumors or other symptoms might be found (Josefsson et al., 2000; Ylitalo et al., 2000). Thus, this nested case-control study found that testing for the amount of HPV 16 DNA during routine gynecologic screenings could greatly improve health care providers' ability to determine whether infections have a high or low risk of evolving into cervical cancer.

does not exist, to conclude there is not an association when one is present, or to simply miscalculate the magnitude of effect for such an exposure (Kelsey et al., 1996). This underscores the importance of planning and conducting studies carefully to minimize potential biases (Chumney & Simpson, 2006; Rothman, 2002). In this section, we briefly discuss three important biases common to cohort and case-control studies: selection bias, information bias, and confounding.

Selection Bias

Selection bias results from systematic errors in the differences in the characteristics of those who were *selected* for inclusion and those who were not, or from those who chose to participate or not to participate (Rothman et al., 2008). One way to minimize selection bias is by randomizing individuals to exposure groups or, where randomization is not possible, carefully selecting the comparison group (i.e., unexposed individuals in cohort studies, nondiseased individual in case-control studies). For example, in occupational cohort studies, selection bias often results from the fact that individuals who are able to work must generally be healthy in order to carry out the duties of their jobs, and nonworking individuals may be unable to work specifically due to illness or disease. (This is often termed the *healthy worker* effect.) An investigator could minimize the possibility of selection bias by comparing workers in one industry to workers in another industry rather than comparing workers to nonworking individuals (Kelsey et al., 1996).

Information Bias

Information bias is a systematic error in the collection of data on study participants that leads to an incorrect estimate of the effect of an exposure on the risk of disease, threatening the internal validity of the study (Gregg, 2008). Recall bias is the most well-known type of information bias that occurs due to differential or inaccurate recollection of a past exposure or experience; this bias is particularly troublesome in case-control studies because cases and controls may recall exposures differently (Rothman, 2002; Rothman et al., 2008). For example, in a case-control study of childhood leukemia, an investigator may wish to interview parents to obtain information about potential exposures in utero and early life that are suspected to be associated with cancer. In an effort to explain what caused a child's cancer, parents of a child diagnosed with leukemia may be more likely than parents of children without leukemia to recall specific exposures such as X-rays the mother received before she knew she was pregnant or that the child received. Parents of a child without leukemia may not recall receiving such an X-ray simply because the event was not salient to them.

Social desirability is another type of information bias that can affect the validity of study findings, especially in studies that involve collection of data on sensitive or personal topics. Social desirability can influence a study participant to respond in a way the participant believes is most acceptable by society and in alignment with cultural norms (Adams et al., 2005; Hebert et al., 1997). In studies about sexual behavior, physical activity, and dietary practices, for example, participants may respond the way they believe researchers want them to respond or that places them in the best possible light. Social desirability can be difficult to measure, however. For example, in a study examining the prevalence of problems with condom use (e.g., breakage, slippage) among patients attending a sexually transmitted infection (STI) clinic and associations with incident gonorrhea and chlamydia, the researchers reported that a limitation of their study was the inability to address potential misclassification of condom use resulting from inaccurate reporting (Warner et al., 2008). They hypothesized that some participants may have been unwilling to admit having unprotected intercourse, instead opting to overreport the frequency of condom use problems; however, they also noted that this type of misreporting would typically bias the association between condom use and incident STI toward the null. Future studies might be able to reduce the likelihood of this type of bias with regard to condom use assessment by incorporating use of objective biologic markers that can detect the presence of semen or other male genital fluids in the vagina (Warner et al., 2008).

In addition to collecting biomarkers, other ways to minimize bias include collecting data as shortly as possible after an event (i.e., keeping the recall period short), using pretested or standardized questionnaires, ensuring interviewers and data collectors are trained to be objective, blinding interviewers to participants' exposure status (in a cohort study) or disease status (in a case-control study) where possible, and obtaining information through reviews of medical and/or insurance records for exposures that occurred prior to diagnosis of the condition (Gregg, 2008; Kelsey et al., 1996; Rothman et al., 2008).

Confounding

Confounding is a bias that occurs when an exposure and an outcome are both associated with a third variable (the confounder) and is of utmost concern in cohort and case-control studies. The primary feature of a confounding variable is that it leads to a spurious (false) finding by distorting the association between exposure and disease. Confounding can lead to a spurious association that overestimates or underestimates the true association, to an association in a direction different from the true direction of the association (harmful instead of beneficial, or vice versa), or to the presence of an association where, in reality, none exists.

To be a **confounder**, a variable must meet three criteria:

1. It must be a risk factor for the disease being investigated in the unexposed group.

2. It must be associated with the exposure being investigated in the source population.

3. It cannot be affected by the exposure or the disease, nor can it lie in the causal path between the primary exposure and the disease of interest. (Rothman et al., 2008)

A study conducted by Stark and Mantel (1966) investigating the relationship between birth order and Down syndrome provides a classic example of potential confounding (Rothman, 2002). Upon examining the data, the investigators observed a strong trend in the occurrence of Down syndrome with higher birth order; however, higher birth order is associated with higher (older) maternal age. Assessment of the relationship between maternal age and the occurrence of Down syndrome revealed an even stronger association. Birth order and maternal age are highly correlated; thus, comparing Down syndrome occurrence in higher versus lower order births is similar to comparing its occurrence in older versus younger mothers (Rothman, 2002). In this example, birth order effects on occurrence of Down syndrome are confounded by the effects of maternal age on Down syndrome (Rothman, 2002; see Figure 7.2). Confounding in observational studies can be effectively minimized through advanced study design (e.g., matching, restriction) and statistical techniques (e.g., stratified analyses, mathematical modeling), the discussion of which is beyond the scope of this chapter. Interested readers are referred elsewhere (Kleinbaum, Kupper, & Morganstern, 1982; Rothman, 2002; Rothman et al., 2008).

Figure 7.2   An Example of Confounding

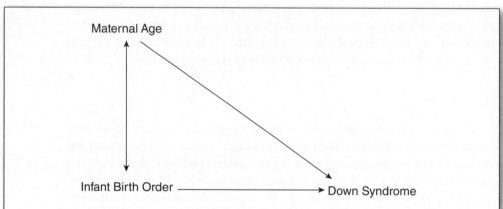

Here, maternal age meets the requirements to be a **confounder** because older maternal age is a risk factor for Down syndrome (outcome) and is associated with infant birth order (exposure), but is not a result of infant birth order (exposure). The double arrow between infant birth order and maternal age denotes a mutual association.

RELEVANCE OF COHORT AND CASE-CONTROL RESEARCH STUDIES TO PUBLIC HEALTH

Cohort and case-control study designs are intuitively appealing to investigators in situations where randomized controlled trials cannot be conducted. The published literature is replete with classic examples of how findings from well-designed observational studies have improved public health through the introduction or removal of an exposure or intervention. Beyond the historic studies mentioned earlier demonstrating the adverse health effects of cigarette smoking (Doll & Hill, 1954) and identifying in utero exposure to DES as the cause of vaginal adenocarcinoma in young women (Herbst et al., 1971), cohort and case-control investigations have yielded many important findings for prevention of both infectious and chronic disease.

Cohort Study Exemplars

Among cohort studies, investigations from the British Doctors Study that followed more than 40,000 male physicians between 1951 and 2001 provided the first compelling evidence of increased risks of heart disease due to smoking (Doll & Hill, 1956) and of lung cancer from occupational exposure to asbestos (Doll, 1955) by comparing disease rates (of heart disease and of lung cancer) between groups of smokers and nonsmokers. The Nurses' Health Studies similarly followed a cohort of more than 100,000 female registered nurses, originally starting in 1976 and adding the Nurses' Health Study II in 1989 among a younger cohort of nurses. The Women's Health Initiative Observational Study began in 1992 and monitored the health of more than 93,000 postmenopausal women between ages 50 and 79 over 15 years. Both of these high-profile cohort studies have yielded important information regarding the health of women in the areas of reproductive cancers, coronary heart disease, and osteoporotic fractures, and have examined the relationships between lifestyle (e.g., smoking, obesity, diet, physical activity) and reproductive factors (e.g., oral contraceptive and postmenopausal hormone use).

Case-Control Study Exemplars

Investigations using case-control designs have also provided important health information regarding the long-term safety of use of oral contraceptives (birth control pills), a product that revolutionized the reproductive health of women when first introduced in the 1960s. While numerous studies have shown that women who use birth control pills have lower risks of both ovarian and endometrial cancers, the evidence regarding the long-term effects on breast cancer has been less conclusive. (The health concern is that a woman's risk of breast cancer may be related to exposure to high hormone levels from oral contraceptives.) One multicenter, population-based case-control study of more than 9,000 women aged 35–64 years, the Women's Contraceptive and Reproductive Experiences Study (Women's CARE), investigated this question by comparing 4,575 women who had a diagnosis of invasive breast cancer (the cases) and 4,682 women who did not (the controls) by exposure to current or former pill use during the reproductive years. Cases were residents identified in one of five sites participating in Women's CARE through field staff or cancer registries. Controls, identified from the same geographic areas as cases, were contacted by telephone if their residential household was selected via random digit dialing. Oral contraceptive use (regardless of type or duration of use) was not associated with a greater odds of later developing breast cancer, providing reassurance to millions of women who have used oral contraceptives and were approaching the age with the greatest lifetime breast cancer risk (Marchbanks et al., 2002). Studies continue to investigate this relationship, with the published literature suggesting that a slightly elevated risk of breast cancer may exist among younger women, which must be balanced against the benefits of pill use.

In another example, it was a historic case-control investigation at the start of the AIDS epidemic—in which 50 gay men with rare infections of Kaposi's Sarcoma or *Pneumocystis carinii pneumonia* were compared to 120 noninfected gay men who were otherwise similar with respect to age, race, and residence—that first identified clear links between risky sexual behavior and illicit substance use and infection (Jaffe et al., 1983). The evidence gained from this and other initial studies led directly to the restriction of high-risk individuals from donating blood, thereby increasing the safety of the blood supply, as well as public health prevention measures promoting safer behavior through avoidance of unprotected sexual activity and needle sharing (CDC, 2011).

One of the most important case-control studies regards the Dalkon Shield, an intrauterine device (IUD) first marketed in the United States in 1971 that, at one time, was used by 2.8 million women (CDC, 1983). Questions about the safety of the Dalkon Shield began to be raised, especially after a survey of physicians suggested that patients who used the product were more likely to experience pregnancy-related complications than users of other IUDs. Further distribution of the device was voluntarily ceased by the manufacturer in 1974 (CDC, 1974). However, a number of small observational studies had also suggested a possible link between IUD use and risk of pelvic inflammatory disease (PID) but were not sufficiently large to examine health risks associated with specific types of IUDs, which was of concern to current IUD users. It was not until a case-control analysis of the large multicenter Women's Health Study was conducted that remaining users of the Dalkon Shield IUD were found to have a five-fold higher risk of PID as compared with women using other IUD types (CDC, 1983). In that definitive study, data on IUD use and IUD type collected during interviews were contrasted between 622 women who were hospitalized with an initial episode of PID and 2,369 women who were also hospitalized but who did not have a history of PID. The finding of this case-control study led CDC and the Food and Drug Administration to jointly recommend in 1983 that women who still were using the Dalkon Shield should have the device removed. Nevertheless, rates of subsequent use of all IUDs plummeted, even though the health risks related to only one type of IUD that was no longer commercially available. Only very recently has the redesigned IUD been making a comeback as a highly effective and safe long-acting reversible contraceptive for women of all ages (Grimes, 2011).

PLANNING, IMPLEMENTING, AND INTERPRETING COHORT AND CASE-CONTROL STUDIES

As noted earlier, cohort and case-control studies differ in their directionality and timing. For cohort studies, investigators follow groups of participants who are free of disease (but at risk) for some defined interval to ascertain disease outcomes (Figure 7.1); participants are selected for follow-up based on their exposure status. Conversely, in case-control studies, participants are selected based on their disease status, and investigators move backward in time to compare histories of exposure between diseased (cases) and nondiseased individuals (controls; Figure 7.1).

Appropriate Uses of Cohort Studies

Cohort studies offer many advantages to the investigator, most notably the ability to ascertain the incidence of a disease in a defined population, assuming that the exposed and unexposed groups were truly disease-free at study outset (Grimes & Schulz, 2002b). The cohort design also allows the temporal sequence between assessment of exposure and onset of outcome to be clearly established—recall that temporality was one of the fundamental components of Hill's (1965) guidance for making arguments for causal associations. Data collected on exposure history in the context of a cohort study generally have higher validity than in a case-control study, given that participants (and, for that matter, investigators) do not know individuals' disease status at the time of assessment. Cohort studies are well-suited to investigate multiple disease outcomes that may arise from a single exposure (e.g., heart disease, stroke, esophageal and oral cancers, and lung cancer, all of which have been attributed to smoking). Additionally, the health effects of exposures that are otherwise rare in the general population, such as occupational exposures to asbestos or radiation, can be assessed with cohort study designs with cooperation of the target population. With a rare exposure, waiting for a sufficient number of exposed individuals to accrue in the general population would otherwise be infeasible.

Cohort studies, however, are generally poorly suited to study rare diseases or conditions with a long induction time because enrollment and follow-up of large numbers of subjects would be necessary. There are exceptions, however. Grimes and Schulz (2002b) note that several large cohort studies, such as the Framingham Heart Study, the British Doctors Study, and the Nurses' Health Study, have successfully provided epidemiologic information on rare diseases due to their sheer size and extended duration of follow-up. Prospective cohort studies are also generally expensive and time-consuming to conduct, as investigators wait for disease outcomes to occur among exposed and unexposed individuals. Retrospective cohort studies, while far less costly and time-consuming, require that suitable records exist with sufficient numbers of both exposed and unexposed individuals and disease outcomes, not to mention ample data quality regarding exposure, outcome, and any potential confounding variables.

Appropriate Uses of Case-Control Studies

Case-control studies can relatively quickly and inexpensively yield important information regarding rare diseases and also diseases with a long latency period. The case-control design is well suited to examine multiple potential causes of a single disease and has proven particularly valuable for hypothesis generation of causes and possible prevention strategies for emerging pandemics (e.g., HIV, SARS). The design is remarkably efficient and requires fewer subjects to be enrolled and their exposure histories assessed.

The relative ease with which case-control studies can be conducted, as compared with cohort studies, comes at a price, however. These studies are unsuitable (and inefficient) for evaluating rare exposures if an insufficient number of cases and controls possess the exposure of interest. Not surprisingly, case-control studies also cannot provide estimates of underlying disease incidence because disease status is the basis on which cases and controls are sampled from the source population. The backward-looking nature of the case-control design, where investigators select subjects based on their disease status and then retrospectively assess their history of exposure, results in an uncertain temporal sequence between exposure and disease. Finally, the design is prone to bias resulting from selection of an inappropriate control group of individuals without disease to compare with the case group. The fact that the exposure history of cases and controls cannot be assessed until study participants (and investigators) know their disease status can introduce recall bias and raise questions about study validity.

Measures of Association in Cohort Studies

As mentioned earlier, cohort studies, whether prospective or retrospective in nature, offer investigators the distinct advantage of being able to calculate incidence rates directly. Comparisons of disease incidence between individuals with the exposure of interest relative to individuals without have been generically termed *relative risks*. Two types of relative risk, risk ratios and rate ratios, can be obtained from cohort studies, and their distinction is important. Use of a **risk ratio**, also known as a cumulative incidence proportion, is an appropriate measure when individuals in the exposed and unexposed cohorts have the same duration of follow-up time. The calculation of a risk ratio from a cohort study can be algebraically presented in a 2 x 2 contingency table designed to assess associations between exposure and disease (Figure 7.3).

Figure 7.3 2 x 2 Contingency Table for a Cohort Study With Count Data

	Diseased	Not Diseased	Totals
Exposed	A	B	A + B *Total Exposed*
Unexposed	C	D	C + D *Total Unexposed*
Totals	A + C *Total Diseased*	B + D *Total Non-Diseased*	N (A + B + C + D) *(Total Participants)*

Proportions of those at risk for disease (incidence of disease)	Exposed	Unexposed
	$\dfrac{A}{A + B}$	$\dfrac{C}{C + D}$

In a cohort study, we calculate the risk ratio, defined as the ratio of the risk (incidence) of developing disease in the exposed to the risk (incidence) of developing the disease in the unexposed.

$$\text{Risk Ratio:} \quad \frac{A / (A + B)}{C / (C + D)}$$

Assuming a study population of size N individuals, the overall incidence of the disease is the sum of the total number of diseased individuals (A + C) divided by the total population: (A + C) / N. Calculated by exposure status, the incidence in the exposed group would equal the number of diseased individuals divided by the total number of exposed individuals, A / (A + B), while the incidence in the unexposed group would similarly be calculated among unexposed individuals, C / (C + D). The risk ratio would therefore be a ratio of the incidence in the exposed divided by the incidence in the unexposed: A / (A + B) ÷ C / (C + D). To determine if the risk ratio is considered statistically significant, epidemiologists typically examine the associated 95% confidence interval. If the confidence interval does not contain the value 1.0, the relative risk is considered to be significant, and not due to chance alone. A hypothetical example of relevant calculations and interpretation of the findings is provided in Figure 7.4.

Figure 7.4   Hypothetical Cohort Study of Asbestos Exposure and Mesothelioma

Cohort Study Example: Asbestos Exposure and Mesothelioma

Investigators are interested in examining whether asbestos exposure is associated with development of mesothelioma (cancer that starts in the cells that line various organs in the body). They enroll 350 participants in their study, none of whom have mesothelioma when the study begins. Of enrollees, 170 have been exposed to asbestos. At the end of the study follow-up period, 97 participants have developed mesothelioma, 69 of whom were exposed to asbestos. Using this information, we can complete the 2x2 table and calculate the risk ratio showing the relationship between asbestos and development of mesothelioma. Statistical software also can be used to generate the risk ratio and 95% confidence interval, though both can also be calculated by hand. (All data below are hypothetical)

	Develop Mesothelioma	Do Not Develop Mesothelioma	Totals
Exposed to asbestos	69	101	69 + 101=170 *Total Exposed*
Not exposed to asbestos	28	152	28 + 152=180 *Total Unexposed*
Totals	69+28=97 *Total who develop Mesothelioma*	101+152=253 *Total who do not develop Mesothelioma*	69 + 101 + 28 + 253 = 350 *Total Participants*

Risk Ratio $\frac{A/(A+B)}{C/(C+D)} = \frac{69/(69+101)}{28/(28+152)} = 2.61$ 95% confidence interval: (1.77, 3.84)

Interpretation: Those exposed to asbestos have more than two and a half times higher risk of developing mesothelioma compared with those not exposed to asbestos. Because the confidence interval does not include 1.0, this association is considered to be statistically significant.

Like risk ratios, rate ratios are used to compare disease incidence between the exposed and unexposed groups from a cohort study. However, **rate ratios** are the preferred measure of association when follow-up time varies considerably between individuals in the exposed and unexposed cohorts. The total person-time at risk (PT), that is, the amount of time each individual is under observation, is summed across individuals in both the exposed (PT_1) and unexposed (PT_0) populations to form the denominators at risk. Assuming the same study population of size N individuals, the rate ratio is calculated as the incidence rate in the exposed (number of diseased individuals divided by the total person-time in the exposed population), $A / (PT_1)$, divided by the incidence rate in the unexposed (number of diseased individuals divided by the total person-time in the unexposed population), $C / (PT_0)$. The rate ratio would correspondingly be calculated as $A / (PT_1) \div C / (PT_0)$. (See Figure 7.5.)

Whether the relative risk measure produced from a cohort study is a risk ratio or a rate ratio, the interpretation remains the same. A relative risk of 1.0 suggests no association with disease, a relative risk exceeding 1.0 indicates that the exposure is associated with higher risk for the disease, and a relative risk between 0 and 1.0 indicates the exposure is associated with a lower risk of disease and may be protective. Remember that it is also important to examine the confidence interval associated with the relative

Figure 7.5 2 x 2 Contingency Table for Cohort Study With Person-Time Data

	Diseased	Not Diseased	Person-years
Exposed	A	–	PT_1 *Total Person-Years for those Exposed*
Unexposed	C	–	PT_0 *Total Person-Years for those Unexposed*
Totals	A + C *Total Diseased*		$PT_1 + PT_0$ *Total Person-Years Contributed*

	Exposed	Unexposed	Study Incidence
Incidence Rates of Disease	$\dfrac{A}{PT_1}$	$\dfrac{C}{PT_0}$	$\dfrac{A+C}{PT_1+PT_0}$

In a cohort study, we calculate the **rate ratio**, defined as the ratio of the incidence rate of developing disease in the exposed to the incidence rate of developing the disease in the unexposed.

$$\textbf{Rate Ratio:} \quad \frac{A/PT_1}{C/PT_0}$$

risk; if the confidence interval does not include 1.0, the finding is considered to be statistically significant.

Measures of Association in Case-Control Studies

Case-control studies cannot yield incidence estimates because of the sampling scheme that gives rise to the cases and controls. Thus, they also cannot produce comparisons of incidence measures, as with the risk ratio and rate ratio in cohort studies. Instead, case-control studies permit comparisons of exposure histories between diseased and nondiseased individuals through an **odds ratio**. With this measure, the odds of exposure among cases is compared with the odds of exposure among controls (see Figure 7.6).

The calculation of an odds ratio can be algebraically derived from the same general 2 x 2 contingency table discussed earlier (Figure 7.6). Again, assuming a study population of size N individuals, the odds of exposure (the probability an event will happen divided by the probability it will not happen) in the case group is ($[A / (A + C)]$ $\div [C / (A + C)]$), while the odds of exposure in the control group is ($[B / (B + D)] \div [D$

Figure 7.6   2 x 2 Contingency Table for a Case-Control Study

1. **Categorize participants based on disease status**

2. Measure exposure	CASES *Ill*	CONTROLS *Well*	Totals
Exposed	A	B	A + B Total Exposed
Unexposed	C	D	C + D Total Exposed
Totals	A + C Total # CASES	B + D Total # CONTROLS	N (A + B + C + D) (Total Participants)

	Cases	Controls
Proportions Exposed	$\dfrac{A}{A+C}$	$\dfrac{B}{B+C}$
Odds of Exposure	A:C or A/C	B:D or B/D

In a case-control study, we calculate the **odds ratio**, defined as the ratio of the odds that the cases were exposed to the odds the controls were exposed.

$$\text{Odds Ratio:} \quad \frac{A/C}{B/D} = \frac{AD}{BC}$$

/ (B + D)]). The odds ratio is the comparison of these two sets of exposure odds and is thus defined as the odds of exposure in the cases divided by the odds of exposure in the controls:

$$\text{Odds Ratio} = \frac{[A / (A + C)] \div [C / (A + C)]}{[B / (B + D)] \div [D / (B + D)]}$$

which reduces nicely to the cross-product multiplier AD / BC. Just as with a risk ratio and a rate ratio, it is important to assess the confidence interval associated with the odds ratio. The criteria remain the same; if the confidence interval does not include the value 1.0, the odds ratio is considered to be statistically significant. Usually, confidence intervals for point estimates (odds ratios, risk ratios, etc.) are obtained as part of a statistical program; however, they can be calculated by hand. The formula for the 95% confidence interval of an odds ratio is

Odds Ratio ± [1.96 x Standard Error of the Point Estimate]

An example of a case-control study, using hypothetical data, is outlined in Figure 7.7. Consider the same hypothetical study of asbestos and mesothelioma noted in the cohort study example (Figure 7.4) and how it might look were it conducted as a case-control study rather than a cohort study. In the case-control study, the researchers enroll 97 cases with mesothelioma and 253 controls without mesothelioma and assess the level of asbestos exposure within each group. Of enrollees, 170 were found to have been exposed to asbestos, 69 from the case group and 202 from the control group.

As with risk and rate ratios, values of 1.0 suggest no association between exposure and case or control status, values greater than 1.0 suggest increased odds of exposure, and values between 0 and 1.0 indicate reduced odds of exposure and possible protective effect. Notably, the odds ratio obtained from a case-control study provides a close approximation of the relative risk when the incidence of disease is "rare" (usually less than 10%; Rothman et al., 2008). In the aforementioned example, the incidence of disease in the cohort study was in fact not rare (97/350, or 28%) and the odds ratio is slightly exaggerated in the direction away from the null.

Interpreting Causation

Interpretation of cohort and case-control study findings is inherently more challenging than interpreting RCT data, given that any relationships detected between exposure and disease reflect association but not necessarily causation. The U.S. Surgeon General's 1964 report on smoking and health (U.S. Department of Health, Education and Welfare, 1964) that declared cigarette smoking "a health hazard of sufficient importance in the United States to warrant appropriate action" was among the first attempts in public health to define when causation could reasonably be inferred from observed associations.

Figure 7.7   Hypothetical Case-Control Study Example

Case-Control Study Example: Asbestos Exposure and Mesothelioma

For this example of a case-control study, we use the same exposure, outcome, and data as we used to compute the risk ratio for the cohort study example. (See Figure 7.4 for details.) In this example, we can complete the 2 x 2 table and then compute the <u>odds ratio</u> and confidence interval. (Study data are hypothetical.)

Mesothelioma

Asbestos Exposure	Cases	Controls	Totals
Exposed	69	202	170
Unexposed	28	152	180
Totals	97 Total # cases	253 Total # controls	69 + 202 + 28 + 152 = 350 (Total Participants)

Proportions exposed

	Cases	Controls
	$\dfrac{69}{69+28}$	$\dfrac{202}{202+152}$

Odds of exposure

69:28 or 69/28	202:152 or 202/152

Odds Ratio $\dfrac{69/28}{202/152} = \dfrac{69 \times 152}{202 \times 28} = 3.71,\ 95\%\ CI: 2.24, 6.15$

Interpretation: The <u>odds</u> of asbestos exposure are 3.71 times higher among those with as compared to those without mesothelioma. Because the confidence interval does not include 1.0, the finding is considered to be statistically significant.

The following year, Sir Austin Bradford Hill (who also worked with Richard Doll on the British Doctors Study) helped further advance thinking about causal interpretation of observational study findings in his President's Address at the Royal Society of Medicine (Hill, 1965). In his written account of that lecture, Hill elaborated on the causal criteria used by the Surgeon General's committee to support its conclusion that smoking was harmful to health and also proposed a few new criteria to define the minimal set of conditions necessary to infer causation from observational studies. Led by strength of association, consistency of findings across studies, and temporality between exposure and outcome, these criteria are now widely referred to "Hill's criteria for causation" (Table 7.1; also, see Chapter 22 for more on the debates over findings about tobacco use and health effects).

Table 7.1 Hill Criteria for Determining Causal Associations

1. **Strength of the association**: The stronger the association, the less likely it is that the association is entirely due to sources of error; conversely, a weaker association does not necessarily mean that there is not a causal effect.

2. **Consistency of the findings**: Consistent findings of the observed association by different persons in different places, circumstances, and times strengthens the likelihood of an effect.

3. **Specificity of the association**: Exposures associated with only one disease in one population with no other likely explanation support likelihood of causal effect.

4. **Temporality**: The cause has to precede the occurrence of the effect.

5. **Biological gradient (dose response)**: Observation that frequency of disease increases with increasing frequency of exposure lends support to causality.

6. **Biologic plausibility of the hypothesis**: Plausible mechanisms that make sense with current biological knowledge regarding observed association help support arguments for causality.

7. **Coherence of the evidence**: Coherence between epidemiological and laboratory findings increases the likelihood of an effect.

8. **Experiment**: Experimental evidence, when in existence, can be useful.

9. **Analogy**: Findings regarding similar factors and diseases may be considered.

Source: Adapted from Kleinbaum et al. (1982). Original source: Hill (1965).

There have been recent concerns that Hill's criteria are being misused in some circles as a simple checklist for evaluating causality, which Hill never intended when he first proposed his general guidance (Rothman, 2002). We refer interested readers elsewhere (Hernan, Hernandez-Diaz, Werler, & Mitchell, 2002; Kleinbaum et al., 1982; Rothman et al., 2008) for further discussion on assessing causal association from observational studies. These concerns, along with the potential for biases to affect results of cohort, case-control, and other observational studies, reemphasize the need for careful attention to the design of a study from the outset. As noted by others, complex statistical analyses (Kleinbaum & Klein, 2002; Rothman, 2008) or larger sample sizes (Grimes & Schulz, 2002a) alone cannot rescue a poorly conceived study.

FUTURE DIRECTIONS

Although the randomized trial is for some scenarios the ideal research design, it is not always possible or ethical to randomize individuals to a particular study exposure. Cohort and case-control studies are two common observational study designs and, when properly executed, can yield important public health findings. A few examples exist in the literature, however, where case-control and cohort studies provided erroneous information regarding the apparent safety (or harm) of a potential public health intervention. Notable egregious examples reported in the media that were later proven false include abortion being linked with an increased risk of breast cancer, and cigarette smoking (despite the well-known adverse effects of smoking on other aspects of health) being associated with an increased likelihood of suicide (Grimes & Schulz, 2012).

To help prevent such misinterpretations of study findings, guidelines have been established regarding the minimal effect sizes needed from cohort and case-control studies to make further investigation for causal association worthwhile (Cohen, 1992; Ellis, 2010; Grimes & Schulz, 2012). Referring back to Hill's (1965) criteria for causation, large associations are more likely to be indicators of a true causal relationship while small associations are more likely to be explained by bias. For cohort studies, recommended credible relationships are generally indicated by a risk ratio or rate ratio exceeding 2 or 3 (i.e., risk of an exposed group acquiring disease is two to three times higher than that of the unexposed group). For case-control studies, which are markedly more prone to bias, the recommended strength of relationship for credibility is more strict, requiring an odds ratio exceeding 3 or 4 (i.e., odds of exposure for diseased individuals being three to four times higher than for nondiseased individuals; Grimes & Schulz, 2012).

To encourage careful planning, conduct, and reporting of cohort, case-control, and other observational studies, standardized reporting frameworks have been issued regarding how investigators should report results from observational studies to peer-reviewed journals. Adapting from guidance successfully established for rigorous reporting of results of randomized trials (otherwise known as Consolidated Standards of Reporting Trials, or CONSORT), guidelines have been recently proposed for reporting of cohort and case-control studies, both for individual studies (Transparent Reporting of Evaluations with Nonrandomized Designs, or TREND; Des Jarlais, Lyles, Crepaz, & TREND Group, 2004; Strengthening the Reporting of Observational Studies in Epidemiology, or STROBE; von Elm et al., 2008) and for meta-analyses (Meta-analysis Of Observational Studies in Epidemiology, or MOOSE; Stroup et al., 2000).

ADDITIONAL RESOURCES

Gordis L. (2009). *Epidemiology* (4th ed.). Philadelphia, PA: Saunders Elsevier.

Gregg, M. B. (2008). *Field epidemiology* (3rd ed.). New York, NY: Oxford University Press.

Kleinbaum, D. G., Kupper, L. L., & Morganstern, H. (1982). *Epidemiologic research: Principles and quantitative methods.* New York, NY: Van Nostrand Reinhold.

Rothman, K. J. (2002). *Epidemiology: An introduction.* New York, NY: Oxford University Press.

Rothman, K. J., Greenland, S., & Lash, T. L. (2008). *Modern epidemiology* (3rd ed.). Philadelphia, PA: Lippincott Williams & Winkins.

World Health Organization. (2013). *Health topics: Epidemiology*. Retrieved from http://www.who.int/topics/epidemiology/en

REFERENCES

Adams, S. A., Matthews, C. E., Ebbeling, C. B., Moore, C. G., Cunningham, J. E., Fulton, J., & Hebert, J. R. (2005). The effect of social desirability and social approval on self-reports of physical activity. *American Journal of Epidemiology, 161,* 389–398. (Erratum in *American Journal of Epidemiology* (2005), *161,* 899)

Centers for Disease Control and Prevention. (1974). IUD safety: Report of a nationwide survey. *Morbidity and Mortality Weekly Report, 23,* 226, 231. With Editorial Note—1997.

Centers for Disease Control and Prevention. (1983). Elevated risk of pelvic inflammatory disease among women using the Dalkon Shield. *Morbidity and Mortality Weekly Report, 32,* 221–222.

Centers for Disease Control and Prevention. (2011). AIDS: The early years and CDC's response. *Morbidity and Mortality Weekly Report, 60*(Suppl), 64–69.

Chumney, E. C. G., & Simpson, K. N. (2006). *Methods and designs for outcomes research.* Bethesda, MD: American Society of Health-System Pharmacists.

Cohen, J. (1992). A power primer. *Psychological Bulletin, 112,* 155–159.

Deeks, J. J., Dinnes, J., D'Amico, R., Sowden, A. J., Sakarovitch, C., Song, F., . . . European Carotid Surgery Trial Collaborative Group. (2003). Evaluating non-randomised intervention studies. *Health Technology Assessment, 7,* iii–x, 1–173.

Des Jarlais, D. C., Lyles, C., Crepaz, N., & TREND Group. (2004). Improving the reporting quality of nonrandomized evaluations of behavioral and public health interventions: The TREND statement. *American Journal of Public Health, 94,* 361–366.

Doll, R. (1955). Mortality from lung cancer in asbestos workers. *British Journal of Industrial Medicine, 12*(2), 81–86.

Doll, R., & Hill, A. B. (1954). The mortality of doctors in relation to their smoking habits. *British Medical Journal, 328,* 1529.

Doll, R., & Hill, A. B. (1956). Lung cancer and other causes of death in relation to smoking: A second report on the mortality of British doctors. *British Medical Journal, 2,* 1071–1081.

Ellis, P. D. (2010). *The essential guide to effect sizes: Statistical power, meta-analysis, and the interpretation of research results.* Cambridge, UK: Cambridge University Press.

Friis, R., & Sellers, T. A. (2004). *Epidemiology for public health practice* (3rd ed.). Sudbury, MA: Jones and Bartlett.

Gordis, L. (2009). *Epidemiology* (4th ed.). Philadelphia, PA: Saunders Elsevier.

Gregg, M. B. (2008). *Field epidemiology* (3rd ed.). New York, NY: Oxford University Press.

Grimes, D. (2011). Intrauterine devices. In R. A. Hatcher, F. Guest, F. Stewart, G. Stewart, D. Kowal, J. Trussell, W. Cates, & M. Policar (Eds.), *Contraceptive technology* (Rev. 20th ed.). New York, NY: Ardent Media.

Grimes, D. A., & Schulz, K. F. (2002a). Case-control studies: Research in reverse. *Lancet, 359,* 431–434.

Grimes, D. A., & Schulz, K. F. (2002b). Cohort studies: Marching toward outcomes. *Lancet, 359,* 341–345.

Grimes, D. A., & Schulz, K. F. (2012). False alarms and pseudo-epidemics: The limitations of observational epidemiology. *Obstetrics & Gynecology, 120,* 920–927.

Hebert, J. R., Ma, Y., Clemow, L., Ockene, I. S., Saperia, G., Stanek, E. J. III, . . . Ockene, J. K. (1997).

Gender differences in social desirability and social approval bias in dietary self-report. *American Journal of Epidemiology, 146,* 1046–1055.

Hennekens, C. H., & Buring, J. E. (1987). *Epidemiology in medicine.* Boston, MA: Lippincott Williams & Wilkins.

Herbst, A. L., Ulfelder, H., & Poskanzer, D.C. (1971). Adenocarcinoma of the vagina: Association of maternal stilbestrol therapy with tumor appearance in young women. *New England Journal of Medicine, 284,* 878–881.

Hernan, M. A., Hernandez-Diaz, S., Werler, M. M., & Mitchell, A. A. (2002). Causal knowledge as a prerequisite for confounding evaluation: An application to birth defects epidemiology. *American Journal of Epidemiology, 155,* 176–184.

Hill, A. B. (1965). The environment and disease: Association or causation? *Proceedings of the Royal Society of Medicine, 58,* 295–300.

Hoover, R. N., Hyer, M., Pfeiffer, R. M., Adam, E., Bond, B., Cheville, A. L., . . . Troisi, R. (2011). Adverse health outcomes in women exposed in utero to diethylstibestrol. *New England Journal of Medicine, 365,* 1304–1314.

Jaffe, H. W., Choi, K., Thomas, P. A., Haverkos, H. W., Auerbach, D. M., Guinan, M. E., . . . Curran, J. W. (1983). National case-control study of Kaposi's sarcoma and Pneumocystis carinii pneumonia in homosexual men: Part I. Epidemiologic results. *Annals of Internal Medicine, 99,* 145–151.

Josefsson, A. M., Magnusson, P. K. E., Ylitalo, N., Sorensen, P., Quarforth-Tubbin, P., Andersen, P. K., . . . Gyllensten, U. B. (2000). Viral load of human papilloma virus 16 as a determinant for development of cervical carcinoma in situ: A nested case-control study. *Lancet, 355,* 2189–2193.

Kelsey, J. L., Whitemore A. S., Evans, A. S., & Thompson, W. D. (1996). *Methods in observational epidemiology* (2nd ed.). New York, NY: Oxford University Press.

Kleinbaum, D. G., & Klein, M. (2002). *Logistic regression: A self-learning text* (2nd ed.). New York, NY: Springer-Verlag.

Kleinbaum, D. G., Kupper, L. L., & Morganstern, H. (1982). *Epidemiologic research: Principles and quantitative methods.* New York, NY: Van Nostrand Reinhold.

Lee, R., Ranaldi, J., Cummings, M., Crucetti, J. B., Stratton, H., & McNutt, L. A. (2011). Given the increasing bias in random digit dial sampling, could respondent-driven sampling be a practical alternative? *Annals of Epidemiology, 21,* 272–279.

Link, M. W., Mokdad, A. H., Stackhouse, H. F., & Flowers, N. T. (2006). Race, ethnicity, and linguistic isolation as determinants of participation in public health surveillance surveys. *Preventing Chronic Disease, 3*(1). Retrieved from http://www.cdc.gov/pcd

Marchbanks, P. A., McDonald, J. A., Wilson, H. G., Folger, S. G., Mandel, M. G., Daling, J. R., . . . Weiss, L. K. (2002). Oral contraceptives and the risk of breast cancer. *New England Journal of Medicine, 346,* 2025–2032.

Miettinen, O. S. (1985). *Theoretical epidemiology: Principles of occurrence research in medicine.* New York, NY: Wiley.

Rothman, K. J. (2002). *Epidemiology: An introduction.* New York, NY: Oxford University Press.

Rothman, K. J., Greenland, S., & Lash, T. L. (2008). *Modern epidemiology* (3rd ed.). Philadelphia, PA: Lippincott Williams & Winkins.

Snow, J. (1965). *On the mode of communication of cholera* (2nd ed.). New York, NY: Hafner. (Original work published 1855)

Stark, C. R., & Mantel, N. (1966). Effects of maternal age and birth order on the risk of mongolism and leukemia. *Journal of the National Cancer Institute, 37,* 687–698.

Stroup, D., Berlin, J. A., Morton, S. C., Olkin, I., Williamson, G. D., Rennie, D., . . . Thacker, S. B. (2000). Meta-analysis Of Observational studies in Epidemiology (MOOSE): A proposal for reporting. *Journal of the American Medical Association, 283,* 2008–2012.

U.S. Department of Health, Education and Welfare. (1964). *Smoking and health report of the Advisory Committee to the Surgeon General of the Public Health Service* (Public Health Service Publication 1103). Washington, DC: U. S. Government Printing Office.

Victora, C. G., Habicht, J.-P., & Bryce, J. (2004). Evidence-based public health: Moving beyond randomized trials. *American Journal of Public Health, 94*, 400–405.

von Elm, E., Altman, D. G., Egger, M., Pocock, S. J., Gøtzche, P. C., Vandenbroucke, J. P., & STROBE Initiative. (2008). The Strengthening the Reporting of Observational Studies in Epidemiology (STROBE) statement: Guidelines for reporting observational studies. *Journal of Clinical Epidemiology, 61*, 344–349.

Warner, L., Newman, D. R., Kamb, M. L., Fishbein, M., Douglas, J. M., Jr., Zenilman, J., . . . Project RESPECT Study Group. (2008). Problems with condom use among patients attending sexually transmitted disease clinics: Prevalence, predictors, and relation to incident gonorrhea and chlamydia. *American Journal of Epidemiology, 167*, 341–349.

Ylitalo, N., Sorensen, P., Josefsson, A. M., Magnusson, P. K. E., Andersen, P. K., Ponten, J., . . . Melbye, M. (2000). Consistent high viral load of human papillomavirus 16 and risk of cervical carcinoma in situ: A nested case-control study. *Lancet, 355*, 2194–2198.

NOTE

1. CDC Disclaimer: The findings and conclusions in this report are those of the authors and do not necessarily represent the official position of the Centers for Disease Control and Prevention.

Designing Randomized Controlled Trials (RCTs)

Theresa Gamble, Danielle Haley, Raymond Buck, and
Nirupama Sista

The previous chapters in this section, covering surveillance, outbreak investigation, and case-control and cohort studies, illustrate the commitment of public health to scientific and systematic methods for the study of health-related issues. In this chapter we cover randomized controlled trials (RCTs), considered the gold standard of clinical research because of their unique ability to link cause and effect. The key elements of randomized controlled trials—probability (randomization), comparison (control), and blinding (control)—work synergistically to create an experiment that can prove this link between an intervention (cause) and its consequences (effect).

The first planned (and documented) controlled clinical trial was conducted in 1743 by James Lind, who found that lemons and oranges were far better at treating scurvy among seamen than several other agents (cider, vinegar, sea water, barley water, and sulfuric acid; Gallin & Ognibene 2007). However, it was another 200 years before the first randomized controlled study began in 1947, in which the antibiotic streptomycin was shown to be better than the standard of care (bed rest only) in treating pulmonary tuberculosis (Bhatt, 2010). Since then, the RCT has become recognized for its scientific rigor, ability to eliminate bias, and capacity to reduce the impact of unknown or extraneous factors. In the pages that follow, we provide an introduction to the critical elements of the RCT, explain its strengths and limitations, and discuss the impact RCTs have on public health. Note that while most of the examples used in this chapter are drawn from biomedical or product-testing trials, RCTs can also be used to test other public health interventions, like smoking-cessation interventions (Bonevski et al., 2011). Since causal chains in public health interventions, especially at the community level, are often complex, other approaches to studying these types of interventions may be more valid (Victora, Habicht, & Bryce, 2004). We refer readers to Bonella and colleagues' discussion of a "realistic" approach to RCTs in these cases (Bonella, Fletcherb, Mortona, Lorencb, & Moorec, 2012).

THE BASICS OF RANDOMIZED CONTROLLED TRIALS (RCTs)

Definition of Randomized Controlled Trial

A randomized controlled trial is a type of experimental clinical study in which participants are randomly assigned to an intervention or control and followed over time. All participants are tracked forward from a well-defined starting point, known as the baseline, and are followed for a predetermined period of time or until they reach a specific outcome. The group of study participants randomized to receive the intervention being evaluated is known as the treatment or intervention group. The group of study participants randomized to receive the placebo, standard-of-care, or existing therapy against which the intervention is being compared is known as the comparison or control group.

RCTs evaluate experimental **interventions** that may consist of either a single approach or a combination of approaches intended to influence the study outcome. Examples of interventions include diagnostic or therapeutic agents (e.g., pharmaceuticals), medical devices, behavior change approaches, and medical procedures (e.g., surgical techniques). It is critical that the intervention is the same (standardized) for all study participants so that the outcomes, or lack thereof, can be attributed to the intervention.

Randomization, a hallmark of RCTs, is the process by which study participants are assigned to either the study intervention or control. Randomization ensures that participants enrolled in the study are as similar as possible across groups. Randomization also ensures that unknown variations within the study population that could affect study outcome are proportionally dispersed through all study groups, and thus will not affect study results. Another key element of RCTs is **blinding**, where the participant (**single-blind**), the participant and the researcher (**double-blind**), or the participant, the researcher, and those analyzing the study data (**triple-blind**) do not know who is receiving the intervention and who is receiving the control. The combination of blinding and randomization is used to lessen the influence of prejudices, both conscious and unconscious, on the part of the participants and/or researchers that can affect the results of a study. The use of comparison groups and randomization are described in more detail later in this chapter.

RCTs are typically used to study the safety, efficacy, or effectiveness of an intervention compared to a control. **Efficacy** studies evaluate the benefit of an intervention as tested under controlled experimental conditions. An example of an efficacy study is the work done in Mali by Thera and colleagues (2011), in which a new vaccine designed to prevent malaria was tested against an existing rabies vaccine. The study found that the new vaccine was not efficacious, meaning it did not prevent malaria any better than the rabies vaccine. **Effectiveness** studies can evaluate the benefits of an intervention in real-world conditions or gather information about long-term side effects (sometimes referred to as **pharmacovigilance**). An example of an effectiveness trial is the study conducted in African American and Latino adults living with Type 2 diabetes in Michigan. Community health workers helped participants manage this chronic condition by providing them with diabetes self-management education, performing regular home visits, and accompanying them to their clinic visits during the 6-month intervention period (Spencer et al., 2011). An earlier trial had shown the intervention to be successful compared to a control group (Two Feathers et al., 2005). This effectiveness study was designed to evaluate the intervention in a real-world community-based setting and demonstrated that those who received the intervention had better glycemic control.

Finally, RCTs can be used to test effective interventions in new populations or with variations in dosing (once a day vs. twice a day) or formulation (immediate vs. time-release capsules). Such trials can be considered a hybrid of both efficacy and effectiveness studies.

Phases of Clinical Research

Clinical research, in which RCTs are commonly used, is often conducted in systematic, step-wise phases. Each phase is designed to answer a different research question, so that smaller, earlier studies inform subsequent larger, more definitive studies (Figure 8.1; ICH E8, 1997).

Figure 8.1   Correlation Between Development Phases and Types of Study

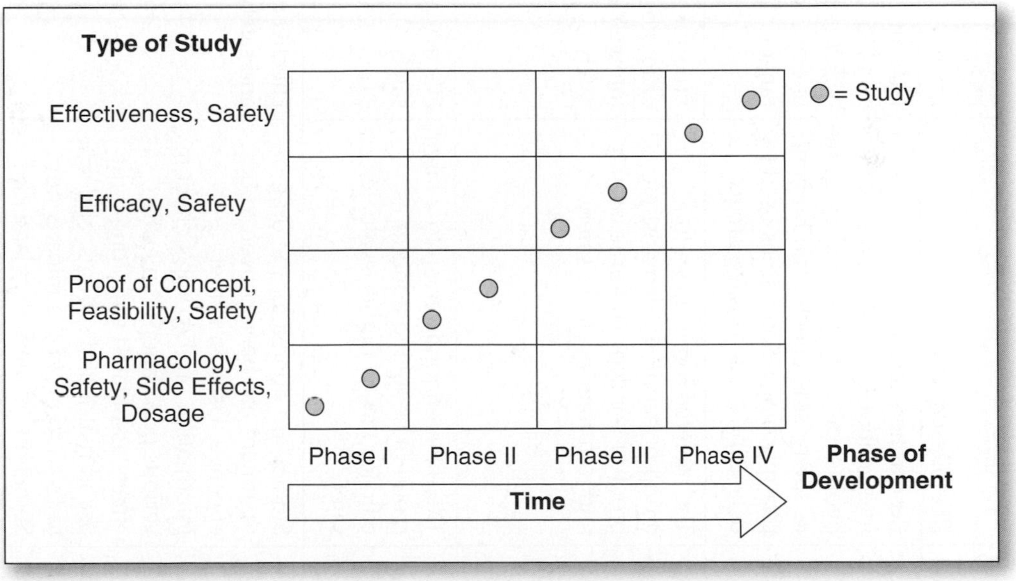

Source: Adapted from ICH E8 (1997).

Table 8.1 The Phases of Clinical Research

Phase	Brief Description	Outcome of Interest	Typical Size	RCT?	Example
I	Researchers test a new intervention in a small group of people for the first time to evaluate its safety, side effects, and human pharmacology. Sometimes used to determine a safe dosage range.	Human pharmacology (safety, side effects, dosage range)	20–80	Possibly	"Phase 1 Study of a Combination AMA1 Blood Stage Malaria Vaccine in Malian Children" (Dicko et al., 2008) This double-blind, dose-escalating RCT evaluated safety and immunogenicity in 36 healthy children aged 2–3 years.
II	The intervention is given to a group of people to demonstrate proof-of-concept and/or feasibility and to further evaluate safety.	Proof-of-concept or feasibility of intervention, safety	100–300	Yes	"A Randomized Controlled Phase 2 Trial of the Blood Stage AMA1-C1/Alhydrogel Malaria Vaccine in Children in Mali" (Sagara et al., 2009) This double-blind RCT evaluated safety, immunogenicity, and biologic impact in 300 healthy children aged 2–3 years
III	The intervention is given to a large group of people to confirm its efficacy and to further evaluate safety.	Efficacy and safety	Hundreds to thousands	Yes	"A Field Trial to Assess a Blood-Stage Malaria Vaccine" (Thera et al., 2011) This double-blind RCT evaluated efficacy in 400 healthy children aged 1–6 years.
IV	Studies are done after the drug or treatment has been proven to be effective. Used to gather information on the drug's effect in various populations, any side effects associated with long-term use in real-world settings, and to test variations of the intervention. Sometimes called postmarket or pharmacovigilance studies or assessments.	Effectiveness and safety	Varies	Possibly	There is no Phase IV study for this vaccine as it was not shown to be efficacious in Phase III.

Source: ClinicalTrials.gov (2012); Friedman, Furberg, and DeMets (2010); ICH E8 (1997).

The word *phase* has both regulatory and developmental meanings and may be used differently across therapeutic areas. For the purposes of this chapter, the phases of clinical research (Table 8.1) refer to guidelines established by the International Conference on Harmonization (ICH) Guidance on General Considerations for Clinical Trials (ICH E8, 1997). These guidelines, used by many countries, including the United States, define the sequence of research required for an intervention to eventually be considered acceptable for widespread use. In other words, the intervention must successfully pass earlier phases in order to undergo further testing. A drug deemed unsafe in a Phase I trial will not continue on the drug development pathway. Similarly, only efficacious interventions will move on to Phase IV effectiveness trials.

As an example, Table 8.1 includes the three clinical trial phases of an experimental malaria vaccine. It should be noted that the table does not include all trials related to the development of this vaccine, but rather the primary Phase I, II, and III studies. A Phase IV trial is not included, as the vaccine did not prove efficacious in Phase III. Treatments must successfully complete Phases I, II, and III to receive approval for use in the general population. While many potentially efficacious interventions fail to complete all three phases, important information gathered in each trial helps to inform future research and development. There are many examples of products that have progressed to Phase IV, or postapproval, clinical trials. For example, broad spectrum antibiotics, such as levofloxacin, have progressed through all four phases and continue to undergo postmarket assessments for use in populations not evaluated in earlier stages of research (U.S. Food and Drug Administration, 2012).

There are many possible designs for collecting the information desired in an RCT: parallel-group, crossover, split-body, cluster, factorial, step-wedge, and adaptive, among others. We explain the most common types, illustrated in Figure 8.2. Purpose, cost, time, ethics, and reliability of results are all taken into consideration when selecting the most appropriate study design. A descriptive analysis of the 616 RCTs indexed in PubMed in December 2006 found that 78% were parallel-group trials, 16% were crossover, 2% were split-body, 2% were cluster, and 2% were factorial (Hopewell, Dutton, Yu, Chan, & Altman, 2010).

The vast majority of RCTs use a **parallel-group** design. In this design, each study subject is randomly assigned to a group, and all the subjects in that group receive the same intervention or the control. All three of the malaria studies included in Table 8.1 (Dicko et al., 2008; Sagara et al., 2009; Thera et al., 2011), as well as the community health worker intervention to improve diabetic self-management cited earlier (Spencer et al., 2011), used a parallel-group design.

In studies with a **crossover** design, subjects are randomized not to one particular intervention but to a sequence of several interventions. Each subject receives multiple interventions or controls in a random sequence and serves as his or her own control. Crossover designs require fewer subjects and are often employed when one wants to reduce the influence of non-intervention-related (confounding) factors. In this type of study design, lingering effects of a prior intervention may affect outcomes of a subsequent intervention, skewing results. This carryover can sometimes be overcome by providing sufficient time (called a **washout period**) between each intervention. A crossover study to determine whether acupuncture can be used to successfully treat

Figure 8.2 Common RCT Design Types

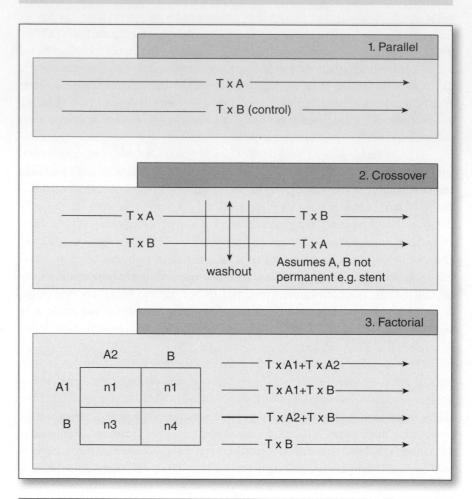

Source: National Institutes of Health, Office of Behavioral & Social Sciences Research (n.d.).

pain (see Figure 8.3) had a 24-hour washout period between treatment with a penetrating needle (acupuncture) and treatment with a nonpenetrating needle (acupressure; Takakura & Yajima, 2009). The results of this study revealed that both acupuncture and acupressure are better than no pain management, but that no difference could be seen between the two techniques.

Split-body is a type of design where the subjects serve as their own control and different body parts (eyes or regions of affected skin, for example) are randomized. For example, Henry and colleagues conducted a split-mouth trial to evaluate the effect of light on tooth whitening (Henry, Bauchmoyer, Moore, & Rashid, 2012). Participants had their front teeth whitened with a 25% hydrogen peroxide in-office whitening system. A light was used on a randomly selected right or left half of the mouth. The opposing side

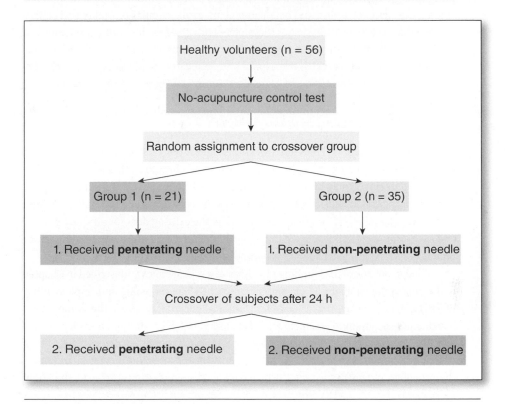

Figure 8.3   Crossover Study Design Comparing Acupuncture (Penetrating Needle) to Acupressure (Nonpenetrating Needle) for Pain Management

Source: Takakura and Yajima (2009).

was whitened only with gel. Tooth shade and tooth sensitivity were measured before, immediately after, and 1 and 2 weeks after whitening. The right and left sides were compared for each participant. The only significant difference between whitening with and without the light was on the teeth in the upper jaw; however, participants could not distinguish this difference themselves.

When the randomization in a parallel or crossover design study is made to preexisting groups of subjects (e.g., villages, schools, physicians), this is usually termed a **cluster** design. Davis and colleagues (2007) describe a trial in which a pop-up prompt in the electronic medical record increased the number of prescriptions written in accordance with the best known evidence for pediatric conditions. In this study, physicians were randomized to either receive or not receive pop-up prompts about the best drugs to prescribe for certain conditions. Data were then collected and analyzed for each physician's patients. The advantage of using a cluster design for this study was that it prevented contamination between the two groups—as physicians were randomized to either always see the pop-up prompts or never to see them—so their patients either consistently benefitted from the additional information or they did not.

Although employed less often, **factorial** designs offer a way to study multiple interventions simultaneously. In such studies, each subject is randomly assigned to a group that receives a particular combination of interventions or noninterventions. The Physician's Health Study was a well-known clinical program with a factorial design that studied the effects of aspirin and beta-carotene on cardiovascular mortality and cancer in more than 22,000 male physicians (Stampfer et al., 1985). In this study, approximately 5,500 subjects were randomized to each of the four treatment arms: (1) active aspirin and active beta-carotene, (2) active aspirin and beta-carotene placebo, (3) aspirin placebo and active beta-carotene, and (4) aspirin placebo and beta-carotene placebo.

Special Ethical Considerations for RCTs

All research must be conducted with the highest ethical standards. As described above, safety is evaluated at all phases of clinical research. Studies that present possible risk to a participant may be monitored by a Data Safety Monitoring Board (DSMB), comprising experts in clinical research as well as the clinical area being studied. DSMBs meet at regular intervals during the study, review the existing data for all study groups, and may recommend study termination if the outcomes are significantly different across groups (which could signal benefit or harm of one treatment versus the other).

Though not one of the founding principles of research ethics as described in Chapter 3, the concept of equipoise is incredibly important when designing and implementing RCTs. Equipoise means that there exists genuine uncertainty about the comparative benefits of each group in a clinical trial (Freedman, 1987). In addition, if evidence confirms that one treatment is superior to the other (based on either the results of other clinical trial results and/or interim analysis), investigators are ethically obligated (under the principles of beneficence and justice) to offer the superior treatment to the study participants. In 2011, an HIV Prevention Trials Network study (HPTN 052) began offering the study intervention to all HIV-infected trial participants when an interim analysis revealed that early initiation of antiretroviral therapy significantly reduced HIV transmission from the HIV-infected individual to his or her sexual partner (Cohen et al., 2011).

Study Objectives and Study Endpoints

A single study cannot answer all the questions associated with an intervention. Such an attempt would exceed resources, encumber implementation, and result in confounding and uninterpretable data. Consequently, RCTs usually define a single primary objective and a limited number of secondary objectives that address specific gaps in knowledge related to the intervention. Clearly defined objectives create the roadmap for determining endpoints, defining study procedures, and interpreting data. With RCTs, defining clear objectives and endpoints is particularly critical to ensure that appropriate meaningful data are collected and analyzed. If the wrong data are collected, it may be impossible or invalid to compare the outcomes between randomized study groups even if data analysis is possible. The absence of clear objectives and endpoints undermines the scientific rigor of the evidence that randomization is designed to provide.

Primary and Secondary Study Objectives

As detailed in Chapter 2, one of the first steps in designing a research study is to determine the research question or hypothesis to be addressed. In RCTs, the research question is outlined by the study objectives; as noted, most RCTs have one primary objective and multiple secondary objectives (Figure 8.4).

Figure 8.4   Primary and Secondary Objectives

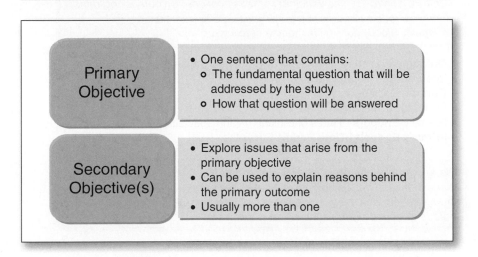

The **primary study objective** should focus on one clearly defined question and include enough information to communicate the study's overall purpose and outcome. The objective defines the key elements of the study:

- the outcome (e.g., efficacy, effectiveness)
- the intervention being evaluated
- the control
- the study population
- the study's duration (e.g., 6 months, 1 year)
- endpoints (which will be measured to determine outcome)

Ideally, a well-defined primary study objective can be expressed as a single, clear sentence that identifies both the research question and how that question will be addressed. **Secondary study objectives** frequently explore issues that arise from the primary question or that may help interpret the outcome of the primary objective. For example, a study whose primary objective is to determine the efficacy of a new drug at the Phase III level will commonly have secondary objectives that address safety, adherence, and quality of life. Although not optimal, some study teams choose to include two primary objectives, often one for efficacy and another for safety. However, usually one of these issues is secondary to the other. For example, in Phase III studies, safety has already been the primary focus of previous studies and efficacy has yet to be determined.

The primary and secondary objectives for the malaria vaccine study cited earlier in this chapter (Thera et al., 2011) could have been written as shown in Figure 8.5.

Figure 8.5   Example of Primary and Secondary Objectives

The **primary objective** is to compare the efficacy of a malaria vaccine versus a control (rabies vaccine) in Malian children by comparing rates of clinical malaria acquisition (fever plus ≥ 2500 parasites per cubic millimeter blood) during six months of follow-up.

- **Outcome**: To determine the efficacy of a new malaria vaccine
- **Intervention**: Malaria vaccine
- **Control**: Rabies vaccine
- **Population**: Malian children
- **Primary Endpoint**: Rates of clinical malaria acquisition
- **Primary Endpoint Time Period**: 6 months

The **secondary objective** is to determine the number of clinical malaria cases that were caused by parasites with the same AMA1 DNA sequence found in the vaccine strain by genotyping all cases of malaria acquired during six months of follow-up.

- **Outcome**: To determine the number of malaria cases caused by parasites with a specific DNA sequence
- **Population**: Malian children
- **Secondary Endpoint**: The genotype of all acquired malaria cases
- **Secondary Endpoint Time Period**: 6 months

Study Outcomes and Endpoints

Each primary and secondary objective should be affiliated with a **study outcome** and a **study endpoint**. In the example above, the outcome of the primary objective is to determine the efficacy of the intervention. To assess the outcome, an endpoint (rate of clinical malaria acquisition) must be measured. Likewise, for the secondary objective, the outcome is the number of cases caused by a specific strain of parasite, which is determined by measuring an endpoint (the genotype of each acquired case of malaria). According to ICH E9 (1998), the primary endpoint should be a variable capable of providing the most clinically relevant and convincing evidence directly related to the primary objective of the study. All endpoints are measurable, and in the literature they are sometimes referred to as outcome measures.

Clinical and Surrogate Endpoints

For many conditions, clear **clinical endpoints** such as survival or the occurrence of a clinical event (e.g., a cardiovascular event) may take place only after many years of therapeutic intervention. In these cases, a biological marker (biomarker) may be used as a substitute or "surrogate" for the clinical endpoint (Strimbu & Tavel, 2010). Common examples of **surrogate endpoints** are cholesterol level for cardiovascular disease, tumor growth for cancer, and viral load and CD4 cell count for HIV/AIDS. The change in a biomarker may not have any immediate or even noticeable clinical effect but, ideally, has been validated to predict changes in clinical outcome.

The use of surrogate endpoints can reduce the size and duration of clinical trials and speed the drug development timeline, such that patients can benefit more quickly from effective treatments. However, the correlation between surrogate endpoints and clinical outcomes can be tenuous. For example, the drug quinidine was shown to help patients with atrial fibrillation maintain a regular heart beat (the surrogate biomarker); unfortunately, long-term use was subsequently linked to a higher rate of death (the clinical outcome) due to cardiac arrest (Coplen, Antman, Berlin, Hewitt, & Chalmers, 1990).

Definition of Control

In an RCT, the control is the point of reference against which the intervention is evaluated. The purpose of the control is to rule out the effects of extraneous factors on outcomes. For example, a study designed to evaluate a new treatment would compare the group receiving the treatment with a control group to ensure that the outcomes measured in the treatment group can be confidently attributed to the treatment and not something unknown. Choosing an appropriate control is very important when designing a trial.

Types of Control

In an RCT, when one group of participants receives an inactive or inert substance, it is considered the placebo control group and is compared with the intervention group. Comparison with a placebo is often the cleanest comparison. A **placebo control** is used when an effective treatment for the indication does not exist or if a commonly used treatment has not been proven to be beneficial or is not well tolerated. In blinded studies, the placebo is identical in its appearance to the intervention. An example of a placebo-controlled study is CAPRISA 004 (Abdool Karim et al., 2010), which evaluated the effectiveness and safety of tenofovir gel, a gel used vaginally to prevent HIV in women. In this study, women were randomized to receive either the tenofovir-containing gel or a placebo gel (gel without any drug). The incidence of HIV was compared between the two groups, and tenofovir gel was found to lower HIV acquisition by 39% compared to placebo gel.

Active Controls

When a proven effective treatment or intervention already exists, the study intervention is usually compared with this known, effective intervention, called an **active control**. In studies involving serious conditions where an approved therapy exists, the use of a placebo would be considered unethical; in these situations active controls are generally considered the best alternative. When the efficacy of an intervention is compared with an active control, the study has to be designed to either demonstrate that the intervention is equivalent to (a **non-inferiority** study) or better than (a **superiority** study) the active control.

An example of an active-controlled study is one that compared apixaban with warfarin to treat atrial fibrillation (Granger et al., 2011). Apixaban was found to be superior to warfarin in preventing stroke or systemic embolism; in addition, apixaban caused less bleeding and lowered mortality in comparison to warfarin.

Standard of Care

For most conditions, the usual care provided in a setting is considered the standard of care and may vary between developed and developing countries. The standard of care may or may not include a therapeutic drug (because it either does not exist or is not available), and is considered a valid comparator group. For example, the effectiveness of a lifestyle intervention on weight loss and reduction of diabetes risk was tested among low-income, Spanish-speaking Latinos at increased risk of diabetes. In this study, participants were randomly assigned to the lifestyle intervention or standard of care (regular visits with no lifestyle interventions) and the incidence of diabetes was assessed (Ockene et al., 2012). The study successfully demonstrated that the intervention could increase weight loss and improve both glycemic control and insulin resistance.

No Intervention at All

In some RCTs, one study group receives no intervention at all. This is useful when analyzing the effect of natural progression and resolution of a condition or disease, and the need to distinguish it from the response to a placebo. An example is a study in asthma patients, where albuterol was shown to improve measured lung function when compared with placebo, sham acupuncture, and no intervention (Wechsler et al., 2011).

Self as Control

In some crossover study designs, individuals are their own controls for a period of time before they receive an intervention; this is described as **self as control.**

Ethical and Design Considerations in the Selection of Controls

Both ethical and design considerations determine the choice of a control. If there is a best therapy, then it may be used as an active control; however, the best therapy may not be chosen as the active control if it is unavailable in the study settings, is cost prohibitive, or cannot be appropriately administered due to lack of infrastructure or trained personnel. In other instances, experts may disagree on the best therapy or approach, so an active control will not be chosen. For these reasons, investigators and ethics committees must thoughtfully consider what the best control should be in a given trial.

Defining the Study Population: Inclusion/Exclusion and Size

Selection of the Study Population

A critical aspect of any RCT is the study population (also known as the study cohort). The defining characteristics of the chosen study population will affect the choice of study design, the feasibility of recruiting eligible participants, the ability to evaluate endpoints, and ultimately, the ability to generalize results. The characteristics of a study population are defined by the study's eligibility criteria. The criteria used to judge whether an individual is appropriate for participation in a study are called inclusion criteria. The criteria used to exclude individuals, either because of a risk to their safety or other factors, are called exclusion criteria. For example, in a study evaluating an anti-hypertensive drug, individuals must have high blood pressure in order to participate (inclusion criterion), but should not be currently taking another anti-hypertensive medication (an exclusion criterion).

Considerations in Defining Study Population

Eligibility criteria critical to evaluation of the intervention must be precisely specified. For example, in a study evaluating an intervention for angina, it may be enough to exclude those with very high blood pressure. In such an example, the exclusion criteria may define a threshold systolic/diastolic pressure above which individuals will be excluded. However, in a study evaluating anti-hypertensive agents, inclusion criteria may need to be more specific, defining how often an individual's blood pressure has been measured at above normal for the person to be eligible for participation.

In a trial evaluating efficacy and safety, eligibility criteria should ensure the safety of the participants while allowing evaluation of the study endpoints. Appropriate criteria permit inclusion of participants who have the potential to benefit from the intervention. For example, in a Phase III study evaluating the efficacy of antiretroviral treatment for HIV, HIV-infected patients must be included in order to evaluate whether the drugs are efficacious in treating HIV. In contrast, HIV-infected individuals with a known resistance to the drugs and/or other health conditions that raise safety concerns may be excluded.

In general, a study's eligibility criteria limit inclusion to a homogenous population, which means the study's participants have similar characteristics. Eligibility criteria that are too restrictive, however, may hinder timely enrollment and impair the ability to generalize results to a larger population for whom the intervention is ultimately intended.

Other Factors That Influence Selection of the Study Population

Questions have been raised about the extent to which the effects of an intervention can be generalized beyond the study population (Berlin & Ellenberg, 2009). Concerns that women and minorities had been underrepresented in important clinical research studies led Congress to mandate that all National Institutes of Health-funded trials provide for valid analysis of whether the variables being studied affect women or members of minority groups differently than other subjects in the trial (NIH Revitalization Act, 1993). The statute allows exceptions when there is substantial evidence of a lack of difference in effects of treatment between subgroups. Pregnant women and women with child-bearing potential have also been excluded from clinical trials, as researchers have been hesitant to expose fetuses to investigational agents. However, this practice has also precluded women from access to needed treatment and limited their ability to make informed risk/benefit choices when deciding whether to use approved treatments (Little, Lyerly, & Faden, 2009). These issues continue to challenge researchers.

Sample Size

Equally critical to defining the study population is determining how many participants are needed to address the primary study objective. The number of participants in a study is called the **sample size**. Sample sizes must be sufficient to demonstrate a statistically significant difference (or lack thereof) between the experimental intervention and the control. The main aim of a sample size calculation is to determine the number of participants needed to detect a clinically relevant treatment effect. The considerations described in this section apply to sample size calculations and hypothesis testing for study designs other than RCTs as well.

In order to calculate the sample size, researchers must have some idea of the results expected in a study. In general, the greater the variability in the outcome variable, the larger the sample size required to assess whether an observed effect is a true effect. On the other hand, the more effective a tested treatment is, the smaller the sample size needed to detect a positive or negative outcome. If the sample size is too small, the study may not be able to detect an important existing effect, whereas samples that are too large may waste time, resources, and money. It is therefore important to optimize sample size (Noordzij et al., 2010).

The statistical practice of hypothesis testing is used to compare interventions in a clinical trial and is the basis for finding its appropriate sample size. Researchers must consider the type of data collected and statistical procedures used for the specified hypothesis tests (see Chapter 18 for a presentation and discussion of these concepts). Despite many choices, the guiding principle is to choose the sample size necessary to minimize the probability that the conclusion drawn from a study is incorrect. Imagine, for the purposes of explanation, that a trial is testing a single intervention against a control. Statistically speaking, the trial has four possible outcomes: (1) the study concludes that the intervention is better than the control, but in reality there is no difference between them; (2) the study concludes that the intervention and control are the same, but in reality they are not; (3) the study concludes that the intervention and control are the same, and in reality they are; (4) the study concludes that the intervention and control have different effects, and in reality they do. Each of these outcomes has a statistical probability of occurring. Researchers must design their trials to minimize the probability that they will come to a mistaken conclusion. When a study concludes that the intervention is better than the control, when in reality their effects are the same, this false-positive conclusion is termed a **type I** error (see Table 8.2) and its associated probability is traditionally called α. The alternate false-negative conclusion, that the treatments have the same effects when in fact they differ, is termed a **type II** error (see Table 8.2) and the associated probability is traditionally called β. The chance of avoiding a false-negative conclusion is referred to as the statistical **power** of the study and is represented by $1-\beta$. For this reason sample size calculations are sometimes called **power analysis**.

Table 8.2   Two Fundamental Errors Associated With Hypothesis Testing

	The two interventions really are the same.	The two interventions really are different.
The study shows that the two interventions are different.	False positive Type I error	True positive Correct outcome
The study shows that the two interventions are the same.	True negative Correct outcome	False negative Type II error

Because both types of errors *will* occur, the goal in choosing the sample size is to balance α (typically 0.05, meaning there is 5% chance that the study will generate a false positive) and β (typically 0.20, meaning there is a 20% chance the study will generate a false negative). If researchers want greater certainty that a new treatment is better than the control, they need to calculate their sample size using a smaller α. However if there was lower cost and no chance of more side effects of a new treatment, then one would want to dramatically increase the power (i.e., reduce β).

Beyond the choices for α and β, the type of data being analyzed and the nature of the hypotheses (superiority vs. non-inferiority), the specific statistical calculations for sample size depend on the number of treatments, expected difference(s) in the analysis endpoint between the treatments, proportion of subjects in each treatment group, and additional factors related to data variability. Details are provided in many statistical and clinical trials texts (Friedman et al., 2010; Julious, 2010). These texts provide specific formulae and sample size tables based on common data analysis assumptions, and a variety of software programs are available for more general analysis considerations.

As a simple example, suppose you were planning an RCT to compare the proportion of subjects who achieve a desired efficacy endpoint. You believe that an increase of 0.10 or 0.15 would represent a clinically meaningful improvement relative to what is achieved with the control. Table 8.3 provides the estimated number of subjects in each treatment group under different treatment effect assumptions and error probability assumptions, while assuming both groups are the same size. The table illustrates the impact of changes in the treatment effect, α, and β on sample size. As can be seen, for the same percentages, reducing α and/or β directly increases the sample size although not to the same extent.

Table 8.3 Example of Sample Size Requirements per Treatment Group

Treatment Effect*	Percentages**		$\beta = 0.20$		$\beta = 0.50$	
	Control	New Treatment	$\alpha = 0.05$	$\alpha = 0.01$	$\alpha = 0.05$	$\alpha = 0.01$
0.10	0.40	0.50	408	597	210	349
0.10	0.80	0.90	219	317	118	189
0.15	0.40	0.55	186	271	99	161
0.15	0.80	0.95	94	126	70	87

*The difference between the effect of the treatment and the effect of the standard of care.

**The percentage of subjects in that group who experience the study endpoint.

Randomization

The key distinguishing feature of the RCT is that subjects are randomly allocated to receive either the intervention or the control(s) in parallel studies, or particular sequences of the intervention and control(s) in crossover studies. In practice, random allocation can be complex, but conceptually, the process is akin to repeatedly tossing a fair coin. The goal is that an unpredictable sequence of study group allocations is generated. This process deliberately introduces an element of chance to help reduce any bias in the selection and allocation of subjects to the study intervention and control(s).

Beyond the reduction of bias, randomization tends to produce study groups in which extraneous factors, both known and unknown, that might influence outcomes are distributed similarly. Thus one is able to deduce that any differences in outcomes can be causally attributed to the difference in treatments. Finally, the use of chance in the randomization provides a statistical basis for quantitative evaluation of the evidence related to treatment effects (e.g., p-values, confidence intervals; Lachin, 1988).

Randomization can be conducted not only for individual subjects, but also for entire groups of subjects that share some physical, social, geographic, or other connection (e.g., clinics, schools, work places, communities). In group-randomized designs, each subject within a group has the same intervention. In these cases, special considerations are taken to compare individuals within the same study group (Murray, Varnell, & Blitstein, 2004).

Typically the numbers of subjects in each study group is nearly the same. However, for certain objectives, unequal allocation of treatments may be desired. For example in initial safety drug trials, a treatment allocation of two actives for each control (2:1) helps to increase overall exposure to the new intervention.

Types of Randomization

The simplest and most common type of randomization, often called an **unrestricted randomization,** uses a (usually computer-generated) process equivalent to repeatedly tossing a coin. If there are two treatments (A and B) that are to be assigned in a 1:1 treatment allocation, (i.e., exactly as many As as Bs) a random sequence of A and B would be generated (ABBAAABB . . .). Eligible subjects would be successively assigned the next treatment in the sequence: the first subject would receive A, the second B, the third B, and so on. The main drawback of such a method is the possibility of imbalanced group sizes in small RCTs, especially if the exact number to be enrolled is not fixed in advance or the trial could end before full enrollment. While the above sequence shows the desired four As and four Bs to this point, it is equally likely that all four As could be assigned first (i.e., AAAABBBB). If there is a possibility that the subjects entering the trial at the beginning are somehow different from those at the end, such an imbalance in the sequence of treatments is highly undesirable.

Randomized block designs avoid such a possibility by enrolling successive blocks (groups) of subjects, with randomization occurring within each block. In this way, balance within treatment groups is maintained over time. For example, a block size of four would have equal numbers of As and Bs within each successive group of four subjects (ABBA, AABB, BBAA, etc.). Unfortunately, an investigator acquainted with this scheme might be able to predict the assignment of subjects toward the end of each block, and thus introduce selection bias. For this reason it is recommended that researchers select the largest practical block size in order to conceal the block size from all investigators, vary the block size under each investigator and within each site, or, for multicenter trials, vary the block size between sites (Wittes, 1998).

Stratified randomization is similar to block randomization and is achieved by performing a separate randomization procedure within each of two or more subsets of study participants. Called **strata**, these subsets share important characteristics that may affect study results. This type of randomization ensures that the number of study subjects receiving each intervention is closely balanced within each subset. Although treatment responses between sites in a multicenter RCT would hopefully be similar, sites are usually treated as a stratification factor for such studies. It is always recommended that the number of stratification factors be small in relation to the number of subjects. While general randomization blocks tend not to be discussed in most analyses of RCTs, in stratified studies the different strata are an important design feature that must be accounted for in all statistical analyses (Breslow, 2006). Additional information about stratified sampling can be found in Chapter 17.

Allocation Concealment

Another process related to randomization and blinding, called **allocation concealment**, is the procedure for protecting the randomization process so that the treatment to be allocated is not known before the patient is entered into the study

(Forder, Gebski, & Keech, 2005). Any effort by an investigator to determine group assignments in order to dictate the assignment of the next patient introduces selection bias and confounding factors (i.e., imbalance in extraneous factors that can affect outcomes), both of which randomization is designed to minimize. Unfortunately, treatment-related side effects or adverse events may be specific enough to reveal allocation to investigators or patients, thereby introducing bias or influencing the reporting of subjective data by investigator or patient. While allocation concealment is maintained to reduce bias and preserve randomization, the assigned treatment information must be readily available in the event of a medical emergency.

Some standard methods of ensuring allocation concealment include opaque-sealed envelopes, sequentially numbered containers, pharmacy-controlled randomization, and central randomization. The methods employed for allocation concealment and randomization disclosure should be decided on prior to study implementation and in any subsequent data reports. Centralized randomization is always recommended for multicenter trials (ICH E9, 1998).

Settings for RCTs

RCTs can take place in a variety of settings such as schools, communities, and clinical settings. These settings will be dictated by the requirements of the study, more specifically the objectives, endpoints, eligibility criteria, and data collection considerations. Setting refers to three general domains: (1) the geographic location where the study takes place, (2) the locale(s) where participants are recruited, and (3) the place where study visits are conducted.

The selection of settings is a critical element in RCT design, as settings affect the ability of the research team to collect high-quality, reproducible measures. Researchers must understand both the social and political climate of any proposed settings to assess the feasibility and acceptability of study implementation at these sites. Involving key stakeholders, such as community members, in the early stages of study development can provide invaluable insight on the realities of study implementation at a site and help identify creative solutions to potential challenges. The role of communities in research is discussed further in Chapter 4.

Geographic Location

Research studies must be conducted in a geographic area where both the endpoint (e.g., disease, behavior) and the study population exist. For example, it is appropriate to test a malaria vaccine in Mali, where malaria is endemic, rather than in the United States, where malaria has been eradicated. Similarly, a randomized controlled trial evaluating a new medication to treat Lyme disease in the United States should focus on geographic regions, such as New Jersey, Massachusetts, and Pennsylvania, with the highest burden of the disease (CDC, 2013).

Recruitment Locales

Once the geographic region is identified, researchers must identify specific areas where eligible potential participants are likely to exist. A study's success depends on the ability to identify eligible participants in a timely manner. Recruitment delays can lead to additional study costs, study closure, or lack of power for analysis. For example, chronic constipation may occur in the general population; however, certain groups are more likely to experience this condition, such as the elderly or individuals using medications known to cause chronic constipation. When designing a study to evaluate the efficacy of a drug for chronic constipation, it may be more efficient to recruit participants from nursing home and hospital settings, where eligible participants are more likely to be found. Similarly, an intervention designed for children may be most effective when delivered in the school setting. Glezen and colleagues describe an intervention evaluating the effectiveness of live attenuated influenza vaccine (LAIV) in school-aged children (Glezen, Gaglani, Kozinetz, & Piedra, 2010). In this trial, the study groups were schools where children were offered LAIV versus inactivated vaccine.

Study Visit Location

When determining the study visit location, it is important to assess a range of implementation considerations, such as confidentiality, clinical procedures, sample collection, processing and storage, location, and infrastructure requirements. The safety of the study participant is paramount, so study visits should be conducted in a location that provides adequate participant privacy and confidentiality. Adequate privacy and confidentiality depend on the nature of the study and the risk of harm to the participant. For example, studies involving treatment of people with HIV may need to consider whether signage at the study visit location may risk revealing someone's HIV status. In addition, the nature of the study procedures may require physical space with four walls and a door for physical exams and interviews involving sensitive topics. In some cases, the process of randomization may require additional confidentiality protections.

Depending on the nature of the study, certain clinical procedures (e.g., blood draw, physical exams) may be needed to assess the study endpoints or participant safety. For example, it may be possible for trained personnel to draw blood in a variety of settings; however, pelvic exams will likely require access to a clinic or similar setting with the necessary equipment, privacy, and personnel. In addition, a variety of biological samples may be collected as part of the study. For example, certain trials may require that the specimens be stored on dry ice or be processed within a certain time frame after collection. In such cases, researchers need to plan ahead and determine whether visit sites need to be within a certain distance of the laboratory.

The items above all speak to site infrastructure and capacity. Although it may be ideal to conduct study visits in community settings, lack of resources (electricity, running water, private space, etc.) may result in changes to implementation or the need to build capacity prior to study initiation. These on-the-ground considerations can influence study timelines, site selection, and even study design.

SPECIAL CONSIDERATIONS FOR RCTS

RCTs have inherent strengths and limitations that are described below and summarized in Table 8.4.

Table 8.4 Strengths and Limitations of RCTs

Strengths	Limitations
• Randomization can balance out factors that cannot be controlled for or are unknown. • Blinding can reduce potential sources of bias. • Results can be applied to populations with characteristics similar to the study cohort.	• The placebo and Hawthorne effects can affect RCT outcomes. • Results cannot be generalized to populations that differ from the study cohort. • RCT outcomes may not be reproducible in real-world settings.

Strengths

Using an RCT to explore a scientific hypothesis offers a number of benefits. At the conclusion of a research trial, it is important to understand the causal relationship between the study intervention and the outcome of interest (and, in particular, to be sure that study results are not due to chance or bias). When well designed and well conducted, RCTs can produce objective and unbiased results, and hence are viewed as the gold standard of clinical research. This is due in large part to the use of randomization, which balances out factors that either cannot be controlled for or are unknown, and the use of blinding (single, double, and triple), which reduces potential sources of bias such as perceived benefit. These design elements ensure that the amount of change attributed to participation in the study is the same across groups. Therefore, change in the outcome of interest can be attributed to the intervention.

A significant advantage of the RCT design is the ability to apply results to members of the broader population with similar characteristics to the study cohort. For example, the Phase I–III malaria vaccine trials (Dicko et al., 2008; Sagara et al., 2009; Thera et al., 2011) described earlier enrolled healthy children in Mali, aged 2–6 years. Had the vaccine proved efficacious, it would be reasonable to assume that the vaccine's efficacy would extend to all children 2–6 years old in malaria-endemic regions.

Limitations

There are several inherent limitations of the RCT design, including the placebo and Hawthorne effects, the negative aspects of generalizability, and the ability to apply successful interventions in real-world settings.

In many clinical trials, a small proportion of participants improve after receiving the placebo (Au, Castro, & Krishnan, 2007). Commonly called the placebo effect, this improvement can be due to the positive impact of the routine care people often receive when they participate in a trial, the self-limiting nature of many disorders that naturally resolve over time, and/or participants reporting positive outcomes in an effort to be perceived as cooperative. If the efficacy of an experimental intervention is low and the placebo effect is strong for a particular population or intervention, an RCT may not be able to detect a difference between the study groups.

Sometimes study participants change their behavior as a result of participating in a research study either because of their perception that they are being monitored or because they are more aware of their behavior. This phenomenon is known as the Hawthorne effect. Fortunately, this effect can usually be controlled for in the design of an RCT by the process of randomization.

Although applicability of the results from the study population to similar members of the overall population is a strength of the RCT design, this feature cuts both ways. The results of RCTs are, in a strict sense, only applicable to those who have the identical characteristics of the study population. Reasons for this include geographical location (what works for one country may not work for another because of cultural or political reasons), demographic features, and disease factors. As mentioned earlier, RCTs may exclude the elderly, women, minorities, and children—and it cannot be automatically assumed that an intervention successful in middle-aged Caucasian men will work in young Black women. In addition, interventions may have very different effects depending on the disease stage (e.g., early vs. late-stage cancer).

Additionally, the intensive, and sometimes unusual or experimental, procedures that are included in RCTs may not be realistically reproducible in the real world. For example, participants in RCTs with biomedical agents often receive extensive behavioral and adherence counseling, which may contribute to the agent's efficacy in an RCT. Such interventions may be resource intensive in a way that cannot realistically be translated to real-world settings. Similarly, an RCT may measure an intervention's effect using a biological assay that is not available in clinical practice or is too expensive to use routinely. Finally, if an RCT's study duration is relatively short, the effectiveness of its intervention in a real-world setting may be different when applied for longer time periods. Chapter 1 (p. 10) contains a text box with further discussion of the merits and limitations of RCTs.

THE RELEVANCE OF RCTS FOR PUBLIC HEALTH

RCTs affect public health in a variety of ways. They can inform decisions on public health policy, spur the creation or revision of guidelines for evidence-based medicine, and provide justification for whether interventions, programs, drugs, and devices are made available to the general public. In addition, RCTs can be used to determine whether an intervention is cost-effective enough to be recommended or implemented by national or international agencies.

Informing Public Health Policy

Sometimes the results of RCTs have a direct influence on public health policy, creating an enabling environment for rapid implementation of new interventions. For example, between 2005 and 2007, three RCTs demonstrated that adult male circumcision reduces the risk of HIV acquisition by approximately 60% (Auvert et al., 2005; Bailey et al., 2007; Gray et al., 2007). As a direct result of these studies, the government of Kenya issued the "National Guidance for Voluntary Male Circumcision in Kenya" (Ministry of Health, Republic of Kenya, 2008). This public health policy provided a national framework for the rollout of safe, accessible, and sustainable adult male circumcision (AMC) services with the goal of reducing the country's incidence of HIV infection. By 2011, this policy resulted in the circumcision of approximately 290,000 adult Kenyan men, primarily in Nyanza Province, an area of the country with the highest HIV burden and a low rate of AMC (Figure 8.6; Mwandi et al., 2011). The impact on HIV incidence is currently under study.

Figure 8.6   Cumulative Circumcisions Done in Kenya 2008–2011

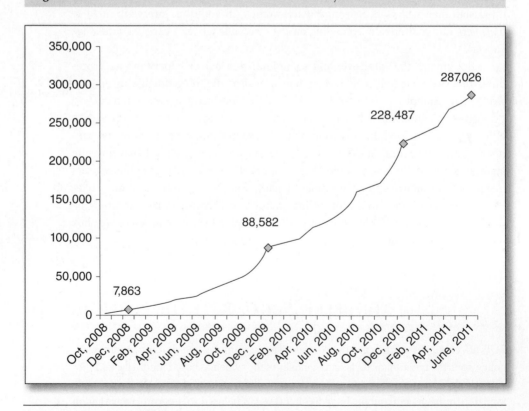

Source: Mwandi et al. (2011).

Guidelines for Disease Prevention and Treatment

The evidence generated from RCTs is often used to develop and update disease prevention and treatment guidelines, enabling individual clinicians to implement the best available scientific evidence in everyday practice (Timmermans & Mauck, 2005). For example, the U.S. Preventive Services Task Force (USPSTF) is an independent panel of experts who review the scientific literature on a broad range of clinical preventive health care services (such as screening, counseling, and preventive medications) and develop recommendations for primary care clinicians. This task force considers data generated from well-designed and well-conducted RCTs to be the highest level of evidence (Figure 8.7; USPSTF, 2008). In May 2012, the USPSTF recommended against prostate-specific antigen (PSA)-based screening for prostate cancer, as it found that the test resulted in little or no reduction in prostate cancer mortality and was associated with harms related to subsequent evaluation and treatment, some of which may be unnecessary (Chou et al., 2011; USPSTF, 2012). The task force based this recommendation on 10 randomized controlled trials, 23 cohort studies, and 6 uncontrolled studies. While not a policy mandate, the new guidelines gave practicing clinicians additional evidence by which to decide whether to recommend PSA testing to their patients.

Figure 8.7   Hierarchy of Research Design Used by the USPSTF

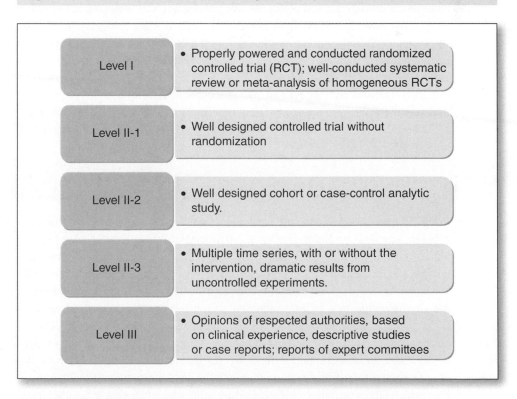

Level I	• Properly powered and conducted randomized controlled trial (RCT); well-conducted systematic review or meta-analysis of homogeneous RCTs
Level II-1	• Well designed controlled trial without randomization
Level II-2	• Well designed cohort or case-control analytic study.
Level II-3	• Multiple time series, with or without the intervention, dramatic results from uncontrolled experiments.
Level III	• Opinions of respected authorities, based on clinical experience, descriptive studies or case reports; reports of expert committees

Source: U.S. Preventive Services Task Force (USPSTF) Procedure Manual. Section 4.3.2.

Making Drugs and Devices Available to the General Public

Many countries or regions have agencies that regulate the use of drugs and devices and assess the safety and efficacy of new therapies. These agencies, for example, the Food and Drug Administration (FDA) in the United States, the Therapeutic Goods Administration (TGA) in Australia, the Pharmaceutical and Medical Devices Agency (PMDA) in Japan, and the European Medicines Agency (EMA), all depend on RCTs to help them decide whether to make drugs and devices available to the general public. In the United States, the FDA typically requires at least two Phase III trials, which are always randomized and controlled, and thus designed to demonstrate drug efficacy and safety, for approval of a new drug.

Determining the Cost-Effectiveness of Interventions

Finally, RCT results can be used to determine the cost-effectiveness of an intervention, which in turn can affect the intervention's accessibility. For example, insecticide-treated bed nets (ITNs) have been shown to be effective in reducing child mortality in regions with high malaria transmission. The data from one RCT was used to determine the cost-effectiveness of ITNs, taking into account the costs associated with the bed nets themselves (purchase, distribution, retreatment with insecticide, etc.), treating sick children (medicine, clinic and doctor fees, etc.), and funerals (Wiseman et al., 2003). The analysis demonstrated ITNs to be a highly cost-effective use of scarce health care resources. Based on this and many other studies, the World Health Organization (WHO) recommended that long-lasting insecticidal bed nets (LLINs) be used in areas where malaria is endemic, and organizations such as The Global Fund made it possible to distribute LLINs at little or no cost to the recipients. According to the 2011 *World Malaria Report* (WHO, 2011), an estimated 50% of households in sub-Saharan Africa now have at least one bed net, and 96% of persons with access to a bed net use it (Figure 8.8).

FUTURE DIRECTIONS

While RCTs are likely to remain the standard for determining the causal relationship between interventions and their effects, two aspects of RCT use may evolve. In cases where a combination of interventions is the best approach, study design may grow more complex and include some subcomponents that are randomized, while other subcomponents use other research methodology. Such complex study designs may also use alternative methods for data collection, such as using aggregate surveillance data instead of data specifically collected for the study. An example of this is HPTN 065, which has five subcomponents and includes both site and individual randomization as well as survey and observational cohort methodology (El-Sadr, Affrunti, Gamble, & Zerbe, 2010).

Another potential change may occur with the development of personalized medicine, which tailors treatment to the individual patient based on genetic or other information. RCTs evaluate the effect of an intervention on an entire study population, not

Figure 8.8   Trend in Estimated Proportion of Households With at Least One ITN in Sub-Saharan Africa, 2000–2011

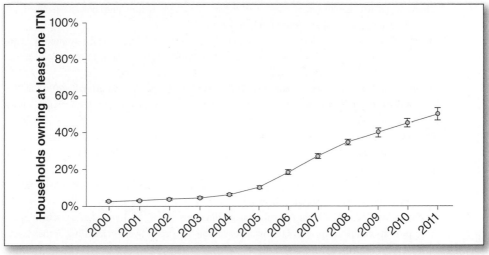

Source: World Health Organization (2011).

specific individuals. If personalized medicine becomes more feasible, methodology other than RCTs, or the adaptation of RCT designs, may occur.

ADDITIONAL RESOURCES

Friedman, L. M., Furberg, C. D., & DeMets, D. L. (2010). *Fundamentals of clinical trials* (4th ed.). New York, NY: Springer.

Portney, L. G., & Watkins, M. P. (2009). *Foundations of clinical research: Applications to practice* (3rd ed.). Upper Saddle River, NJ: Pearson Prentice Hall.

Stone, J. (2010). *Conducting clinical research: A practical guide for physicians, nurses, study coordinators, and investigators* (2nd ed.). Cumberland, MD: Mountainside MD Press.

REFERENCES

Abdool Karim, Q., Abdool Karim, S. S., Frohlich, J. A., Grobler, A., Baxter, C., Mansoor, L., . . . Taylor, D. (2010). Effectiveness and safety of tenofovir gel, an antiretroviral microbicide, for the prevention of HIV infection in women. *Science, 329,* 1168–1174.

Au, D. H., Castro, M., & Krishnan, J. A. (2007). Selection of controls in clinical trials: Introduction and conference summary. *Proceedings of the American Thoracic Society, 4,* 567–569.

Auvert, B., Taljaard, D., Lagarde, E., Sobngwi-Tambekou, J., Sitta, R., & Puren, A. (2005). Randomized, controlled intervention trial of male circumcision for reduction of HIV infection risk: The ANRS 1265 Trial. *PLoS Medicine, 2*(11), e298.

Bailey, R. C., Moses, S., Parker, C. B., Agot, K., Maclean, I., Krieger, J. N., . . . Ndinya-Achola, J. O. (2007). Male circumcision for HIV prevention in young men in Kisumu, Kenya: A randomised controlled trial. *Lancet, 369*, 643–656.

Berlin, J. A., & Ellenberg, S. S. (2009). Inclusion of women in clinical trials. *BMC Medicine, 7*, 56.

Bhatt, A. (2010). Evolution of clinical research: A history before and beyond James Lind. *Perspectives in Clinical Research, 1*(1), 6–10.

Bonella, C., Fletcherb, A., Mortona, M., Lorencb, T., & Moorec, L. (2012). Realist randomised controlled trials: A new approach to evaluating complex public health interventions. *Social Science & Medicine, 75*, 2299–2306.

Bonevski, B., Paul, C., D'Este, C., Sanson-Fisher, R., West, R., Girgis, A., . . . Carter, R. (2011). RCT of a client-centred, caseworker-delivered smoking cessation intervention for a socially disadvantaged population. *BMC Public Health, 11*(1), 70.

Breslow, N. E. (2006). Clinical trials—I. In S. Kotz, N. Balakrishnan, C. B. Read, & B. Vidakovic (Eds.), *Encyclopedia of statistical sciences* (Vol. 2, 2nd ed., pp. 981–989). Hoboken, NJ: Wiley-Interscience.

Centers for Disease Control and Prevention. (2013). *Lyme disease data*. Retrieved from http://www.cdc.gov/lyme/stats/index.html

Chou, R., Croswell, J. M., Dana, T., Bougatsos, C., Blazina, I., Fu, R., . . . Lin, K. (2011). Screening for prostate cancer: A review of the evidence for the U.S. Preventive Services Task Force. *Annals of Internal Medicine, 155*, 762–771.

ClinicalTrials.gov. (2012). *Learn about clinical studies*. Retrieved from http://clinicaltrials.gov/ct2/info/understand

Cohen, M. S., Chen, Y. Q., McCauley, M., Gamble, T., Hosseinipour, M., Kumarasamy, N., . . . Fleming, T. R. (2011). Prevention of HIV-1 infection with early antiretroviral therapy. *New England Journal of Medicine, 365*, 493–505.

Coplen, S. E., Antman, E. M., Berlin, J. A., Hewitt, P., & Chalmers, T. C. (1990). Efficacy and safety of quinidine therapy for maintenance of sinus rhythm after cardioversion: A meta-analysis of randomized control trials. *Circulation, 82*, 1106–1116.

Davis, R. L., Wright, J., Chalmers, F., Levenson, L., Brown, J. C., Lozano, P., & Christakis, D. A. (2007). A cluster randomized clinical trial to improve prescribing patterns in ambulatory pediatrics. *PLoS Clin Trials, 2*(5), e25.

Dicko, A., Sagara, I., Ellis, R. D., Miura, K., Guindo, O., Kamate, B., . . . Doumbo, O. K. (2008). Phase 1 study of a combination AMA1 blood stage malaria vaccine in Malian children. *PLoS One, 3*(2), e1563.

El-Sadr, W. M., Affrunti, M., Gamble, T., & Zerbe, A. (2010). Antiretroviral therapy: A promising HIV prevention strategy? *Journal of Acquired Immune Deficiency Syndrome, 55*(Suppl 2), S116–S121.

Forder, P. M., Gebski, V. J., & Keech, A. C. (2005). Allocation concealment and blinding: When ignorance is bliss. *Medical Journal of Australia, 182*(2), 87–89.

Freedman, B. (1987). Equipoise and the ethics of clinical research. *New England Journal of Medicine, 317*(3), 141–145.

Friedman, L. M., Furberg, C., & DeMets, D. L. (2010). *Fundamentals of clinical trials* (4th ed.). New York, NY: Springer.

Gallin, J. I., & Ognibene, F. P. (Eds.). (2007). *Principles and practice of clinical research* (2nd ed.). Burlington, MA: Academic Press.

Glezen, W. P., Gaglani, M. J., Kozinetz, C. A., & Piedra, P. A. (2010). Direct and indirect effectiveness of influenza vaccination delivered to children at school preceding an epidemic caused by 3 new influenza virus variants. *Journal of Infectious Diseases, 202*, 1626–1633.

Granger, C. B., Alexander, J. H., McMurray, J. J. V., Lopez, R. D., Hylek, E. M., Hanna, M., . . . Wallentin, L. (2011). Apixaban versus warfarin in patients with atrial fibrillation. *New England Journal of Medicine, 365,* 981–992.

Gray, R. H., Kigozi, G., Serwadda, D., Makumbi, F., Watya, S., Nalugoda, F., . . . Wawer, M. J. (2007). Male circumcision for HIV prevention in men in Rakai, Uganda: A randomised trial. *Lancet, 369,* 657–666.

Henry, R. K., Bauchmoyer, S. M., Moore, W., & Rashid, R. G. (2012). The effect of light on tooth whitening: A split-mouth design. *International Journal of Dental Hygeine, 11,* 151–154.

Hopewell, S., Dutton, S., Yu, L. M., Chan, A. W., & Altman, D. G. (2010). The quality of reports of randomised trials in 2000 and 2006: Comparative study of articles indexed in PubMed. *British Medical Journal, 340,* c723.

ICH E8. (1997). International harmonised tripartite guideline: General considerations for clinical trials: E8. *Federal Register, 63,* 66113–66119.

ICH E9. (1998). International conference on harmonisation: Guidance on statistical principles for clinical trials; availability—FDA. Notice. *Federal Register, 63*(179), 49583–49598.

Julious, S. A. (2010). *Sample sizes for clinical trials.* Boca Raton, FL: CRC Press/Taylor & Francis.

Lachin, J. M. (1988). Statistical properties of randomization in clinical trials. *Controlled Clinical Trials, 9,* 289–311.

Little, M., Lyerly, A. D., & Faden, R. (2009). Pregnant women and medical research: A moral imperative. *Bioethics Forum, 2,* 60–65.

Ministry of Health, Republic of Kenya. (2008). *National AIDS/STD Control Programme: National guidance for voluntary male circumcision in Kenya.* Nairobi, Kenya: Author.

Murray, D. M., Varnell, S. P., & Blitstein, J. L. (2004). Design and analysis of group-randomized trials: A review of recent methodological developments. *American Journal of Public Health, 94,* 423–432.

Mwandi, Z., Murphy, A., Reed, J., Chesang, K., Njeuhmeli, E., Agot, K., . . . Bock, N. (2011). Voluntary medical male circumcision: Translating research into the rapid expansion of services in Kenya, 2008–2011. *PLoS Medicine, 8*(11), e1001130.

National Institutes of Health, Office of Behavioral & Social Sciences Research. (n.d.). *Clinical trials.* Retrieved from http://www.esourceresearch.org/tabid/198/Default.aspx

NIH Revitalization Act. (1993). Subtitle B. Part 1, PL 103-43.

Noordzij, M., Tripepi, G., Dekker, F. W., Zoccali, C., Tanck, M. W., & Jager, K. J. (2010). Sample size calculations: Basic principles and common pitfalls. *Nephrology, Dialysis, Transplantation, 25,* 1388–1393.

Ockene, I. S., Tellez, T. L., Rosal, M. C., Reed, G. W., Mordes, J., Merriam, P. A., . . . Ma, Y. (2012). Outcomes of a Latino community-based intervention for the prevention of diabetes: The Lawrence Latino Diabetes Prevention Project. *American Journal of Public Health, 102,* 336–342.

Sagara, I., Dicko, A., Ellis, R. D., Fay, M. P., Diawara, S. I., Assadou, M. H., . . . Saul, A. (2009). A randomized controlled phase 2 trial of the blood stage AMA1-C1/Alhydrogel malaria vaccine in children in Mali. *Vaccine, 27,* 3090–3098.

Spencer, M. S., Rosland, A. M., Kieffer, E. C., Sinco, B. R., Valerio, M., Palmisano, G., . . . Heisler, M. (2011). Effectiveness of a community health worker intervention among African American and Latino adults with type 2 diabetes: A randomized controlled trial. *American Journal of Public Health, 101,* 2253–2260.

Stampfer, M. J., Buring, J. E., Willett, W., Rosner, B., Eberlein, K., & Hennekens, C. H. (1985). The 2 x 2 factorial design: Its application to a randomized trial of aspirin and carotene in U.S. physicians. *Statistics in Medicine, 4*(2), 111–116.

Strimbu, K., & Tavel, J. A. (2010). What are biomarkers? *Current Opinions in HIV and AIDS, 5,* 463–466.

Takakura, N., & Yajima, H. (2009). Analgesic effect of acupuncture needle penetration: A double-blind crossover study. *Open Medicine, 3*(2), e54–e61.

Thera, M. A., Doumbo, O. K., Coulibaly, D., Laurens, M. B., Quattara, A., Kone, A. K., . . . Plowe, C. V. (2011). A field trial to assess a blood-stage malaria vaccine. *New England Journal of Medicine, 365,* 1004–1013.

Timmermans, S., & Mauck, A. (2005). The promises and pitfalls of evidence-based medicine. *Health Affairs (Millwood), 24*(1), 18–28.

Two Feathers, J., Kieffer, E. C., Palmisano, G., Anderson, M., Sinco, B., Janz, N., . . . James, S. A. (2005). Racial and Ethnic Approaches to Community Health (REACH) Detroit partnership: Improving diabetes-related outcomes among African American and Latino adults. *American Journal of Public Health, 95,* 1552–1560.

U.S. Food and Drug Administration. (2012). *Postmarket drug safety information for patients and providers.* Retrieved from http://www.fda.gov/Drugs/DrugSafety/PostmarketDrugSafety InformationforPatientsandProviders/default.htm

U.S. Preventive Services Task Force. (2008). *Procedure manual.* Retrieved from http://www.uspreventiveservicestaskforce.org/uspstf08/methods/procmanual.htm

U.S. Preventive Services Task Force. (2012). *Screening for prostate cancer.* Retrieved from http://www.uspreventiveservicestaskforce.org/prostatecancerscreening.htm

Victora, C. G., Habicht, J. P., & Bryce, J. (2004). Evidence-based public health: Moving beyond randomized trials. *American Journal of Public Health, 94,* 400–405.

Wechsler, M. E., Kelley, J. M., Boyd, I. O., Dutile, S., Marigowda, G., Kirsch, I., . . . Kaptchuk, T. J. (2011). Active albuterol or placebo, sham acupuncture, or no intervention in asthma. *New England Journal of Medicine, 365,* 119–126.

Wiseman, V., Hawley, W. A., ter Kuile, F. O., Phillips-Howard, P. A., Vulule, J. M., Nahlen, B. L., & Mills, A. J. (2003). The cost-effectiveness of permethrin-treated bed nets in an area of intense malaria transmission in western Kenya. *American Journal of Tropical Medicine and Hygiene, 68*(4 Suppl), 161–167.

Wittes, J. (1998). Randomized treatment assignment. In P. Armitage & T. Colton (Eds.), *Encyclopedia of biostatistics* (Vol. 5, pp. 3703–3711). Chichester, NY: Wiley.

World Health Organization. (2011). *World malaria report.* Geneva, Switzerland: Author. Retrieved from http://www.who.int/malaria/world_malaria_report_2011/9789241564403_eng.pdf

PART III

Structural and Operational Research

9

Using Secondary Data

Sarah Boslaugh

Analysis of secondary data plays a key role in modern public health research. This is not surprising, given the emphasis in public health on understanding health and disease at the population level, and the extensive data sets required to study health at this level. It's the rare researcher who can afford to collect data to represent a national population, much less the populations of multiple nations or over multiple years. Fortunately, such data sets are regularly collected by governments and nongovernmental organizations, and made available to researchers, often free of charge.

People are sometimes confused by the terms *primary* and *secondary data analysis*, because the distinction lies not in the data set itself, but in the relationship between the data set and the person analyzing it. With primary data analysis, the person analyzing the data was also part of the original research team conducting the project or study for which the data were collected; with secondary data analysis, the analyst was not part of the original research team. So in Figure 9.1, if Sarah leads a research team that collects data about childhood vaccination rates in Georgia, and her team analyzes that data set, they are doing primary data analysis. If anyone outside Sarah's research team analyzes that data set, they are doing secondary analysis (for instance, if Sally finds it in an archive and has permission to use it).

Often when people think of secondary data analysis, they think of large data sets collected by governments, international organizations, and so on, such as the U.S. Census or the Global Health Observatory Data Repository available from the World Health Organization. These are secondary data sets to both Sarah and Sally, because neither was involved in their collection; any use they make of them will be secondary analysis.

Certainly you can combine primary and secondary data in the same study, and in fact this is done quite often. You might call it having the best of both worlds: You can

Figure 9.1   Primary vs. Secondary Analysis of Data

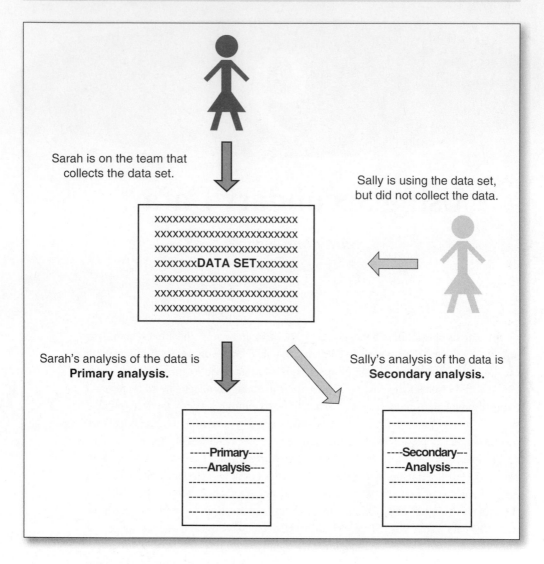

focus your resources on collecting the data needed to answer your specific research question (that's the primary data), while also incorporating secondary data into your analysis to take advantage of the work done by others. That's the approach my colleagues and I took when we studied the relationship between neighborhood characteristics and physical activity (Boslaugh, Luke, Brownson, Naleid, & Kreuter, 2004). This study is discussed further in the text box below, but briefly, it was a multilevel analysis of the influence of individual and neighborhood factors on people's opinions of how safe and pleasant their neighborhoods were as places to perform physical activity. The individual factors were primary data collected by the lab in which I worked; the neighborhood factors were secondary data, drawn from the U.S. Census.

A STUDY COMBINING PRIMARY AND SECONDARY DATA: NEIGHBORHOOD CHARACTERISTICS AND PHYSICAL ACTIVITY

An appropriate level of physical activity is considered an important factor in a healthy lifestyle, and the health benefits of physical activity have been heavily promoted in campaigns by the Centers for Disease Control and Prevention and other public health organizations. Yet many American adults do not participate in any leisure-time physical activity. Many reasons have been proposed to explain this paradox, but one obvious factor is whether a person has a safe, pleasant, and convenient place to participate in physical activity. This study, conducted in St. Louis, Missouri, used a hierarchical linear model to look at the relationships among individual and neighborhood characteristics on an individual's perception of his or her neighborhood as a venue for physical activity (Boslaugh et al., 2004). We built two models, one to explain perceived neighborhood pleasantness for exercise and one to explain perceived neighborhood safety for exercise.

The individual characteristics in the final models—race and income—were primary data, collected through a survey conducted by the research group in which I was working at the time. The neighborhood characteristics in the final models were drawn from secondary data, collected by the U.S. Census: the percentage of African American residents, the percentage of residents living in the same house as 5 years prior, the percentage using public transportation to get to work, the percentage that walked or bicycled to work, and the median house value.

Why did we use Census data rather than simply asking our respondents about their home value, their use of public transportation, and so on? Because we wanted the data to characterize the *neighborhoods* our respondents lived in, not merely their individual characteristics; to collect data at the neighborhood level, we would have had to do another survey including each neighborhood represented in the study. That would have been prohibitively expensive and also a duplication of effort, since fairly recent data were available from the Census.

We had to make one compromise in order to use the Census data in this study: We used ZIP codes to define neighborhoods, an imperfect choice because ZIP code areas are established for the convenience of the post office rather than on the basis of any historical or social characteristics defining a neighborhood. However, ZIP codes were the Census level of aggregation that seemed the closest to the common perception of a neighborhood, and we felt this was a reasonable compromise.

ADVANTAGES AND DISADVANTAGES OF SECONDARY DATA ANALYSIS

There are many advantages to using secondary data in public health, and several of them are particularly germane to students. Table 9.1 summarizes these, along with some disadvantages.

Table 9.1 Advantages and Disadvantages of Secondary Data Analysis

Advantages	Disadvantages
• Broad scope of data available (national, international, multiple years) • Savings in time and money: no need to collect the data yourself • Many people can analyze the same data set, so studies can be replicated, research questions refined, and so on • Data collection usually planned and executed by experts	• Can only use the data that are available; may not be optimal for your needs • Time and effort required to learn how to use the data • Methods used for collecting and processing the data may be unknown or may be less precise than is desirable • May be more difficult to get funding for secondary analysis projects

The first advantage has already been broached: Secondary data sets often contain data of a scope greater than what a typical individual researcher (or student) could hope to collect. Extant secondary data sets allow you to examine issues at the national and international level, and to study changes over multiyear periods. Even if you had substantial funding and a team of experienced researchers already in place, it would be difficult to collect data at the scope comparable to what is available, for instance, from the U.S. Census or the Centers for Disease Control and Prevention (CDC). Researchers around the country—and around the world—can benefit from the efforts of others by using data already available.

A second advantage of using secondary data is economy, in terms of both money and time. Analyzing secondary data usually represents a substantial savings compared to collecting and analyzing your own data, because you avoid the expenses associated with data collection. Many secondary data sets are available for free. For those that are fee-based, it is still nearly always cheaper to use data already collected than to collect data yourself. A related advantage is the time savings: With secondary data, you get to skip over the planning and data collection stages of research and begin your work with analysis of the data. You may be able to complete several analyses using secondary data in less time than you could collect and analyze a single data set, and as an additional benefit, sequential analyses may take you deeper into the data and help you identify more interesting and important questions and findings.

A third advantage is that, because many researchers can analyze the same secondary data set, it is much easier to replicate results. When multiple people from different places work on the same data, hypotheses can be refined and results become more definitive.

A fourth advantage is that secondary data sets, particularly at the national and international levels, are usually collected observing the highest standards of research professionalism, by staff who are specialists and work full-time in their field. In the best-case scenario, the results from secondary data sets are highly reliable and generalizable because the data have been collected using complex sampling plans, designed so the sample can be weighted to be representative of the population in question; by data collectors trained to achieve consistency; and with missing data already imputed (i.e., plausible values have replaced the missing data, using one of several generally accepted methods).

Not surprisingly, there are also disadvantages associated with analyzing secondary data. One major drawback is that you have to settle for the data that are available, rather than designing a data collection plan to optimally address your specific research questions. Sometimes this means making compromises (see the text box above for an example related to the use of ZIP codes to define neighborhoods).

A related problem is that the variables in the secondary data set may not have been defined exactly as you would have chosen, had you collected the data yourself. Perhaps you want exact figures for income, and the secondary data set offers income information only in categories, or you are interested in current smoking habits and the secondary data set only includes data on lifetime smoking. Definitions are particularly a problem when trying to compare data across countries or time periods. Even the same survey may change the wording of a question in ways that change its meaning or change the number of ethnic and racial categories used, while different countries may define characteristics such as "current smoker" differently, making comparisons difficult. And even if you can find a data set that comes close to addressing your research question, it may be several years old or it may not cover exactly the geographic region you wish to study.

A second major drawback with using secondary data is that you may need to spend a substantial amount of time learning about the data set, including how it was collected and how it is organized, and this may eat into the time and effort savings otherwise achieved by analyzing secondary data. When you analyze primary data, you have the advantage of being familiar with the goals of the project, the methods used to collect the data, how problems such as nonresponse were dealt with, and so on. With secondary data, if you are lucky this will all be documented and you need only invest the necessary time and effort to get up to speed on the data; if not, you may have to invest more energy in locating this information (e.g., contacting someone involved in the data collection effort) or simply do the best you can with the information available.

A third drawback, particularly when using secondary data from sources not designed for research purposes (e.g., hospital billing records), is that the methods by which the data were collected and processed may not be well documented, and the methods used and/or their execution may not have been up to the standards customary for research data. In this case, the researcher is responsible for learning as much as possible about how the data were collected and any limitations to them.

A fourth drawback is less significant, but still worth mentioning. It's often harder to secure funding to analyze secondary data than it is for projects that will collect new data. And relatedly, publications based on secondary data may not carry as much prestige. The latter point may seem petty, but it is worth considering given today's competitive work environments. You may wish to consult with someone more senior in your field to get a feeling for how analyses based on secondary data are valued in your particular specialty.

HOW TO DO SECONDARY DATA ANALYSIS

The intellectual process involved in conducting a secondary data analysis is not really different from that necessary to conduct a primary data analysis. You formulate a research question, analyze relevant data, and draw your conclusions based on the results of the analyses. Of course, the specifics differ quite a bit, because with primary data analysis you have to collect the data yourself, while with secondary data analysis you use data someone else has already collected.

There are two ways to begin a secondary data analysis: You can start with a question, then look for a data set to analyze, or you can begin with the data set and think of some interesting questions to ask of it. Both are acceptable, although the first is probably more common, because we tend to think in terms of questions we are interested in and to seek answers through analysis. On the other hand, sometimes researchers do begin with an existing data set and think of questions that could be answered by analyzing it; this approach is particularly common just after a major new data set has been released.

To keep things simple for our purposes, let's assume you will begin with your research question. In this case, we can look at the process of secondary data analysis as having five steps (see Figure 9.2).

Figure 9.2 The Five Steps of Secondary Data Analysis

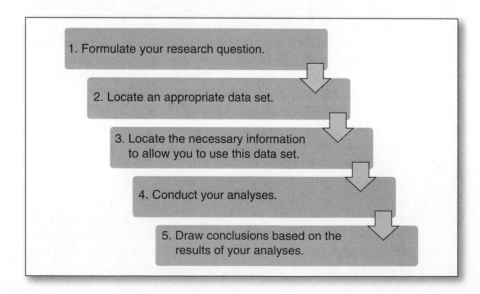

1. Formulate your research question.

2. Locate an appropriate data set.

3. Locate the necessary information to allow you to use this data set.

4. Conduct your analyses.

5. Draw conclusions based on the results of your analyses.

Students and new researchers often begin with very general areas of interest—perhaps you are interested in the relationship between poverty and health, the benefits of physical activity for children, or the health effects of being uninsured. As with primary data analysis, such general topics need to be narrowed down to a specific question. A literature review and expert advice from more experienced researchers can be invaluable in this process.

The next step, locating an appropriate data set, is specific to secondary data analysis. View this as a mini-research project and use all the resources available to you to find an appropriate data set for your question; finding the right data is crucial to the success of your analysis and any publications you may hope derive from it. The data sets listed later in this chapter may be helpful, as may other references (e.g., Boslaugh, 2007; Smith et al., 2010), expert advice from senior researchers and reference librarians, and Internet searches. Before you start the process, it may be helpful to make a list of the important characteristics of the data you are seeking, including specific variables that must be included, how you would (ideally) like them defined, the time period of interest, the population classes of interest (e.g., age, gender, race/ethnicity), the geographic area of interest, and any other important characteristics (e.g., Do you need longitudinal data? Do you need clustered data?). A checklist is helpful in clarifying what your main needs are and may help if you have to choose between several data sets, none of which are exactly right for your needs.

LOCATING APPROPRIATE SECONDARY DATA: A CASE STUDY

In 2008, Pearce and colleagues at University College London conducted a survey of existing U.K. data sets to assess their usefulness in monitoring trends in childhood obesity, physical activity, and diet (Pearce, Jenkins, Kirk, & Law, 2008). Their work offers a useful perspective on the process of finding and evaluating secondary data sets to investigate a topic of interest (note: the purpose of this study was not to conduct an analysis, but to see what data were available to address a particular set of questions).

Pearce and colleagues located a total of 96 data sets that met their initial criteria (sufficient sample size, 1990 or newer, accessible, not limited to a specific population). However, only 11 of the 96 could be used to assess trends over a time period from 2 to 10 years. In addition, only 8 of the 11 data sets included physical activity data; 8 included data about diet; and 3 included data about obesity. Sample sizes of the 11 data sets (for a single year) ranged from about 500 to over 14,000.

Measurement issues were most obvious for data about diet and physical activity, and least for obesity data. Obesity was measured in all three data

(Continued)

(Continued)

sets by height and weight, taken by a trained health worker, and sometimes waist-to-hip ratio and skinfold thickness were recorded as well. On the other hand, all the measures of physical activity and diet were self-reported, and it was not always clear if the methods used to collect these data had been validated. A variety of measures were used to assess physical activity, with three primary categories of activity recorded: participation in recreational leisure activity, participation in travel activity (e.g., cycling to school), and sedentary activity. Measures used to assess diet were also diverse and fell into five categories: household food purchases, breakfast, fruit and vegetable consumption, other food consumption, and consumption of soft drinks and sweets. Most of the data sets included sufficient information to compare demographic groups (e.g., gender, ethnicity, socioeconomic status) and geographical regions.

The third step is to become familiar with your chosen data set. This may be more time-consuming than you expect, but it's an effort that will pay dividends. If the data were obtained through a survey, find the actual questionnaire so you know how the questions were worded and also to see what skip patterns were used. If a complex sampling plan was used, find documentation of this and learn how to correctly apply sample weights in your analysis. You need to find out how missing data were handled; for instance, were different reasons for missing data recorded (e.g., declined to answer, didn't know, not applicable), and if imputation was used, how was it executed? If data were collected through physical measurements, how exactly was this done; for instance, if blood pressure was measured, was it taken on a single occasion, or were several measurements taken and averaged? Fortunately, the major secondary data sets are usually well documented. Don't be shy about seeking help; particularly in the case of data collected by government agencies, there are often personnel whose job includes assisting researchers who use agency-collected data. It is often helpful to search PubMed (www.ncbi.nlm.nih.gov/pubmed) and other relevant databases to see what has been published about the data set you are planning to use and what analyses have already been published using the data.

The fourth and fifth steps, doing the analysis and drawing your conclusions, are much the same whether you are working with primary or secondary data. This should be encouraging, because you don't need to learn different statistical techniques to work with secondary data or to write them up. Also encouraging should be the fact that once you have become familiar with your chosen data set, you can probably think of other questions you could ask of it, so you can spend more time doing analyses and publishing your results and less time hunting down data sets and information about them.

A FEW WORDS ON SKIP PATTERNS

A skip pattern in a survey or questionnaire means that some questions will not be asked of all respondents, based on their personal characteristics or their answers to other questions. For instance, in the 2011 Behavioral Risk Factor Surveillance System (BRFSS; CDC, 2011), an annual survey conducted in the United States, respondents were asked if a health professional had ever told them that they had a heart attack; the possible answers were *yes, no, don't know/not sure,* and *refused*. Respondents who answered *yes* were asked an additional question about whether they went to outpatient rehabilitation after their heart attack; for those who did not answer *yes*, the follow-up question was skipped.

This may seem like an obvious point, but many a researcher has panicked upon realizing that most of the data for a particular variable were missing, not recognizing that this was simply due to a skip pattern in the questionnaire.

Skip patterns may also be due to personal characteristics of the respondent. To take another example from the 2011 BRFSS, respondents who were female and under 45 years of age were asked a series of questions about preconception health and family planning; those questions were skipped for men and for women age 45 or older. Again, this may seem like an obvious point, but it demonstrates how important it is to understand how the data were collected, including the specific questionnaire used and the instructions to the data collectors.

THE IMPORTANCE OF READING THE QUESTIONNAIRE

There are many ways to get information about a topic, and when working with data collected through surveys, it's crucial to see exactly what question was asked to elicit the information recorded. Suppose you are interested in studying the health and well-being of gay and lesbian adolescents, and you decide to conduct a secondary data analysis examining this issue. Fortunately, you discover that several fairly recent surveys of adolescent health have collected information about sexual orientation; unfortunately, the questions used to obtain information about sexual orientation vary significantly from one survey to another. This means that your ability to compare results from different surveys will be limited and that you need to decide exactly what you mean by

(Continued)

(Continued)

"sexual orientation" and choose a data set whose questions match the way you conceptualize it. These issues are discussed at further length in Saewyc et al. (2004), from which the examples here are drawn, and in a report from the Williams Institute (2009; which includes recommendations for best practices in asking about different aspects of sexual orientation).

Some surveys include questions about sexual behavior. For instance, the 1986 Minnesota Adolescent Health Survey includes the questions "Have you ever had any kind of sexual experience with a male?" and "Have you ever had any kind of sexual experience with a female?" (both with answer options *yes/no*), while the 1998 *Minnesota Student Survey* includes the question "During the past 12 months, with how many different male partners have you had sexual intercourse?" and the equivalent question about female partners, both with answer options from *none* to *6 or more persons*. Even though both surveys are asking about sexual behavior, one asks about lifetime experience, the other about experience in the past 12 months, and thus their results are not strictly comparable.

Other surveys ask questions about identity or attraction. For instance, the 1999 Seattle Teen Risk Survey asked, "How would you describe your sexual orientation?" and offered these choices:

- 100% heterosexual (attracted to persons of the opposite sex)
- mostly heterosexual
- bisexual (equally attracted to men and women)
- mostly homosexual
- 100% homosexual (gay/lesbian; attracted to persons of the same sex)
- not sure

Another aspect of sexual orientation is attraction or intention, and this aspect was targeted by a question on the 1990 National American Indian Adolescent Health Survey—"Which of the following best describes your feelings?"—with these answer choices:

- "I am *only* attracted to people of the *same* sex as mine, and I will only be sexual with persons of the same sex."
- "I am *strongly* attracted to people of the same sex, and most of my sexual experiences will be with persons of the same sex as mine."
- "I am *equally* attracted to men and women both and would like to be sexual with both."
- "I am *strongly* attracted to persons of the opposite sex, and most of my sexual experience will be with persons of the opposite sex."

- "I am *only* attracted to persons of the opposite sex, and I will only be sexual with persons of the opposite sex."

These are all valid approaches (and there are others as well) to measuring sexual orientation, but the different questions address different aspects of sexual orientation and could produce different responses even from the same person. It is not correct to assume that sexual identity, sexual behavior, and sexual attraction or intention are always perfectly aligned, and this makes comparing results from different surveys problematic.

SOME ISSUES IN SECONDARY DATA ANALYSIS

Complex Survey Designs

Many common statistical procedures assume that data analyzed are from a simple random sample drawn from an essentially infinite population, an assumption that is not always upheld with large secondary data sets. Instead, often these data sets are collected using a complex sampling plan, typically a multistage process using one or more advanced techniques such as stratification, cluster sampling, and unequal probability sampling. There are several reasons for using these techniques, including economy and the ability to oversample relatively small population groups of particular interest so that accurate parameter estimates can be calculated for them. Data collected using a complex design must be weighted in order to have the estimates calculated on the sample accurately represent the target population. One of the tasks necessary when working with this type of data is learning how to apply the weights correctly. These issues may be clearer if we consider a particular example: the National Health and Nutrition Examination Survey (NHANES).

The purpose of the NHANES is, in the broadest sense, to measure and monitor the health of the U.S. population and of subgroups within the population (National Center for Health Statistics, 2012). Data for the NHANES are collected using a complex, multi-stage probability sampling design, both for reasons of economy (the data collection process includes a physical examination and collection of laboratory samples as well as an interview, and NHANES employees must travel to each location where data are collected) and because a complex design allows oversampling of specific population groups. The details of the NHANES sample design have changed over the years, but the basic principles have remained consistent (National Center for Health Statistics, 2012, 2013; CDC, 2013). In the current system, the Primary Sampling Units (PSU) are counties; segments (e.g., city blocks) are selected within counties, households within segments, and individuals within households. Different subgroups have been oversampled in different years, including Mexican Americans, persons age 60 and older, adolescents, and women of childbearing age.

Because of this complex design, in order to analyze NHANES data and produce correct parameter estimates for the U.S. population, the data must be weighted. The National Center for Health Statistics (2012) identifies five reasons weights were calculated for NHANES data:

1. To compensate for differential probabilities of selection among population subgroups

2. To reduce nonresponse bias (bias due to the fact that respondents may differ on other characteristics from nonrespondents)

3. To make the weighted sample match target population totals, as determined by the U.S. Census Bureau

4. To compensate for problems with the sampling frame (e.g., omission of people without a known address)

5. To reduce variance using auxiliary information

The calculation of these sampling weights can be extremely complex (see, e.g., National Center for Health Statistics, 2012), but fortunately all the *user* of NHANES or any other data set collected using a complex design needs to know is how to apply the weights correctly, and in most cases ample documentation exists that explains how to do that. The analyst is responsible for learning to use one of the software packages that can produce a correct analysis of data collected using a complex design, such as SUDAAN (RTI International, 2013), SAS (Berglund, 2002; SAS Institute 2013a, 2013b), or R (Lumley, 2010). Procedures intended for a simple random sample (e.g., SAS REG) will not produce correct results with a complex sample. Fortunately, several textbooks (e.g., Brogan; 2006; Heeringa, West, & Berglund, 2010) as well as conference papers and online documentation are available to make this task easier.

Changes in Measurement

One appeal of secondary data analysis is that it facilitates studies of change in some factor over time. For instance, you might be interested in looking at how the percentage of the American population without health insurance has changed over the years 1990–2010. You would need a time machine as well as considerable resources to collect that information yourself today, but fortunately the National Health Interview Survey, a program of the CDC, has already collected those data and made them available to researchers (CDC, 2012). However, one problem with using secondary data sets collected in different years is that the definitions of variables, and the questions used to collect them, often change, making the data from different years less comparable than you might wish.

For instance, many public health studies include race or ethnicity as a variable, but the categories used to define race and ethnicity, as well as the specific questions asked to obtain this information, have varied substantially over the years. In the United States, many public health surveys use the categories and definitions for race and ethnicity established by the Office of Management and Budget for the U.S. Census. Table 9.2 details the changes in categories and definitions for race and ethnicity from 1980 through 2010.

Table 9.2   Changes in U.S. Census Categories for Race and Ethnicity, 1980–2010

In 1980 and 1990, four racial categories were offered:

- White
- Black
- American Indian and Alaskan Native
- Asian and Pacific islander

A separate question has been included in the Census since 1980, inquiring if the person was of Hispanic origin.

In 2000, six categories were offered, and for the first time individuals were also allowed to indicate that they were multiracial by checking more than one of the boxes offered. The six racial categories offered on the 2000 Census:

- American Indian and Alaska Native
- Asian
- Black or African American
- Native Hawaiian and Other Pacific islander
- White
- Some other race (Lee, 2001)

In 2010, both the Hispanic origin question and the race question became more detailed. The Hispanic origin question included clarification that Hispanic origin was a separate question from race, and it offered the following categories, first for Hispanic origin, then for race:

- No, not of Hispanic, Latino, or Spanish origin
- Yes, Mexican, Mexican American, Chicano
- Yes, Puerto Rican
- Yes, Cuban
- Yes, another Hispanic, Latino, or Spanish origin (with a space to specify)
- White
- Black, African American, or Negro
- American Indian or Alaska Native
- Asian Indian
- Chinese
- Filipino
- Japanese
- Korean
- Vietnamese
- Native Hawaiian
- Guamanian or Chamorro
- Samoan
- Other Pacific Islander
- Some Other Race (Humes, Jones, & Ramirez, 2011)

Sources: Lee (2001, March); Humes et al., 2011, March).

Causation

Everyone knows that correlation does not prove causality, and this is as true for secondary data analysis as it is for primary data analysis. In fact, causation may be a greater issue in secondary data analysis, because many secondary data sets are cross-sectional. This means that the data were collected at a single point in time, and thus it is difficult if not impossible to establish an order of events (did smoking marijuana put you on the road to juvenile delinquency, or were you introduced to marijuana after you were already launched on your career as a juvenile delinquent?), and the lack of a clear order of events militates against drawing causal inferences.

Causal inference is a complex topic that can only be mentioned here; for a more in-depth discussion, see Pearl (2009, 2010); Rothman, Greenland, and Lash (2008); Parascandola and Weed (2001); and Phillips and Goodman (2006). When you observe that A and B are correlated, this does not establish that A causes B. In the absence of any further information, it is also possible that B causes A or that the observed relationship between them is due primarily to the influence of a third variable, C. Establishing an order of events can help to clarify causality (although it is not sufficient to establish it), and longitudinal data are useful in this regard. It may also be possible to establish the order of events by considering the logical sequence in which some things happen. For instance, data recorded on a birth certificate are often considered cross-sectional because they are collected at a single point in time, but order can be deduced logically for some events—for instance, prenatal care by definition occurred before the birth and so can be evaluated as a causal factor in birth outcomes.

DOMESTIC SOURCES

The United States is particularly rich in terms of secondary data sets relating to public health. This provides great opportunities for researchers, but also poses challenges for locating the right data set to address a particular question because so many different governmental and nongovernmental entities are working in the field. In addition, studying matters related to health and health care in the United States is complex because the country does not have a system of national health or an integrated system of patient records. Space constraints limit discussion here to a few major data sources, while further guidance is available from published sources (e.g., Boslaugh, 2007; Smith et al., 2010), reference librarians, colleagues, and Internet searches.

Behavioral Risk Factor Surveillance System (www.cdc.gov/brfss)

This is the main website for the BRFSS, an annual health and health behavior survey conducted in the United States since 1984; data are available for each state, selected metropolitan areas and counties, and the country as a whole. In addition to the data sets, resources on the website include the questionnaires, codebooks, and documentation for each year, as well as a searchable question archive. Each year's survey includes a set of core questions included on all surveys (although the specific core questions change from year to year) and optional questions asked in some states but not in others. If you want to go straight to the data sets, they are available at www.cdc.gov/brfss/annual_data/annual_data.htm.

CDC Wonder (wonder.cdc.gov)

This site is a portal to public health statistical reports and data sets from the CDC. Many of the data sets can be queried online, with options to download the data or use software provided on the website to produce tables, maps, and charts without going through the download process. Data may be located through a text search, by topic (organized into the broad categories of Chronic Conditions, Communicable Diseases, Environmental Health, Tools, Health Practice & Prevention, Injury Prevention, Occupational Health, and Reference Data), or through a detailed subject and data set index (from AIDS Public Use Data to Youth Risk Behavior Surveillance System).

Data.gov (www.data.gov)

This data portal is designed to make it easy to locate and download data generated by the executive branch of the U.S. federal government; this site is particularly useful if you need some nonhealth data (e.g., about employment or household income) for your research. Data can be located by text search, by browsing through different "communities" (Education, Health, Law, Safety), or by agency. A map interface contains links to U.S. cities and 34 states that make their data publicly available. The Health community (www.healthdata.gov) is the community most immediately relevant to public health, although other communities could also provide useful information. Within the Health community, data sets can be located by text search and filtered by agency or subagency, date updated, collection frequency, geographic granularity (e.g., state, county, ZIP code), date released, media format (e.g., CSM, XLS), or subject (Administrative, Biomedical Research, Children's Health, Epidemiology, Health Care Cost, Health Care Providers, Medicaid, Medicare, Population Statistics, Quality Measurement, Safety, Treatments, or Other).

FedStats (fedstats.gov)

A web portal created in 1997, FedStats provides links to downloadable statistical data and statistical reports from over 100 U.S. federal government agencies. As with Data.gov, this website is particularly useful if you are looking for nonhealth data (for health data, CDC Wonder is a more logical starting point). Data sets may be located through text search, by browsing through the topic list (from Adoption to Women), by an index of topics within programs (e.g., the Administration for Children and Families includes the topics of adoption, child abuse, child care, child support enforcement, foster care, and the Head Start program), or by the agency index (e.g., Centers for Medicare and Medicaid

Services, National Cancer Institute). A separate index allows you to locate data by the agency that collected it (including the National Center for Health Statistics). Statistical profiles for smaller levels of aggregation (state, county, city, congressional district, or federal judicial district) can be accessed by a map interface or dropdown menu.

Inter-university Consortium for Political and Social Research (ICPSR; www.icpsr.umich.edu)

The ICPSR is a digital archive of over 500,000 data files in social science fields, including public health and medical care; both U.S. and international data are included. Some ICPSR data sets are available for free download by anyone, while other data are available free only to students, faculty, and staff at member institutions (including about 700 universities, governments agencies, etc.) or by payment of a fee of $500 per data set. Data files may be located by text search, by using the subject thesaurus, or through indexes by topic, geography, investigator, or series (e.g., Medicare Current Beneficiary Survey Series, National Survey of Family Growth series). Although much of the data in the ICPSR are available elsewhere, the ICPSR presents information about each data set on an index page that makes it easy to decide quickly if a data set will be useful for your purposes. The information provided varies somewhat by data set, but usually includes a detailed study description, links to documentation files, and links to published literature using the data. Some ICPSR data sets may be analyzed online using the Survey Documentation Analysis (SDA) tool; of these data sets, SDA capability for some is available to everyone, for others only to those affiliated with ICPSR institutions.

National Center for Health Statistics (NCHS): Data Access (www.cdc.gov/nchs/data_access.htm)

This website provides download access to public-use data files, questionnaires, and documentation from eight NCHS surveys and data collection systems:

- National Health and Nutrition Examination Survey
- National Health Care Surveys
- National Health Interview Survey
- National Immunization Survey
- National Survey of Family Growth
- National Vital Statistics System
- Longitudinal Studies of Aging
- State and Local Area Integrated Telephone Survey

It also contains information about NCHS data linkage programs (e.g., linking mortality data and Medicare enrollment and claims data with data from the National Health Interview Survey).

Partners in Information Access for the Public Health Workforce: Heath Data Tools and Statistics (phpartners.org/health_stats.html)

This website provides a compendium of links to public health data and information collected at the local, state, national, and international levels. The links are a mix of downloadable data, ranking and visualization tools (e.g., CDC Interactive Atlas of Heart Disease and Stroke), statistical reports, and others. The most useful aspects of this site for the secondary data researcher are the collection of state and local links and the topical pages bringing together links to subjects such as bioterrorism, dental public health, and public health genomics.

Society of General Internal Medicine (SGIM): Public Datasets (www.sgim.org/communities/ research/dataset-compendium)

This website provides a compendium of links to the websites of secondary data sets of particular interest to those wanting to do research in the fields of health services research, clinical epidemiology, and medical education. It includes links to 46 "featured" data sets that are generally available for free or upon payment of a fee, and 8 proprietary data sets controlled by SGIM members who have indicated their willingness to collaborate in research with junior investigators or fellows. Information provided for each data set includes the years of data collection, sample size and geographic location, purpose of the study, overview of the data, links to publications based on the data, and cost (if any). A topical grid for the featured data sets identifies those relevant to five topics: health systems medical education; health behaviors; access, costs, and social concerns; health status; and health care. The website also includes advice about using secondary data and links to other data repositories and compendia.

INTERNATIONAL SOURCES (AND SPECIAL CHALLENGES OF WORKING WITH THEM)

Working with international sources of secondary data can pose a number of challenges. First of all, there's the language barrier: The language of mathematics may be universal, but human languages are not, and excellent language skills may be required to understand a given study and its documentation. An even greater challenge may be posed by cultural context—every culture has its unstated assumptions, and understanding these may hold the key to understanding the data. Categorizations of racial and ethnic groups differ across countries, as do the meaning of even such basic terms as *family*. Norms regarding matters such as appropriate gender roles, the age at which a child becomes an adult, or what constitutes a good diet can also vary markedly from one culture to another. Doing the background research is key; you need to be able to understand what the data set means in its original context, rather than simply viewing it through your own.

Having said that, working with international secondary data sets allows the researcher to examine many important questions that would be difficult or impossible to address if primary data had to be collected. In addition, English is becoming the dominant language in international public health, and if you have serviceable skills in one or more other languages as well (French and Spanish are particularly useful), you will be able to access an even wider variety of data sets.

Global Health Data Exchange (ghdx. healthmetricsandevaluation.org)

This website provides a compendium of links to data sets relevant to global health, maintained by the Institute for Health Metrics and Evaluation, a health research center at the University of Washington focused on determining effective ways to improve global population health. Data sets may be searched by keyword, geographical name, type (e.g., census, disease registry, epidemiological surveillance), and series (e.g., Contraceptive Prevalence Survey, Global Youth Tobacco Survey). For each data set, the website provides a brief description, including geographic area and years covered, and a link to the organization providing the data.

MEASURE DHS: Demographic and Health Surveys (www.measuredhs.com)

This web portal provides access to data collected by the Monitoring and Evaluation to Assess and Use Results Demographic and Health Surveys (MEASURE DHS), a project funded by the U.S. Agency for International Development. MEASURE DHS has conducted more than 300 surveys in over 90 countries; most fall into one of five main survey types. Demographic and Health Surveys are nationally representative household surveys gathering information about health, nutrition, and social and economic factors. AIDS Indicator Surveys provide information about HIV prevalence, knowledge, attitudes, and behavior. Service Provision Assessments focus on health service delivery in a country. Malaria Indicator Surveys collect data on internationally recognized malaria indicators, including ownership and use of mosquito nets, malaria prevention during pregnancy, indoor insecticide use, and occurrence and diagnostic blood testing of children under 5 with high fevers. Key Indicators Surveys briefly cover five topics: family planning, maternal health, child health, HIV/AIDS, and malaria prevention. Data may be downloaded or examined online, and documentation, questionnaires, and reports using the data are also available for download.

Health and Social Care Information Centre: Find Data (www.hscic.gov.uk/searchcatalogue)

In this repository of data from the National Health Service of England, data sets are organized into 10 categories: audits and performance (e.g., clinical audits, NHS Outcomes Framework Indicators), health and lifestyles (e.g., alcohol, contraception, immunization, smoking), hospital care (e.g., accident and emergency statistics, hospital episode statistics, summary hospital-level mortality indicator), mental health (e.g., mental health surveys, specialist mental health services), population and geography (e.g., vital statistics, neighborhood statistics), primary care (e.g., prescriptions, general practice, pharmacies), screening for breast cancer and cervical cancer, social care (e.g., disability; social care for children, adults, and older adults), workforce (e.g., NHS staff numbers, earnings, and turnover), and facilities (data from the Patient Environment Action Team, an annual assessment of inpatient healthcare sites). Health data may also be accessed through the Public Health Indicator Portal at indicators.ic.nhs.uk/webview, which allows variables to be selected from an indexed list.

OECD.StatExtracts (stats.oecd.org)

This is a compendium of core data from countries belonging to the Organisation for Economic Co-operation and Development (OECD) and selected nonmember countries. Data may be accessed by keyword search, through a thematic index (one category is Health Status), or through an alphabetical index of topics and indicators. Data sets may be customized and downloaded, and charts may be created online. A data set of key health indicators for OECD countries for 2013 may also be downloaded from www.oecd.org/els/health-systems/oecdhealthdata2013-frequently requesteddata.htm.

Statistics Canada: Health (http://www.statcan.gc.ca/ start-debut-eng.htm)

This is the home page for health data from Canada's federal statistical agency, which is responsible for providing statistical data for both the country as a whole and each province. This website provides access to data through keyword search, an alphabetical subject list, and a categorized subject list: health (general), disability, diseases and health conditions, environmental factors, health care services, life expectancy and deaths, lifestyle and social conditions, mental health and well-being, pregnancy and births, and prevention and detection of disease. The website also provides links to numerous reports, working papers, and the *Canada Year Book (Health)*.

World Bank: Data (data.worldbank.org)

This is a portal to World Bank data sets, which may be located by keyword search or by indexes of countries, topics, and indicators; the latter two indexes are organized into categories including gender, health, and social development. In addition, the Microdata Library includes data from over 700 surveys conducted by the World Bank and ancillary documents such as sampling plans and questionnaires used.

World Health Organization: Global Health Observatory Data Repository (http://apps.who.int/gho/data/view.main)

This portal provides access to over 50 global data sets on health topics, including mortality, burden of disease, the Millennium Development Goals (maternal and child health, HIV/AIDS, malaria, TB, etc.), epidemic-prone diseases, noncommunicable diseases, health systems, environmental health, and violence and injuries. Data may be searched by keyword or accessed through a topical index, and custom data sets may be built and exported from the online interface. Most information is provided at the country level, with some also available at higher levels of aggregation.

World Health Organization: Regional Office for Europe: Data and Evidence (www.euro.who.int/en/what-we-do/data-and-evidence/databases)

This is a collection of databases for the 53 countries in the European Region of the World Health Organization, including the European Health for All Database (HFA-DB). The HFA-DB is designed to facilitate international comparisons among European Region countries and includes core demographic and health statistics, including risk factors, health status, and health care resources, utilization, and expenditures. Two databases allow analyses of mortality: the Mortality Indicator Database includes information dating back to 1980 and allows analysis of mortality trends by gender, age, broad disease groups, and 67 specific causes of death; the European Detailed Mortality Database includes data back to 1990 and allows more detailed analysis (mortality is coded by three-digit ICD codes). The European Hospital Morbidity Database reaches back to 1999 and provides hospital discharge information by detailed diagnosis, age, and sex. The Centralized Information System for Infectious Diseases is Europe's main surveillance database and includes information on immunization, communicable diseases, and recent outbreaks. The Tobacco Control Database includes information on tobacco control and smoking prevalence. Two inventories provide access to policy initiatives on violence and injury prevention and case studies on physical activity promotion. The data sets may be downloaded or queried and analyzed online.

OTHER TYPES OF DATA

Administrative Data

Often, data are collected by an organization for administrative purposes—for instance, hospitals generally maintain extensive records of the services they provide to individual patients as well as billing and payment records. Although these records are usually not designed for research purposes, they can often be useful to researchers. Advantages of administrative data include that they represent the regular operations of an organization, as opposed to special conditions existing for the purpose of an experiment; that the data sets are often quite large, facilitating subgroup analyses; that the data are often available for multi-year periods, facilitating longitudinal studies; and that they are often already in electronic form, making access relatively easy. Disadvantages of administrative data include the fact that they were not designed with research in mind and may have peculiarities related to their purpose (e.g., diagnostic codes in hospital billing records may be chosen to maximize reimbursement); that they represent the operation of a particular organization (like a private hospital) and selection factors may make the patients included not representative of the larger community or population; and that desired information may not be included in the data because it was not relevant to the administrative purpose or may have been removed in order to preserve confidentiality.

Hall, Hirbe, Waterman, Boslaugh, and Dunagan (2007) compared actual versus risk-adjusted mortality in patients undergoing surgical procedures at an academic teaching hospital, using two risk-adjustment methods: one based on a review of medical records (i.e., chart reviews) and the other based on administrative records. They found that results were comparable using either system, and they suggest that the lower cost of using preexisting administrative records, as opposed to chart reviews, provides a case for further research into the use of algorithms based on administrative records.

Vital Statistics

Vital statistics are a type of administrative data often used in public health research. Vital statistics collect information about births and deaths, and sometimes other information such as marriages and divorces as well. Vital statistics are collected in nearly every country in the world, are meant to include the entire population (although that goal may not be achieved in practice), and are used to compute basic statistics, such as infant mortality, that are used to compare the quality of health services between countries. However, different types of information are included in different countries, and the definition of key terms such as *live birth* can also vary from one country to another, complicating efforts to make comparisons across national boundaries.

In the United States, birth certificates include demographic data on the infant and parents, and about maternal and infant health. Kistka and colleagues (2007) took advantage of this fact to study the relationship between race and preterm birth, using a maternally linked database from the Missouri Department of Health containing records of all births in Missouri between 1989 and 1997. They found that recurrent preterm birth was significantly more common among Black mothers than White mothers, even after adjusting for maternal medical and socioeconomic factors, and also that successive preterm births to the same mother tended to have very similar gestational ages, suggesting that genetic factors were at least part of the explanation.

Another analysis of the same data set, by Palomar, DeFranco, Lee, Allsworth, and Muglia (2007), found that paternal Black race was also significantly associated with increased risk for preterm birth. Both studies capitalized on the availability of a large, inclusive administrative data set, but both were also limited by the information available from birth certificate data—for instance, being a Medicaid recipient stood in as a definition of poverty, and the necessity of using socially defined racial categories as a stand-in for the genetic makeup of the parents studied.

Ecological Data

Ecological data are reported at the group, rather than individual, level. Because many statistics are reported at the country level by international organizations such as the World Health Organization and the World Bank, conducting analyses at the ecological level is relatively easy and is often a starting point for more detailed research. Although it is incorrect to assume that relationships observed at the group level also hold true at the individual level (this assumption is known as the *ecological fallacy*), ecological data can often suggest hypotheses that can then be tested at the individual level.

Many contemporary studies of the relationship between diet and health can be traced back to observations made in the 1950s that there seemed to be a relationship between diet and serum cholesterol levels: People living in regions where the ordinary diet included a high intake of animal fat had higher levels of cholesterol, as compared to those living in regions with diets richer in vegetable fats. The relationship between fat intake and cholesterol has since been tested at the individual level in many experiments, and although this relationship is not yet fully understood, current medical opinion favors the interpretation that the type, rather than the amount, of fat consumed does relate to cholesterol level—consumption of saturated and trans fats are associated with elevated cholesterol, while consumption of monounsaturated and polyunsaturated fats are not.

CURRENT ISSUES AND FUTURE DIRECTIONS

Data Sharing

Secondary data analysis is only possible when people and organizations are willing to share their data. While a substantial amount of secondary data is already available publicly from governmental sources or international organizations, individual researchers have been slower to share their data. Public health has lagged behind some other fields, such as biology, in this regard, but various ventures are underway to promote data sharing. One of the most significant is the Joint Statement of Purpose developed by the World Health Organization and the Wellcome Trust (a global charity based in the United Kingdom and focused on improving human health).

The signatories of the Joint Statement include a number of major governmental organizations and large funders of health research, including the Bill and Melinda Gates Foundation, the World Bank, the CDC, the Canadian Institutes for Health Research, and the U.K. Medical Research Council (Wellcome Trust, n.d.-b). The signatories agree to promote greater access to data, in an equitable, ethical, and efficient manner, that is collected through research that they fund. Intermediate goals of the Joint Statement include developing standards for data management and use of secondary data, including giving appropriate credit to the original collectors of the data. Long-term aspirations include archiving data sets used in peer-reviewed articles and making them available to other researchers (Walport & Brest, 2011).

Although no major journal currently requires authors to share their data as a condition of publication, two major journals now require authors to indicate their willingness to share data, and under what conditions they will share. Since 2009, *BMJ* (formerly the *British Journal of Medicine*) requires authors to publish a statement declaring what, if any, of their data is available to other researchers (Wagner, 2009). The *Annals of Internal Medicine* (2013) also requires authors to indicate their willingness to share their study protocol, computer code, and data sets, and a statement regarding their willingness to share is published with each article. Several other leading journals have published editorials in favor of increased data sharing, including the *New England Journal of Medicine*, *Nature*, and *PLoS Medicine* (Wellcome Trust, n.d.-a).

ADDITIONAL RESOURCES

Boslaugh, S. (2007). *Secondary data sources for public health: A practical guide.* New York, NY: Cambridge University Press.

Cooke, C. R., & Kwashyna, T. J. (2013). Using existing data to address important clinical questions in critical care. *Critical Care Medicine, 41*, 886–896.

Doolan, D. M., & Froehlicher, E. S. (2009). Using an existing data set to answer new research questions: A methodological review. *Research and Theory for Nursing Practice, 23*, 203–215.

Smith, A. K., Ayanian, J. Z., Covinsky, K. E., Landon, B. E., McCarthy, E. P., Wee, C. C., & Steinman, M. A. (2010). Conducting high-value secondary dataset analysis: An introductory guide and resources. *Journal of General Internal Medicine, 26*, 920–929.

REFERENCES

Annals of Internal Medicine. (2013). *Information for authors.* Retrieved from http://annals.org/public/authorsinfo.aspx

Berglund, P. A. (2002, April). *Analysis of complex sample survey data: Using the SURVEYMEANS and SURVEYREG procedures and macro coding.* Paper presented at the SAS Users Group International 27th annual convention, Orlando, FL. Retrieved from http://www2.sas.com/proceedings/sugi27/p263-27.pdf

Boslaugh, S. (2007). *Secondary data sources for public health: A practical guide.* New York, NY: Cambridge University Press.

Boslaugh, S. E., Luke, D. A., Brownson, R. C., Naleid, K. S., & Kreuter, M. W. (2004). Perceptions of neighborhood environment for physical activity: Is it "who you are?" or "where you live?" *Journal of Urban Health, 81*, 671–681.

Brogan, D. J. (2006). *Survey data analysis using software: SUDAAN, SAS, STATA, and SPSS.* Hoboken, NJ: Wiley.

Bulmer, M. I. A., Sturgis, P. J., & Allum, N. (2006). *The secondary analysis of survey data.* Thousand Oaks, CA: Sage.

Centers for Disease Control and Prevention. (2011). *2011 Behavioral Risk Factor Surveillance System questionnaire.* Retrieved from http://www.cdc.gov/brfss/questionnaires/pdf-ques/2011brfss.pdf

Centers for Disease Control and Prevention. (2012). *Trends in current cigarette smoking among high school students and adults, United States, 1965–2010.* Retrieved from http://www.cdc.gov/tobacco/data_statistics/tables/trends/cig_smoking/index.htm

Centers for Disease Control and Prevention. (2013). *Continuous NHANES web tutorial.* Retrieved from http://www.cdc.gov/nchs/tutorials/NHANES/index_continuous.htm

de Vaus, D. A. (2002). *Surveys in social research* (5th ed.). London, UK: Routledge.

Hall, B. L., Hirbe, M., Waterman, B., Boslaugh, S., & Dunagan, W. C. (2007). Comparison of mortality risk adjustment using a clinical data algorithm (American College of Surgeons National Surgical Quality Improvement Program) and an administrative data algorithm (Solucient) at the case level within a single institution. *Journal of the American College of Surgeons, 205*, 767–777.

Heeringa, S. G., West, B. T., & Berglund, P. A. (2010). *Applied survey data analysis.* Boca Raton, FL: Chapman & Hall/CRC.

Humes, K. R., Jones, N. A., & Ramirez, R. R. (2011). *Overview of race and Hispanic origin: 2010.* Washington, DC: U.S. Census Bureau. Retrieved from http://www.census.gov/prod/cen2010/briefs/c2010br-02.pdf

Kistka, Z. A., Palomar, L., Lee, K. A., Boslaugh, S. E., Wangler, M. F., Cole, F. S., . . . Muglia, L. J. (2007). Racial disparity in the frequency of recurrence of preterm birth. *American Journal of Obstetrics and Gynecology, 196*(2), 131.e1–6.

Lee, S. M. (2001). *Using the new racial categories in the 2000 census.* Baltimore, MD: Annie E. Casey Foundation. Retrieved from http://www.prb.org/pdf/census2000_usingnewracialprofiles.pdf

Lumley, T. (2010). *Complex surveys: A guide to analysis using R.* Hoboken, NJ: Wiley.

National Center for Health Statistics. (2012). The National Health and Nutrition Examination Survey: Sample design, 1999–2006. *Vital Health Statistics, 2*(155). Retrieved from http://www.cdc.gov/nchs/data/series/sr_02/sr02_155.pdf

National Center for Health Statistics. (2013). *Analytic guidelines: The National Health and Nutrition Examination Survey.* Retrieved from http://www.cdc.gov/nchs/nhanes/nhanes2003-2004/analytical_guidelines.htm

Palomar, L., DeFranco, E. A., Lee, K. A., Allsworth, J. E., & Muglia, L. J. (2007). Paternal race is a risk factor for preterm birth. *American Journal of Obstetrics and Gynecology, 197*(2), 152.e1–7.

Parascandola, M., & Weed, D. L. (2001). Causation in epidemiology. *Journal of Epidemiology and Community Health, 55*, 905–912.

Pearce, A., Jenkins, R., Kirk, C., & Law, C. (2008). An evaluation of UK secondary data sources for the study of childhood obesity, physical activity and diet. *Child: Care, Health and Development, 34*, 701–709.

Pearl, J. (2009). *Causality: Models, reasoning, and inference* (2nd ed.). New York, NY: Cambridge University Press.

Pearl, J. (2010). An introduction to causal inference. *International Journal of Biostatistics, 6*(2), 7.

Phillips, C. V., & Goodman, C. J. (2006). Causal criteria and counterfactuals: Nothing more (or less) than scientific common sense. *Emerging Themes in Epidemiology, 3*(5). Retrieved from http://www.ete-online.com

Rothman, K. J., Greenland, S., & Lash, T. (2008). *Modern epidemiology* (3rd ed.). Philadelphia, PA: Lippincott Williams & Wilkins.

RTI International. (2013). *Online help manual for SUDAAN 10.* Retrieved from http://www.rti.org/sudaan/page.cfm/Support

Saewyc, E. M., Bauer, G. R., Skay, C. L., Bearinger, L. H., Resnick, M. D., Reis, E., & Murphy, A. (2004). Measuring sexual orientation in adolescent health surveys: Evaluation of eight school-based surveys. *Journal of Adolescent Health, 35*(4), e1–e15.

SAS Institute. (2013a). *SAS/STAT(R) 9.22 user's guide: The SURVEYMEANS procedure.* Retrieved from http://support.sas.com/documentation/cdl/en/statug/63347/HTML/default/viewer.htm#surveymeans_toc.htm

SAS Institute. (2013b). *SAS/STAT(R) 9.22 user's guide: The SURVEYREG procedure.* Retrieved from http://support.sas.com/documentation/cdl/en/statug/63347/HTML/default/viewer.htm#surveyreg_toc.htm

Smith, A. K., Ayanian, J. Z., Covinsky, K. E., Landon, B. E., McCarthy, E. P., Wee, C. C., & Steinman, M. A. (2010). Conducting high-value secondary dataset analysis: An introductory guide and resources. *Journal of General Internal Medicine, 26,* 920–929.

Wagner, E. (2009). *BMJ Ethics Committee annual report 2009.* Retrieved from http://www.bmj.com/about-bmj/advisory-panels/ethics-committee/bmj-ethics-committee-annual-report-2009

Walport, P., & Brest, P. (2011). Sharing research data to improve public health. *Lancet, 377,* 537–539.

Wellcome Trust. (n.d.-a). *Development of the joint statement of purpose.* Retrieved from http://www.wellcome.ac.uk/About-us/Policy/Spotlight-issues/Data-sharing/Public-health-and-epidemiology/WTDV030691.htm

Wellcome Trust. (n.d.-b). *Signatories to the joint statement.* Retrieved from http://www.wellcome.ac.uk/About-us/Policy/Spotlight-issues/Data-sharing/Public-health-and-epidemiology/Signatories-to-the-joint-statement/index.htm

Williams Institute. (2009). *Best practices for asking questions about sexual orientation in surveys.* Retrieved from http://williamsinstitute.law.ucla.edu/wp-content/uploads/SMART-FINAL-Nov-2009.pdf

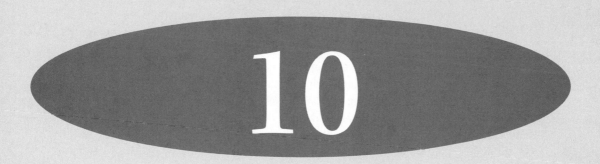

Economics of
Population Health

*Emma McIntosh, Lyndal Bond, Cam Donaldson, Kenny
Lawson, and Helen Mason*

I n this chapter, we introduce readers to key concepts of health economics, with particular relevance to the role of economic evaluation in population health. The material here was derived from a contemporary series of blogs on the economics of
population health (www.gcph.co.uk/latest/blogs) with the aim of facilitating fresh thinking on key matters of importance in the economics of population health.

WHAT IS HEALTH ECONOMICS?

The past three decades have seen a rapid growth in the discipline of health economics
particularly in the area of economic evaluation of health care interventions. **Economics**
has been defined as

> the study of how men [*sic*] and society end up choosing, with or without the use of
> money, to employ scarce productive resources that could have alternative uses, to
> produce various commodities and distribute them for consumption, now or in
> the future, among various people and groups in society. It analyses the costs and
> benefits of improving patterns of resource allocation. (Samuelson, 1948)

Health economics is the discipline of economics applied to the topic of health (Mooney, 1992). If a perfectly competitive market of health care consumers existed, patients or members of the population would present as fully informed, knowledgeable customers weighing the costs and benefits of health care relative to other normal goods such as cars, shoes, and food. Consumers would spend the amount of money on health care that maximizes their well-being. Indeed, such transactions would result in the appropriate amount of resources being allocated to health care overall and to different types of health care. However, for a large number of reasons outlined by Donaldson and Gerard (1993), while no markets work perfectly, *none* of the ideal assumptions of perfect markets work in the case of health care, and as a consequence, extensive government intervention is often required to efficiently allocate health care resources in populations. Health economics provides the tools by which scarce resources can be allocated in the most efficient manner to generate the most "health gain" to society.

Economic evaluation is a mechanism which aims to replace the "missing market" and facilitates the comparison of the costs and outcomes of particular goods, services, or interventions with a view to providing evidence on the best possible use of those resources. Economic evaluations also try to account for the more complex notions of equity and fairness which, in large part, lie behind why we have publicly funded systems in the first place: Some interventions and services may not be reaching the most disadvantaged. We argue that it is likely to be cost-effective in the long run to pay greater attention to addressing the social determinants of health within and outside of the healthcare system. This approach often uses the term *upstream*, which relates to the social determinants of health and to factors that relate to but are larger than health specifically, such as housing, neighborhood, and working conditions. As identified in the report *Securing Good Health for the Whole Population*, a key challenge to improving population health and reducing health inequalities is the "lack of information about *cost-effectiveness* of interventions, which hinders priority setting at local level" (Wanless, 2004). Such statements provide the justification for pursuing sound economic evaluation of population health initiatives.

THE NEED FOR ECONOMIC EVALUATION IN POPULATION HEALTH: SCARCITY AND VALUE

All societies have to limit what they spend on the health of their population. Some spend more than others, but, at some level, such limits imply a value on life or health and raise difficult questions: Should we be providing drugs for people with mild dementia? What about extending life for people with terminal cancer? Should general practitioners check the blood pressure of every adult who visits their clinic? Are the costs of early years parenting interventions justified by the resulting outcomes? Do housing regeneration schemes improve population health? These are examples of frequently asked questions about who should do what to whom, with what health care resources, and with what relation to other services or government budgets. The recent economic recession emphasizes that a society has to limit what it spends on population health, whether interventions originate from within the health sector or, for more upstream cases, other areas of the public sector. Underlying this is the notion of scarcity in the sense that we do not have enough resources to meet all of society's needs. Scarcity has always been with us, but, in the good times, we focus less on it. Good management of scarcity is required to maximize lives saved and health gained. Scarcity simply means that there is an inevitability of choice, whereby in choosing to use resources to meet one need, we give up the opportunity to use those resources to meet some other need. This means that we are forced, as a society, to place values on health interventions. It also means we are either implicitly or explicitly placing values on life and health in different contexts.

For most commodities, these notions of value are played out in the marketplace within a typical competitive market. Yet there are basic and persistent characteristics of health and well-being interventions (such as risk and uncertainty associated with contracting illness) which make them susceptible to market failure and thus more efficiently financed through the public purse. Most advanced economies of the world have recognized this. Table 10.1, using Organization for Economic Co-operation and Development (OECD) data, illustrates that the vast majority of health spending in such countries comes from the public purse.

Table 10.1   Total Health Expenditure and Percentage of Total Which Is Public (Selected OECD Countries, 1990 and 2010)

Country	1990 total health expenditure US$ PPP*	% Public	2010 total health expenditure US$ PPP	% Public	Absolute % change
Australia	1,195	66	3,670	69	+ 3
Canada	1,735	75	4,445	71	− 4
France	1,444	77	3,974	77	0
Germany	1,798	76	4,338	77	+ 1
Netherlands	1,414	71	5,056	86	+ 15
New Zealand	985	82	3,022	83	+ 1
Sweden	1,594	90	3,758	81	− 9
United Kingdom	960	84	3,433	83	− 1
United States	2,851	39	8,233	48	+ 9

Source: OECD Health Data 2012.

*PPP is a form of currency conversion.

The question still remains, however, about how to achieve maximum value from this spending and from other public and private resources that contribute to health and well-being. The examples outlined earlier emphasize that, even within public sector budgets, societies often focus on drugs and gadgets when prioritizing what should be provided by publicly funded systems. Public health tends to receive less attention, especially in times of "fiscal tightness," and even less so in the case of upstream interventions which are more about improving people's life circumstances and environments than providing individualized prevention services. Upstream interventions are also complex in the sense of being multi-sectoral, aimed at prevention, and having long-term perspectives and a focus on reducing health inequalities. Furthermore, we know that health is determined by many different factors. For example, Figure 10.1 shows that the Czech Republic spends almost five times less on health care than the United States does but has equivalent healthy life expectancy, highlighting the need to better map the complexities of resource inputs and resulting health outcomes.

Figure 10.1 Does Spending More Improve Health Outcomes?

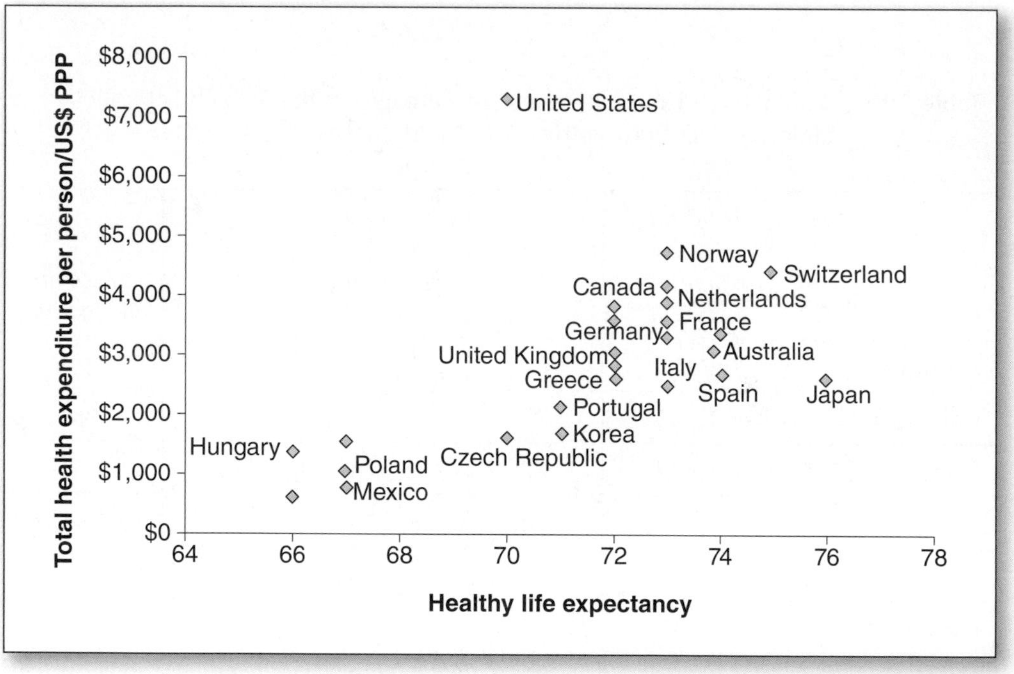

Sources: OECD Health Data 2009 and World Health Organization.

Despite much support for acting on health determinants, evidence regarding both effectiveness and value for money is still seriously lacking. For these reasons population health interventions cannot be exempt from the scrutiny of economic evaluation.

BASIC CONCEPTS IN ECONOMIC EVALUATION

Cost-Effectiveness Analysis and Cost-Utility Analysis

How can information on costs and benefits be used to help make health care decisions? A simple framework is proposed here, starting from the consideration that all health authorities and hospitals currently deploy resources in some way or other. Any change in the way care is delivered is likely to have an impact on both health outcomes and costs. By first deriving and then linking estimates of relative costs and outcomes of alternative procedures under consideration, it should be possible to determine whether a change (e.g., replacing current care with a new procedure) results in

- lower costs and the same or better outcome as current care, in which case the change would be judged to be a better use of health care resources (i.e., more technically efficient); or
- higher costs and better outcome than current care, in which case a judgment would have to be made about whether the extra cost is worth the gains in health achieved (an allocative efficiency question, as treating the same number of patients by some different option will mean using more resources for this group and having fewer available for another group).

The first of these questions is often addressed through what economists call cost-effectiveness analysis (CEA), while the second can be addressed using methods such as cost-utility analysis (CUA) or cost-benefit analysis (CBA). Whichever economic evaluation label is used, it is the case that in any context, information on outcomes and costs can be summarized in a matrix format to aid in the judgment about whether a new procedure is preferable to the current situation. In Figure 10.2 we can see that, relative to the status quo, a new procedure could achieve (1) greater outcome, (2) the same level of outcome, or (3) less outcome. In terms of cost, a new procedure could (A) save costs, (B) result in no difference in costs, or (C) increase costs. For further reading on economic evaluation methods, see Drummond, Sculpher, Torrance, O'Brien, and Stoddart (2005); for specific details on using CBA in health care, see McIntosh, Clarke, Frew, and Louviere (2010).

For any procedure, where a new treatment is in square A1 of the matrix (i.e., it would both save costs and have greater health outcomes relative to current care), then it is clearly superior to current care. In fact, in squares A1, A2, and B1, the new procedure is more efficient than current care and is assigned a ✓ in response to the question of whether it is to be preferred to current care. In squares B3, C2, and C3, the new procedure is less efficient than current care and thus receives an ✗ response. In squares A3 and C1 a judgment would be required as to whether extra health benefits justify the extra costs (C1) or the cost savings justify the lost benefits (A3). For example, in square C1 there is a cost involved, in the sense that the extra resources required to implement the new procedure would have to come from some other group of patients. In both A3 and C1, economics can highlight the magnitudes of extra resources required and outcomes gained. There is, however, a judgment required beyond that as to whether the extra benefits might justify the extra costs involved.

As we will discuss, all economic evaluation procedures, whether for planning services where there are multiple competing alternatives or for evaluating single interventions relative to current practice (or the status quo), are versions of operationalizing this decision matrix, aimed at providing decision makers with a tangible means of weighing service options with regard to both technical and allocative efficiency. Of course, sometimes costs will fall on multiple agencies and outcomes might also be multidimensional. Table 10.2 demonstrates how, to some extent, these issues can be accommodated.

Table 10.2 Matrix Linking Effectiveness With Cost

			Improving outcome →		
			1	*2*	*3*
Compared with the control treatment, the new treatment has:			*Evidence of greater outcome*	*Evidence of no difference in outcome*	*Evidence of less outcome*
Decreased Cost	A	Evidence of cost savings	✓	✓	JR
	B	Evidence of no difference in costs	✓	✗ ✓	✗
	C	Evidence of greater costs	JR	✗	✗

✓ = Yes; ✗ = No; ✓✗ = Indifferent; **JR**= judgment required.

Source: Adapted from the Cochrane Collaboration Handbook (see www.cochrane.org).

Cost-Consequence Approach

Another approach to economic evaluation, which may be more pertinent to population health interventions, is the cost-consequence approach (CCA). This is similar to cost-effectiveness analysis in terms of the questions addressed, but is applied to evaluate interventions with more than one multidimensional outcome. In this way the CCA approach can be entirely societal in perspective (as opposed to a health service–only perspective). In CCA, for each alternative the evaluation computes total (and component) costs and measures change along each of the relevant outcome dimensions (Kelly, McDaid, Ludbrook, & Powell, 2005). The cost and outcome results would need to be reviewed by decision makers, and the different outcomes valued and compared with costs. While this approach has theoretical problems, as it does not synthesize benefits and costs, it can be used to look at issues of changing behavior that are so crucial to population health interventions. CCA does not attempt to combine measures of benefit into a single measure of effectiveness, so it cannot be used to rank interventions. Nevertheless it is a systematic technique that allows decision makers to weight and prioritize the outcomes of an evaluation. This approach has been recommended as ideally suited to the economic evaluation of population health interventions due to its pragmatic framework and its ability to capture the layered outcomes of such interventions (Kelly et al., 2005).

Two Key Aims: Efficiency and Equity

When setting the economic objectives of health care systems, both efficiency and equity notions must be taken into account (see Table 10.3 for operational definitions). As mentioned briefly earlier, efficiency can be sought at two levels: **allocative efficiency** determines the worthwhileness of programs, and **technical efficiency** the best ways of producing worthwhile programs (Donaldson & Gerard, 1993). The key rule to allocative efficiency is simply to undertake activities where benefits outweigh the costs. In allocative efficiency, a broad social perspective should be taken for economic evaluations (i.e., as opposed to a narrower health service–only perspective). Such a broad perspective ensures that due account is taken of all costs and benefits of interventions, regardless of whether they fall within or outside the health care sector. Allocative efficiency, with such a broad scope, is therefore ideally suited to the evaluation of upstream population health interventions where the costs and outcomes may stretch beyond the health service and into housing, education, criminal justice, and employment. Technical efficiency, on the other hand, asks, "Given that some activity is worth doing, what is the best way of doing it?" This perspective combines costs with outcomes and involves the selection between alternative means of achieving the same ends. An example of technical efficiency would be identifying the most cost-effective way of treating a patient with advanced Parkinson's disease: drug therapies or surgery? A key rule for achieving technical efficiency is this: If one means of achieving a given end is less (or more) costly and produces the same amount of output, then this option should (or should not) be preferred.

Table 10.3   Operational Definitions of *Efficiency* and *Equity*

Allocative efficiency	Pursuing health care programs that are worthwhile (benefits exceed costs)
	For programs that are worthwhile, expand up to the point where marginal benefits equal marginal costs
Technical (or operational) efficiency	For worthwhile programs, ensure that the best use is made of scarce resources to meet the program's objective
Horizontal equity criteria	• Equal expenditure for equal need • Equal utilization for equal need • Equal access for equal need • Equal health/reduced inequalities in health
Vertical equity criteria	• Unequal treatment for unequal need • Progressive financing based on ability to pay

Source: Adapted from Donaldson and Gerard (1993).

In most societies there exists a concern that health care resources and outcomes should be distributed in some fair or just way. The guiding principles underlying each health care system give an indication of the relative concern for equity (Donaldson & Gerard, 1993). A useful way of summarizing the possible dimensions of this idea is in terms of horizontal equity and vertical equity. **Horizontal equity** is concerned with equal treatment of equals. **Vertical equity** addresses the question of the extent to which individuals who are unequal in society should be treated differently (see Table 10.3). For a more comprehensive summary of these issues, see Donaldson and Gerard (1993).

Health Care Evaluation Versus Evaluations of Health Interventions

Because health economics has been so successful in becoming used in health care settings, many health economics debates are focused on health care evaluation. This ignores the challenge of the multi-sectoral nature of many upstream population health interventions, in the sense that what might be efficient for one funder is not necessarily so for another, making implementation even more challenging. Figure 10.2 outlines the main determinants of population health (Dahlgren & Whitehead, 1991) and reveals the many cross-sector impacts that would have to be considered in some population health evaluations. The diagram is limited in that the interaction between the various drivers is not captured and nor is the life course, where an individual's early years development can influence his or her adult outcomes. Nonetheless, it is a commonly used and helpful illustration that health is not simply the product of health care.

Figure 10.2   The Main Determinants of Health

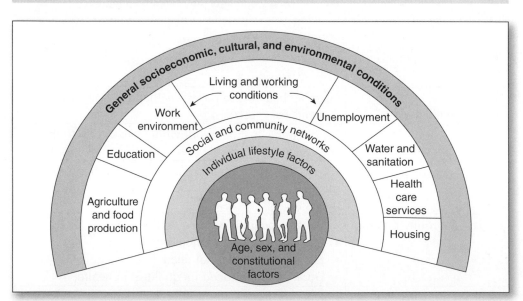

Source: Dahlgren G, Whitehead M. (1991). Policies and Strategies to Promote Social Equity in Health. Stockholm, Sweden: Institute for Futures Studies.

Opportunity Cost and Marginal Analysis

An economic approach to priority setting in public health (Lawson, Mason, McIntosh, & Donaldson, 2014) has to adhere to two key economic concepts: opportunity cost and the margin. **Opportunity cost** refers to having to make choices within the constraint of limited resources; some opportunities will be taken while others must be forgone. Hence, the benefits of the forgone opportunities are termed opportunity costs, and it is these displaced benefits which reflect the true cost of investing in one program and not another. Thus, we need to know the costs and benefits from various activities.

Marginal analysis refers to the focus on the benefit gained from the next unit of resources or the benefit lost from having one unit less. If the marginal benefit per pound, dollar, or euro spent on, say, an elective heart operation program is greater than that for an elective hip replacement, then resources should be taken from hips and given to hearts. But where does this allocation process stop? Should the hips program be removed completely? This is best answered by use of the sequence of diagrams in Figures 10.3a–d. Let us assume we can measure both costs and benefits (i.e., health gains) from treating patients in Program A (who might be heart patients) under and in Program B (say, hips patients) in terms of money, as on the vertical axis (Figure 10.3a).

A further assumption in Figure 10.3a is that these programs and all others are operating at maximum technical efficiency; that is, there is no waste in the system, as achieved by approaches such as "lean thinking." Minimization of technical inefficiencies would obviously be a desirable first step, but is assumed for now for purposes of illustration. We invoke the standard economic principle of diminishing marginal benefit, where patients differ in their potential to benefit from treatment, and then make the reasonable assumption that health professionals prioritize patients according to potential to benefit. Thus, those who can gain most from the procedure in program A will be treated first.

Accordingly, if we increase the number of patients that are treated over a set period of time, we are adding patients that benefit less and less from the procedure, leading to the downward sloping marginal benefit line for A and a corresponding one for Program B; although note the Program B line has a different slope.

Now moving to Figure 10.3b, we assume that the marginal cost of each procedure is constant and equal for all patients receiving either procedure. With the assumed starting levels of service provision shown in Figure 10.3c, it can be seen that the ratio of marginal benefits to marginal cost is great for A than for B. This implies that, to enhance benefits without spending more in total, resources should be taken from B and given to A. Then, cutting back on B from its starting point (Figure 10.3c) will increase its ratio of marginal benefit per pound spent, while expanding Program A will diminish its equivalent ratio (i.e., we will get less and less return in terms of health gain for each additional pound invested in A).

To maximize total patient benefit derived from the combined budgets of the two programs, the process of reallocation should continue until the ratios of marginal benefit to marginal cost for the programs are equal (Figure 10.3d).

Thus, service elimination is never really considered, although it remains a possibility. Rather, through examining changes "at the margin," the application of economics becomes about the balance of services.

Figure 10.3   Marginal Analysis in Action

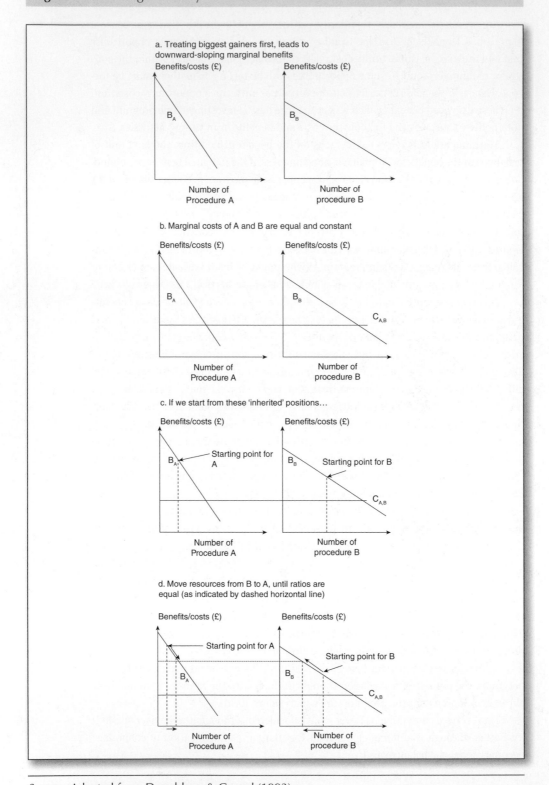

Source: Adapted from Donaldson & Gerard (1993).

*Operationalizing Opportunity Cost: An Economic
Framework for Needs Assessment*

Program budgeting and marginal analysis

An economic approach to needs assessment might use the methodology of Program Budgeting and Marginal Analysis (PBMA), which requires answering five questions:

1. What resources are available in total?

2. In what ways are these resources currently spent?

3. What are the main candidates for more resources and what would be their effectiveness?

4. Are there any areas of care in the program which could be provided to the same level of effectiveness but with fewer resources, so releasing those resources to fund candidates from 3?

5. Are there areas of care which, despite being effective, should have more resources because a proposal (or proposals) from 3 is (are) more effective for the resources spent?

The PBMA framework provides a structured approach to planning service delivery either at the (micro) level of a program (e.g., diabetes) or services for a whole population (a more macro approach). Note that the starting point here is *resources*, not need, the latter being the natural starting point for many health professionals. The important result to emerge from this process of thinking, however, is that need met from available resources will be maximized. Indeed, the wider the range of services covered (e.g., with health and social services under one budget), the better the result.

Program budgeting comprises the first two questions, while the last three pertain to marginal analysis. The underlying premise of program budgeting is that we cannot know where we are going if we do not know where we are. If our budget is fixed, opportunity cost is accounted for by recognizing that the candidates for more resources (question 3 in the process) can be funded only by taking resources from elsewhere (questions 4 and 5). Resources can be obtained from elsewhere by being more technically efficient (e.g., doing things differently so we achieve the same health outcomes at less cost, as addressed by question 4) or more allocatively efficient (e.g., doing entirely different things for different people to achieve a greater health outcome at the same cost, as addressed by question 5). Possibilities under question 4 are more desirable, while question 5 is more difficult to address because it involves taking resources from some groups of patients to give to others (robbing Peter to pay Paul).

However, the key is that all of this can be done at the margin by considering the amounts of different services provided. Although, in reality, quantitative data on marginal benefits are often lacking in many areas of health care, it is the clear and logical way of thinking underpinning the framework that is of prime importance. The more technical ways of estimating costs and benefits are outlined later. Although some readers may think that top priorities for service development could always be funded from annual resource increases from government, such increased funds are unlikely to cover all proposed growth areas (i.e., scarcity still exists). Thus, the elements of the economic approach to needs assessment actually apply in principle to the whole base budget spent on health in the National Health Service (NHS) and elsewhere in the public sector, an issue which will be increasingly recognized in forthcoming years.

Portfolio Approach

One way in which the economics approach to needs assessment in population health could be improved is to adopt the idea of portfolio theory (Bridges, Stewart, King, & van Gool, 2002) from the world of financial investment. Using this approach, investors allocate, as part of a portfolio, some level of their budget to high-risk ventures for which there may be little certainty as regards success, but for which the payoffs would be high if such success is achieved. In priority setting, with respect to allocating resources to health interventions, it might be that many upstream population health interventions could be seen as high-risk ventures. Decision makers could start from these to assess what levels of intervention in such ventures would be acceptable. Portfolio theory, as applied in health economics, highlights the trade-offs that exist between the returns on investments in health care and the risk associated with the outcomes (both costs and effects; Sendi, Gafni, & Birch, 2003).

CONSIDERATIONS FOR ECONOMIC EVALUATION OF POPULATION HEALTH INTERVENTIONS

As outlined earlier, the premise of economic evaluation is to capture everything of value. So we should start by generating a "balance sheet" that audits all the major outcomes, with benefits on one side and costs on the other. But then we may have a huge number of different outcomes—some positive, some negative. So the key next step is to take this social accountancy exercise further by valuing these outcomes where possible. For that, we need some generic measure of final outcome to map everything onto. This enables economists to compare the overall value of different kinds of interventions, with the aim to inform policy as to the "best buys." The main problem with this approach is choosing which generic outcome measure(s) to use; those choices will be guided by the guiding perspective of the evaluation.

Perspective

Funder Perspective

If we adopt a funder (or decision maker) perspective, while recognizing that some interventions are statutory in nature, then the decision makers' objectives regarding what they wanted to achieve from the intervention are made explicit. Only these benefits and costs are valued, and we ignore the other outcomes on the balance sheet. This is a relatively narrow approach, but typically the approach used in health technology assessment (HTA). The UK's National Institute for Clinical Excellence (NICE) has a reference case (essentially a how-to manual) which guides economic evaluators to look primarily at quality-adjusted life years (QALYs) and the costs to the NHS and personal social services.

Unfortunately, population health interventions that originate from, and usually affect, multiple sectors do not always fit with the narrow approach used by HTA organizations. For instance, a funder of housing and regeneration interventions may be primarily interested in the number and quality of houses. If so, then any health outcomes arising from such regeneration activities are really a by-product of the intervention and may not influence the decisions to build new homes. However, there are examples where the broader impacts of such activities (or regeneration) are being considered. In Glasgow, UK, there is a 10-year research program underway, GoWell (Beck et al., 2010), which evaluates the wider impacts (including health) of housing and regeneration. GoWell is funded across multiple sectors, including the Glasgow Housing Association, NHS, and Scottish Government, and includes an economic evaluation.

Societal Perspective

A wider approach to economic evaluation is to take a societal perspective and try to value all the different outcomes separately on the balance sheet, akin to the CCA approach outlined earlier. Outcomes of interest may include health, education, well-being, employment, empowerment, and so on. Time horizon is very important in this context—enough time for all outcomes and costs/savings to manifest themselves.[1] To then value all outcomes on a consistent basis, societal preferences are elicited. We contend that economic evaluations need to reflect a societal perspective which will better reflect the multi-sectoral basis of many population health interventions, and methods need to be developed that not only reflect such a perspective but can be applied locally as well as nationally.

Health Perspective

Finally, we could adopt a health perspective. In this case, the observed outcomes listed in the balance sheet would be projected onto expected long-term health consequences. We would also consider the long-term consequences for net costs. Returning to the housing example, it may take a long time for health impacts to properly manifest themselves (even over a generation). Specialized research groups spend considerable time trying to work out the impacts of different policies on health, while health economists try to do the same with a focus on measuring health outcomes.

Measuring the Benefits of Population Health Interventions

As outlined earlier, when evaluating any intervention it is just as important to consider the benefits that arise as it is to consider the costs. This raises the question of how to measure benefits (or outcomes or consequences) in economic evaluation. In a perfectly competitive market, consumers would simply pay for a good and this payment would reflect its value; however, for reasons alluded to earlier, such traditional market mechanisms do not work perfectly in health. We need to reconstruct the missing market somehow. The following section outlines two popular methods for valuing outcomes in economic evaluation in health care (QALYs and willingness to pay) and one method used in global health (disability adjusted life years).

Quality-Adjusted Life Years

In the early days of health economic evaluation, the benefits of interventions were measured in clinical outcomes, usually within a CEA framework. This limited comparisons between interventions for different conditions. Then came the QALY, which was developed in the mid-1980s (Williams, 1985) as a measure of benefit that was conceptually easy to understand, easy to calculate, and, importantly, comparable across interventions. Such comparability is often claimed to be important for purposes of resource allocation. The QALY is a summary measure of health gain that takes into account length of life *and* quality of life. In the calculation of QALYs, the number of life years over which an individual will experience a particular condition is combined with an assessment of his or her quality of life during those years. Quality of life in the calculation of QALYs is measured on a 0 to 1 scale, where 0 is equated to *being dead* and 1 is *full/normal health*. Values between 0 and 1 are known as health state utilities. By reflecting different degrees of impairment across different dimensions of health, these utilities can be interpreted as judgments of how good or bad different conditions are.

To calculate the number of QALYs for any health state, the utility or value of that state (measured on a scale where 0 = *death* and 1 = *full health*) is multiplied by the number of life years. For example, 2 years in a health state valued at 0.5 would be 1 QALY (i.e., 2 x 0.5). If people experience multiple states over time, the respective QALYs for time spent in each state would simply be added up. This can be illustrated using a hypothetical example, as illustrated in Figure 10.4. Imagine a patient with chronic renal failure. The standard treatment is dialysis, which would allow the patient to live for 10 years with a quality-of-life measurement at 0.6, so this person would have 6 QALYs. An alternative to dialysis is to have a kidney transplant. If a patient has a transplant, let's say this would increase life expectancy by 10 years (from 10 years to 20 years) and would return the patient to full health (i.e., a utility value of 1)—a success which we assume for purposes of exposition, recognizing that many will suffer from background morbidity. A person who had a transplant would have 20 QALYs.

The QALY gain from having a transplant over continuing dialysis is therefore 14 QALYs (shown by the shaded area). If, however, instead of quality of life on dialysis being valued at 0.6 it was 0.8, this would give a gain of 12 QALYs; the values attached to quality-of-life gains are therefore very important.

The QALY has arguably been the biggest contribution of health economics to the evaluation of health policy. However, like any measure, there are limitations to its use, especially in the evaluation of population health interventions. It may be obvious from the name, but QALYs measure values only for health-related quality of life, which are

Figure 10.4   QALYs for a Hypothetical Kidney Failure Patient, for Transplant
Relative to Dialysis

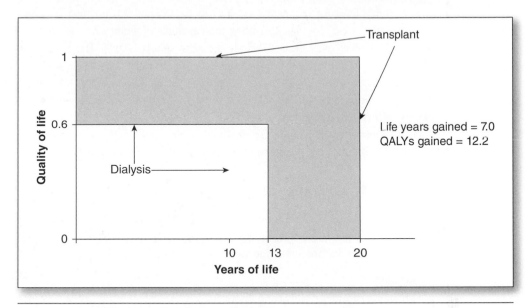

Source: Adapted from Donaldson & Gerard (1993).

then multiplied by the number of years lived. In the case of population health interventions, are QALYs an appropriate measure? Yes, if health is the main outcome of a policy,
such as a mass screening program for the prevention of, say, cardiovascular disease.
However, population health interventions often include other areas of the public sector
beyond the health system, resulting in nonhealth benefits such as reducing crime levels
or raising education levels. To capture these effects, one possible approach is to measure
nonhealth QALYs and then combine these with *health QALYs* to create a more comprehensive generic measure of well-being. However, despite some previous attempts to do
this for crime interventions, this particular research area is not well advanced.

Willingness to Pay

The concept behind willingness to pay (WTP) is straightforward: The benefit (or utility)
that an individual gains from an intervention can be valued by the maximum amount he or
she would be willing to pay for that intervention (Donaldson, Farrar, Mapp, Walker, &
MacPhee, 1997). To measure WTP, individuals are presented with a description of an intervention and the outcomes that would be associated with that intervention (Donaldson et al.,
1997). For example, if we were evaluating a screening service, the description would include
information like what the screening test would involve, how often it would occur, where it
would take place, and what potential information would be given following the screening
test. After reading this description the respondent would then be asked, hypothetically, the
maximum amount he or she would be willing to pay for the service described.

CALCULATING QALYS

The methods used for calculating QALYs can be categorized into two main groups: generic and condition specific. A good example of a generic measure is the EQ-5D, which was devised by the EuroQol group (2011). The EQ-5D (EuroQol Group, 1990) has five dimensions, each of which has three levels (although a new five-level version has been developed which will be more sensitive to changes in health), and there is a corresponding index of quality-of-life scores for the United Kingdom which has been developed to score all potential combinations of levels (Dolan, Gudex, Kind, & Williams, 1995). Figure 10.5 provides an excerpt from the descriptive system of the EQ-5D instrument.

Figure 10.5 EQ-5D Descriptive System

By placing a tick in one box in each group below, please indicate which statements best describe your own health state today.

Mobility

I have no problems in walking about ☐

I have some problems in walking about ☐

I am confined to bed ☐

Self-Care

I have no problems with self-care ☐

I have some problems washing or dressing myself ☐

I am unable to wash or dress myself ☐

Usual Activities (e.g., work, study, housework, family, or leisure activities)

I have no problems with performing my usual activities ☐

I have some problems with performing my usual activities ☐

I am unable to perform my usual activities ☐

Pain/Discomfort

I have no pain or discomfort ☐

I have moderate pain or discomfort ☐

I have extreme pain or discomfort ☐

Anxiety/Depression

I am not anxious or depressed ☐

I am moderately anxious or depressed ☐

I am extremely anxious or depressed ☐

Source: ©EuroQol Group (1990).

While generic QALY measures can be applied to any group of interest, condition-specific measures focus directly on the characteristics of the condition being evaluated. For condition-specific methods we generally start by producing a description of the condition being evaluated, including items like symptoms.

Whether generic or condition-specific, health state descriptions then need to be valued. The two main methods to do this are the standard gamble and the time trade-off. In the standard gamble technique, people are asked to choose between two alternatives—Alternative A is a certain outcome of remaining in the health state as described (so in the kidney disease example, dialysis for the rest of the person's life), while Alternative B is some form of treatment that has two possible outcomes: a return to full health for remaining life with a probability p or immediate death with a corresponding probability $1 - p$ (see Table 10.4). That is, Alternative B comes in the form of a gamble.

Figure 10.6   Standard Gamble Format

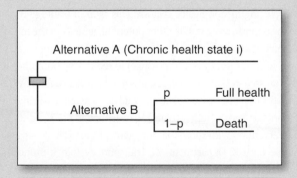

Source: Adapted from Donaldson & Gerard (1993).

The respondent makes a series of choices in which the probabilities for Alternative B are varied until the individual is indifferent (finds it difficult to choose) between Alternatives A and B. The utility of the description (in this case "being on dialysis") is then taken as p. The time trade-off approach involves a similar iterative process, but asks people to choose between living in the health state described for a given period of time t or in full health for a shorter period of time x. The period of time in full health is varied until the individual is indifferent between the two and the corresponding utility score is calculated as x/t.

This can be quite a difficult task as many people (covered by public or private insurance) have never thought about paying for health care, so following the description of the intervention there is often some type of additional prompt for respondents to help them think about what their maximum WTP would be. This can take the form of a set of payment cards respondents are given, each with different amounts of money printed on them, and respondents decide if they would pay the amount shown to help them narrow down what their WTP would be. Alternatively, people could be given one monetary amount and asked if they would pay the amount shown in a straightforward yes/ no response (this requires much larger sample sizes and could lead to bias through respondents' temptations to answer yes when they do not really mean it). There are a number of methodological works describing the various payment vehicles that can be used in WTP studies (or studies including a cost attribute within discrete-choice experiments; McIntosh et al., 2010; Slothuus Skjoldborg & Gyrd-Hansen, 2003).

WTP for population health interventions

The context for the intervention description is important in all WTP studies, but in the evaluation of population health interventions there are a few additional key features we need to consider. One is the time horizon associated with the elicitation of population health WTP values, with the benefits of interventions typically occurring and then extending much further into the future. Another is to outline all outcomes, including those which may be non-health benefits occurring in non-health sectors. This is an advantage over QALYs in that individuals have the opportunity to value other potential benefits of the intervention beyond health gain. This may especially be useful in the evaluation of population health interventions where we may not want (or it may not be possible) to reduce the outcomes into a change in health status as expressed in QALY terms. The more holistic approach of WTP could help us in valuing the benefits of these services. The other advantage of measuring the benefits of an intervention in monetary terms (rather than QALYs) is that, in principle, it allows us to compare the health intervention with those that are being proposed in other areas of the public sector. For example the UK Department for Transport evaluates proposed interventions using WTP to measure the benefits, as does the Department for Environment, Transport and Rural Affairs. This is useful when thinking about resource allocation across the public sector. If other areas of the public sector, such as transport or environment, use WTP as the most common measure of benefit in economic evaluation, why has WTP not taken off in health?

Fundamentally, many people are not comfortable assigning monetary values to things which they believe are incommensurate with monetary valuation, such as human life or health. However, decision makers are already implicitly doing this; whenever they make a decision to limit the extent of availability of an intervention, a value is placed on health or life. Even for those who do feel comfortable using monetary valuation, another frequently cited concern with WTP is its association with ability to pay and the implications of this for equity. Indeed, when asking people to give their WTP responses, we encourage them to think about their current income because if they are not trading with an amount which is within their capacity, their response has no meaning. So what does this mean for equity? Many population health interventions are targeted at the most deprived, who have a low ability to pay. If we surveyed only those at whom the intervention is directly targeted, this could result in a benefit-to-cost ratio which is not a true reflection of the intervention. WTP values should be elicited from a representative sample of the general public, which would include the full income distribution.

Once WTP values have been estimated for a particular intervention it is important to examine whether people in higher income groups tend to choose one option more frequently than those in lower income groups, and whether the WTP values of those in the higher group distort the overall value given for one or other option. If so, distributional weights can be applied in adjusting the raw values. The overall average WTP would then be applied to all regardless of income status—as is the case in work that has been conducted on using WTP to value lives and QALYs saved by safety and health interventions. It is also worth noting that QALYs, through deriving their values from risk and time trade-off questions, also suffer from a similar distributional problem as WTP.

Disability-Adjusted Life Years: Measuring Health in a Global Context

The World Health Organization (WHO) published its first Global Burden of Disease (GBD) report in August 1996 (Murray & Lopez, 1996). The GBD approach is a systematic, scientific effort to quantify the comparative magnitude of health loss due to diseases, injuries, and risk factors by age, sex, and geography over time. The GBD provides systematic epidemiological estimates for 150 health conditions and introduced a new metric for measuring and valuing health, the disability-adjusted life year (DALY), developed by Murray and Lopez (1996). The DALY is based on years of life lost from premature death and years of life lived in less than full health. One DALY can be thought of as one lost year of healthy life. The sum of these DALYs across the population, or the burden of disease, is a measurement of the gap between current health status and an ideal health situation where the entire population lives to an advanced age, free of disease and disability (DALYs for a disease or health condition are calculated as the sum of the years of life lost (YLL) due to premature mortality in the population and the years lost due to disability (YLD) for incident cases of the health condition:

DALY = YLL + YLD

YLL correspond to the number of deaths multiplied by the standard life expectancy at the age at which death occurs. The basic formula for YLL for a given cause, age, and sex is as follows:

YLL = N x L

where:

- N = number of deaths
- L = standard life expectancy at age of death in years

The basic formula for YLD (without applying social preferences) is:

YLD = I x DW X L

where:

- I = number of incident cases
- DW = disability weight
- L = average duration of the case until remission or death (years)

DALYs have been recommended by WHO for use in generalized cost-effectiveness analysis (Tan-Torres Edejer, et al., 2003). The Global Burden of Diseases, Injuries, and Risk Factors Study 2010 recently reported the DALYs for 291 diseases and injuries in 21 regions (Murray et al., 2013). DALYs are conceptually similar to QALYs but differ in key theoretical ways, most notably the methods used to estimate the disability weights and the use of age weights by DALYs. For a review of the DALY approach, and critiques by economists, see Fox-Rushby (2002).

Costing "Rules" for Multi-Sectoral Population Health Interventions

To this point, we have paid attention to important theoretical concepts, such as scarcity and opportunity cost, and methods for measuring and valuing outcomes, including QALYs, WTP, and DALYs. The aim of this section is to move away from the outcomes side to the often-neglected but equally important cost side of the economic evaluation equation. Economists perceive the true cost of any intervention in relation to the forgone benefits of investing those resources in their next best alternative use. For example, in population health, the opportunity cost of investing in a home visit intervention for vulnerable infants could be the QALYs that could have been gained through investing these same resources in, say, reducing asthma through improved housing ventilation. Although such forgone benefits are often difficult to measure in practice, opportunity cost represents a useful mode of thought as it makes explicit the trade-offs made when investing in one intervention and not another. It also emphasizes that it is resources which have opportunity costs and thus require valuation. While in theory the opportunity cost is the correct "price," in practice, most economists use market prices (at least as a starting point) to value the majority of resource items in an economic evaluation.

Costing has three elements: identification; measurement, and valuation. Identification of costs requires consultation with service users, professionals delivering a service, and, where possible, detailed research of the scope of possible costs and effects (Drummond et al., 2005). In population health interventions where the scope of costs and cost savings are likely to be broader than a clinical evaluation, this identification stage is highly important and contact with stakeholders in all affected sectors should be established early on in the evaluation. There is a range of cost determination methods (Figure 10.7), each of which has advantages and drawbacks to consider.

Measurement of the quantities of resource use is the next stage. Within the confines of a well-designed evaluation, it is likely that for some interventions the costs will be readily measured in terms of, say, number of home visits, costs of access to sports facilities, or costs of telephone advice for smoking cessation. However, it may become more complex when a new swimming pool is built to increase leisure activity within a population. To ensure accuracy, these "lumpy" one-off built costs should ideally be measured at the stage when budget information on spending is available, as would be the case for, say, regeneration of housing stock. Without good dialogue or the use of common cost language with stakeholders in such sectors, accurate cost information may be difficult to obtain. It may also be the case that lumpy items of cost may have to be shared between more than one population health intervention and costs apportioned between programs accordingly.

Figure 10.7   Cost Determination Methods and Precision (U.S. Context)

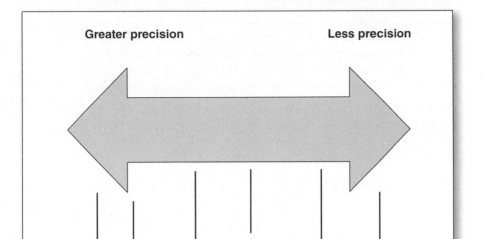

Source: Adapted from U.S. Department of Veterans Affairs (2013).

The second stage to the measurement of costs is deciding the appropriate unit of analysis: Per person? Per household? Per community? The unit of analysis on the cost side should eventually be aligned with the appropriate unit of analysis on the outcome side, such that a decision maker can identify the resources required for achieving a given level of outcome. The key issue is that we estimate the total cost arising from any particular policy proposal, and the unit of analysis essentially gives us the rate at which costs are incurred. Note that the unit of analysis will influence the ultimate cost per unit of outcome and the final economic recommendation may be sensitive to changes in the unit of analysis. Table 10.5 lists several categories and examples of possible resource use for inclusion in population health interventions; see also Weatherly et al. (2009).

The final stage is the valuing of costs, namely, the process of attaching relevant unit costs or prices to the measured costs. It may be the case in population health interventions that typical unit costs of the type used in health sector economic evaluations are not relevant, as outlined in the example of the costs of building a swimming pool or housing regeneration. For these large-scale lumpy costs, their values will be derived from available spending data on these items, and this may be an accounting exercise. The opportunity cost of such large items can, however, be reported alongside the monetary

---

Table 10.5   Examples of Resource Use in Population Health
Interventions

Health sector resources: hospital stay, outpatient appointments, staff time, drugs, consumables, theater time, equipment, capital items, overheads, community-based health care (e.g., general practitioner appointments), paramedic and emergency ambulance services

Community health and personal social service resources: community-based social care (e.g., social workers), occupational therapy services, nursing home, residential care, community-based health care staff, day care, foster care services

Patient and family resources: travel time and expenses, out-of-pocket costs such as over-the-counter medications, opportunity cost of leisure time, childcare costs, domestic resources (e.g., cleaning and yard maintenance costs due to ill health)

Other government sector costs: housing, employment, education, environmental, home affairs and justice, social welfare, transport

Productivity gains/losses: value of changes in productivity (patient and caregivers)

---

price to identify potential benefits forgone. In the instance of extended time horizons which may occur with preventive interventions such as smoking cessation or childhood interventions, lumpy costs will require annuitization over the expected life span of the intervention using a recommended discount rate (currently UK's NICE recommends 3.5% and more recently 1.5% for public health economic evaluations) as well as some consideration of the throughput or cost per use. Alternatively, a more practical approach may be to leave these costs in their lumpy total cost format and report the various consequences alongside in a cost-consequence approach.

A further point to note here is that, as Pearce (1971) outlines in his discussion of CBA, "the basic decision rule in CBA requires that benefits and costs be expressed in monetary units over the economic life of the project." This is especially important for population health interventions, as it is a reminder that, with many costs in population health interventions being front-loaded (e.g., investment in housing, preventive health measures) with benefits likely to be longer term, appropriate consideration of the relevant time horizon for costs and cost savings is crucial. Economic evaluation over longer time horizons will allow longer term effects to fully manifest themselves.

As mentioned, a broad societal perspective is recommended in population health interventions to permit all costs, cost savings, and effects to be measured and valued within each affected sector. By reporting the results of economic evaluations in population health in this way, decision makers can easily see where the effects occur. This may be challenging where costs/savings occur across sectors, because identifying units of analysis that can be aggregated meaningfully across sectors may be difficult. Attribution of costs and benefits is also a technical challenge. Consider a home visiting intervention that aims to improve outcomes in infants: The costs incurred are to the health and social services sector, yet the cost savings may be accrued in the educational sector (improved attainment, less truancy and reduced costs of monitoring), the justice sector (reduced crime), the housing sector (with increased educational outcomes there may be less requirement for a government housing subsidy), and so on. A narrow health care perspective in this instance would have overlooked these valuable spillover effects to the other sectors.

The Role of Modeling in Economic Evaluation

Policymaking is difficult because uncertainty is inevitable. There is imperfect information regarding the consequences of decisions, limited capacity as human beings to process complex information, and the policy arena is a contested process, with competing objectives and value judgments. Nonetheless, decisions need to be made and policies set. Modeling (if done well) can help us cope with complexity and guide us through the evaluation and decision-making process.

What Is a Model?

Models are simulations, a simplification of reality designed to focus on the essentials of a particular situation. Models vary in sophistication, from a satellite navigation system, with programed geographical maps to give us the best route home, to macroeconomic models, which program economic theory about how the economy works, to estimate the impact of changes in interest rates on house prices. Figure 10.8 shows the Alzheimer Association's model of costs for Alzheimer's care over the next several decades.

Benefits of Modeling I: Facilitating Longer Term Evaluation

Evaluation periods are usually relatively short, whereas the impacts of interventions may be fully realized only over the longer term. If health economists limit evidence gathering on benefits and costs to a within-trial evaluation, there is a risk of misrepresenting an intervention and drawing erroneous conclusions. Modeling can help project the best estimate about long-term impacts. In HTA, economists build models by simulating an underlying disease process, incorporating the relevant epidemiology and statistics, and collaborating in relevant multidisciplinary teams. For instance, in cardiovascular disease (CVD), health economists can model from CVD risk factors (e.g., blood pressure, cholesterol) to estimate future CVD events (e.g., heart attacks, stroke) and estimate the consequences for life expectancy. For instance, a statin trial might estimate the impact on reducing cholesterol, and models can then convert this information into projections of the change in (quality-adjusted) life expectancy and health service costs.

Benefits of Modeling II: Helping to Choose Between Interventions

Given scarce resources health economists need to make choices between different kinds of interventions. This may be a complicated task if different evaluations have collected information on different outcome measures or over different time periods.

Figure 10.8 Projected Costs of Care for People With Alzheimer's Disease in the United States

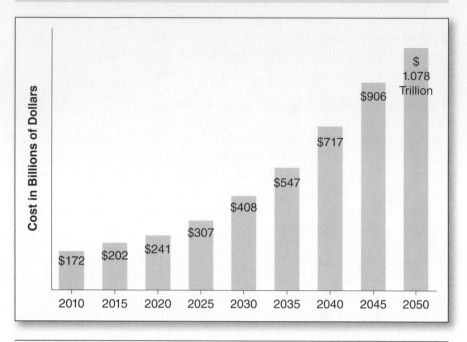

Source: Alzheimer's Association (2010).

Models can help with this process by

- encouraging decision makers to make explicit their objectives and budget,
- collating the information on different intervention options, and
- taking us through an "option appraisal" process to point to the interventions promising best value for money

This process requires larger generic models to allow many different interventions to be compared. For instance, we ideally want a CVD model that can simulate the likely impacts of both individually targeted (e.g., statins, exercise regimes) and population-wide interventions (e.g., a smoking ban). These kinds of models permit policymakers to develop and evaluate packages of interventions.

Multi-Criteria Decision Analysis

Another form of modeling is multi-criteria decision analysis (MCDA). which can be seen as a framework for organizing information for making choices. Part of the process for MCDA involves defining a range of outcomes, placing weights on their relative importance and, where data are not available, on the extent to which such outcomes have been achieved by the various interventions being assessed in order to devise some sort of scoring mechanism instead. When scored and weighted outcomes have been combined with cost data, the interventions can be ranked in terms of benefit achieved for resources expended, with options nearer the top of the list receiving priority. Of course, such systems are not perfect, but the scoring and weighting systems can be "played with" to examine how sensitive the final ranking would be to different values. Furthermore, such rankings merely serve to inform a discussion about what the final set of priorities should be. The important factor is that the process is explicit and this is better than having no process at all.

Economic Models in Population Health

Economic evaluation of upstream population heath interventions to date has been rare, especially for interventions such as welfare reform, housing improvements, or urban regeneration. However, the need for modeling here can be even more important than for clinical evaluations. For instance, the impact of upstream interventions will only be fully realized in the distant future, perhaps intergenerationally, while the upfront costs can be considerable. The challenge is to work with other social scientists and interventionists to develop testable intervention theories to be used as a basis for modeling. For example, it is common for social interventionists to create logic models (Baxter, Killoran, Kelly, & Goyder, 2010) that harness expert opinion and map out the intended impacts of interventions. Such an approach would prove very useful for economic evaluations of population health interventions. The collective challenge is to turn these into formal causal models to be tested using evaluation data. In application, models can convert intervention impacts seen in short-run evaluations into longer term projections.

In short, models are there to compensate for lack of perfect information. Models can help get the most out of short-term evaluations and can help economic evaluation outline the possible consequences of different policy options. Ideally, a model should be as simple and user-friendly as possible. Decision making and evaluation in an uncertain world is difficult, and models are there to help make the best choices given the available data.

CASE STUDIES

Keep Well: Scotland's Targeted CVD Primary Prevention Program

To illustrate some of the concepts presented in this chapter, we will use two case studies. First, we introduce Keep Well, Scotland's primary prevention program (www.healthscotland.com), which aims to prevent the premature onset of CVD, reduce associated health service costs, and reduce health inequalities. Keep Well is (at present) focused on the most deprived 15% of areas of Scotland. Individuals aged 45–65 are screened using the ASSIGN risk score (Woodward, Brindle, & Tunstall-Pedoe, 2007) to assess the risk of an event in the forthcoming 10 years. The risk factor is composed of nine variables, a mixture of modifiable variables, such as systolic blood pressure and cholesterol, and nonmodifiable variables, such as age, sex, and a measure of socioeconomic deprivation to detect the underlying social gradient in the incidence of CVD. High-risk individuals, defined as those with a risk score of ≥ 20%, are referred to tailored multifactorial programs, including pharmaceutical and behavioral interventions.

No existing economic models were equipped to evaluate the impact of the Keep Well program, so important policy context was incorporated into the Scottish CVD Policy

Model, funded by the Chief Scientist Office in Scotland. The model was built using the same longitudinal data set used to create the ASSIGN 10-year risk score. But rather than estimate the relationship between the ASSIGN risk factors and CVD over 10 years, the health economic analysis estimated how risk factors predict QALYs and lifetime health service costs. The model could then be used to readily estimate the impacts of interventions (single or multiple) on changing QALYs and costs. Further, given the inclusion of a measure of deprivation, the model also estimates the impact on health inequalities.

To date, there has not been a comprehensive evaluation to assess whether the Keep Well program is reducing the incidence of CVD. In the absence of evidence, the model used secondary data sources on the efficacy of interventions (e.g., statins, smoking cessation) and expert opinion. Through a sensitivity analysis, the model illustrated why the program may not actually be cost-effective and highlighted key areas of uncertainty (e.g., adherence to medication, behavior change) and made the unequivocal case that a robust economic evaluation is needed if scarce health service resources are to be used efficiently. The good intentions of the program may not be matched by the reality of effectiveness and cost-effectiveness.

The Cost-Effectiveness of Salt Reduction

Eating a diet high in salt increases a person's risk of high blood pressure, which in turn increases risk of a cardiovascular event such as a heart attack or stroke. Reducing the amount of salt the population consumes has the potential to reduce the overall level of CVD in a country. One study designed to evaluate policies to reduce dietary salt intake was the MedCHAMPS project, which covered four Eastern Mediterranean countries (http://research.ncl.ac.uk/medchamps). The starting point was an epidemiological model which explains CVD trends across a population based on a number of risk factors, including obesity, smoking, cholesterol, and blood pressure (the IMPACT CHD model). This information had to be incorporated with identification of policies to reduce salt intake and the effect these policies would have on blood pressure. Two policies selected were: a health promotion campaign highlighting the health effects of a diet high in salt; and a reformulation of food products.

As is the case in most models, estimates from the literature on the effectiveness of each policy to reduce blood pressure were used. The expected reduction of current salt consumption for each policy was estimated, and this estimate was then translated into a change in blood pressure. Change in blood pressure was used to estimate the number of deaths prevented or postponed. The number of life years gained and the number of deaths prevented or postponed were estimated. Costing these different policy options involved bringing together data from a number of sources; existing comparable policies, data from ministries of health and, for the cost of reformulation, from the food manufacturers. Health care costs of CVD events were also incorporated and data were taken from standard hospital records. Finally, data on the costs of introducing each policy were combined with the effectiveness information generated by the epidemiological model. It was estimated that in Palestine, for example, the health promotion policy would save PPP$4 million, with 97 life years gained across the population, while the reformulation campaign would result in an incremental cost of PPP$2 million and 479 life years gained.

CONCLUSION

The aim of this chapter was to introduce some key economic concepts such as scarcity, value, marginal analysis, and opportunity cost and to develop the notion of economic evaluation in a population health context. If you plan to work on economic evaluation of population health, we recommend taking a broad societal perspective, incorporating all sectors where costs and effects might occur and ensuring the time horizon for evaluations is sufficient to capture long-term effects. The methods used to carry out these economic evaluations are, in the main, very well established, and guidance on how to employ them is readily accessible. We encourage researchers working in this area, however, to go beyond cost-effectiveness analysis and into the realms of environmental or transport economics, where the use of broader evaluative techniques such as cost-benefit analysis and discrete-choice experiments are common.

ADDITIONAL RESOURCES

Donaldson, C., & Gerard, K.. (1993). *Economics of health care financing: The visible hand.* London, UK: Macmillan.

Kelly, M. P., McDaid, D., Ludbrook, A., & Powell, J. (2005). *Economic appraisal of public health interventions.* London, UK: Health Development Agency.

McIntosh, E., Clarke, P., Frew, E., & Louviere, J. J. (2010). *Applied methods of cost benefit analysis in health care.* Oxford, UK: Oxford University Press.

Weatherly, H., Drummond, M. F., Claxton, K., Cookson, R., Ferguson, B., Godfrey, C., . . . Snowden, A. (2009). Methods for assessing the cost-effectiveness of public health interventions: Key challenges and recommendations. *Health Policy, 93*(2–3), 85–92.

REFERENCES

Alzheimer's Association. (2010). *Changing the trajectory of Alzheimer's disease: A national imperative.* Retrieved from http://www.alz.org/alzheimers_disease_trajectory.asp

Baxter, S., Killoran, A., Kelly, M. P., & Goyder, E. (2010). Synthesizing diverse evidence: The use of primary qualitative data analysis methods and logic models in public health reviews. *Public Health, 124*(2), 99–106.

Beck, S., Hanlon, P., Tannahill, C., Crawford, F., Ogilvie, R., & Kearns, A. (2010). How will area regeneration impact on health? Learning from the GoWell study. *Public Health, 124*(3), 125–130.

Bridges, J., Stewart, M., King, M., & van Gool, K. (2002). Adapting portfolio theory for investment in health with a multiplicative extension for treatment synergies. *European Journal of Health Economics, 3*(1), 47–53.

Dahlgren, G., & Whitehead, M. (1991). *Policies and strategies to promote social equity in health.* Stockholm, Sweden: Institute for Future Studies.

Dolan, P., Gudex, C., Kind, P., & Williams, A. (1995). A social tariff for EuroQol: Results from a UK General Population Survey (Discussion Paper 138). York, UK, University of York, Centre for Health Economics.

Donaldson, C., Farrar, S., Mapp, T., Walker, A., & MacPhee, S. (1997). Assessing community values in health care. *Health Care Analysis, 5*(1), 7–29.

Donaldson, C., & Gerard, K. (1993). *Economics of health care financing: The visible hand.* London, UK: Macmillan.

Drummond, M. F., Sculpher, M. J., Torrance, G. W., O'Brien, B., & Stoddart, G. L. (2005). *Methods for the economic evaluation of health care programmes* (3rd ed.). Oxford, UK: Oxford University Press.

EuroQol Group. (1990). EuroQol: A new facility for the measurement of health related quality of life. *Health Policy, 16,* 199–208.

EuroQol Group. (2011). *EQ-5D-5L user guide. Version 1.0.* Rotterdam, Netherlands: Author.

Fox-Rushby, J. (2002). *Disability adjusted life years (DALYs) for decision making? An overview of the literature.* London, UK: Office of Health Economics.

Kelly, M. P., McDaid, D., Ludbrook, A., & Powell, J. (2005). *Economic appraisal of public health interventions.* London, UK: Health Development Agency.

Lawson, K., Mason, H., McIntosh, E., & Donaldson, C. (2014). Priority setting in public health. In R. Cookson & M. Suhrcke (Eds.), *Encyclopaedia of health economics.* London, UK: Elsevier.

McIntosh, E., Clarke, P., Frew, E., & Louviere, J. J. (2010). *Applied methods of cost benefit analysis in health care.* Oxford, UK: Oxford University Press.

Mooney, G. (1992). *Economics, medicine and health care* (2nd ed.). Harvester, UK: Wheatsheaf.

Murray, C. J. L., & Lopez, A. D. (1996). *The global burden of disease: A comprehensive assessment of mortality and disability from diseases, injuries and risk factors in 1990 and projected to 2020.* Cambridge, MA: Harvard University Press.

Murray, C. J. L., Voss, T., Lozano, R., Naghavi, M., Flaxman, A. D., Michaud, C., . . . Memish, Z. A. (2013). Disability-adjusted life years (DALYs) for 291 diseases and injuries in 21 regions, 1990–2010: A systematic analysis for the Global Burden of Disease Study 2010. *Lancet, 380,* 2197–2223.

Pearce, D. W. (1971). *Cost-benefit analysis.* London, UK: Macmillan.

Samuelson. P. (1948). *Economics.* New York, NY: McGraw-Hill.

Sendi, P. A., Gafni, A., & Birch, S. (2003). Optimizing a portfolio of health care programs in the presence of uncertainty and constrained resources. *Social Science and Medicine, 57,* 2207–2215.

Slothuus Skjoldborg, U., & Gyrd-Hansen, D. (2003). Conjoint analysis: The cost variable: An Achilles' heel? *Health Economics, 12,* 479–491.

Tan-Torres Edejer, T., Baltussen, R., Adam, T., Hotubessy, R., Acharya, A., Evans, D. B., & Murray, C. J. L. (2003). *WHO guide to cost-effectiveness analysis.* Geneva, Switzerland: World Health Organisation.

U.S. Department of Veterans Affairs. (2013). *Methods for cost determination.* Retrieved from http://www.herc.research.va.gov/methods/methods_cost.asp

Wanless, D. (2004). *Securing good health for the whole population: Final report.* London, UK: HM Treasury.

Weatherly, H., Drummond, M. F., Claxton, K., Cookson, R., Ferguson, B., Godfrey, C., . . . Snowden, A. (2009). Methods for assessing the cost-effectiveness of public health interventions: Key challanges and recommendations. *Health Policy, 93*(2–3), 85–92.

Williams, A. (1985). Economics of coronary artery bypass grafting. *British Medical Journal (Clinical Research Edition), 291,* 326–329.

Woodward, M., Brindle, P., & Tunstall-Pedoe, H. (2007). Adding social deprivation and family history to cardiovascular risk assessment: The ASSIGN score from the Scottish Health Health Extended Cohort (SHHEC). *Heart, 93,* 172–176.

NOTE

1. These future outcomes are discounted using standard discount rates to represent their present value; the current recommended discount rate used in UK economic evaluations is 3.5% for both costs and outcomes and 1.5% for economic evaluations of public health interventions.

IN FOCUS

COST ANALYSIS FOR INTERVENTIONS
Rick Homan

In public health we are often faced with the challenge of scare resources. Many potential interventions can be considered to improve health of a population, but there are rarely sufficient resources to support all of the things we would like to do. Being able to assess the cost of undertaking a program or intervention helps guide decisions about whether a program or intervention is affordable given current resources and can assist in resource mobilization efforts to advocate for a program or intervention.

Estimating Costs

This section provides a quick overview of how you can begin to estimate the costs of a program or intervention. A useful starting point is a logic model which describes a program or intervention with respect to inputs, process, outputs, and outcomes (IF Figure 1). Logic models are often created during the development of monitoring and evaluation plans, but if a logic model does not already exist for an intervention, it is a useful exercise to assist in the cost estimation.

IF Figure 1 Logic Model for Program or Intervention

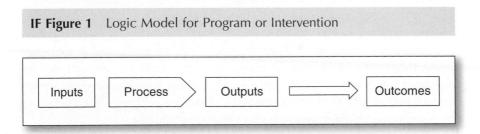

Costs are used to represent the flow of resources used over time to support a program or intervention. It is important to note that costs are not the same as expenditures because not every resource used will require a financial transaction (e.g., volunteer labor, donated inputs), and some financial transactions may be for resources that will have a longer useful life than the time period of interest (e.g., infrastructure). The implication of this is that no matter how tempting it may be, we cannot ask the program accountant to tell us how much a program costs.

The approach we use for costing is closely related to activity-based costing and follows a four-step process. The first step is to **identify** the resources being used in a program or intervention. These are typically what we see as inputs in IF Figure 1. When seeking to identify resources, it is often helpful to answer the following question: Who is doing what, with what supplies and equipment, and where are they doing this? A generic template to assist in the costing of a program or intervention can be found in IF Table 2.

The second step in costing is to **measure** the quantity of each resource used in its natural units over the time period of interest (e.g., hours of labor, units of supplies, pieces of equipment, square footage of physical space). By measuring resources in their natural units, we are able to introduce the flexibility to make resource substitutions (e.g., change a health worker for a nurse) or adjust the volume of resources required (e.g., change the amount of drugs used) without having to change input prices. Note that resource requirements refer to a specific time period (usually a year) but as this can change, it is important to state in your analysis what time period is being used.

The third step requires assigning a unit cost **value** to each identified resource. The appropriate unit cost will depend on the perspective used for the analysis. Typically we use a payer perspective, but sometimes we may be interested in costs from a donor or social perspective. The unit cost can vary with perspective, so it is important to state in your analysis which perspective you are using. Assigning a value to equipment, trainings, and infrastructure that have a useful life beyond the time period of interest requires that we compute the annualized value of these resources. The data required for this calculation include the expected useful life of a resource (measured in years) and a discount rate.[1] The typical discount rate used for analyses in developed countries is 3%. For developing countries, you can use the return rate on recent Treasury bill sales usually reported on the Internet by that country's Central Bank. It is important to document where your unit cost values are coming from so others can evaluate their appropriateness if they wish to review your results.

The final step in the cost estimation is to multiply the quantity of each resource used by its associated unit cost and then **aggregate** across all resources to obtain an estimated annualized total cost for the program or intervention. The value of resources required to support a program or intervention can then be compared to the expected impact or outcome of the program or intervention (last box in IF Figure 1) to assess the relative cost-effectiveness of the program (Gold, Siegel, Russell, & Weinstein, 1996). This information on the value of resources required and expected outcomes for a program or intervention is useful when trying to choose between alternative uses for scarce resources. It is important to note that just because an intervention is judged to be cost-effective, this in no way guarantees that it is affordable.

As implied above, the value of resources being used to support a program or intervention is not the same as the financial investment required to support the program or intervention. If the goal is to assess the affordability of a program or intervention, then we need to adjust the estimate to reflect the time in which the costs are incurred. Specifically, we would no longer annualize investments such as trainings, equipment purchases, or infrastructure improvements. Rather, we would use their full cost in the valuation step. Often it is useful to provide two data points on the costs required to support a program or intervention. The first estimate is typically for the first year of operation, which would include the full cost of training workers in new skills or bringing in a new cadre of workers, equipment, and capital investments (e.g., buildings, vehicles) as well as the costs of service provision in that first year. In addition to this estimate, an estimate for subsequent program years in which the capital and up-front investments are no longer required is useful. This information can then be used by the decision maker to decide whether this program is affordable given the resources available. This presentation can also help with resource mobilization as a donor can see how an investment may pay off over time.

IF Table 2 Generic Template to Assist in Costing of Program or Intervention

Resources Used by Type (a)	Quantity Used per Year (b)	Quantity Metric (c)	Cost per Unit (d)	Total Annual Cost (e) = (b) x (d)
Labor				
List by cadre		Person hours		
Subtotal				
Supplies[1]				
List by item		Units		
Subtotal				
Equipment[2]				
List by item		Piece		
Subtotal				
Infrastructure				
Buildings/space		Square footage		
Utilities		Actual cost or % of building cost		
Subtotal				
Consultants				
List by purpose		Person days		
Subtotal				
Trainings/ meetings/ special events				
List each type by purpose		Event		
Subtotal				
Total				

[1] Supplies with a monthly cost of < $50 are not worth tracking in most cost exercises.

[2] Equipment includes items with an expected useful life of > 1 year. Only include equipment with a unit cost of > $100.

Summary

This is a very basic overview of some of the key elements in a cost analysis. Before undertaking a cost analysis, it is critical to understand what question you are trying to answer, who the audience for the information is, and how that will impact the valuation of resources and presentation of your analysis results (Drummond, Sculpher, Torrance, O'Brien, & Stoddart, 2005). Ideally you will be able to work closely with the program implementers to gain a complete understanding of how resources are being used and the outputs and outcomes associated with a program as you work through the analysis to ensure the results you generate are accurate and a true reflection of the program.

Additional Resource

UNAIDS. (2011). *Manual for costing HIV facilities and services.* Geneva, Switzerland: Author. Retrieved from http://www.unaids.org/en/media/unaids/contentassets/documents/document/2011/20110523_manual_costing_HIV_facilities_en.pdf

References

Drummond, M. F., Sculpher, M. J., Torrance, G. W., O'Brien, B. J., & Stoddart, G. L. (2005). *Methods for the economic evaluation of health care programmes* (3rd ed.). Oxford, UK: Oxford University Press.

Gold, M. R., Siegel, J. E., Russell, L. B., & Weinstein, M. C. (1996). *Cost-effectiveness in health and medicine.* New York, NY: Oxford University Press.

Note

1. For example, if we have a piece of equipment that costs $10,000 to acquire new today, and the equipment is expected to last 15 years, then using a 3% discount rate, the annualized cost of the equipment would be computed as: Annualized Cost = Cost Today * $(r / (1 - ((1 + r)^{-n})))$ where r is the discount rate and n is the number of years. In our example, annualized cost = $10,000 * (.03 / (1 - ((1 + .03)^{-15})))$ or $10,000 * 0.083767 = 837.67. Note that if we multiply this figure by expected life (15 years) we obtain $12,565, and the excess represents the time value of money tied up in the equipment that is not available for other uses.

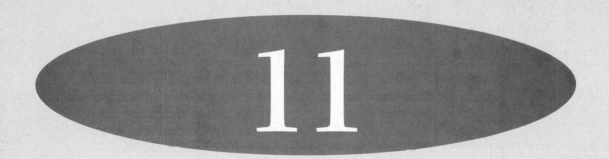

Health Services Research

Heidi W. Reynolds

In the last chapter, we saw how health economics contributes to public health by offering approaches to examine issues of efficiency and cost-benefit analyses in the context of health, healthcare, and health policy. Health services research (HSR) can include elements of health economics, but it looks at broader operational questions about how services are organized, financed, and delivered, and addresses the supply, demand, and quality of health services (Colby, 2008; Field, Tranquada, & Feasley, 1995). An oft-cited definition of health services research is from Lohr and Steinwachs (2002, p. 16): HSR is a "multidisciplinary field of scientific investigation that studies how social factors, financing systems, organizational structures and processes, health technologies and personal behaviors affect access to health care, the quality and cost of health care, and ultimately our health and well-being." In other words, HSR is multidisciplinary and applied. It studies the effects of costs, quality, accessibility, planning, delivery, distribution, organization, provision, and financing of health care services on health care outcomes (Institute of Medicine, 1995; Shi, 2008).

A BRIEF HISTORY

HSR is a young field relative to other disciplines, but by the 1960s the term and practice were in wide use. Many authors point to the establishment of Medicare and Medicaid in 1965 and the increasing involvement of the federal government in the financing, provision, regulation, and planning of health care services as events that established HSR as an academic discipline in its own right (Colby, 2008; Colby & Baker, 2009; Shi, 2008). The increasing cost of health care in the United States since the late 1960s (Figure 11.1) underscored the need for research to understand factors driving up costs and to identify solutions to contain costs with new payment methods (Colby & Baker, 2009). The most recent major policy in health care reform, the Patient Protection and Affordable Care Act (P.L. 111-148), passed in March 2010, introduces a whole new set of questions for health service researchers about how to translate the policy into effective programs.

Figure 11.1   Total Expenditure on Health as a Percentage of Gross Domestic Product in the United States From 1960–2010

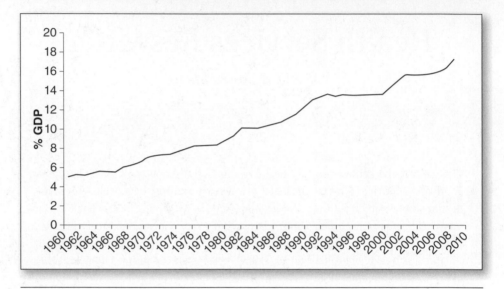

Source: Organization for Economic Co-operation and Development (2013).

GLOBAL CONTEXT

Of course, the benefits of HSR extend well beyond the United States and its unique health care system. People in all countries need basic primary care services such as maternal and child health care, and as more countries move through the epidemiological transition, chronic health problems such as cancer and cardiovascular diseases increase. Similarly, protection from the financial risks associated with seeking and paying for health care is a major global issue. Global health and health care also have political implications. Poverty and disease can destabilize countries and entire regions, and on the other hand, improving health indicators have many positive externalities such as improving women's access to education, participation in political leadership, and positive effects on the environment (Ross & Lurie, 2004). A global perspective within HSR means that challenges, methods, tools, and research findings can be shared internationally so that solutions to improving public health can be found more efficiently.

BENEFICIARIES OF HEALTH SERVICES RESEARCH (HSR)

Just as HSR can be applied to local, national, or international health issues, it varies too in its focus on actors and level of decision making (E.H. Bradley et al., 2011). The audience for the results of HSR can be the individual health consumer or patient, care providers, communities, employers or payers of health care coverage, professional societies engaged in guideline development or recommendations, or the government and regulatory agencies engaged in policymaking (Eden, Wheatley, McNeil, & Sox, 2008). HSR results can be used by these groups to inform their choice of health care and insurance plans, their health behaviors, their provision of care, their coverage and financing of care and procedures, and/or their policies and guidelines.

THE INTERDISCIPLINARY NATURE OF HSR

To address varied objectives for a range of audiences, HSR draws on a number of different disciplinary perspectives to address health services problems and is not defined by any one discipline or disease (Agency for Healthcare Research and Quality, 2009; E. H. Bradley et al., 2011; Ricketts, 2009). The disciplines more commonly involved in HSR are depicted in Figure 11.2 and described below.

Figure 11.2   Disciplinary Perspectives Used in Health Services Research

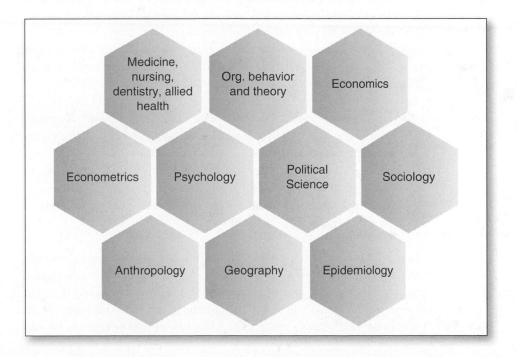

- Medicine, nursing, dentistry, and allied health (Agency for Healthcare Research and Quality [AHRQ], 2009), often serve as the disciplines from which health care questions arise, although the actual provision of care and the clinical trials of drugs and procedures fall outside the scope of HSR.
- Organizational behavior and theory addresses both the dynamics in the organization, such as staff functioning, and between organizations and how different organizations interact with each other and their environment (E. H. Bradley et al., 2011).
- Economics brings perspectives on provider payments and incentives, market regulation, and competition. Economists have tools for modeling policy choices and tradeoffs and models of decision making (E. H. Bradley et al., 2011).

  ○ Econometrics is housed within economics and refers to the study of empirical economic problems and using statistical techniques to solve them (Kennedy, 1998). Often economic questions do not lend themselves to randomization or controlled experiments, so econometrics tackles the challenges posed by the violations to traditional statistical assumptions. Thus, econometrics are increasingly important to health service researchers as much of HSR cannot be experimentally controlled, but still needs to yield unbiased and reliable results.

- Psychology provides insights into human motivation and theories of health behaviors (E. H. Bradley et al., 2011).
- Political science addresses the political side of health care policies and governance (E. H. Bradley et al., 2011).
- Sociology is concerned with social and community structures that influence health behaviors of patients, providers, and organizations. Social network theory (see Chapter 14) is a specific subset of sociology that contributes to understanding how social and organizational networks influence behavior patterns, power, and distribution of health information and services (E. H. Bradley et al., 2011).
- Anthropology addresses the cultural contexts in which service delivery takes place and provides an understanding of the social reality of patients (E. H. Bradley et al., 2011).
- Geography is also highly interdisciplinary, but it brings a spatial perspective to the social, cultural, political, and environmental aspects of health (Dummer, 2008). Understanding the physical location of health services relative to the population and their health needs is an important aspect of HSR.
- Epidemiology and biostatistics are the basic sciences of public health. Epidemiology studies groups of people, not individuals, to understand the determinants and distribution of disease. Biostatistics is the application of methods to analyze data (Hebel & McCarter, 2006).

Different disciplines have different ways of approaching scientific study (Aboelela et al., 2007). For the physical and social sciences, a positivist or postpositivist method of inquiry is typical, where research is hypothesis driven and understanding is gained through experimentation (Robson, 2011). The humanities disciplines often use critical theory or constructivist methods of study where reality is defined by experiencing and observing it through either real time or history; study within these fields is usually not hypothesis driven. The interdisciplinary nature of HSR therefore puts this full range of theories and methods at researchers' disposal, to look at the issues outlined in the definition of HSR, including

- the organizing and financing of health services,
- access to health care,
- quality of care,
- behavior of providers and patients,
- clinical evaluation and outcomes research, and
- informatics in measurement and decision making (Field et al., 1995).

In the remainder of this chapter, we discuss each of these research areas in more detail, review the tools and techniques used to study those concepts, and offer guidance on how to implement HSR.

CONTRIBUTIONS OF HSR TO PUBLIC HEALTH

Organizing and Financing of Health Services

This area of research looks at the relationships among costs, charges, health insurance, and organization of care (Field et al., 1995; Thaul, Lohr, & Tranquada, 1994). Also included here are studies of the effects of health insurance structures, like the move from fee-for-service to managed care and market-based strategies to control health care costs (Shi, 2008). A primary—and complex—research question for HSR is how to integrate the structures of funding, administration, and clinical and organizational service delivery to improve access to and quality of care and to gain efficiencies (Kodner, 2009). Another question is whether and how public-private (or government-commercial) partnerships can control costs and build partnership capacity while maximizing individual and community health outcomes (Bagnell Stuart, Thornton Walker, & Minzner, 2011).

In the United States, the hot topic for research on the organization and financing of health services is the design of health insurance. When people have health insurance, they pay fees to a company that pools these funds across all people who have paid in to the plan (Knickman, 2011). A minority of people will need costly health care, and a majority of people are healthy and will use little care. The pooling of funds enabled by insurance coverage allows the amount that an individual has to pay to be constant and predictable, even though her or his actual health care expenses may vary widely from year to year.

There are many types of insurance, and insurance coverage in the United States has evolved to be largely employer based and of voluntary participation (Capretta & Miller, 2010), though some public funding provides coverage to the elderly and the poor through Medicare and Medicaid (Schoen et al., 2010). The U.S. health insurance structure poses risks to continuing insurance coverage when employment status changes (Baicker, 2008;

Capretta & Miller, 2010), because if a person loses or changes jobs she or he risks losing health insurance. The most recent estimates from the U.S. Census Bureau (2012) show that in 2011, 15.7% (48.6 million) of Americans were without health insurance.

Because the U.S. health insurance system has historically been voluntary, an individual can decide whether to obtain health insurance. One of the risks is that people, especially healthy people, will decide not to buy health insurance, thereby creating insurance pools that have a disproportionate share of sick or high risk people (Parmet, 2011). The system has had checks in place to avoid this "adverse selection," that is, the practice of buying insurance only when you are sick (Capretta & Miller, 2010). These checks include denial of coverage for people with preexisting conditions or setting insurance premiums based on an individual's health status ("underwriting"; Capretta & Miller, 2010). Thus, the number of uninsured includes healthy people who choose not to buy health insurance and people who want health insurance but are excluded due to preexisting conditions or because they cannot afford it. The Patient Protection and Affordable Care Act (ACA) will begin to change that (see box below).

THE U.S. PATIENT PROTECTION AND AFFORDABLE CARE ACT

The Patient Protection and Affordable Care Act (ACA), passed in 2010, is a landmark event in health care reform and is designed to enable uninsured citizens to obtain health insurance. The "insurance mandate," which requires all citizens to enroll in a plan or face a financial penalty each year, is one of the implementation strategies of the ACA. Similarly, employers with 51 or more employees must provide coverage or face fines. Another strategy is for states to expand Medicaid by lowering the eligibility requirements and by creating new "insurance exchanges" to enable low-income families not eligible for Medicaid to purchase subsidized private insurance (Knickman, 2011). The Affordable Care Act also requires that insurance companies offer insurance to all people, including those with preexisting conditions, and prohibits lifetime limits on coverage. Finally, the law provides for adults up to age 26 to be covered under their parents' plan.

The individual insurance mandate is intended to increase the number of healthy people who enroll in health insurance, balancing out the sick people who will join the pool when the provisions go into effect—including people with preexisting conditions or who join the insurance exchanges (Parmet, 2011). The Affordable Care Act in general, and the individual mandate specifically, have sparked fierce debates in the United States. Some argue that the mandate will fail to broaden risk pools because the financial penalty is too low (i.e., some people—and more likely healthy people—will choose to pay the penalty rather than enroll in health insurance). Others argue against the mandate not on public health grounds, but on its constitutionality. In June 2012, the Supreme Court ruled to uphold the constitutionality of the ACA, arguing, surprisingly to many, Congress's right to collect taxes (Jost, 2012). The Court did not uphold the expansion of Medicaid, however, deeming it unconstitutional to make states expand Medicaid under the threat of losing existing Medicaid funding because it was coercive.

Over the next decade, health services researchers will be investigating to what extent the ACA increased the number of people with health insurance, whether overall health indicators improved, and whether health care costs are contained. The ACA also has provisions for studies of payment policy reforms such as bundled payments, improved information technology and increased use of electronic medical records, and comparative effectiveness research to identify less costly treatment strategies (Billings, Cantor, & Clinton, 2011).

Similarly, in the international arena, it is a priority to find mechanisms to protect people from financial hardship when they seek care. The World Health Organization (WHO; 2012a) estimates that 100 million people are pushed into poverty each year as a result of health care expenses that they pay for out of pocket. This raises questions, particularly for developing countries, about how to move from out-of-pocket payments to pre-payment financing mechanisms with pooled risk, and how to identify those mechanisms that are also equitable and efficient. Accompanying questions include how to improve methods for measuring and analyzing the benefits and costs of health financing practices, revenue collection, pooling, and provision or purchasing of services (WHO, 2005). For example, in Ghana, South Africa, and Tanzania, the public health sector has an important role in the provision of services, but there are inequities based on geography. Ghana and Tanzania have adopted health insurance schemes, but large portions of the workforce are in the informal sectors. Questions remain about how to extend coverage to those individuals (Mills, Ally, Goudge, Gyapong, & Mtei, 2012).

Access to Health Care

In order for an individual to have access to care, services must be available and there must be enough of those services available to meet demand. Availability is defined as "the physical availability of a specified range of health care services, health infrastructure, health service workforce, medical goods and products, and the timely provision of affordable and adequate services" (Scheil-Adlung & Bonnet, 2011, pp. 23–24). But availability of services is only one aspect of access to care. Clients may not be able to access available services due to a variety of barriers such as inability to pay for care; problems with the organization of care that affect clients' ability to navigate or gain access to care; lack of transport or other logistical supports; lack of culturally appropriate care and fear of mistreatment, stigma, or discrimination; or lack of individual readiness, perceived susceptibility, or knowledge of service availability (Rosenstock, 2005). Thus, the concept of access to care is a composite of making care available and offering care that is also affordable, physically accessible, acceptable, timely, and appropriate (Gulliford et al., 2002; Figure 11.3). This theme includes the study of cultural, organizational, and financial barriers to accessing care in order to find solutions to overcome the barriers.

An individual's access to health care requires three steps: (1) enter into the health system, (2) get to sites where health care services are available, and (3) find providers who meet patients' needs (AHRQ, 2012). In the United States, people from racial and ethnic minorities or of low socioeconomic status face more challenges accessing health care at all steps along the way. Some of these disparities can be traced to the fact that minorities and the poor are less likely to have health insurance or go longer times without health insurance (AHRQ, 2012). They are less likely to have access to a usual source of care (e.g., a provider or facility where one regularly receives care) or a primary care provider (AHRQ, 2012). However, there is recognition that these disparities exist even after taking into account health insurance and other co-factors, because the disparities are based in broader historical and social inequality (Nelson, 2002). To promote more equitable access to health care, the Institute of Medicine (IOM) has recommended strategies such as the use of evidence-based guidelines, more equitable payment systems, improved communication and trust between providers and patients, use of financial incentives to reduce barriers, use of language interpretation services, and use of community-based health workers (Nelson, 2002). Each of these strategies poses questions for health services researchers to examine.

Figure 11.3 Illustration of the Concept of Access to Care

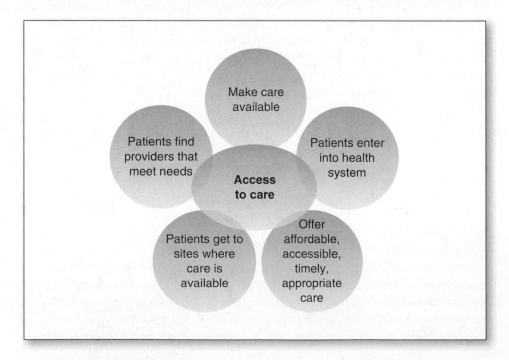

Quality of Care

IOM's (1991) definition of quality of care refers to health services that improve health outcomes and are consistent with the most current medical evidence. There are two elements central to quality of care (Donabedian, 1988): One is the health care provider's technical performance in terms of knowledge of medical strategies and judgment to implement those strategies. The other element is the provider's ability to manage the interpersonal interaction with the client, particularly communicating information about diagnoses and treatment. Assessments of quality of care focus on

- the structure or setting in which care occurs, such as the health facility, equipment, human resources, and administrative procedures and organization;
- the process of giving (the provider's role) and receiving (the client's role) care; and
- the effect of that care on health outcomes (Donabedian, 1988).

Health outcomes include both the clinical measures of disease and clients' reports of health status and satisfaction with health services (Steinwachs & Hughes, 2008).

Quality of care has been a central focus of international family planning programs for decades. Family planning programs in the 1970s and 1980s were characterized by a focus on curbing population growth, and attention was focused on achieving goals and targets for contraceptive use. In worst cases, this led to coercive practices and violations of women's rights. The focus shifted to the quality of family planning programs following calls for those programs to emphasize clients' health, needs, and rights over meeting targets (Seltzer, 2002). The International Conference on Population and Development in 1994 emphasized women's rights to reproductive autonomy. In the United States specifically, the Tihart Amendment in 1998 emphasized voluntary and informed contraceptive choice (Seltzer, 2002). Today, all international family planning programs are grounded in the six elements of quality of care defined in the Bruce framework from 1990: (1) provide a wide range of methods, (2) provide information about the methods to inform clients' choice, (3) ensure providers' clinical and technical competence, (4) promote a private and confidential relationship between providers and clients, (5) ensure mechanisms to encourage continuity of method use, and (6) ensure that services are convenient and acceptable to clients (Bruce, 1990).

Quality of care is a central focus in HSR; thus, there exist numerous standardized questionnaires for measuring it. Internationally, the Service Provision Assessments (SPA) measure service availability, readiness, compliance with standards of care, and provider and client satisfaction (MEASURE DHS, n.d.), and the content is consistent with international service readiness indicators (WHO, 2012b). In the United States, there is an entire National Quality Forum (NQF) that receives funds from private and public sources. Since 2009, the NQF worked with the Department of Health and Human Services to develop quality and efficiency measures. One standardized survey endorsed by the NQF is the Hospital Care Quality Information from the Consumer Perspective Survey (HCACPS or CAHPS Hospital Survey) for measuring patients' perspectives on hospital care.

Behavior of Providers and Patients

HSR is concerned with understanding the factors that affect patient health behaviors such as seeking care for prevention or when ill, engaging in preventive behaviors, and ensuring adherence to treatment and therapy. Deeper understanding of these issues can be translated into strategies to improve care. Rosenstock argues that, for preventive behavior, an individual will not take action until he or she is psychologically ready to take action, which is related to how susceptible the person feels to getting the condition and the perceived seriousness of its consequences (Rosenstock, 2005; see the Appendix in this volume for more on this theory). The person also has to believe that the preventive action (e.g., test, behavior) is feasible and appropriate and would reduce his or her susceptibility or severity. Finally, an internal (e.g., perceived change in the body) or external (e.g., advertisement, interpersonal interaction) cue or trigger is necessary in order to initiate the behavior. Understanding behaviors are important to inform and tailor education and awareness campaign messages and efforts.

Because of the face-to-face contact providers have with patients, providers can be important motivators of clients' behaviors. Providers' delivery of care for their clients is influenced by the environment in which they work, their professional training, and their socialization and underlying sensitivities or biases toward clients (Thaul et al., 1994). HSR seeks to understand the factors that influence provider decisions related to care and to study the effect of interventions to improve the care given by providers.

Pay-for-performance (P4P) is an intervention that aims to incentivize providers to improve care practices. Under the Affordable Care Act, P4P strategies feature prominently. P4P seeks to reimburse providers based on achievement of certain specified outcomes (e.g., quality, cost), rather than just on services rendered (Trisolini, 2011). P4P is a young field and is still evolving. The theory of P4P is that it will improve quality in general, while also reducing some of the inequities in quality observed in the United States by region and across similar types of providers (Trisolini, 2011). Interventions vary widely based on the type of pay incentive, the type of provider targeted for care, and the performance outcome measure of interest to change (Van Herck et al., 2010). The effect of pay-for-performance interventions has been examined on clinical effectiveness, access and equity of care, coordination and continuity of care, patient centeredness, and cost-effectiveness. Studies have found that successful interventions tend to have more influences on process (e.g., appropriate tests or drugs administered) than outcome (e.g., death, quality of life, satisfaction) variables, that successful interventions tend to promote purely positive financial incentives rather than competitive ones (where someone wins or loses), and that successful interventions tend to be targeted at the individual or team rather than a bigger group (e.g., a hospital; Van Herck et al., 2010). Many research gaps remain.

Clinical Evaluation and Outcomes Research

While clinical trials of drug and intervention efficacy fall outside the HSR domain (see Chapter 8), clinical evaluation and outcomes research examine the effectiveness of drugs and interventions in applied settings—or how they improve health status within the context of "typical use"—in order to inform clinical practice guidelines and policy. Often HSR is engaged in understanding the comparative effectiveness of different interventions and their acceptability and interest to patients and providers. HSR also develops methods for assessing health outcomes in order to compare health outcomes across studies. Comparative effectiveness studies seek to understand the relative effectiveness of different treatments, taking into account patient characteristics (Steinwachs & Hughes, 2008).

Comparative effectiveness research (CER) has many vocal supporters and critics. The IOM was mandated by Congress in 2009 through the American Recovery and Reinvestment Act (ARRA; P.L. 111-5), to compile a list of the most pressing CER questions. According to the legislation, CER covers "research that compares the clinical outcomes, effectiveness, and appropriateness of items, services, and procedures that are used to prevent, diagnose, or treat diseases, disorders, and other health conditions" (IOM, 2009, p. 1). The group prioritized 100 topics, the largest number of which focused on the health care delivery system and increasing the effectiveness of care, rather than on a particular disease area (Iglehart, 2009). The second and third most common priorities to be addressed were racial and ethnic disparities and patients' functional limitations and disabilities, respectively. CER is championed as an evidence-based approach for identifying efficiencies in the health care system; that is, places where the system can spend less if less expensive interventions and treatments are at least as effectives as more costly ones (Henry J. Kaiser Family Foundation, 2009). Critics contend that CER will not sufficiently consider individual differences and that it represents rationing of access to expensive but effective therapies and government intrusion into the patient-provider relationship (Iglehart, 2009; Rich, 2009).

In 2010, the Affordable Care Act also touched CER, essentially renaming it "patient-centered outcomes research" (PCOR). This move reflects an increasing interest in measuring outcomes of health care in terms of the patient's perspective (Wu, Snyder, Clancy, & Steinwachs, 2010). Traditionally, outcomes have been measured from a clinical perspective (e.g., physiological measures such as blood pressure, events such as death). Patient reports add the patient perspective to health care and can provide insight into patients' experiences of physical functioning such as pain or ability to walk, social and role function such as being able to dress oneself or carry a child, and psychological health such as depression (Wu et al., 2010). Patients can also report on their symptoms, their satisfaction with care, their use of care services, and their health behaviors, all of which can inform treatment and care options. The patient perspective is important too because patients might be required to make decisions about their treatments and care that have tradeoffs in terms of survival, pain experience, or physical function (Clancy & Eisenberg, 1998). Current HSR is focusing on how to best measure patients' perspectives, along with increasing use of patient outcome measures in clinical studies.

Informatics in Measurement and Decision Making

Informatics is receiving attention for its role as a strategy to make information more readily available in a way that is user-friendly but protective of sensitive information.

Informatics refers to computer-based information systems, whether static or mobile, used for a variety of purposes, including

- To run clinical decision support tools such as electronic medical records and tools that use data to calculate risk factors or alternative treatment strategies,
- To facilitate prescribing and reduce drug interactions,
- To remind providers or patients to follow up or make appointments,
- To link computer-based records across databases for analyses or to link medical records with clinical measurements to facilitate diagnosis, and
- To share and disseminate best practices in the medical evidence to providers and the general public (C. J. Bradley, Penberthy, Devers, & Holden, 2010; Lovell & Celler, 1999).

Additionally, a review of information communication technologies (ICT) in developing countries found that programs were using ICT for the following purposes:

- To combat health care worker shortages by extending geographic coverage and limiting the distance between provider and patients through telemedicine (e.g., videoconference, helplines, instant messaging)
- To facilitate communication with patients outside regular clinic visits, including providing health education and encouraging compliance
- To enable less skilled workers to improve diagnosis and treatment through real-time assistance from other skilled providers
- To improve data management through data collection with mobile devices and share data remotely for analysis
- To facilitate financial transactions to pay for care
- To prevent fraud and abuse by being able to verify products, identities, and transactions (Lewis, Synowiec, Lagomarsino, & Schweitzer, 2012)

The review found that phones, followed by computers, were by far the most popular type of devices. As the technologies develop, so do the challenges and questions about how to protect the confidentiality of health information and avoid the misuse of that information.

PROGRAM INPUTS, OUTCOMES, EFFICACY, AND EFFECTIVENESS

As you think about how to design and conduct HSR, you will need to understand some key terms that apply to many types of research, but that are particularly relevant to HSR. Across the areas of study outlined above, the field of HSR is interested in understanding the effect of program inputs (e.g., finances, personnel, equipment and supplies, policies and guidelines) on direct program outputs, intermediate effects, and ultimate effects (Veney & Kaluzny, 1998). **Direct outputs** are the items produced by the program and are the combination of its inputs. Outputs can usually be quantified, and in health care they may be the number of specific tests, immunizations, contraceptive methods, screenings, or so forth provided. **Intermediate effects** (or intermediate outcomes) follow from the direct outputs. They are the result of the outputs, such as a proportion of a population reached with a test, immunization, or method. For example, in a malaria program, insecticide-treated bed nets may be distributed to prevent malaria transmission. The number of nets distributed is the direct output, while the intermediate effect or outcome is the proportion of children under 5 years old who slept under a net the previous night. **Ultimate effects** (long-term outcomes or impact) are the definitive effects the program is trying to achieve, such as improved health status, equity, and quality of life and reduced rates of disease and death. In the malaria example, the ultimate effect may be reduced proportion of deaths attributed to malaria among children under 5. Figure 11.4 shows the linear relationship between program inputs, outputs, and effects.

Figure 11.4   Relationship Between Program Inputs, Outputs, and Effects

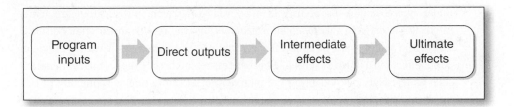

Health services research studies are often conducted to understand whether a health services intervention has an effect on a predetermined outcome. **Health outcomes** broadly include clinical measures of disease, patient-reported health and functioning, patient-reported satisfaction with services or quality of life, and health service costs (Steinwachs & Hughes, 2008). Health service researchers might also be interested to know if the program or intervention was implemented as designed (**program monitoring**) and use that information to make program improvements. Then they might move on to assessing whether the program achieved its desired outputs and intermediate and ultimate effects.

During the research design process (see Chapter 2), health services researchers identify a **primary outcome** of interest and its associated measure. In clinical trials (Chapter 8), a primary outcome is that end point which represents the greatest therapeutic benefit of the drug or therapy being tested (Sedgwick, 2010). While health service researchers are not conducting randomized controlled drug trials, they are still trying to identify the end point variable that is expected to change the most given the theoretical effect of the program or intervention being tested. In choosing a primary outcome, there are also pragmatic considerations of what is feasible to measure given the funding, logistic, and ethical parameters.

Researchers usually identify other outcomes that they also expect to be influenced by the program or intervention. These are called **secondary outcomes**. For example, in a study of the effectiveness of care for HIV-exposed infants in an integrated care model or a referral model, the primary outcome was rates of care attendance (in other words a measure of loss-to-follow-up; Ong'ech et al., 2012). The secondary outcome was receipt of immunization at 14 weeks. The variables of interest for secondary outcomes may range widely from clinical measures of health and reports of patient health, functioning, or satisfaction, to other measures such as side effects or unanticipated effects.

The concepts of efficacy and effectiveness are program characteristics important for HSR because they address the relationship between intervention resource inputs and their effect on outcomes. **Efficacy research** is interested in understanding the expected benefit of a drug, procedure, or other intervention under ideal conditions of use. Its goal is to achieve high internal validity so that researchers have confidence that the independent variables (e.g., the use of the drug, intervention, or technology) resulted in changes in the outcome of interest (e.g., health status), rather than other factors. This means that researchers control as much as possible the procedures and environment, and subjects are randomly assigned into a treatment or control group.

Effectiveness research is also interested in testing a drug, procedure, or other intervention, but the goal is to understand the expected benefit of the intervention under typical conditions of use. In effectiveness research, investigators are more interested in external validity, or how generalizable the results are to other settings. Would the same results be found if the study was conducted again with a different population or in a different setting? Effectiveness research is also concerned with issues such as feasibility of conducting the intervention in the setting, acceptability of the intervention to the beneficiaries, and assurance that the intervention can continue after the study is finished if it has been found to be beneficial (Hohmann & Shear, 2002).

Oftentimes, intervention effectiveness will vary compared with what was found in the clinical setting. In the typical setting, intervention effectiveness is influenced by factors that normally are controlled in the clinical setting, factors such as the patient's underlying health, behaviors, adherence, or demographics or the setting of the intervention, such as the care setting, providers' skills and training, and timing (Eden et al., 2008).

Effectiveness research is also concerned with identifying the correct study population. In other words, the research aims to determine whether the population targeted for the intervention is the population that is most likely to benefit from the intervention and is the population that is most likely to receive the intervention on scale-up. Complementary considerations include the available care setting, availability and training of providers, and how other factors associated with how care is delivered might influence the interventions. Finally, it is important to consider that the outcomes measured will yield the most useful information about the intervention effect.

These considerations translate into questions to consider when planning an effectiveness study (Hohmann & Shear, 2002): Who should be in the study? What is the appropriate sample size needed? What population characteristics need to be documented, such as sex, age, ethnicity, socioeconomic status, or health status? What are the appropriate outcomes to be measured? What are the proximate factors to study, factors that work to influence the ultimate outcomes?

DATA COLLECTION METHODS IN HSR

Health services research involves observation, hypothesis formulation, experimentation, and modification and retesting of hypotheses. Many of the steps in the process of developing a HSR project are found in Chapter 2. These steps include problem identification, research question development, using theory and conceptual models, reviewing the literature, study designs, sampling, data collection methods, data management and analysis, and communicating results.

Other chapters in this book cover data collection methods that are commonly used in HSR, particularly randomized control trials (Chapter 8), using secondary data (Chapter 9), health economics (Chapter 10), surveys (Chapter 12), and qualitative methods (Chapter 15). Therefore, this section touches on some data collection methods that are not addressed elsewhere, including mystery client or simulated client methods, methods to measure staff time, and service provision assessments.

Mystery Client or Simulated Client Methods

Mystery client or simulated client methods (SCM) have been used to study quality of care and interactions with providers and staff. They are also called "mystery shoppers" in the pharmaceutical literature (Watson, Norris, & Granas, 2006). Mystery clients (MCs) or simulated clients are "trained people (usually community members) who visit program facilities in the assumed roles of clients, and then report (by completing a survey or through an interview) on their experience" (Boyce & Neale, 2006, p. 3). The approach can rely on MCs who are actually affected by the illness for which they are seeking treatment or who are interested in receiving care (Madden, Quick, Ross-Degnan, & Kafle, 1997). The other approach is to rely on MCs who are trained to act in a certain way when they are using care or to have them pretend they are seeking care on behalf of a friend or family member. In these situations there is usually a predetermined scenario or story that the MC follows. This has the advantage of standardizing the data collection, but also helps the MC appear more natural in his or her role (because he or she will not have to come up with fictional symptoms or responses on the spot).

The simulated or mystery client methods are more covert than other data collection techniques. They have the advantage over staged methods (e.g., the use of role play or vignettes which test providers' knowledge and behavior in simulated scenarios) of engendering the providers' natural responses, since they do not know they're being observed. Although informed consent may be obtained from a clinic manager who gives permission for the study to take place over some period of time (but who does not know who the MCs are), clinic staff may feel deceived. Ethical review of studies using SCM is imperative, and committees will thoroughly review the proposed procedures for recruiting and training MCs, for conducting observations, and for consent and provider protection provisions.

A review of the use of simulated clients in pharmacy practice found that the method could be used to assess provision of counseling and advice, treatment of major and minor illnesses, and health activities of pharmacy and drug store staff (Watson et al., 2006). In one example, SCM was used to study retail drug shops to determine whether drugs were dispensed with a prescription and to assess the drugs and advice provided (Madden et al., 1997). SCM has also been used in studies of family planning services in developing countries to understand the quality of care offered by staff (Madden et al., 1997). Table 11.1 lists the advantages and disadvantages of this method.

Table 11.1 Advantages and Disadvantages of the Simulated Client Method

Advantages	Disadvantages
• Record unselfconscious provider behavior from the client's perspective, thus avoiding bias • Measure actual provider behavior and practices • Useful for assessing and improving quality of services • Can gather enough observations even if the actual volume of clients is low • Practical	• Involves misrepresentation • Recruitment may be difficult in small communities where the mystery client may be recognized by the staff • Dependent on mystery client recall • Needs methods to increase reliability between mystery clients, such as thorough training, clear criteria on rating, or mystery client providing explanations for ratings • Difficult to generalize to health problems or symptoms outside the mystery client scenarios

Source: Adapted from Boyce and Neale (2006); Madden et al. (1997).

The decision to use SCM is made in the same way that any other method is selected: if it is the most relevant and feasible method that will yield the information needed to answer the research questions. Similarly, the selection of clinics and providers and the number of observations are all determined by decisions made during the study design, sampling frame definition, and sample size calculations steps. The study protocol will describe the rationale for the design and method, including the data collection instrument, and be approved by one or more ethical review committee. Figure 11.5 details the steps for conducting mystery client interviews once those details are determined and permissions obtained (adapted from Boyce & Neale, 2006; more information is available on the web).

Figure 11.5 Process for Conducting Mystery Client Technique

Data collection instruments are developed
- With or without input from the mystery clients.
- Standardized data collection instruments help improve reliability.

Identify and recruit potential mystery clients
- Select with education level, sex, age, ethnic group, or other factors that may influence the quality of care in mind.
- Consider seeking variation in these variables among MC characteristics, or in keeping them consistent. Both have advantages/disadvantages.

Train mystery clients
- Provide an orientation to the overall study.
- Inform them of the role they will be playing.
- Provide stories and illnesses that mirror their real life, or prepare scenarios ahead of time that they are going to adopt.

Set clear rules about MC roles
- Include things like not revealing to anyone that they are an MC, not telling anyone their real name.
- Ask them to record the time they enter and leave the clinic, to collect educational materials, and observe or ask about what interventions they can and cannot receive (e.g., counseling on family planning methods but not undergoing a pelvic exam).

Role play and pilot test
- Provide an opportunity for MCs to practice their roles through role play or mock visits in pilot settings (clinics not involved in the real study).
- If there is an interviewer who debriefs the MC after the study, that person also takes part in the training, role play, and pilot.

Obtain informed consent, usually from the clinic manager
- Provide the rationale for the study, and associated informed consent description (risks and benefits).
- Do not provide a list of dates and times that the MC will be visiting.

Collect data
- MCs go to assigned clinics according to a pre-determined schedule.
- Typically MCs do not record data during the visit, but immediately after, out of view of the clinic and providers.
- Debrief with an interviewer (if applicable) as soon as possible after the visit to improve recall of events.

Analyze data and present results
- Include MCs in preliminary interpretation of results, since they were the eyes and ears who collected the data.

Source: Adapted from Boyce & Neale (2006).

Data from SCM may be quantitative, qualitative, or mixed. Quantitative results can be useful for understanding changes in quality and provider behavior before and after an intervention or between intervention and control groups. Results can be compared to standard operating procedures or other standards of care, or results can be assessed by experts (Madden et al., 1997). Qualitative results can be useful for a deeper understanding of behaviors and provide information about clinic operations and communication.

Because people who act as mystery clients have different strengths and the method relies on recall, reliability (where results are reproducible at different times or by different observers) and validity (data measure what they are actually supposed to measure) are issues of concern. As mentioned above, thorough training, standardized questionnaires, clear scenarios, and criteria and explanations for ratings can help to mitigate some of this concern. Other techniques such as audio or video recording or the use of two MCs at the same time to monitor behavior and cross-check results have been proposed to increase reliability and validity (Madden et al., 1997; Watson et al., 2006). On the other hand, it has been argued that what the client remembers or understands is equally, if not more, important because it may reflect the information that typical clients retain. Another recommendation is for studies to include detection methods to improve the facility validity of the simulated clients (Watson et al., 2006). In other words, providers who suspect that they have been visited by a simulated client have a mechanism to report this to the study team.

Methods to Measure Staff Time

Understanding how health personnel spend their day is important in HSR because it has implications for organizing health services in a way that optimizes costs without compromising quality of care provided to clients. In general there are four approaches to measuring staff time: (1) time motion study, (2) patient flow analysis, (3) provider interviews, and (4) self-administered time sheets (Bratt et al., 1999; see Table 11.2). Data on how providers use their time combined with information about staff costs (e.g., salaries and benefits obtained from other data collection methods) make it possible to calculate the average cost per unit of output, such as cost per medical test conducted. The information can be useful for program management to understand whether there is excess or under capacity of staff. Understanding the amount of "unproductive" time, or time not spent in client care or on administrative activities, can help program managers make better use of existing capacity and save costs. This information can be used in projections of resources to satisfy future demand, such as if a service is being scaled up and it is necessary to plan for staffing. Where resources are limited, criteria for selecting sites could be developed based on those that are thought to be operating at full capacity in order to define standards of contact and administrative time. These methods can also be applied before and after an intervention to see how providers' time use has changed.

Health Facility and Service Provision Assessments

Health services researchers often want to know what health care services are provided; the quality of those services; the infrastructure and resources available to provide services, including the physical space, availability of supplies and equipment, and staffing; and client and provider satisfaction with services and environment. Thus, a service provision assessment that observes the facility and includes provider and client interviews and other data collection methods is warranted. A well-known assessment

Table 11.2   Methods for Measuring Clinician Time Use

Method	Description	Pros	Cons
Time motion study	Measures the amount of time health personnel spend on various types of activities (e.g., contact with clients, administrative work, down time). Specially trained data collectors directly observe how staff spend their time. Observers records activities every 3 minutes using a precoded form.	Considered gold standard. Generates an accurate estimate of providers' time use. Yields information about what providers do during their shifts, including time not with clients.	Time and resource intensive. Require skilled observers. Presence of observer may distort provider behavior.
Patient flow analysis	Documents how patients flow through clinics and contact with providers and other personnel. Clients get precoded form to carry during visit. Staff record times of contacts and types of contact. For clients, measures total visit length, length of each contact, types of contact, and waiting time. For providers, measures time spent with clients.	Observational, does not rely on self-reporting by providers. Can consistently estimate client contact time compared with TM.	Does not record what providers do when they are not with clients. May underestimate providers' total shift time. May underestimate providers' nonproductive time.
Provider interviews	Interviews with staff at the end of each shift to understand time spent on specific activities. Routine program statistics can be used to help providers' recall activities. Providers estimate average duration of client contact.	Less resource intensive in terms of data collection, possibly less burden on providers.	Weakest method since it may underestimate nonproductive time and overestimate total shift time and time spent with clients.
Self-administered time sheets	Providers get a log book to record all activities during shift.	May consistently measure client contact time if contacts have discrete beginning and ending times.	May underestimate total shift time. May underestimate nonproductive time.

Source: Adapted from Bratt et al. (1999).

used in many developing countries to assess services for maternal and child health, HIV, malaria, tuberculosis, family planning, and treatment for sexually transmitted infections is the Service Provision Assessment (SPA; MEASURE DHS, n.d.). The SPA is a product of the MEASURE DHS project funded by the U.S. Agency for International Development and managed by IFC International. The questionnaires introduce an inventory to measure types of services available, staff coverage, infrastructure, communication, water and electricity sources, waste management, equipment processing, drugs, and laboratory capacity. There are also questionnaires for observing care consultations and conducting provider interviews and exit interviews with clients.

Patient interviews, provider interviews, patient-provider interaction observations, and patient records offer various advantages and disadvantages in HSR (see Table 11.3). The choice of method needs to be determined based on the study purpose and primary outcome measure, in addition to other factors such as study budgets, feasibility and logistics considerations, and ethical considerations.

Table 11.3 Advantages and Disadvantages of Interview and Observation Methods

Method	Advantages	Disadvantages
Patient interviews	• Provides patient perspective • Good level of agreement with observations (but depends on question)	• Courtesy bias • Recall bias • Clinic experiences (e.g., waiting time, stress, fatigue) or client characteristics (e.g., education) may affect reliability
Provider interviews	• Helpful to assess skills, knowledge, and attitudes, especially those that are not easily observed	• Not as reliable as observations
Patient provider interaction observations	• Good agreement with patient record	• Hawthorne effect (improved performance due to observation)
Patient records	• Provides information about treatment provided	• No patient perspective • May not indicate accuracy of diagnosis • May not indicate counseling content • May underreport patient provider encounters

Source: Adapted from Bessinger and Bertrand (2001); Franco, Franco, Kumwenda, and Nkhoma (2002).

Systematic Reviews and Meta-Analysis

Systematic reviews deserve mention in the context of HSR because often synthesis of the evidence makes a more powerful argument for changing policy and practice or for defining and prioritizing new areas for research than a single study or two on a topic (Gilson, 2012). Systematic reviews are different from literature reviews in that they comprehensively cover the available literature; assess the quality of the evidence; and use a transparent and explicit set of rules to search, include, and review the literature (Robson, 2011). The Cochrane Review, mentioned in Chapter 1, is a well-known source for systematic reviews of health care and health policies.[1]

Meta-analyses also systematically review and synthesize research studies, but they focus on summarizing the effect sizes of studies of the same or similar intervention on a standardized outcome (Bamberger, Rugh, & Mabry, 2012; Robson, 2011). Meta-analyses employ sophisticated statistical models to aggregate data across studies and reanalyze it. Some attempts have been made to conduct meta-analysis with qualitative data (Robson, 2011).

Systematic reviews can be used to change national U.S. policy and recommendations. These national-level changes affect what health insurance companies will cover and messages that providers convey to patients. In 2009, for example, U.S. guidelines for cervical and breast cancer screening and prevention were updated based on the results of systematic reviews of literature and modeling of screening strategies. Screening for cervical and breast cancer are some of the more common prevention interventions in the United States. In 2008, 76% of women 18 years and older had had a Papanicolaou (Pap) Test in the last 3 years and 67% of women over age 40 and 70% of women over age 50 had had a mammogram in the last 2 years (National Center for Health Statistics, 2010). The new guidelines suggest the need for less screening: The recommendations are for mammogram screening for breast cancer to start at age 50 and for cervical cancer screening by the Pap Test to be conducted every 3 years, if there have been three previous negative screens (Davisson, 2011). This sparked a major debate between politics and science, with some claiming that this was "rationing care" and others defending the need to balance benefit and harm (Davisson, 2011). Calls for doing less can be difficult to accept, especially when use of an established technology is at issue. There are economic considerations for those who make money on providing mammography and cervical examinations (Gusmano & Gray, 2010), and there were also political ramifications because of opposition to the Affordable Care Act. Controversies such as these create confusion for providers and clients. Insight into the public's understanding of the benefits of certain procedures are crucial to better inform the way the changes are communicated (and received).

Scaling Up

Scaling up a health service intervention has been characterized as the process of making health interventions available to more people (Yamey, 2011). While studies of clinical efficacy and research on effectiveness help refine and improve interventions with targeted samples of participants, scale-up is focused on expanding the implementation of an intervention to a wider population such as a state, district, or country.

Yamey (2011) has identified a number of factors that need to be present to facilitate the scale-up of interventions:

- The tool or service being scaled is relatively simple.
- The policies related to the intervention are informed by good science.
- There is strong leadership to support the intervention.
- There is support from local implementers and key stakeholders.
- There is careful consideration of the appropriate approach to scale up (e.g., using diffusion of innovation theory, cascade implementation).
- The community targeted for the intervention has favorable attitudes toward the intervention.
- A final important aspect is to use research to guide the scale-up process and help learn how to adapt the intervention to the setting.

While HSR is instrumental in identifying interventions that should be scaled, the methods and approaches used in HSR are also relevant as they provide information to inform and refine interventions as they are scaled up. Information from HSR studies inform clinical guidelines and standard operating procedures, identify at what level of the health system interventions should be delivered (e.g., hospital, facility, community), inform human resources training needs and numbers, identify requisite equipment and supplies, and detail intervention inputs and costs to inform planning for scale-up.

For instance, in developing countries with high HIV prevalence, clinical trials of adult male circumcision showed dramatic reductions in acquisition of HIV among men who were circumcised compared with those who were not (Bailey et al., 2007; Gray et al., 2007). Subsequent studies have suggested that adult male circumcision can reduce HIV risks to women and reduce risks of high-risk human papillomavirus and genital ulcer disease (WHO, 2010). In light of widespread international support to scale up male circumcision, studies have been conducted to estimate the costs and impact of scaling up male circumcision services in 14 countries. Scale-up is being facilitated by robust national leadership and the development of national policies, quality assurance systems, monitoring and evaluation systems, communication campaigns, and provider training initiatives (WHO, 2010).

HSR approaches and methods can also be used to answer questions about the scale-up of male circumcision interventions. Examples include research related to appropriate site and staffing models, studies of effectiveness and safety of task shifting (where a less educated medical professional performs similar duties as a more educated one, e.g., from a doctor to a nurse) to expand the number of providers who can implement the intervention, and studies of strategies to reach hard to reach populations (e.g., older men in the case of male circumcision) or other communities or cultures (Mwandi et al., 2011).

CURRENT ISSUES AND FUTURE DIRECTIONS

A number of current issues and recent policies and laws, in particular the Patient Protection and Affordable Care Act, have been peppered throughout this chapter and will shape HSR priorities for years to come. The Henry J. Kaiser Family Foundation maintains an interactive timeline showing the changes that have taken place and are intended to be implemented (see http://kff.org/interactive/implementation-timeline). HSR in the United States will continue to be concerned with how to control costs while maintaining and improving quality. Patient-centered outcomes research, also mentioned earlier, seems to be an emerging trend in HSR as well.

Additionally, the field of health policy and systems research has emerged and claims to focus on a broader field of work than "older" HSR, since health services are but one of the elements of health systems. Health system functions such as governance, health workforce, informatics, financing, and medical products, in addition to health services, play an important role in the success or failure of achieving national health goals. Health policy and systems research, therefore, takes a wider view and acknowledges the "fuzzy boundaries" between health system elements (Gilson, 2012).

Co-emerging with an attention to the broader health system is recognition that most interventions take place in complex environments. Since HSR study designs and research methods are more flexible than the traditional randomized controlled trial and yield information more rapidly, HSR may be increasingly looked to for research questions across fields of public health. Using theory and developing hypothesized causal pathways become increasingly important strategies to manage and explain complex interventions (Gilson, 2012). On the other hand, complex interventions mean that the simple independent-dependent variable, left-to-right, and linear relationship conceptual model may not apply.

ADDITIONAL RESOURCES

AcademyHealth: www.academyhealth.org

Agency for Healthcare Research and Quality: www.ahrq.gov

Alliance for Health Policy and Systems Research: www.who.int/alliance-hpsr/en

American Health Quality Association: www.ahqa.org

Centers for Medicare & Medicaid Services: www.cms.gov

Henry J. Kaiser Family Foundation: www.kff.org

Institute of Medicine: www.iom.edu

National Center for Health Statistics: www.cdc.gov/nchs

Patient-Centered Outcomes Research Institute: www.pcori.org

Robert Wood Johnson Foundation: www.rwjf.org

Barton, P. L. (2010). Understanding the U.S. health services system (4th ed.). Chicago, IL: Health Administration Press.

Health Services Research, 46(6.2). Issue dedicated to the topic of global health services research.

REFERENCES

Aboelela, S. W., Larson, E., Bakken, S., Carrasquillo, O., Formicola, A., Glied, S. A., . . . Gebbie, K. M. (2007). Defining interdisciplinary research: Conclusions from a critical review of the literature. *Health Services Research, 42,* 239–346.

Agency for Healthcare Research and Quality. (2009). *Preparing for a career in health services research: Opportunities for minority students* (AHRQ Publication No. 09-P009). Rockville, MD: Author. Retrieved from http://archive.ahrq.gov/fund/minortrg.pdf

Agency for Healthcare Research and Quality. (2012). *National healthcare disparities report 2011.* Rockville, MD: Author. Retrieved from http://www.ahrq.gov/research/findings/nhqrdr/nhqr11/nhqr11.pdf

Bagnell Stuart, J., Thornton Walker, J., & Minzner, A. (2011). *A critical review of partnership capacity and effectiveness: Moving from theory to evidence.* Bethesda, MD: Abt Associates.

Baicker, K. (2008). Formula for compromise: Expanding coverage and promoting high-value care. *Health Affairs, 27,* 658–666.

Bailey, R. C., Moses, S., Parker, C. B., Agot, K., Maclean, I., Krieger, J. N., . . . Ndinya-Achola, J. O. (2007). Male circumcision for HIV prevention in young men in Kisumu, Kenya: A randomised controlled trial. *Lancet, 369,* 643–656.

Bamberger, M., Rugh, J., & Mabry, L. (2012). *RealWorld evaluation: Working under budget, time, data and political constraints* (2nd ed.). Thousand Oaks, CA: Sage.

Bessinger, R. E., & Bertrand, J. T. (2001). Monitoring quality of care in family planning programs: A comparison of observations and client exit interviews. *International Family Planning Perspectives, 27*(2), 63–70.

Billings, J., Cantor, J. C., & Clinton, C. (2011). Access to care. In V. D. Weisfeld, S. Jonas, A. R. Kovner, & J. Knickman (Eds.), *Jonas and Kovner's health care delivery in the United States* (10th ed., pp. 151–180). New York, NY: Springer.

Boyce, C., & Neale, P. (2006). *Using mystery clients: A guide to using mystery clients for evaluation inputs.* Watertown, MA: Pathfinder International. Retrieved from http://www2.pathfinder.org/site/DocServer/m_e_tool_series_mystery_clients.pdf

Bradley, C. J., Penberthy, L., Devers, K. J., & Holden, D. J. (2010). Health services research and data linkages: Issues, methods, and directions for the future. *Health Services Research, 45,* 1468–1488.

Bradley, E. H., Fennell, M. L., Wood Pallas, S., Berman, P., Shortell, S. M., & Curry, L. (2011). Health services research and global health. *Health Services Research, 46,* 2019–2028.

Bratt, J. H., Foreit, J., Chen, P. L., West, C., Janowtiz, J., & de Vargas, T. (1999). A comparison of four approaches for measuring clinician time use. *Health Policy and Planning, 14,* 374–381.

Bruce, J. (1990). Fundamental elements of quality of care: A simple framework. *Studies in Family Planning, 21*(2), 61–91.

Capretta, J. C., & Miller, T. (2010). How to cover pre-existing conditions. *National Affairs, 4,* 110–126.

Clancy, C. M., & Eisenberg, J. M. (1998). Outcomes research: Measuring the end results of care. *Science, 202,* 245–246.

Colby, D. C. (2008). Health services research. In S. L. Isaacs & D. C. Colby (Eds.), *To improve health and health care* (Vol. XI, pp. 1–15). San Francisco, CA: Jossey-Bass.

Colby, D. C., & Baker, L. C. (2009). HSR in 2020: An assessment of the field's workforce needs. *Health Services Research, 44,* 2193–2197.

Davisson, L. (2011). Rational care or rationing care? Updates and controversies in women's prevention. *West Virginia Medical Journal, 107,* 2–32.

Donabedian, A. (1988). The quality of care. How can it be assessed? *Journal of the American Medical Association, 60,* 1743–1748.

Dummer, T. J. B. (2008). Health geography: Supporting public health policy and planning. *Canadian Medical Association Journal, 178,* 1177–1180.

Eden, J., Wheatley, B., McNeil, B., & Sox, H. (Eds.). (2008). *Knowing what works in health care: A roadmap for the nation* (pp. 25–41). Washington, DC: National Academies Press. Retrieved from http://www.nap.edu/catalog/12038.html

Field, M. J., Tranquada, R. E., & Feasley, J. C. (1995). Overview of health services research. In *Health services research: Work force and educational issues.* Washington, DC: National Academy Press. Available from http://www.nap.edu/catalog/5020.html

Franco, L. M., Franco, C., Kumwenda, N., & Nkhoma, W. (2002). Methods for assessing quality of provider performance in developing countries. *International Journal for Quality in Health Care, 14*(Suppl 1), 17–24.

Gilson, L. (Ed.). (2012). *Health policy and systems research: A methodology reader.* Geneva, Switzerland: World Health Organization.

Gray, R. H., Kigozi, G., Serwadda, D., Makumbi, F., Watya, S., Nalugoda, S., . . . Wawer, M. J. (2007). Male circumcision for HIV prevention in men in Rakai, Uganda: A randomised trial. *Lancet, 369,* 657–66.

Gulliford, M., Figueroa-Munoz, J., Morgan, M., Hughes, D., Gibson, B., Beech, R., & Hudson, M. (2012). What does access to health care mean? *Journal of Health Services Research Policy, 7*(3), 186–188.

Gusmano, M. K., & Gray, B. H. (2010). Evidence and fear: Navigating the politics of evidence-based medicine. *Academy Health Reports, 38*(1), 4–5.

Hebel, J. R., & McCarter, R. J. (2006). *The study guide to epidemiology and biostatistics* (6th ed.). Sudbury, MA: Jones and Bartlett.

Henry J. Kaiser Family Foundation. (2009). *Explaining health reform: What is comparative effectiveness research?* Retrieved from http://www.kff.org/healthreform/upload/7946.pdf

Hohmann, A., & Shear, M. K. (2002). Community-based intervention research: Coping with the "noise" of real life in study design. *American Journal of Psychiatry, 159,* 201–207.

Iglehart, J. K. (2009). Prioritizing comparative effectiveness research—IOM recommendations. *New England Journal of Medicine, 361,* 325–328.

Institute of Medicine. (1991). *Improving information services for health services researchers.* Washington, DC: National Academy Press.

Institute of Medicine. (1995). *Training and work force issues. Health services research: Workforce and education issues.* Washington, DC: National Academy Press.

Institute of Medicine. (2009). *Initial national priorities for comparative effectiveness research.* Washington, DC: National Academy Press.

Jost, T. S. (2012). The affordable care act largely survives the Supreme Court's scrutiny—but barely. *Health Affairs, 31,* 1659–1662.

Kennedy, P. (1998). *A guide to econometrics* (4th ed.). Cambridge, MA: MIT Press.

Knickman, J. R. (2011). Health care financing. In V. D. Weisfeld, S. Jonas, A. R. Kovner, & J. Knickman (Eds.), *Jonas and Kovner's health care delivery in the United States* (10th ed., pp. 47–66). New York, NY: Springer.

Kodner, D. (2009). All together now: A conceptual exploration of integrated care. *Healthcare Quarterly, 13,* 6–15.

Lewis, T., Synowiec, C., Lagomarsino, G., & Schweitzer, J. (2012). E-health in low- and middle-income countries: Findings from the Center for Health Market Innovations. *Bulletin of the World Health Organization, 90,* 332–340.

Lohr, K. N., & Steinwachs, D. M. (2002). Health services research: An evolving definition of the field. *Health Services Research, 37*(1), 15–17.

Lovell, N. H., & Celler, B. G. (1999). Information technology in primary health care. *International Journal of Medical Informatics, 55,* 9–22.

Madden, J. M., Quick, J. D., Ross-Degnan, D., & Kafle, K. K. (1997). Undercover careseekers: Simulated clients in the study of health provider behavior in developing countries. *Social Science and Medicine, 45,* 1465–1482.

MEASURE DHS. (n.d.). *SPA overview.* Retrieved from http://www.measuredhs.com/What-We-Do/Survey-Types/SPA.cfm

Mills, A., Ally, M., Goudge, J., Gyapong, J., & Mtei, G. (2012). Progress toward universal coverage: The health systems of Ghana, South Africa, and Tanzania. *Health Policy and Planning, 27,* i4–i12.

Mwandi, Z., Murphy, A., Reed, J., Chesang, K., Njeuhmeli, E., Agot, K., . . . Bock, N. (2011). Voluntary medical male circumcision: Translating research into the rapid expansion of services in Kenya, 2008–2011. *PLoS Medicine, 8,* 11.

National Center for Health Statistics. (2010). *Health, United States, 2009: With special feature on medical technology.* Hyattsville, MD: Author.

Nelson, A. (2002). Unequal treatment: Confronting racial and ethnic disparities in health care. *Journal of the National Medical Association, 94,* 666–668.

Ong'ech, J. O., Hoffman, H. J., Kose, J., Audo, M., Matu, L., Savosnick, P., & Guay, L. (2012). Provision of services and care for HIV-exposed infants: A comparison of maternal and child health clinic and HIV comprehensive care clinic models. *Journal of Acquired Immune Deficiency Syndrome, 61*(1), 83–89.

Organization for Economic Co-operation and Development. (2013). *OECD health data 2013—Frequently requested data.* Retrieved from http://www.oecd.org/els/health-systems/oecd-healthdata2013-frequentlyrequesteddata.htm

Parmet, W. E. (2011). The individual mandate: Implications for public health law. *Journal of Law, Medicine & Ethics, 39,* 401–413.

Rich, E. C. (2009). The policy debate over public investment in comparative effectiveness research. *Journal of General Internal Medicine, 24,* 752–757.

Ricketts, T. C. (2009). Preparing the health services research workforce. *Health Services Research, 44,* 2227–2241.

Robson, C. (2011). *Real world research* (3rd ed.). West Sussex, UK: Wiley.

Rosenstock, I. M. (2005). Why people use health services. *Milbank Quarterly, 83*(4), 1–32.

Ross, A. C., & Lurie, N. (2004). Global health services research: Challenging the future. *Health Services Research, 39,* 1923–1926.

Scheil-Adlung, X., & Bonnet, F. (2011). Beyond legal coverage: Assessing the performance of social health protection. *International Social Security Review, 64*(3), 21–38.

Schoen, C., Osborn, R., Squires, D., Doty, M. M., Pierson, R., & Applebaum, S. (2010). How health insurance design affects access to care and costs, by income, in eleven countries. *Health Affairs, 29,* 2323–2334.

Sedgwick, P. (2010). Primary and secondary outcome measures. *BMJ, 340,* c1938.

Seltzer, J. R. (2002). *The origins and evolution of family planning programs in developing countries.* Santa Monica, CA: RAND.

Shi, L. (2008). *Health services research methods* (2nd ed.). Clifton Park, NY: Delmar Cengage Learning.

Steinwachs, D. M., & Hughes, R. G. (2008). Health services research: Scope and significance. In R. G. Hughes (Ed.), *Patient safety and quality: An evidence based handbook for nurses* (pp. 1-163–1-177). Rockville, MD: Agency for Healthcare Research and Quality.

Thaul, S., Lohr, K. N., & Tranquada, R. E. (1994). *Health services research: Opportunities for an expanding field of inquiry.* Washington, DC: National Academy Press.

Trisolini, M. G. (2011). Introduction to pay for performance. J. Cromwell, M. G. Trisolini, G. C. Pope, J. B. Mitchell, & L. M. Greewald (Eds.), *Pay for performance in health care: Methods and approaches* (pp. 7–32). Research Triangle Park, NC: Research Triangle Institute. Retrieved from http://www.rti.org/pubs/bk-0002-1103-mitchell.pdf

U.S. Census Bureau. (2012). *Health insurance: Highlights, 2011.* Retrieved from http://www.census .gov/hhes/www/hlthins/data/incpovhlth/2011/highlights.html

Van Herck, P., De Smedt, D., Annemans, L., Remmen, R., Rosenthal, M. B., & Sermeus, W. (2010). Systematic review: Effects, design choices, and context of pay-for-performance in health care. *BMC Public Health Services Research, 10,* 247. Retrieved from http://www.biomedcentral .com

Veney, J. E., & Kaluzny, A. D. (1998). *Evaluation and decision making for health services* (3rd ed.). Chicago, IL: Health Administration Press.

Watson, M. C., Norris, P., & Granas, A. G. (2006). A systematic review of the use of simulated patients and pharmacy practice research. *International Journal of Pharmacy Practice, 14,* 83–93.

World Health Organization. (2005). *Resolution on sustainable health financing, universal coverage and social health insurance.* Retrieved from http://www.who.int/health_financing/documents/ cov-wharesolution5833/en/index.html

World Health Organization. (2010). *Towards universal access: Scaling up priority HIV/AIDS interventions in the health sector: Progress report 2010.* Geneva, Switzerland, Author.

World Health Organization. (2012a). *10 facts on universal health coverage.* Retrieved from http:// www.who.int/features/factfiles/universal_health_coverage/en

World Health Organization. (2012b). *Measuring service availability and readiness.* Geneva, Switzerland: Author. Retrieved from http://www.who.int/healthinfo/systems/SARA_ ServiceReadinessIndicators.pdf

Wu, A. W., Snyder, C., Clancy C. M., & Steinwachs D. M. (2010). Adding the patient perspective to comparative effectiveness research. *Health Affairs, 29,* 1863–1871.

Yamey, G. (2011). Scaling up global health interventions: A proposed framework for success. *PLoS Medicine, 8*(6), e1001049.

NOTE

1. For more information about Cochrane Reviews, see www.thecochranelibrary.com/view/0/ AboutCochraneSystematicReviews.html.

PART IV

Behavioral and Social Science Research

12

Survey Design and Implementation

Kathy Hageman, Andrea Kim,
Travis Sanchez, and Jeanne Bertolli

Disclaimer: The findings and conclusions in this report are those of the authors and do not necessarily represent the official position of the Centers for Disease Control and Prevention.

It is fitting that this section on behavioral and social science approaches begins with survey research, since surveys arc likely familiar to every reader, if not from public health, then from marketing, political science, or another field of social and behavioral inquiry. Survey research is the systematic method of gathering information with the use of questionnaires to draw quantitative conclusions about the respondents' attitudes, beliefs, opinions, and behaviors. One of the earliest types of survey and perhaps the most well known is the population census, often conducted by governments (Groves, Fowler, Couper, Lepkowski, & Singer, 2009) to systematically collect "demographic, economic and social data pertaining ... to all persons in a country" (United Nations, 2013). Charles Booth, acknowledged by some as the originator of the modern-day survey, recognized that surveys could also be used to investigate social problems (Groves et al., 2009). In addition to quantifying the percent of Londoners living in poverty in the 1890s, Booth sought to understand the *reasons* for poverty. By the end of the 19th century, European social theorists had defined public health as a social science, calling attention to social determinants as a fundamental cause of health and illness (Coreil, 2008). Since then, public health has come to recognize that some of the greatest challenges for improving health at the individual, population, and structural levels are related to social, cultural, and behavioral change. Yet much remains to be investigated, understood, and overcome.

USE OF SURVEYS TO INVESTIGATE SOCIAL AND BEHAVIORAL HEALTH DETERMINANTS

The use of surveys to investigate social issues led to collaboration with social science research and ultimately the development of survey methodology as a science (Groves et al., 2009). By investigating behaviors, knowledge, attitudes, or beliefs of individuals, survey research is able to provide insight into such things as attributes of a population, social issues, public opinion, changes in health trends, and why people do the things they do. This investigation of social issues brings us back to behavioral epidemiology (Chapter 1), a framework used to conceptualize the link between behavior and health. Two methodological approaches have embodied the behavioral epidemiology framework: the more traditional behavioral etiology perspective that a behavior can lead to a disease (e.g., smoking leads to lung cancer) and the social-ecological approach that seeks to investigate the "distribution and determinates of behaviors that are linked to disease" (e.g., why does someone start and/or continue to smoke; Raymond, 1989, p. 284). An increase in health conditions of "substantial behavioral etiology," such as cardiovascular and pulmonary diseases, diabetes, cancers, and HIV, required an understanding of the relationship between behavior and disease (Sallis, Owen, & Fotheringham, 2000).

CONTRIBUTION OF SURVEYS TO PUBLIC HEALTH RESEARCH AND PRACTICE

Purposes of Surveys

Surveys are designed to answer key questions of interest to health care policy-makers, public health professionals, and researchers and may be used to

- identify and assess the extent of a health problem and its impact on the functional health and well-being of the population;
- understand the differences in health across subpopulations linked with social or economic disadvantage (health disparities);
- identify risk factors and provide an evidence base for future interventions;
- inform decision making and the distribution of resources among people or programs (resource allocation) to shape a public health response; and/or
- evaluate progress with or impact of programs, refine or improve programs, measure the delivery and uptake of interventions.

Because surveys can focus on health issues that are important social concerns, they can provoke and encourage public discourse. Statistics from surveys anchor newspaper stories, provide topics for TV talk shows, spark public policy debates, and inspire government initiatives.

Surveys, which can range from large national surveys to smaller projects that may focus on one community or a specific subpopulation, seek to assess the frequency and distribution of health-related population characteristics or experiences, health-related behaviors, and knowledge and attitudes, as well as monitor changes in the health status of a group. These uses distinguish surveys from qualitative methods (Chapter 15). For example, a survey might be designed to quantify the percentage of a population always wearing seatbelts while riding in a car; a qualitative study might seek to identify nuances in the reasons people give for using or not using seatbelts.

The Importance of Survey Data and Examples of Their Use

Surveys serve an important role in guiding public health action by providing data that can directly impact prevention and intervention efforts and policy decision making. Given space constraints, we will highlight only a few critical ways in which surveys have directly affected public health action. These include describing the national health status, evaluating the impact of public health campaigns, identifying factors associated with health disparities, and monitoring health disparities.

Describing the National Health Status

Some health surveys are so important to our public life, they are mandated by law. The United States National Health Survey Act of 1956 provided for the establishment of a continuing National Health Survey to obtain information about the health status of individuals residing in the United States, including the services received. This legislation authorized the National Health and Nutrition Examination Survey (NHANES), perhaps the largest and oldest national source of objectively measured health and nutrition data, which began in 1959. In 1999, NHANES became an annual survey with the flexibility to meet emerging trends (see Chapter 9).

The potential to link NHANES to other related health and nutrition surveys of the U.S. population, including the National Health Interview Survey (NHIS) and the U.S. Department of Agriculture's Continuing Survey of Food Intakes by Individuals increases its value. By combining and integrating the data from these large, population-based surveys, a more comprehensive evaluation of the current health and nutritional status of the U.S. population can be made.

NHANES has contributed substantially to several areas of public health, as described in the text box titled "Outcomes of the National Health and Nutrition Examination Survey" on page 344.

Evaluating the Impact of Public Health Campaigns

The high-profile campaign against childhood obesity, Let's Move, launched in February 2010 and championed by First Lady of the United States Michelle Obama, provides a more recent example of the use of national survey data to identify and raise awareness of a public health problem, shape the public health response, measure the delivery and uptake of interventions, and evaluate the impact of intervention programs. According

OUTCOMES OF THE NATIONAL HEALTH AND NUTRITION EXAMINATION SURVEY

- NHANES, along with NHIS, has been the source of anthropometric data for the development of growth charts used by pediatricians and health clinics across the United States and around the world.
- NHANES has aided in the determination of population groups at nutritional risk and spawned measures to address these nutritional inadequacies. For example, findings from the first two NHANES surveys indicated insufficient amounts of iron in the diets of women of childbearing age, young children, and the elderly. This information led to the practice of fortifying grain and cereal products with iron. NHANES data also helped to confirm the connection between folate intake and neural tube defects, information that led to folate fortification of grain and cereal products.
- Early NHANES data provided the first solid evidence of high blood levels of lead among Americans. As a result, the Environmental Protection Agency announced restrictions on production and sales of consumer goods containing relatively large amounts of lead, such as gasoline and household paints.

Source: Centers for Disease Control and Prevention (2011).

to NHANES data, between the survey periods 1976–1980 and 2007–2008, obesity more than tripled among children and adolescents, rising from 5% to 17% (Ogden & Carroll, 2010). Let's Move is a national public awareness campaign that is central to an interagency plan overseen by the Task Force on Childhood Obesity to solve the problem of childhood obesity within a generation (White House Task Force on Childhood Obesity, 2010). The plan includes an objective of returning to a childhood obesity rate of just 5% by 2030, with interim objectives that by 2015 there will be a 2.5% reduction in each of the current rates of overweight and obese children, and by 2020 a 5% reduction. Progress on these main objectives will be charted through the NHANES survey, and nine other surveys will track key indicators to monitor progress (see Table 12.1).

Table 12.1 Selected Examples of Objectives, Indicators, and Survey Data Sources for the Let's Move Campaign

Objective	Indicator	Data Source
The average child will score 65 on the U.S. Department of Agriculture's (USDA's) Healthy Eating Index by 2015.	Number of children eating a healthy diet	National Health and Nutrition Examination Survey
Half of babies are breastfed for at least 9 months by 2015 (increased from 30%).	Initiation and duration of breastfeeding	National Immunization Survey

Objective	Indicator	Data Source
All elementary and secondary schools will offer meal options that meet standards for total fat and saturated fat by 2015.	Number of elementary and secondary schools offering meal options that meet standards for total fat and saturated fat	School Nutrition Dietary Assessment Study
Increase the percentage of parents who use food labels.	Number of parents who notice, understand, and use food labels	Health and Diet Survey
Increase the number of high school students who participate in daily PE classes to 40% by 2015 and 50% by 2030.	Percentages of high school students who participate in daily PE classes	Youth Risk Behavior Survey
Increase the percentage of schools that offer recess to all students and grades in elementary schools to 95% by 2015.	Percentage of elementary schools that offer recess to all students and grades	School Health Policies and Practices Survey

Source: White House Task Force on Childhood Obesity (2010).

Identifying Factors Associated With Disparities in Healthcare Quality

Health insurance

Surveys also help to describe access to and use of health care as well as the distribution of factors associated with access to care, such as health insurance status. This information is useful for understanding disparities in healthcare quality and to guide action to address them. Examples of surveys pertinent to health disparities are listed in Table 12.2.

As shown in Table 12.2 the Medical Expenditure Panel Survey (MEPS), is a set of large-scale surveys designed to provide timely information about changes in the U.S. health care system, including changes in insurance coverage. Further detail to flesh out the picture of health insurance coverage is available from the most recent Commonwealth Fund Health Insurance Tracking Survey. Surveys like MEPS and those sponsored by the Commonwealth Fund provide the basis for laws and policies to increase access to care. For example, the finding that uninsured lower-income adults are more likely than insured adults in the same income group to cite factors other than medical emergencies as reasons for going to the emergency department (Collins, Robertson, Garber, & Doty, 2012), coupled with an analysis that showed that hospital emergency departments could save $4.4 billion annually if more visits took place at alternative care sites (Weinick, Burns, & Mehrotra, 2010), illustrates the power of information to shift policy. To address healthcare inequities, some of which are described above, starting in 2014 options for affordable health care coverage will be

Table 12.2 Surveys Monitoring Healthcare Disparities and Their Underlying Causes

Survey	Focus	Methods
Medical Expenditure Panel Survey[a]	Changes in the U.S. health care system	Annual subsample of households that participated in the most recent previous National Health Interview Survey, supplemented by surveys of medical and health insurance provider
Commonwealth Fund Health Insurance Tracking Survey	Health insurance coverage	Telephone interviews of a random, nationally representative sample of adults living in the continental United States
Commonwealth Fund, 2004	Health care quality	Nationally representative sample of adults in Australia, Canada, New Zealand, the United Kingdom, and the United States

[a] See Agency for Healthcare Research and Quality (n.d.).

available through implementation of the Affordable Care and Patient Protection Act of 2010. To track the impact of this law, a series of three nationally representative online surveys is planned by the Commonwealth Fund. The longitudinal surveys will follow randomly selected panels of adults over the next several years to examine changes in their health insurance coverage and health care as the law is implemented.

Assessing health care quality

Surveys have been used to compare patients' experiences of their health care systems in the United States and other countries. Surveys by the Commonwealth Fund in 2004 and 2005, which yielded a score reflecting the quality of each country's health care, showed that although the U.S. system ranked first on effectiveness, it ranked last on other dimensions of quality, especially on measures reflecting equitable, safe, efficient, and patient-centered provision of care. Yet the other countries spend much less on health care per person and as a percentage of gross domestic product than the United States. Findings like these have helped to spur discussions about performance improvement and additional health services research (see Chapter 11).

Monitoring Health Outcome Disparities

Surveys can also be used to monitor disparities in health outcomes directly. One of the challenges in measuring disparities in health is achieving large enough numbers of the group of people intended to be studied, or the target population, to draw statistical conclusions (discussed in Chapter 17). An example of how this can be overcome is to utilize data from a variety of surveys to investigate or monitor a public health issue. Together, the National Comorbidity Survey Replication, the National Survey of American Life, and the National Latino and Asian American Study provide information on the mental health of racial and ethnic subgroups, including immigrant populations. Before these surveys, data on the mental health of groups like U.S. Caribbean Black populations were limited, and studies of the mental health of heterogeneous groups like Latinos and Asian Americans had insufficient statistical power to examine within-group differences. The capacity to analyze health disparities among diverse populations has been increased through common core data components across these national surveys (Boyce & Cain, 2007).

DEVELOPING AND CONDUCTING SURVEYS

To provide practical guidance regarding survey design and implementation, we divide this section into two phases: initial considerations and planning. Although we present the steps in a linear fashion, good survey research demands the flexibility to adapt to new information and changing environments.

Initial Considerations

As discussed in Chapter 2 generally, two important initial considerations for survey research are (1) what are the research objectives and research questions and (2) is a survey the most appropriate approach for meeting the research objectives and answering the research questions. Adequate attention to each consideration will increase the survey's scientific integrity as well as minimize challenges to successful implementation.

Developing Research Objectives and Research Questions

The objectives of the survey should be clearly stated and justified. Deciding on the purpose of the study and research objectives will lead to the development of the research questions. You will need to clearly articulate what exactly you would like to know, how you plan to measure it, and how the data will be used to improve the health of the population. Failure to provide clear objectives of the survey may lead to wasted resources and lost opportunities in the data collection phase. This process should be largely guided by local needs and context and a review of the literature.

Considering a Survey Approach

Be careful not to assume that all topics can be investigated via a survey; another of the primary data collection approaches discussed in this book may be more appropriate, or survey data from other sources may be available to address the research question.

Using existing (secondary) data has many advantages related to minimizing cost, time, impact on resources, and so on (see Chapter 9). However, existing data collected for another purpose may not answer the questions of interest as well as a survey that has been specifically tailored to the research questions. If you determine that primary data collection is necessary, consider whether a survey is feasible. Answering the questions provided in the following text box can help inform your decision-making process.

CONSIDERING A SURVEY APPROACH: KEY QUESTIONS

Population-related

   a. Is the target population definable?
   b. Is the target population accessible?
   c. Is the target population willing to complete a survey? To answer questions of a potentially sensitive nature?
   d. Who are the gatekeepers of the target population? Are gatekeepers accessible? Open to the study?

Study-related

   a. What are the ethical considerations for the target population? (potential benefits and harms)
   b. Can protection of privacy be ensured for all respondents?
   c. Can a team of experts be identified?
   d. Will the local environment (e.g., laws, politics, culture) be accepting of the survey?
   e. Whose permission is needed to conduct the study? (e.g., gatekeepers, community, governing officials)
   f. Is the necessary infrastructure available to support the study's needs? (e.g., staffing, technical expertise, laboratories, data infrastructure, logistical support)

Population-related considerations

Two critically important considerations in determining whether a survey is an acceptable approach is determining whether the target population is definable and accessible. Research on HIV infection in mobile populations, such as migrant workers or illegal immigrants, provides an illustrative example. For such research, it is important to consider whether there is sufficient information to define the population clearly enough to allow a survey to be conducted. Yet some populations that can be clearly defined may not be accessible to researchers. For example, sex workers may be reluctant to participate in research if they fear the legal consequences of engaging in sex work. Additional questions to consider related to accessibility are whether it will be feasible to recruit a sufficient number of survey respondents to complete the survey and whether it will be necessary to prescreen potential respondents for specific eligibility criteria (e.g., age, race, behavior) to ensure the appropriate persons are recruited. Once accessibility has been determined, it is important to assess the willingness of the target population to participate in the survey, particularly if the survey contains sensitive issues. To help with community engagement, identify gatekeepers (individuals capable of facilitating access to a community or group) to inform about the survey and discuss any concerns or potential barriers to participation to help ensure community acceptance.

Study-related considerations

As discussed in Chapter 3, it is important to also consider the ethics of conducting the survey and the possible benefits and risks to the respondent. Will the respondent be put at risk if contacted or asked sensitive questions by a member of the research team? Can the research team provide a safe place to take the survey? How do ethical issues differ by data collection format, for example, electronic versus paper and pen? As discussed in Chapter 3, the answers to such questions determine the ethical considerations and how the research team can minimize harm to respondents. Along with the ethics experts of the Institutional Review Board, it is helpful to engage experts in survey research design, measurement and questionnaire design, sampling, statistical analysis, and the subject matter specific to the survey's topic. If the survey is computer-administered, then a computer programmer will also be needed.

Also assess community-level resources: Does the community have the necessary infrastructure (e.g., staffing, technical expertise, laboratories, data management systems, logistical support) to conduct the survey?

Planning the Survey

Most, if not all, decisions made during the planning stage will directly affect the survey's data quality and its implementation success. We cover a variety of topics to be considered, ranging from the use of qualitative research to guide survey development, to data preparations, to piloting the survey to ensure successful implementation.

Conducting Formative Qualitative Research

Qualitative research can provide valuable formative information for the development of surveys or as an adjunct to surveys. Chapter 15 discusses qualitative research in detail, and Chapter 19 covers mixed methods designs that incorporate both qualitative and quantitative components; therefore, this section focuses on how qualitative research intersects with survey designs and implementation. Qualitative methods may contribute to the following activities:

- Developing the study's methods, such as for sampling and recruitment, or logistics
- Exploring characteristics of the target population, which can be useful for developing the recruitment approach and for maximizing the number of individuals who complete the survey (response rate)

- Guiding survey designers in understanding the context of a survey—which might influence what questions are asked and how they are asked, as well as how the survey should be described to respondents and the topics to be covered in the survey (domains) to satisfy stakeholders; some surveys employ ongoing collection of qualitative data to guide implementation (Allen, Finlayson, Abdul-Quader, & Lansky, 2009)
- Guiding questionnaire design (e.g., the development of response sets for closed-ended questions that include responses that are likely to be most frequent or important, or to explore the need for follow-up questions), including a specific type of qualitative research—cognitive interviewing, in which potential survey questions are asked and answered by respondents, followed by questions about how the respondent interpreted the questions

The National HIV Behavioral Surveillance System (NHBS) comprises annual risk group–specific surveys designed to characterize sexual and injection drug use behaviors that place respondents at risk of HIV infection. Before data are collected, local staff in 20 U.S. cities conduct formative research that may include key informant interviews and focus groups with professionals and members of the target population to identify potential barriers to implementation and explore possible solutions. Information collected during formative research also helps to ensure that the interviewers are aware of local terminology for behaviors and geographic areas to ideally obtain more accurate responses for the survey (Nichter, Quintero, Nichter, Mock, & Shakib, 2004).

Conducting a Pre-Survey Assessment of Needs

A pre-survey assessment, or a needs assessment, can also be a useful tool for planning a survey and may involve qualitative methods, literature review, expert consultations, or other information-gathering methods. An assessment can provide insight for defining the population and eligibility criteria for respondent selection, assist with identifying an appropriate sampling strategy, and guide implementation logistics. We provide examples of questions to help investigate each topic in the text box below.

CONDUCTING A PRE-SURVEY ASSESSMENT: SUGGESTED QUESTIONS

Defining the target population and eligibility criteria

   a. What characteristics can be used to identify the target population and its members?

   b. What are the behaviors or demographic characteristics of the target population?

   c. Can the target population be divided by differences in their behaviors and organization? If so, does it affect who would be eligible and who would not be eligible for the study? Will a screening process or screening questions be needed to determine whether a respondent is eligible?

Investigating sampling strategies

    a. Is the size of the target population known?

    b. Does a list of the target population exist?

If yes (probability sample is an option):

- What type of contact information is available for the persons on this list?
- What other information is available for the persons on this list that would permit sampling within subgroups?

If no (probability sample is not an option):

- How can the target population be accessed?
- Does a high proportion of the target population gather at identifiable locations that can be listed, and are they accessible through those locations? Is it possible to identify the members of the subpopulation at the locations where they gather? Is venue-based sampling an option?
- Do group members know each other? Are they part of a network? Can the same individuals be found at more than one location? Is respondent-driven sampling an option?

Ensuring successful implementation

Population-related considerations

    a. What will it take to access and recruit the target population? (e.g., mailing costs, advertising, reimbursement for study participation)

    b. What literacy accommodations (e.g., flashcards, visual aids) may need to be made to ensure that respondents are able to complete the survey?

    c. What is the preferred language(s) of the target population? Can language-specific versions of the questionnaire be developed that retain the nuances of the original survey?

    d. What will be the best times of the day to find target population for recruitment and study participation? Are certain subgroups (e.g., the employed) available at certain times, but not others?

Study-related considerations

    a. What survey type is likely to yield the highest response rate?

    b. Does the topic of the survey demand attention to respondents' privacy? What are the possible locations where data could be collected where privacy will be ensured?

    c. What interviewer characteristics would ensure the most valid reporting from the respondents?

(Continued)

(Continued)

    d. Who can manage the survey process and make sure it runs smoothly and without disruption?

    e. What practical problems could field workers come across? (e.g., ensuring privacy and safety, monitoring for possible scams for study inclusion or reimbursements)

    f. What is needed to administer the survey? (e.g., survey materials, computers, software, website, servers)?

    g. What is the minimum time (e.g., weeks, months, years) needed by the researchers to implement the survey?

    h. What is the estimated time for respondents to complete the survey? Will the estimated time be acceptable to the target population?

Selecting a Survey Type

Surveys can be classified according to how the interview is administered, how frequently the survey is conducted (periodicity), and whether a one-time survey is conducted among the population (cross-sectional study) or repeatedly involves the same individuals (longitudinal or panel survey). Surveys can be self-administered or interviewer-administered. They can also involve direct measurements of something without interviews, such as the Centers for Disease Control and Prevention's HIV Family of Surveys, which involved conducting HIV testing on remnant blood from pregnant women (Davis et al., 1998). Surveys may also include direct physical measurements (e.g., height, weight, blood pressure) or obtain biological specimens (e.g., blood, hair, urine).

Within self- and interviewer-administered surveys there are various subtypes. Self-administered surveys may include the following:

- mail surveys in which the respondent returns a paper questionnaire
- telephone surveys, in which the respondent calls a toll-free number and enters responses using touchtone data entry (TDE) after hearing recorded questions
- computer-assisted self-interview (CASI) and audio computer-assisted self-interviews (ACASI), in which survey staff provide a computer that displays the questions on screen, and the respondent reads the questions or the computer plays audio recordings of the questions and the respondent records his or her own responses
- telephone ACASI (T-ACASI), in which survey staff telephone the respondent and switch him or her over to an automated recording of the questions; the respondent enters responses with the telephone keypad or by responding verbally

- computerized self-administered questionnaires (CSAQ) such as web-based surveys, in which the respondent may have minimal or no interaction with study staff but may participate in all of the survey procedures in an entirely automated and self-guided environment
- two-way phone texting, in which the respondent replies to survey questions in the form of text messages sent to the respondent's phone. The global expansion of cell phones has allowed for more efficient and real-time data collection, particularly in geographic areas that may not traditionally have the staff or technological resources to implement a survey

Interviewer-administered interviews may include the following:

- paper-and-pencil, face-to-face interviews in which the interviewer reads and records responses
- computer-assisted personal interviews (CAPI) or handheld-assisted personal interviews (HAPI), in which the computer displays the questions on screen; the interviewer reads the questions aloud and records the responses on the computer; CAPIs are typically conducted with computers, laptops, and tablets, while HAPIs are conducted with handheld computer devices such as personal digital assistants (PDA)
- telephone interviews, such as computer-assisted telephone interviewing (CATI), in which the interviewer places a telephone call to the respondent and reads questions to him or her from a computer screen and records the responses

The pros and cons of self-administered and interview-administered surveys are listed in Table 12.3. Your choice of a survey type can be driven by considerations of the target population, the availability of a sampling frame and the ability to obtain up-to-date contact information for the persons selected from this frame, the feasibility of locating those selected for participation and whether they are widely dispersed, the content of the survey, and the need for anonymity. Depending on the characteristics of the population the survey is intended to reach, there may not be a list (sampling frame) from which to sample respondents, in which case investigators may employ venue-based sampling (specific days and times are identified when the target population gathers at specific venues) or respondent-driven sampling (respondents recruit other respondents). If there is a list, the availability of up-to-date mailing or email addresses or telephone numbers, whether the respondents are reachable by mail, email, telephone, or the Internet may determine the survey type. For example, persons who are unemployed and have applied for unemployment benefits may be identifiable through a list but may not be reachable by mail, telephone, or web-based surveys. Even if address information is available, it may not be feasible for interviewers to conduct interviews face to face with respondents if the respondents are widely dispersed.

With advancements in technology, options beyond paper-based tools exist for more efficient approaches in data collection. Electronic data capture tools (e.g., personal digital assistants, ACASI, web-based surveys, two-way text messaging) have significant benefits that can, in theory, help to expedite data collection data management and analysis, and improve the overall quality of the data collected. (Additional information on electronic data collection is provided in Chapter 21.)

Cost is an important consideration in choosing a survey type. Mail, email, and web-based surveys are the cheapest way to reach large numbers of people. They also increase the opportunity for respondents to remain anonymous, which may be their strongest advantage. However, if the enrollment request is considered junk mail or spam, this may lead to poor response rates and potential bias. Data quality may also be affected by differences in the capabilities of respondents' computers.

No one mode of data collection is best in all circumstances. Mixing modes may help to compensate for weaknesses of individual modes. For example, paper surveys may also be distributed to people without Internet or email access or a phone with texting capabilities for surveys that employ these methods; similarly, both mail and telephone modes of contact may be used in the same survey. However, mixing modes can also lead to some challenges. For example, people may respond differently depending on the mode of data collection. To preserve consistency in your survey, it is typically inadvisable to mix modes of administration (self-administered or interviewer-administered) as responses to questions administered through these two methods can be considerably different.

The choice of mode should be made within the context of the public health purpose and objectives, available resources and infrastructure, and the characteristics of the target population. In addition, the mode of survey administration is also guided by the relative importance of measurement, nonresponse, and coverage error, which will be discussed below.

Table 12.3 Advantages and Disadvantages of Self-Administered and Interviewer-Administered Survey Types

Survey Type	Advantage	Disadvantage
SELF-ADMINISTERED	May be less prone to biased responses due to social desirability than are interviewer-administered	Does not allow explanation of questions, exploring responses, observations; incomplete responses
Mail	Is relatively inexpensive, allows anonymity	Mailing addresses may not be available, potential bias from low response rate, not an effective mode of administration for survey with complex skip patterns, slow, requires data entry, difficult to know whether person responding is sampled (eligible) person

Survey Type	Advantage	Disadvantage
Interviewer-assisted telephone	Potentially better response rate than T-ACASI, may be less expensive than ACASI, suitable for complex surveys	Telephone numbers may not be available; those reachable by telephone may be a biased sample, especially if limited to land lines; more expensive than methods not involving interviewer assistance; vulnerable to programming errors of the automated questions and responses; difficult to know whether person responding is sampled (eligible) person
T-ACASI	Potentially less prone to social desirability bias, less expensive than methods involving an interviewer	Same as above; potentially lower response rate than for interviewer-assisted telephone interviewing
ACASI	Quicker results than methods that require data input; reasonable chance of ensuring the respondent who they say they are; same advantages as for other computerized methods (see CAPI)	Requires respondents to be tech-savvy (comfortable with computers), is more expensive than methods not involving purchase of computers and interviewer assistance, is vulnerable to programming errors, requires uploading the data from the data collection computers to a server
Web-based	Relatively inexpensive, rapid development and deployment of survey, does not require a specific address, allows anonymity, effective for complex surveys, same advantages as CAPI	Can be difficult to reach target population, requires respondents to be comfortable with computers, may be a biased sample (self-selection bias and biased toward those with technology access and literacy), difficult to verify that respondents are who they say they are
Mobile technology/ two-way texting	Relatively inexpensive; rapid development and deployment of survey; does not require land line phone, Internet access, or address;	Can be difficult to reach target population, sampling frame is harder to determine, survey design must be simple

(Continued)

(Continued)

Survey Type	Advantage	Disadvantage
	other advantages like those of CAPI; acceptable to younger populations; capable of real-time data collection	
Email	Very inexpensive; effective for complex surveys, quick results	Requires respondents to be comfortable with computers; target population may not have email addresses, or a list of email addresses for the population may not exist; those reachable by email may be a biased sample; survey requests may be identified by email provider as junk or spam and may not reach the target population; potentially low response rate
INTERVIEWER-ADMINISTERED	Allows explanation of questions, exploring response; more complete responses; reasonable chance of ensuring that respondents are who they say they are; ability to tailor recruitment strategies; allows personal observation and use of visual aids (e.g., flashcard) to aid comprehension or memory	Expensive, need interviewer training, respondents may be influenced by the interviewer (interviewer bias)
Paper and pencil	Same as above	Requires data entry; not effective for surveys with complex skip patterns; interviewer influence may be greater than for interviewer-administered interviews by telephone; errors, missing data may be more frequent than for programmed questionnaire applications

Survey Type	Advantage	Disadvantage
CAPI	Same as for self-administered surveys; does not require data entry; effective for complex surveys; reduced errors relative to noncomputerized methods; allows possibility of real-time data transfer; enhanced data security and confidentiality via verification, authentication, and encryption	Vulnerable to programming errors
Telephone	Less expensive than face-to-face methods	Requires data entry, difficult to ensure that the person responding is the sampled (eligible) person

Understanding Sampling

A complete discussion of sampling is provided in Chapter 17, including description of probability and nonprobability samples. We focus here on how sampling intersects specifically with survey designs and implementation.

The mode of data collection for a survey depends on whether the sampling method permits contact with respondents to administer the survey face to face or via telephone, text, or Internet, so survey type and coverage of the target population are also linked. In a survey with probability sampling, if a sampling frame permits contact through only land line telephone, the survey coverage will be limited to those reachable by land line telephone. The proportion of households with land line telephones in the United States was about 94% in 2006; however, the rapid rise in use of cell phones (many of which are not included in telephone listings) has reduced reliance on land line telephones, which may impact surveys that sample from telephone directories. Though many cell phones also allow for text messaging and Internet access through which survey data may be collected, identifying appropriate sampling frames for these uses may be difficult. Household surveys that require a complete listing of household members for random selection usually have fewer coverage errors because they are completed face to face. The choice of a survey type is a critical one that in turn influences other survey design decisions. Area-probability sampling frames will necessitate face-to-face contact; face-to-face is expensive and is therefore almost always used with clustered sampling, whereas mail and web surveys do not gain advantages by clustered sampling.

Sample

The sample is the actual group that will be recruited to respond to the survey. The type of sampling used will depend on whether the study aims to yield representative estimates of health status or factors related to health status for a population or simply to document the existence or types of certain health conditions or health-related factors or behaviors. The type of sampling might also be determined by what is feasible. For example, an investigator aiming to describe health care needs of migrant workers may find it infeasible and unnecessary to employ probability-based sampling. In contrast, an investigator seeking to estimate the prevalence of a health-related behavior in a city would not be able to achieve the survey objective without probability sampling.

In a hypothetical situation in which the study objective requires a population-representative sample, and everyone in a population had the same characteristics and experiences as everyone else, a sample of one would perfectly mirror the population. Given that this will never be the case, the next best thing might be to make estimates of health status with a known degree of accuracy, for example, to know that 79% of Americans (+/– 6 percentage points) are satisfied with their health (Clifton & Gingrich, 2007).

Sample size

As discussed in Chapters 17 and 18, ensuring adequate sample size is important to be able to satisfy the statistical needs to detect significant differences within a probability-based sample. To determine how large of a sample will be needed, it is necessary to decide how much sampling error, or the error derived from observing a sample versus the entire population, is acceptable; to know the size of the population from which the sample will be drawn; to determine the variability in the population with regard to measured parameters (e.g., mean, variance); and to determine the desired confidence level for estimates of these parameters (Dillman, 2007). For nonprobability sampling methods, from which study findings cannot be generalized to the target population, sample size can be based on feasibility. Specifically, how many of the individuals from the target population can be recruited to participate, and how many survey respondents are needed to provide acceptable levels of precision of power to answer the research question.

How Errors and Biases Affect Surveys

Several sources of error can create bias and affect the ability to generalize the findings from a survey to the larger population. These include coverage, nonresponse, and measurement error. Coverage error results when some part of the target population is not on the sampling frame and, therefore, not included among respondents. Bias can result if the subpopulation not included has characteristics that are not represented in the sample. For example, a survey designed to describe the health of HIV-infected patients receiving medical care based on a sampling frame including only patients who received care during the first few months of the year would be biased if the sampling frame overrepresented patients with AIDS, with public or private insurance, on antiretroviral therapy, and with more favorable immunological and virological profiles (Sullivan et al., 2011). Coverage is important, but coverage has to be balanced against other factors. For some surveys, the data collected will not be useful if delayed, so coverage has to be balanced against speed.

Nonresponse error stems from nonparticipation of individuals in the survey. This type of error can be thought of as the statistical difference between results when only those who respond are included, and the results that might have been had the nonrespondents participated. Nonresponse errors can produce selection bias, a type of error caused when one group of people is selected or participates more than other groups in the study.

Measurement error results when respondents misinterpret questions, intentionally give a response that misrepresents the truth, or selectively refuse to answer questions. These types of errors can result in response bias. The following are types of response bias:

- acquiescence bias, a tendency of respondents to agree with all questions or concur with a particular position
- extremity bias, a tendency of respondents to choose extreme responses
- interviewer bias, when the interviewer influences responses
- auspices bias, when respondents are influenced by the organization conducting the survey
- social desirability bias, a tendency of respondents to misrepresent answers to avoid social stigma (e.g., to appear intelligent, to conceal information that would compromise the respondent's social position, to avoid embarrassment)

Other biases can result from the following administrative errors:

- sample selection errors (e.g., improper sampling design execution of sample selection)
- interviewer errors (e.g., unintentional misreporting of responses not in agreement with the interviewer's own opinions or perceptions, deliberate falsification, failure to ask questions that make the interviewer uncomfortable)
- questionnaire design errors (e.g., faulty skip patterns in an electronic questionnaire application)

Methods to minimize error and characterize bias

As mentioned above, error from nonresponse can affect the quality of survey results. Fortunately, some design features can reduce nonresponse. Making multiple contact attempts on different days at different times can increase the chances of successful contact. Other ways to help minimize refusal rates include providing a prenotification to the community that explains the study, offering reimbursement for study participation, obtaining a sponsorship or endorsement that increases legitimacy, tailoring recruitment efforts to address respondent concerns, and matching interviewer characteristics to respondent characteristics. It is important to recognize, though, that efforts to reduce bias, if done incorrectly, can actually increase bias. For example, reimbursement for study participation in the form of free food may be more appealing to some subpopulations (e.g., people who are homeless or of a low socioeconomic status), resulting in greater participation than the general population of interest. Efforts to reduce bias can be a delicate balancing act that warrants careful consideration during the planning stages.

Although it is not possible to prevent error from nonresponse, it is advisable to build in ways to characterize nonrespondents as completely as possible. For example, demographic information for nonrespondents, when compared with similar information from respondents, helps investigators characterize and understand the potential for bias in survey findings and can help boost their credibility if, for example, nonrespondents are not so very different from respondents with regard to key characteristics.

Developing a Survey Plan

Decision-making process for content and survey items

Deciding on the survey's content and design can be a challenging process. Ideally, the research team, literature, local needs and context, and research objectives will guide survey development. Researchers have the option to use existing survey items or develop their own. There are pros and cons to both.

Developing survey items

A successful survey depends on good questions, yet developing questions can often be rushed due to investigators' competing study preparation demands. The research team should include an expert who understands measurement as well as the key concepts to be measured (e.g., behaviors, knowledge, attitudes, intentions). Measurement is the *assignment of numerals* to topics being investigated and their attributes (Di Iorio, 2005) so that responses are useful for quantitative analysis. Measurement allows researchers to describe a population or assess change over time within a population.

Two key concepts of measurement are reliability and validity. As discussed more generally in Chapter 2, a measure that is reliable is one that is consistent. For example, if a person steps onto a weight scale multiple times and the scale reports a different weight each time, the scale is not consistent and therefore has low reliability. If the weight scale reports the same weight every time, then the scale has high reliability. Validity assesses the degree to which the question measures what it is intended to measure. Keeping with the example of a weight scale, if a weight scale is valid, it does a good job of measuring the true weight of the individual. It is important to note that a weight scale can be reliable without being valid, but it cannot be valid without being reliable. The goal is to have survey questions that have high reliability and high validity. Reliability and validity are illustrated in Figure 12.1 by a series of targets.

Reliability can be evaluated through testing and retesting, comparing results with other questions that measure the attribute or underlying concept, and testing

Figure 12.1   Understanding Reliability and Validity Using a Weight Scale Example

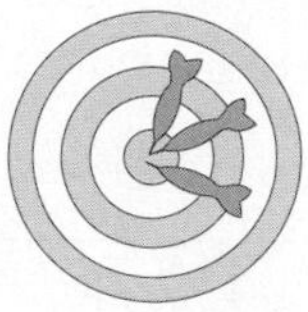	Reliable and valid	This weight scale measures the same weight for a person each time and measures the weight accurately.
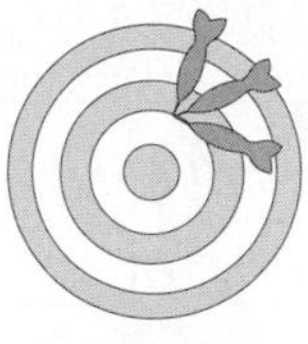	Reliable, not valid	This weight scale adds 5 pounds (2.3 kg) to a person's actual weight; the scale is reliable because it measures weight consistently, but it is not valid because the weight measurement is always 5 pounds greater than the true weight.
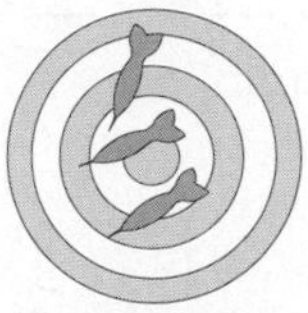	Unreliable and not valid	This weight scale measures a person's weight differently each time and therefore also cannot be valid.
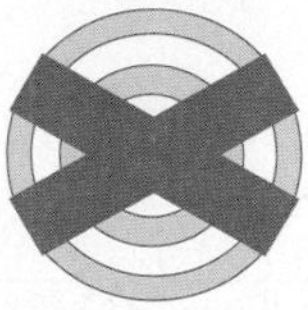	Unreliable but valid	This scenario is not possible, as a scale that measured the person's weight differently each time (unreliable) cannot accurately measure the person's weight (valid).

whether questions designed to measure the same attribute or concept yield consistent results. Measurement validity can be evaluated on a variety of dimensions. For example, validity might be evaluated based on impressions of whether "on the face of it" a question seems to be a good measure of the attribute or concept of interest, whether a question reflects the definition of what is being measured, whether responses to the question accurately predict something that theory indicates should be predictable, or whether responses are able to distinguish between groups as would be expected on a theoretical basis. Methods of evaluating reliability and validity are covered in more detail in Chapter 13.

Another important aspect of developing a survey is deciding whether questions will allow closed- or open-ended responses, or both. Closed-ended responses are used when findings from previous studies, either qualitative or quantitative, have defined a range of responses that accurately capture the necessary information. Open-ended responses allow respondents to answer the question without predetermined response options and can provide a great depth of information to the study. Open-ended responses are typically used (1) when previous research identified too many potential response options to be listed on a survey or (2) when greater detail from the respondents is desired to answer the research question(s). Table 12.4 provides examples of open- and close-ended questions.

Table 12.4 Example Survey Questions for an Assessment of Public Transportation Attitudes and Usage

1. **[Open-ended]** When you think about public transportation in your city, what is the first thought that comes to your mind?

   _____

   _____

   _____

2. **[Close-ended: True/false]** In the past 24 hours, have you used any form of public transportation?
   No........☐ 0 *(Skip to #4)*
   Yes........☐ 1 *(Go to #3)*

3. **[Close-ended: Multiple choice/checklist]** What forms of public transportation have you used in the past 24 hours?
   Taxi............... ☐ 1
   Bus/minivan.....☐ 2
   Subway...........☐ 3
   Train...............☐ 4
   Airplane......... ☐ 5
   Other.............☐ 6
   None............ ☐ 7

4. **[Close-ended: Likert scale]** The next question asks about your feelings regarding public transportation in your neighborhood. The response options are *strongly disagree, disagree, neutral, agree,* or *strongly agree*. Circle the number that represents your response to the question:

   Having convenient public transportation options is important to me when I am deciding where to live.

Strongly disagree	Disagree	Neutral	Agree	Strongly agree
1	2	3	4	5

Using Existing Survey Items

Identifying existing survey questions applicable to the research objectives can be advantageous for many reasons. Perhaps the most important is that previously used questions may have been extensively tested for reliability and validity. Identifying questions with high reliability and validity can be invaluable to a survey, yet their use needs to be considered carefully, specifically with regard to the applicability to the proposed study's populations of interest, local and cultural context, intended use of findings, and so on. For example, an item that measures attitudes toward sexual behavior that has been found to have high reliability and validity when used with married adults may not have comparable reliability and validity when used to collect sexual behavior information from a different population, such as adolescents and teens.

In addition to investigating an existing question's measurement properties, it is also important to consider such things as whether the previously used question is suitable to the mode of survey administration (e.g., self- or interviewer-administered, pencil-and-paper, or electronic data collection) and the sample population, and whether the sample size will allow for reliable measurement. A disadvantage of using existing survey questions is that they may not be fully applicable or do not provide an exhaustive list of response options for the target population, context, or purpose. In such situations, it may be necessary to adapt or modify a previously used question to make it applicable for the proposed survey (University of Michigan, 2011). When applicable questions have been identified, they can greatly reduce the time, money, and other resources needed to prepare the survey.

Pretesting and Evaluation of Survey Questions

It is important to pretest new and previously used survey questions to identify potential problems for the interviewers or respondents prior to finalization of the questionnaire (Presser et al., 2004). Problems may include questions that can be misunderstood or interpreted in different ways, cannot be answered accurately, or do not collect the intended information (Collins, 2003). Pretesting also provides an opportunity to assess acceptability and, if applicable, the translation of the questionnaire into secondary languages. Pretesting may include cognitive interviews, statistical analyses, and review by survey experts (Collins, 2003; Di Iorio, 2005; Presser et al., 2004; Willis, 1999). The extensiveness of pretesting varies by study and will be influenced by budget, resources, and length and/or complexity of the survey. It is beyond the scope of this chapter to provide details regarding the different methods of pretesting, but there are many resources available. in addition to those mentioned above (Collins, 2003; Di Iorio, 2005; Presser et al., 2004; Willis, 1999).

Preparing for Interviewing

Interviewer selection

In addition to considering experience and skill when selecting interviewers, it may be necessary to make selections that take into consideration the specifics of the local context, cultural and social norms, and language fluency. For example, it may not be appropriate for a younger person to interview an older person or an interviewer of the opposite gender to interview a respondent about sensitive topics such as sexual behavior, drug use, family planning, and so on. If a respondent is not comfortable with the interviewer administering the survey, interviewer bias may be introduced. During formative work, it is important to investigate the type of interviewers with whom different respondents would and would not feel comfortable in order to minimize bias as much as possible.

Interviewer training

Training of individuals administering the survey is an essential component to the survey process for multiple reasons. The first is to achieve standardization of survey delivery by all interviewers. Standardization is important to ensure data quality. Standardization means that respondents have very similar experiences regardless of where or by whom they are interviewed. Although a respondent will have the same past behaviors and experiences regardless of interviewer or location of interview, *what* she or he chooses to report during an interview can be very different depending on the interviewer or setting. These differences cause measurement error and bias. Second, to increase the quality of the data collected, interviewers should be trained on the techniques of nonjudgmental and unbiased interviewing, particularly when asking sensitive questions. The respondents comfort level, the nature of interactions with and demeanor of project staff, distractions during the interview, and privacy-related concerns may influence how a respondent chooses to answer a question.

Interviewer training typically includes the following steps, although this list may not be exhaustive: (1) review each item in the survey to ensure that interviewers understand the context and meaning of the question, (2) conduct practice interview sessions so interviewers become familiar with administering the survey, and (3) evaluate interviewers to improve interviewing skills. The use of a standardized evaluation form helps to ensure that each interviewer has mastered the needed skills and that the interviewers are standardized in their administration of the survey, which is critical for reducing measurement error. Interviewers should not start data collection until they have successfully demonstrated the skills outlined on the evaluation form (See Figure 12.2.).

Interviewer monitoring

After data collection has begun, the investigators should systematically monitor interviewers administering the survey to ensure that the performance standards established during training are maintained. Over time, project staff, even those with extensive experience, may drift from the standards established during interviewer training. Conducting standardized performance evaluations on a regular basis will promote standardization and data quality throughout data collection. The importance of ongoing evaluations cannot be overstated. Staff should undergo retraining when they fail to maintain performance standards.

Automated interviewing monitoring

Although automated interviewing, such as that employed in Internet surveys, does not require training or monitoring of interviewers, it does require additional processes for development and testing of the survey site prior to implementation. Once implemented, incoming data should be monitored closely to identify potential problems early in the process and make appropriate adjustments to the automation (e.g., correcting skip patterns).

Data quality monitoring

A key part of any survey is to monitor the data quality and identify problems in the survey. Typically this is done during the first few weeks of the survey so problems

Figure 12.2 Example Interviewer Evaluation Form

General Instructions

- Permission should be obtained from the potential respondent before an evaluator joins an interview.
- The evaluator typically interrupts the interview only for major issues, is discreet when doing so, and directs questions to the interviewer.
- Shaded areas are examples of recommended performance standards.

Interviewer:

Evaluation Date:

Evaluator:

Rating instructions: Circle the number that corresponds with your evaluation for each criterion. For criteria that do not apply, check the N/A box.

☐ **Pre-implementation Evaluation**
☐ **Ongoing Evaluation**

Time to Complete Survey	Time		
1. Eligibility screener (if applicable)	Start: _____	End: _____	Length: _____
2. Consent process	Start: _____	End: _____	Length: _____
3. Core questionnaire	Start: _____	End: _____	Length: _____

Set-up	Rating				
	1 Not at all	2	3 Some	4	5 Fully
4. All necessary materials were prepared prior to starting (flashcards, consent forms, prevention materials, referral information, pens, etc.).	1 Not at all	2	3 Some	4	5 Fully
5. Was knowledgeable of safety procedures.	1 No				5 Yes
Consent Process					
6. All aspects of informed consent were followed per local IRB requirements (e.g., read as written if required, covered all relevant points if summarized).	1 No				5 Yes
7. Provided the respondent with a copy of the consent form to follow along.	1 No				5 Yes
8. Offered the respondent a copy of the consent form to keep.	1 No				5 Yes

Item	1	2	3	4	5
9. Provided an opportunity for questions about the project and consent process.	No				Yes
10. Obtained consent for the interview.	No				Yes
11. Obtained consent for specimen storage or additional testing. □ N/A	No				Yes
12. Pace of reading the consent was . . .	Too slow		Too fast		Just right

Eligibility and Questionnaire Administration

Item	1	2	3	4	5
13. Oriented the respondent by reading each introductory statement.	Never	Rarely	Sometimes	Usually	Always
14. Read each question as written.	Never	Rarely	Sometimes	Usually	Always
15. Read response options as written when instructed to read aloud.	Never	Rarely	Sometimes	Usually	Always
16. Did not read response options when instructed not to read aloud.	Never	Rarely	Sometimes	Usually	Always
17. Reread and clarified instructions, questions, and responses as needed. □ N/A	Never	Rarely	Sometimes	Usually	Always
18. Recognized inconsistent responses, clarified with respondent, and corrected data as needed. □ N/A	Never	Rarely	Sometimes	Usually	Always
19. Probed incomplete, implausible, unclear responses. □ N/A	Never	Rarely	Sometimes	Usually	Always
20. Used neutral probes (i.e., probed without influencing response).	Never	Rarely	Sometimes	Usually	Always
21. The amount of time given for responses was . . .	Too short		Too long		Just right
22. Pace of reading the screener was . . .	Too slow		Too fast		Just right
23. Pace of reading the questionnaire was . . .	Too slow		Too fast		Just right

Flashcards ☐ N/A

	1	2	3	4	5
24. Used flashcards when instructed.	Never	Rarely	Sometimes	Usually	Always
25. Oriented the respondent to the flashcard response options (i.e., pointed to responses as being read).	Never	Rarely	Sometimes	Usually	Always
26. Read the flashcards as written.	Never	Rarely	Sometimes	Usually	Always

Establishing and Maintaining Rapport

	1	2	3	4	5
27. Established and maintained a good yet neutral rapport with respondent (i.e., demonstrated interest, empathy, appropriate tone, and, if needed, refocused respondent).	Not at all	Poorly	Okay	Well	Very well
28. Maintained eye contact with respondent throughout interview.	Not at all	Poorly	Okay	Well	Very well
29. Provided neutral feedback throughout the interview.	Never	Rarely	Sometimes	Usually	Always
30. Remained engaged with respondent and his or her responses throughout the survey.	Not at all	Poorly	Okay	Well	Very well
31. Demonstrated a professional demeanor.	Never	Rarely	Sometimes	Usually	Always

Criterion #	Skill Description, Recommendations, Accolades, and Additional Comments

Recommended steps for the evaluator:
☐ Review evaluation form with the interviewer and provide time for interviewer to ask questions.
☐ Provide the interviewer with recommendations for improvement.
☐ If applicable, briefly described how each skill was below standard and provide recommendations for meeting the standard.

can be fixed before a majority of the surveys have been completed. With the speed in which automated interviewing can take place, the majority of surveys may be completed within days, therefore creating the opportunity for problems in the survey to go unnoticed, and unresolved, prior to the completion of the survey. For surveys with potential rapid uptake by respondents, it is important to monitor the data as much as possible in real time to ensure that problems are noticed and fixed in an appropriate amount of time.

Preparing for Data Management and Analysis

Data management and analysis plans

Surveys may employ more than one method of collecting data (e.g., collection on paper, via a computer), and data management plans should specify how data collected through each method will be managed. The investigators should design the data management plan so that data confidentiality is addressed at every step in the process, including plans for protecting or removing identifying information (e.g., name, date of birth, home address), specifying who can have access to the data and how, and how data will be stored and for how long.

Developing a data analysis plan (discussed in Chapter 2) before the actual data collection begins will provide the investigators with an opportunity to clarify how the analysis of the collected data will meet the research objectives; it can also help point toward any last-minute changes to the data collection instrument or methods that might be necessary to achieve the objectives.

Data ownership and access

Data ownership refers to the possession of and responsibility for the data collected through a survey. Data ownership can be a particularly sensitive issue for surveys in which investigators and collaborators are from different agencies or even countries. The data from surveys that engage multiple participating institutions or agencies may have a single or multiple owners. Investigators should discuss data ownership during the early planning stages of a survey and come to an agreement about data ownership that is documented in writing. Factors that can influence ownership are funding, where data were collected, level of engagement, and who will be creating policy based on the data. After a data ownership agreement has been completed, the owners of the data typically decide how data will be shared, whether data can be accessed for analysis by external groups, as well as the process to gain access to the data and to publish the data. Decisions regarding data ownership and publication should be documented. In some settings, a memorandum of understanding between groups collaborating on the survey research may be worthwhile or required.

Piloting Study Procedures and Conducting Practice Interviews

Prior to implementation of the survey, investigators and study staff should conduct a full run-through of the study procedures, including recruitment, interviewing, data collection, data entry, data analysis, and, if applicable, specimen collection. A pilot study provides the opportunity to

- test the procedures for selecting and recruiting survey respondents,
- ensure any problems or concerns regarding the survey questions have been resolved,
- estimate how many interviews can be conducted in a day and help assess whether the time and resources budgeted will be sufficient to complete the survey, and
- ensure that all methods for data collection and data entry, including data entry software, can be implemented successfully and efficiently, whether they involve paper, a laptop, a handheld or mobile device, the Internet, biometric devices, or specimen collection.

After a pilot study of survey procedures, investigators should allow adequate time for adjustments to be made and discussions with study staff and stakeholders about lessons learned. Rushing to launch a survey without a solid research design, valid and reliable measurement instruments, and feasible procedures may seriously impact data quality.

USING REPORTING GUIDELINES TO HELP PLAN SURVEY RESEARCH

The EQUATOR Network (Enhancing the Quality and Transparency of Health Research) provides a variety of reporting guidelines for publication of health research to promote transparency and accurate reporting (EQUATOR Network, 2011). Although the guidelines are written to advise the reporting of research, they can also help researchers in the planning stages of a study to envision reporting their findings and guide them to take steps that will enable a thorough and accurate report later (Gallo et al., 2011). For example, the STROBE statement (Strengthening the Reporting of Observational Studies in Epidemiology) can help guide survey planning. A similar checklist, CHERRIES (Checklist for Reporting Results of Internet E-Surveys), is available for reporting of Internet survey research (Eysenbach, 2004).

COLLECTION OF BIOLOGICAL SPECIMENS AS PART OF SURVEY DATA COLLECTION

Many surveys collect biologic specimens to determine physiologic parameters (e.g., cholesterol, nutrient levels, blood lead levels) or the occurrence of a biological pathogen (e.g., HIV, sexually transmitted infections, malaria) among the study population and individual-level factors associated with these parameters or pathogens. The ability to link demographic and behavioral survey data to a respondent's biological specimen greatly increases options for analyses and has become the gold standard for survey data collection.

Collection of Biologic Specimens

A number of factors are involved in determining which biologic tests should be included. Characteristics of the population or survey setting and the test should be considered. It may be difficult to obtain some types of specimens from certain respondents if, for example, respondents are distrustful of research, if they fear invasive procedures like drawing blood, if they are concerned about privacy, or if they do not perceive the testing to be of benefit to them. In all cases, team members should be well trained to inform respondents about the purpose of specimen collection, risks involved in providing specimens, benefits to the respondent and to the public, and how the information from biologic testing will be used. Every effort should be made to ensure that the standard of care is met for returning test results in a study or providing linkages to other testing services that can provide results to the respondent. Plans for the collection of respondents' contact information and the returning of test results should follow national guidelines and be included in the study's protocol for review by the Institutional Review Board.

Develop a Biological Specimen Analysis Plan

A specimen analysis plan is typically required for surveys that conduct biologic testing. This plan outlines the processing, testing, and storage of specimens as well as plans for linkage to demographic and behavioral data for analysis purposes. The specimen analysis plan should include how data from the laboratory conducting the analysis will be merged with the interview survey data.

CONDUCTING SURVEYS IN INTERNATIONAL SETTINGS

Careful planning is required for any survey, and surveys conducted internationally may require extra time, particularly for obtaining required approvals. In the international context, pre-survey assessments are useful to improve understanding of the local context, to determine capacity required for conducting the survey, and for other factors critical to successful implementation.

Understanding Local Context and Garnering Community Support

To ensure that the survey addresses the local context, consider these strategies:

- Review local laws pertaining to research to identify any legal impediments to the survey and whether options, if any, exist to overcome the challenges. Be aware of the particular provisions in a country's laws that may (1) complicate participation by certain individuals (e.g., the age of legal adulthood may prohibit surveys of respondents younger than a certain age), (2) require reporting of individuals discovered to have communicable diseases, and (3) minimize risk to respondents (e.g., laws that protect study results, including risk behavior, from dissemination).
- Engage individuals who are directly influential in the community (e.g., community leaders, political representatives, public health officials) and/or those who will be directly involved in the survey (e.g., target population) throughout the planning, implementation, and analysis process to maximize community support as well as the usefulness of the collected and analyzed information to the community (see also Chapter 4).
- Use respected mechanisms of communication in the community to build consensus and credibility for a survey.
- Conduct formative assessment to gain a greater understanding of the issues of local concern and to identify barriers to be resolved before implementation (see also Chapter 15).

Logistical Considerations

Attention to logistics is necessary to maximize the survey's success. In most cases, surveys will take longer than anticipated due to unexpected delays. In resource-constrained settings, the infrastructure and systems required for setting up and implementing a study may contribute to greater delays. Challenges may include identifying a sufficient number of staff with the necessary technical skills or a lack of electricity to power the electronic devices used for data collection, analysis, or refrigeration of biologic specimens. An important step in the planning stage is to try to identify the variety of challenges that may arise over the course of the study to ensure that adequate time and financial resources are allotted to manage the challenges. If the survey requires use of equipment that must be purchased or imported, one should factor in time for delays in procurement and receipt of these commodities.

For aspects of the study that require specialized experience or training, such as qualitative research skills or survey programming, investigators should consider the time and cost needed to identify and hire staff with the appropriate skills and experience. Likewise, if a survey requires field work to collect data, external factors such as extreme weather, rough terrain, civil insecurity, and political activity can cause considerable delays or interruptions in data collection. In areas where access to bank accounts is limited or nonexistent, a financial management plan must also be developed. Further, fluctuations in exchange rates can significantly affect the cost of a survey.

Data Collection and Technology

As mentioned in the Planning the Survey section of this chapter, advancements in technology have helped make data collection more efficient while reducing biases. Whereas the benefits of electronic data collection are encouraging, survey settings will require the infrastructure to enable it. Common challenges in resource-constrained settings include frequent electricity outages, unreliable cellular networks, and spotty or nonexistent wireless networks. Electronic data collection may result in catastrophic loss of data if backup plans are not in place should the systems fail. Where infrastructure is limited, it is important to consider paper-based data collection.

CURRENT ISSUES AND FUTURE DIRECTIONS

Survey design and implementation—indeed, all aspects of information collection, use, and exchange-are in the midst of a dramatic paradigm shift from paper-based to electronic data collection. These changes are driven by the general public's thirst for information and technology–based interactions between individuals. As of 2013, 39% of the world's population was online (International Telecommunication Union, 2013) with more than half utilizing social networking websites (Pew Research Center, 2013). By 2014, the number of mobile phones is expected to exceed the world's population of seven billion (International Telecommunication Union, 2013). Market researchers first capitalized on this shift to increased technology use and interconnectedness by developing an entirely new set of survey research support tools. These tools initially appeared as stand-alone computer programs (often on large institutional computers), but now run on the full spectrum of information technology from text messaging devices to web-based survey servers. This shift to more technology use in our personal and professional environment is also occurring in an era of increased globalization and decreased resources for public health.

This environment produces unique challenges and opportunities for public health surveys related to resource conservation, data quality, scope, periodicity, technology-biology, and privacy.

Resource Conservation

Public health practice, including surveys, is constrained by limited resources—time, human, and financial. These constraints necessitate more efficient ways to collect, analyze, and disseminate high-quality public health survey data. Resource conservation can occur in many ways, such as streamlining data collection to reduce burden. For example, the U.S. government enacted the Paperwork Reduction Action of 1995, implemented by the Office of Management and Budget, which requires federal agencies to implement effective and efficient methods to reduce the paperwork burden imposed on private business and citizens. The Paperwork Reduction Act is designed to conserve resources by (1) ensuring net benefits over costs of data collection, (2) minimizing respondent burden, and (3) avoiding redundant data collection.

The use of technology can also increase the efficiency of data collection. Initial technological tools for surveys were often complex and expensive, but there are now many off-the-shelf solutions for complex surveys administered through many different modalities. There is also a rapidly growing base of highly skilled human resources for custom programming of data collection instruments, resources that are driving down cost and time required for completion. The improvements to data quality, scope, periodicity, and information sharing also reduce the resource needs for each survey collection (Evans & Mathur, 2005). Yet technological tools, even those using readily available web-based technology, do not entirely eliminate resource needs. In addition to the up-front costs associated with getting a survey programmed and tested, maintaining the survey system and ensuring the security of the data can be costly. Technological-based surveys also require hardware (e.g., computers, cell phones) with associated initial investments and costs for maintenance and usage if purchased by the research team. (See the In Focus at the conclusion of Chapter 21 for more on technology in data collection.)

Data Quality

One of the initial drivers of the switch to technology-supported surveys was the need for improvements in data quality. Data errors could be better addressed through the use of preprogrammed checks of logic and consistency. However, the validity and bias introduced by technology-based surveys is difficult to describe, particularly as surveys use more self-administered technology-driven modes of administration (e.g., computers, text messaging on smartphones, the web) rather than paper-based interviewer-administered surveys For example, people who take surveys on a computer or on the web may be more willing to accurately answer sensitive questions than during a conversation with an interviewer. Researchers developing self-administered computer or web surveys need to take extra care in crafting questions that are easily understood without the assistance of an interviewer and must employ technologies that are either familiar or easy to learn for survey respondents (Chang & Krosnick, 2010). Self-administered technology-based surveys often also require additional effort to ensure equal access to those with sensory disabilities (e.g., vision impairment, hearing loss) or lower literacy.

Some electronic data collection may impose constraints on the sampling method that can be employed and the representativeness of that method. For instance, surveys administered on the web probably allow for the most flexibility in survey question design (e.g., multimedia questions, complex logic checks) and the most data management functions (e.g., centralized data storage, automated monitoring) but may also be limited to the survey population with access to this technology. Surveys administered through cell phone text messaging may be feasible, even in emergency situations and resource limited settings, but may also have limitations with respect to quality controls such as logic checks and additional questions to validate responses (i.e., limited response options and survey length; Magee, Isakov, Paradise, & Sullivan, 2011; Zurovac, Talisuna, & Snow, 2012). New technological solutions are also being developed for monitoring and adjusting sampling methods while surveys are underway—with the objective of improving the quality of the final data (Axinn, Link, & Groves, 2011).

Scope

The topical scope of public health surveys has historically been limited by resources. Survey content (complexity and length) was proportionally related to time and costs for development, implementation, analysis, and dissemination. Even in situations where public health problems may share common causes or may exist in similar populations (HIV, other sexually transmitted infections, some viral hepatitis), resource constraints limited the ability to efficiently collect survey data in an integrated fashion. With technology tools, these resource constraints are diminished through improvements in efficiency at all levels. The challenge to balancing this improved efficiency is that surveys may become overly long, complex, and unwieldy, to the point of producing survey fatigue among respondents. The ease and potential scope of surveys is also producing a growing need to compete against other personal and professional electronic interactions that are engaging respondents' attention and their growing expectation of succinct communication and ease to use.

Increased geographic scope is also a boon and a bane for public health surveys using technology. Surveys collected in person involve finite geographic scope, while surveys collected with technological tools, such as through the Internet or text messaging systems, allow for surveys to be collected from very wide geographic areas using standardized methods and in a very short time frame (Schmidt et al., 2012). Investigators should carefully consider the necessary geographic scope of a survey, how the scope is related to the public health purpose of the survey, and how the scope will be determined and controlled. For example, it is now technologically feasible to collect survey data about sexual behaviors from an Internet sample of hundreds of thousands of persons in dozens of countries, all in a matter of months, but how will these data be used in each country or across countries? What is the smallest geographic unit at which measures are stable? If the ultimate purpose of public health surveys is to inform public health action, how will the geographic scope of the survey relate to the geographic scope of future public health interventions?

Periodicity

Periodicity, the frequency with which a survey is conducted, is also undergoing changes during the paradigm shift. As technological tools reduce resource constraints and increase the scope of public health surveys, there is also an increased capacity for repeated measurement and increased frequency of recurring surveys. In many cases the ability to collect data more often produces advantages in monitoring trends in population health, but it does not come without additional costs, both monetary and scientific. Increased periodicity of public health surveys is occurring in an environment of increased scope and a preponderance of general survey research. This means that some populations could be exposed to multiple surveys on seemingly similar topics all in a short period of time. For individual survey respondents, there may also not be a notable difference between surveys for public health purposes and surveys for marketing or political research purposes. This could result in survey fatigue, which may lead to reduced response rates, selection bias, and response biases. These problems may also not be entirely mitigated by reduced survey length (Cape, 2010).

Technology-Biology Connection

Many public health surveys have historically combined collection of data with biologic information or specimens for laboratory testing. Although technology can be used to efficiently collect and record some biomarker information (e.g., weight, height, facial features, fingerprints), respondents who are remotely accessing the survey may not be available to provide the full complement of biologic information and specimens desired. For in-person surveys, biomarker data are often collected from a large proportion of respondents (USAID, 2012), but remote collection of surveys (e.g., Internet-based) may result in only a subset of respondents providing this information, raising concerns about selection bias. In addition to new technologies available for remote biometry (e.g., blood pressure, blood glucose, activity levels), health researchers are exploring self-collection of biologic specimens (Huppert et al., 2012; Soni & White, 2011). The application of these newest techniques is still within the realm of research, but may have utility for future technology-based surveys in which the respondent and survey team may either not be able to have or be interested in an in-person interaction (e.g., because of geographic distance).

Confidentiality

Public health surveys must preserve the privacy and confidentiality of data. Even in situations where survey data are anonymous, the sensitivity of health information dictates that steps should be taken to protect privacy during survey administration and unauthorized access and release of survey results. Breaches of privacy and confidentiality can potentially occur regardless of how the data were collected and stored, but the shift to technological tools has increased the potential scope of these breaches. Just as the technology has improved the scope of surveys, it has also made it harder to verify respondents' and administrators' access to surveys and made it easier to collect vast amounts of sensitive information in centralized locations. Technological tools to collect survey information may also inadvertently carry information about how the data were collected (metadata; e.g., location, time, user IDs) that could be potentially identifying for individual respondents. With increasingly complex and accessible survey analysis tools, it may also be possible to reconstruct identities from seemingly "anonymous" data (Electronic Privacy Information Center, n.d.).

The use of connected technology for surveys (e.g., networks, Internet, mobile services) has also increased the pool of people who might potentially gain unauthorized access to survey data. Most breaches of public health data that have been reported have seemingly resulted from carelessness, but there are some instances in which concerted attempts have been made to gain unauthorized access (Kaplan, 2009). Public health surveys are also building on the constantly developing field of information security by using commercially available survey tools that incorporate industry-standard security (e.g., SurveyMonkey, www.surveymonkey.com; SurveyGizmo, www.surveyverisigngizmo.com) or by using commercially available information security verification on custom surveys (e.g., VeriSign, www.verisigninc.com; GeoTrust, www.geotrust.com). However, the wide availability and use of these commercial tools may also increase vulnerability to attacks.

CONCLUSION

Surveys continue to serve an important role in guiding public health action. New opportunities to expand the content and geographic scope of public health surveys are arising with advances in technology, as are new challenges for implementation. Yet as survey methods change to accommodate new technology, some tried and true advice for survey researchers continues to apply. Careful planning is necessary to establish scientific credibility, meet ethical obligations, and ease implementation of a survey. Formative work such as literature review and preliminary data-gathering activities (such as pre-survey assessments to define the target population, investigate survey feasibility, guide choice of survey type and implementation logistics, or pilot test methods and instruments) can provide critical information for planning.

ADDITIONAL RESOURCES

Di Iorio, C. K. (2005). *Measurement in health behavior: Methods for research and education.* San Francisco, CA: Jossey-Bass.

Dillman, D. A. (2007). *Mail and Internet surveys: The tailored design method.* New York, NY: Wiley.

EQUATOR Network. http://www.equator-network.org/home

Eysenbach, G. (2004). Improving the quality of web surveys: The Checklist for Reporting Results of Internet E-Surveys (CHERRIES). *Journal of Medical Internet Research, 6*(3), e34.

Groves, R. M., Fowler, F. J., Couper, M. P., Lepkowski, J. M., & Singer, E. (2009). *Survey methodology* (2nd ed.). Hoboken, NJ: Wiley.

University of Michigan, Institute for Social Research, Survey Research Center. (2011). *Guidelines for best practice in cross-cultural surveys* (3rd ed.). Retrieved from http://www.ccsg.isr.umich.edu/pdf/FullGuidelines1301.pdf

REFERENCES

Agency for Healthcare Research and Quality. (n.d.). Medical Expenditure Panel Survey. Retrieved from http://meps.ahrq.gov/mepsweb

Allen, D. R., Finlayson, T., Abdul-Quader, A., & Lansky, A. (2009). The role of formative research in the National HIV Behavioral Surveillance System. *Public Health Reports, 124*(1), 26–33.

Axinn, W. G., Link, C. F., & Groves, R. M. (2011). Responsive survey design, demographic data collection, and models of demographic behavior. *Demography, 48*, 1127–1149.

Boyce, C. A., & Cain, V. S. (2007). Disentangling health disparities through national surveys. *American Journal of Public Health, 97*(1), 10.

Cape, P. (2010). *Questionnaire length, fatigue effects and response quality revisited.* Shelton, CT: Survey Sampling International.

Centers for Disease Control and Prevention. (2011). *National Health and Nutrition Examination Survey: Data accomplishments.* Retrieved from http://www.cdc.gov/nchs/nhanes/DataAccomp.htm

Chang, L., & Krosnick, J. A. (2010). Comparing oral interviewing with self-adminstered computerized questionnaires. *Public Opinion Quarterly, 74*(1), 154–167.

Clifton, J., & Gingrich, N. (2007). Are citizens of the world satisfied with their health? *Health Affairs, 26*, W545–W551.

Collins, D. (2003). Pretesting survey instruments: An overview of cognitive methods. *Quality of Life Research, 12*, 229–238.

Collins, S., Robertson, R., Garber, T., & Doty, M. (2012, February). The income divide in health care: How the Affordable Care Act will help restore fairness to the U.S. health system. *Tracking Trends in Health System Performance.* Retrieved from http://www.commonwealthfund.org/~/media/Files/Publications/Issue%20Brief/2012/Feb/1579_collins_income_divide_tracking_brief.pdf

Coreil, J. (2008). Social science contributions to public health: Overview. In S. Quah & K. Heggenhougen (Eds.), *International encyclopedia of public health* (Vol. 6, pp. 101–114). San Diego, CA: Elsevier.

Davis, S. F., Rosen, D. H., Steinberg, S., Wortley, P. M., Karon, J. M., & Gwinn, M. (1998). Trends in HIV prevalence among childbearing women in the United States, 1989–1994. *Journal of Acquired Immune Deficiency Syndromes and Human Retrovirology, 19*(2), 158–164.

Di Iorio, C. K. (2005). *Measurement in health behavior: Methods for research and education.* San Francisco, CA: Jossey-Bass.

Dillman, D. A. (2007). *Mail and Internet surveys: The tailored design method.* New York, NY: Wiley.

Electronic Privacy Information Center. (n.d.). *Re-identification.* Retrieved from http://epic.org/privacy/reidentification

EQUATOR Network. http://www.equator-network.org/home

Evans, J. R., & Mathur, A. (2005). The value of online surveys. *Internet Research, 15*(2), 195–219.

Eysenbach, G. (2004). Improving the quality of web surveys: The Checklist for Reporting Results of Internet E-Surveys (CHERRIES). *Journal of Medical Internet Research, 6*(3), e34.

Gallo, V., Egger, M., McCormack, V., Farmer, P. B., Ioannidis, J. P. A., Kirsch-Volders, M., . . . Vineis, P. (2011). STrengthening the Reporting of OBservational studies in Epidemiology—Molecular Epidemiology STROBE-ME: An extension of the STROBE statement. *Journal of Clinical Epidemiology, 64*, 1350–1363.

Groves, R. M., Fowler, F. J., Couper, M. P., Lepkowski, J. M., & Singer, E. (2009). *Survey methodology* (2nd ed.). Hoboken, NJ: Wiley.

Huppert, J. S., Hesse, E. A., Bernard, M. C., Bates, J. R., Gaydos, C. A., & Kahn, J. A. (2012). Accuracy and trust of self-testing for bacterial vaginosis. *Journal of Adolescent Health, 51*, 400–405.

International Telecommunication Union. (2013). T*he world in 2013: ICT facts and figures.* Retrieved from http://www.itu.int/en/ITU-D/Statistics/Pages/facts/default.aspx

Kaplan, D. (2009, May 5). Hackers seek payment after break-in on state health care site. *SC Magazine*. Retrieved from http://www.scmagazine.com

Magee, M., Isakov, A., Paradise, H. T., & Sullivan, P. (2011). Mobile phones and short message service texts to collect situational awareness data during simulated public health critical events. *American Journal of Disaster Medicine, 6*, 379–385.

Nichter, M., Quintero, G., Nichter, M., Mock, J., & Shakib, S. (2004). Qualitative research: Contributions to the study of drug use, drug abuse, and drug use(r)-related interventions. *Substance Use & Misuse, 39*, 1907–1969.

Ogden, C., & Carroll, M. (2010). Prevalence of obesity among children and adolescents: United States, trends 1963–1965 through 2007–2008. *National Center for Health Statistics Health E-Stats*. Retrieved from http://www.cdc.gov/nchs/data/hestat/obesity_child_07_08/obesity_child_07_08.pdf

Pew Research Center. (2013). *Pew Internet: Social networking*. Retrieved from http://pewinternet.org/Commentary/2012/March/Pew-Internet-Social-Networking-full-detail.aspx#

Presser, S., Couper, M. P., Lessler, J. T., Martin, E., Martin, J., Rothgeb, J. M., & Singer, E. (2004). Methods for testing and evaluating survey questions. *Public Opinion Quarterly, 68*(1), 109–130.

Raymond, J. S. (1989). Behavioral epidemiology: The science of health promotion. *Health Promotion, 4*, 281–286.

Sallis, J. F., Owen, N., & Fotheringham, M. J. (2000). Behavioral epidemiology: A systematic framework to classify phases of research on health promotion and disease prevention. *Annals of Behavioral Medicine, 22*, 294–298.

Schmidt, A. J., Weatherburn, P., Hickson, F., Berg, R., Breveglieri, M., Fernández-Dávila, P., . . . Marcus, U. (2012, July). *Advancing methods in Internet-based HIV prevention gay community research projects: EMIS, the European MSM Internet Survey in 38 countries*. Paper presented at the International AIDS Conference, Washington, DC. Retrieved from http://www.emis-project.eu/sites/default/files/public/publications/ias2012_thpe252_emismethods_a3.pdf

Soni, S., & White, J. A. (2011). Self-screening for Neisseria gonorrhoeae and Chlamydia trachomatis in the human immunodeficiency virus clinic—High yields and high acceptability. *Sexually Transmitted Diseases, 38*, 1107–1109.

Sullivan, P. S., Juhasz, M., McNaghten, A. D., Frankel, M., Bozzette, S., & Shapiro, M. (2011). Time to first annual HIV care visit and associated factors for patients in care for HIV infection in 10 US cities. *Aids Care-Psychological and Socio-Medical Aspects of AIDS/HIV, 23*, 1314–1320.

United Nations. (2013). *Population and housing censuses*. Retrieved from http://unstats.un.org/unsd/demographic/sources/census/alternativeCensusDesigns.htm

University of Michigan, Institute for Social Research, Survey Research Center. (2011). *Guidelines for best practice in cross-cultural surveys* (3rd ed.). Retrieved from http://www.ccsg.isr.umich.edu/pdf/FullGuidelines1301.pdf

USAID. (2012). *Biomarker field manual: Demographic and health surveys methodology*. Retrieved from http://www.measuredhs.com/pubs/pdf/DHSM7/DHS6_Biomarker_Manual_9Jan2012.pdf

Weinick, R. M., Burns, R. M., & Mehrotra, A. (2010). Many emergency department visits could be managed at urgent care centers and retail clinics. *Health Affairs, 29*, 1630–1636.

White House Task Force on Childhood Obesity. (2010). Solving the problem of chilhood obesity within a generation. Retrieved from http://www.letsmove.gov/sites/letsmove.gov/files/TaskForce_on_Childhood_Obesity_May2010_FullReport.pdf

Willis, G. B. (1999). *Cognitive interviewing: A "how to" guide*. Paper presented at the Annual Meeting of the American Statistical Association.

Zurovac, D., Talisuna, A. O., & Snow, R. W. (2012). Mobile phone text messaging: Tool for malaria control in Africa. *PLoS Medicine, 9*(2), e1001176.

13

Scale Development and Validation

Glenn Gamst, Lawrence S. Meyers, Holly McClain Burke, and A. J. Guarino

You may be familiar with scales or scaling from exposure to health surveys or from mention in the previous chapters. Scales are simply "measurement instruments that are collections of items combined into a composite score . . . intended to reveal levels of theoretical variables not readily observable by direct means" (DeVellis, 2011, p. 11). We need scales to measure phenomena like attitudes, self-efficacy, or social support that we believe exist (based on theory), but that are not directly observable. For instance, we do not need a scale to measure body temperature. We can use an appropriate instrument—a medical thermometer—to take a measurement of one's temperature and then compare that reading to another. Depression, by contrast, has no such observable measurement. It is a construct, or latent variable, which we believe to exist and are trying to assess. It may have clinically recognized symptoms, but a scale constructed of items related to these manifestations is necessary to *measure* the degree or severity of depression.

Scales are used in many areas of public health research, including HIV prevention (Rhodes et al., 2011), tobacco cessation (Wegmann, Bühler, Strunk, Lang, & Nowak, 2012), obesity prevention (Singh et al., 2011), and public health organizational readiness (Stamatakis et al., 2012). A few examples of scales that have been used in public health are listed in Table 13.1, to give readers a sense of what types of constructs are amenable to scaling. Note that this list is not meant to be exhaustive, nor is it an endorsement or evidence for a scale's validity. Validity should be examined each time we use a scale in a new context (including a later time) or with a new population.

Additionally, many of the scales listed in the table have been refined or adapted for use in other than the original contexts and populations, and have been used to answer different research questions since they were first developed. Another option for researchers is to search for preexisting scales in a compendium of scales such as *Measuring Health: A Guide to Rating Scales and Questionnaires* (McDowell, 2006), and the *Handbook of Sexuality-Related Measures* (Fisher, Davis, Yarber, & Davis, 2011). These books report on the reliability and validity of scales and provide references for more information.

Table 13.1   Some Examples of Scales Used in Public Health Research

Scale	Source
AIDS Information Survey	DiClemente, Boyer, and Morales (1988)
Health Days Measure	Centers for Disease Control and Prevention (2011)
Gender-Equitable Men Scale	Pulerwitz and Barker (2008)
Health Locus of Control Scale	Wallston, Wallston, Kaplan, and Maides (1976)
Levenson Multidimensional Locus of Control Inventory	Levenson (1981)
Mastery	Pearlin and Schooler (1978)
Perceived AIDS-Related Stigma	Kalichman et al. (2005)
Rosenberg Self-Esteem Scale	Rosenberg (1965)
UCLA Multidimensional Condom Attitudes Scale	Helweg-Larsen and Collins (1994)
WHO Quality of Life Scale	World Health Organization (1993)

THE ESSENTIAL ELEMENTS OF SCALES

Constructs

We mentioned earlier that depression is a construct. **Constructs** are the abstract ideas, themes, and characteristics of people that researchers and program evaluators in public and community health, behavioral medicine, psychology, and related fields routinely speak of and theorize about. For example, we may attempt to determine the self-esteem level of a certain group of individuals or we might wish to assess the satisfaction of patients with their health care system. Self-esteem and patient satisfaction are constructs, and it is these sorts of phenomena that we describe in our research and explicate in our models.

Because constructs are abstractions or, more technically, *latent* variables, they are not directly measured. We must therefore assess them indirectly by (directly) measuring other variables that indicate or point to them. These directly measured variables are instances, exemplars, or specific aspects of the more general constructs. And that is where scales come in.

We estimate how much of the construct individuals possess by administering a scale or inventory to them, usually in written or electronic form but sometimes even orally. The responses to the items on the scale constitute our direct measurement. For example, to assess the construct of satisfaction with health care providers, we can ask patients how easy it was to make an appointment with their physician, how completely their physician answered their questions, and so on. These item responses are values on our measured variables and these values can be (statistically) bound together (e.g., by computing a total or an average score for the item responses) so as to achieve a composite or scale score. This scale score may then be used to represent the level of the construct for the average respondent, for example, the degree to which patients are satisfied with their health care provider.

Not everything we measure is a construct; some objectives can be measured directly, as in the body temperature example above. In public health, even our broader outcomes are often directly measurable (measuring the prevalence of a disease or condition). However, our efforts to influence these outcomes sometimes require us to modify human behavior: persuading people to stop smoking, use condoms, wear seat belts, or engage in exercise. Such attempts to influence behavior are often guided by health behavior theories (Glanz, Rimer, & Viswanath, 2008). In the process of applying these theories to create appropriate intervention strategies, we usually need to assess constructs concerning attitudes, beliefs, and motivations toward smoking, condom use, and so on by using scales developed for the particular purpose.

Scales of Measurement

Stevens (1946) defined measurement as "the assignment of numerals to objects or events according to rules" (p. 677). He identified four scales of measurement representing an escalating set of rules governing how these values were assigned to objects, and his general treatment of this topic became one of the cornerstones underlying data collection and analysis. The four measurement scales Stevens identified are, very briefly, as follows:

- *Nominal measurement* represents sorting entities into categories (e.g., categorizing drugs into seven schedules). The values are the category labels (e.g., Schedule III), and the entities are those drugs meeting the criteria for the category (e.g., Vicodin and Tylenol with codeine are classified as Schedule III drugs). This represents *qualitative* measurement.
- *Ordinal measurement* represents a rank ordering of entities on some quantity, thus permitting *greater than* and *less than* statements. We can say, for example, that Patient A appears to be the most energetic, Patient B appears to be next most energetic, Patient C is less energetic than Patient B, and Patient D appears to be the least energetic of the group.

- *Interval measurement* represents a status of quantitative measurement that we often approximate in the scales that we use. At this level of measurement, the intervals between values are constant across the scale but the zero point is arbitrary (zero does not mean the absence of the quantity). The most common example of an interval scale is temperature, where the difference in heat between 101 and 102 degrees is equal to the difference between 102 and 103 degrees. Because the zero value (on a Fahrenheit or Centigrade scale) does not reflect the absence of temperature, we cannot assert any judgments of ratio or proportion (we cannot legitimately assert that 80 degrees is twice as hot as 40 degrees). A summated response format (e.g., a 5-point response format with 1 representing *very little* and 5 representing *very much*), used extensively in public health-related scales, approximates interval measurement. A host of statistical computations (e.g., means, standard deviations) can be meaningfully performed on interval or approximately interval scales.

- *Ratio measurement* represents the highest level of quantitative measurement. In ratio measurement, the intervals between values are constant across the scale (as is true for interval measurement) but the zero point does indicate the absence of the quantity. Time and distance are two examples of ratio scales. Because the zero value is absolute (e.g., zero distance means no distance), we can derive ratio judgments from the measurement. For example, we can legitimately say that someone who is 6 feet tall is twice as tall as someone who is 3 feet tall. The range of statistical computations applied to interval scales can also be meaningfully performed on ratio scales.

Validity of the Inferences Drawn From the Scale Score

Validity as the Weight of Evidence

Validity is the benchmark we strive to meet when we develop scales. The simplest expression of validity with reference to scales is that a scale measures what it is presumed to measure (CDC, 2011). A somewhat more explicit definition is that validity "refers to the degree to which evidence and theory support the interpretations of test scores" (American Educational Research Association [AERA], American Psychological Association [APA], & National Council on Measurement in Education [NCME], 1999, p. 9). Within this approach, we marshall evidence from a variety of sources, such as the reliability or measurement error associated with a set of scale items and the correlation of the scale score to measures of other related constructs, to make the case for the validity of our inferences. High-quality scales clearly and directly focus on their target construct with a minimum of measurement error and permit us to draw valid inferences from the scores.

Validity evidence also serves to set limits on the generalizability of our inferences. For example, Geary, Burke, and Wedderburn (2006) found that the widely popular Rosenberg Self-Esteem Scale was not applicable in a study of Jamaican adolescents aged 12 to 14 years. Without psychometric and validation information, it is not possible to know if we are accurately measuring the construct we think we are measuring. When public health decisions are made based on research results using inappropriate measurements, incorrect conclusions may be drawn, leading to inefficient use of scarce resources or to a mischaracterization of the dynamics underlying the behaviors we want to influence.

Validity Drives the Generation of Scale and Subscale Scores

Which scale items are combined to generate a score is not an arbitrary decision on the part of researchers. Rather, such a decision is based on validity evidence relating to the internal (statistical) structure of the scale. When the validity evidence permits us to combine all of the items into a single overall score, we speak of a *unidimensional* scale that assesses the construct as a whole; the total or average of the full item set is labeled as a *scale* value. When items assess two or more themes underlying the general construct, we speak of a *multidimensional* scale. In a multidimensional scale, each item is associated with just one of the themes, and we separately combine together only the responses of the subset of items representing each theme; the total or average of each item subset is labeled as a *subscale* value.

THE SCALE DEVELOPMENT PROCESS

Development of high-quality validated scales entails a series of ordered steps. The following, based in part on strategies suggested by Clark and Watson (1995), Dawis (1987), DeVellis (2011), Reise, Waller, and Comrey (2000), and Worthington and Whittaker (2005), represents one way to organize the scale development process and forms the structure of the remaining portion of this chapter:

- conceptualizing the construct
- selecting the response format
- developing the item pool
- reviewing the item pool
- selecting validation scales
- selecting the sample
- preliminary statistical evaluation of the items
- performing a structural analysis
- assessing the quality of measurement
- assembling validation evidence
- adopting a multicultural perspective

Conceptualizing the Construct

An appropriate starting point in any scale development project is to conceptualize the target construct by placing it in theoretical context. Further, it is necessary to specify the degree of construct specificity that will be assessed; that is, whether the scale is to be a relatively broad measure (e.g., a measure of health practitioner self-perceived cultural competence) or a narrow-band gauge of some behavior, attitudes, or values (e.g., a measure of health practitioner culturally competent interviewing skills).

Any construct conceptualization must be informed by a careful literature review, which should provide clarification of the construct's range of content, identification of problems with existing measures, and indications of whether a new scale is actually needed (Clark & Watson, 1995). Such a review should assess how others have conceptualized and operationalized the particular construct targeted for scale development as well as other related constructs. Theory helps put into context what is gleaned from the literature review; it delineates the conceptual boundaries of what the construct comprises and what it addresses (Dawis, 1987). A theory-driven literature review will also identify, early on, potential convergent and divergent patterns of correlation among other variables and constructs.

Historically, at least three types of (variously labeled) strategies have been suggested to facilitate how the construct to be scaled can be conceptualized (see, e.g., Brown, 1983; Downing & Haladyna, 2006; Edwards, 1970; Friedenberg, 1995; Worthington & Whittaker, 2005). A *rational* strategy uses the intuition and personal judgment of the scale developers to determine items representing the target construct. A *theoretical* strategy utilizes public health theory (or some other theoretical domain) to guide the development of an item pool. These strategies typically are integrated into an *empirical* strategy that often takes into account the results of research studies to generate items and uses statistical analysis to select and structure the items that will make up the scale. Clark and Watson (1995) recommend as a construct conceptualization exercise to generate a brief thesis statement describing the construct under development. This statement would address construct specificity in the form of the range of behaviors, values, or attitudes along the continuum represented by the construct.

Selecting the Response Format

Some Commonly Used Response Formats

There are several ways to format or structure the manner in which respondents affirm or endorse the items on an inventory. Table 13.2 presents examples of several of the available item formats that are used by researchers. Clark and Watson (1995) suggest that Likert (summated response) rating scales (with three or more options) and dichotomous scales (*yes-no*, *true-false*) are the two dominant response formats in modern scale construction.

Type represents the kind of data that are generated by the format: *bipolar* measurement represents a quantitative graded response measure in that there are a limited number of response choices (usually 5 or 7) based on a bipolar continuum (the anchors are opposite ends of the continuum); *analogue* measurement allows respondents to place a mark on a continuum (usually depicted by a line) to express the strength of their endorsement of the item content; *dichotomous* measurement allows respondents to either endorse or not endorse the content referred to in an item; and *graded response* measurement represents limited jumps in the endorsement of an item (the anchors represent very little or a good deal of endorsement of the content of the item).

Table 13.2 Examples of Several Item Formats

Format	Type	Stem	Response Mode
Semantic Differential	Bipolar	My personal physician is:	Cold ▯ ▯ ▯ ▯ ▯ ▯ ▯ Warm
Visual Analogue	Quantitative	My personal physician is:	Cold _____ Warm
Checklist	Dichotomous	My personal physician is:	Warm ▯
Summated Response	Graded Response	My personal physician warmly interacts with me:	Very Little 1 2 3 4 5 6 7 Very Much
Summated Response	Bipolar	My personal physician warmly interacts with me:	Disagree 1 2 3 4 5 6 7 Agree
Binary Rating	Dichotomous	My personal physician warmly interacts with me:	Yes ▯ No ▯

Semantic differential

The semantic differential technique, developed by Osgood, Suci, and Tannenbaum (1957; see also, Heise, 2010; Osgood, May, & Miron, 1975), was designed to measure the connotative meaning of concepts. Respondents are asked to choose where their feeling lies on a multiple-point response scale between two bipolar adjectives (e.g., *strong-weak, active-passive, good-bad*).

Visual analogue

The visual analogue response format measures subjective characteristics or attitudes that have respondents specify their level of agreement to an item by marking a position along a continuous line between two end-points. This continuous line or analogue is unique and distinct from the more common Likert (summative) or discrete psychometric scales. Recent computer-based Internet survey methodologies are increasing the popularity of this technique (Reips & Funke, 2008).

Checklists

Checklists permit respondents to examine a list of items and check or mark only those items that are applicable to them within a particular context. This approach, while easy to use, has garnered increasing criticism for its susceptibility to response bias effects (Clark & Watson, 1995; Green, Goldman, & Salovey, 1993).

Summated ratings

Summated response formats measure attitudes or characteristics by asking respondents to rate statements about a construct in terms of the extent to which they endorse its content (Likert, 1932; Likert, Roslow, & Murphy, 1934). Likert's original *strongly approve-strongly disapprove* anchors (labels defining the rating continuum) have given way to many others addressing issues of construct frequency (*infrequently-frequently*), degree or extent (*very little-very much*), similarity (*very similar-very dissimilar*), and agreement (*agree very little-agree very much*), but what is common to this sort of measurement is that there are graded (ordered) fixed-choice response options typically using from 4 to 7 scale points. These types of scales have become one of the most widely used scaling methods in behavioral and social science research (Monette, Sullivan, & DeJong, 2011). Although summated rating scales do not necessarily have equal intervals between their scale points, it is meaningful to compute means and standard deviations on the responses, and most researchers treat these scales as sufficiently interval-like to perform a full range of parametric statistical analyses (e.g., factor analysis, multiple regression) on such data.

Dichotomous or binary ratings

As the name implies, dichotomous items have two possible response options (e.g., *yes-no*, *true-false*, *agree-disagree*) and are very frequently used for knowledge assessment (e.g., multiple-choice items scored *correct-incorrect*) in educational and licensure/certification testing. One disadvantage of dichotomous items is that they restrict the range of item variance; respondents have only a pair of response choices (DeVellis, 2011). As a result, longer lists of dichotomous items are usually needed to at least partly compensate for the lack of variation. The dichotomous item format was extensively used in the middle portion of the 20th century (e.g., personality testing in psychology), but has since given way in many fields to summative response scales.

With dichotomously scored items, statistical procedures based on assumptions of the general linear model requiring at least approximately normal distributions of item data cannot be appropriately used. For example, linear factor analysis and principal components analysis are routinely used in the scale development process for a summated response format, but we instead should perform a full-information (nonlinear) factor or bifactor analysis for dichotomous items (Cai, Yang, & Hansen, 2011; McLeod, Swygert, & Thissen, 2001; Reise, Morizot, & Hays, 2007; Reise et al., 2011; Wirth & Edwards, 2007).

Developing the Item Pool

At the start of this step, the target construct has been conceptually elaborated, the content arenas subsumed by the construct have been identified, and the item format has been determined. Actual scale construction can now begin by developing a relatively large pool of items to be evaluated and trimmed down in statistical analyses to a manageable number that in combination will best assess the construct. The primary goal of developing an item pool is to ensure a systematic sampling of all content areas of the latent construct (Netemeyer, Bearden, & Sharma, 2003) while identifying the fewest items that explain the most variance.

Item Content

Each item that is developed should reflect some aspect of the underlying latent construct. In effect, item development can be thought of as sampling from a large domain of possible content depicting the construct under scrutiny. This sampling results in a sample of items from the domain that, individually and in combination, have adequate psychometric characteristics to permit us to draw a justifiable inference from the scale score.

Initial items are developed by the scale authors, are drawn or modified from the existing literature (without violating copyrights), and are suggested by expert judges or panel members (DeVellis, 2011; Netemeyer et al., 2003). These items should exhibit evidence of *content validity* of the various aspects of the targeted construct; that is, the items should align themselves with the content domain subsumed by the construct. In addition, Clark and Watson (1995), following the initial lead of Loevinger (1957), argue for proportional representation of items: More important or salient content areas should have more items, while narrower or less salient content topics should be represented by fewer items. Furthermore, *face validity,* or the appearance to respondents that the items are practical, pertinent, and related to the target construct, can be enhanced through careful consideration of the instrument reading level, clarity of items, and utility of response formats (Netemeyer et al., 2003; Nevo, 2005).

Number of Items

There is no minimum number of items to be included in an initial item pool. Typically, large item pools are desirable because they increase the odds of strengthening potential internal consistency reliability of the items (DeVellis, 2011). Perhaps the most important consideration is that scale developers provide a sufficient number of items of each content domain to ensure the survival of that representational facet in the final version of the scale. Item *redundancy* in the initial item pool development process should be expected and can help to ensure that a particular domain is captured (DeVellis, 2011).

Item Writing

Sources for item writing guidelines include Aiken (1997), Fowler (1995), and Kaplan and Saccuzzo (2012), and all agree that the ultimate goal is item clarity. Scale questions or statements should always be simple, clear, and unambiguous. To accomplish this, scale developers should use language that is straightforward and target the item at the appropriate reading level (Clark & Watson, 1995; Fry, 1977, 2002). Lengthy items are also to be avoided; the extra wording makes the reading level too high and often camouflages the gist of the issue being addressed.

Double-barreled items express two or more ideas simultaneously (Sudman & Bradburn, 1982) and should not be used. For example, consider the following hypothetical item: "Culturally competent health practitioners understand their own cultural biases and share a progressive political outlook with their clients." Some respondents who agree with the first part of this statement may have trouble answering the second part, or vice versa. Here, if both elements are important to assess, they should be addressed in separate (and thus simpler) items. A rule of thumb is that if an item contains an *or* or *and*, it likely needs to be split into two items.

One of the primary goals to be achieved by an item is to differentiate respondents from one another (assessed, in part, by a measure of item variability such as the standard deviation). To accomplish this goal, items should be written to maximize variability of endorsement across respondents. For example, we suspect that most respondents would select 5 (on a 5-point *disagree-agree* scale) in response to "My physician is some-times attentive to my concerns." To the extent that this happens, the variance of that item is close to zero (it supplies little information in differentiating respondents), its correlations with all other variables would be close to zero, and thus the item would not fare well in the item evaluation process. Such items ordinarily require editing before being used. In the above example, the word *sometimes* is likely driving respondents toward the higher response category because even rare events sometimes happen, and removing that word should increase the variance exhibited by the item.

Item *polarity* is an important consideration in the scale development process as well. It is natural, especially when initially developing items, to phrase them positively with respect to the construct. For example, if the construct is the quality of physician care, one aspect of it might be the attention given to patients drafted as the item "My physician is attentive to my concerns." Greater levels of endorsement of this item would presumably reflect a higher quality of physician care.

If all of the scale items are positively worded, and this is especially true for lengthy questionnaires, respondents can slip into *response sets* (patterns of responding) that increase measurement error. One such response set is *acquiescence bias,* where respondents tend to endorse items regardless of their content (Robinson, Shaver, & Wrightsman, 1991). A similar bias happens when respondents become careless, coming to believe that they no longer need to read (or carefully read) the items but simply record responses consonant with those they have provided to earlier items.

One way to guard against acquiescence and carelessness biases is to word some of the items *negatively* or in a *reverse* direction with respect to the construct (e.g., "My physician is *not* attentive to my concerns"). Such wording requires respondents to use both sides of the response scale across the range of inventory items in order to consistently reflect their standing on the construct rather than respond with values at one end of the scale (DeVellis, 2011). This will tend to break an acquiescence bias and will "catch" those who are no longer (carefully) reading the items. By incorporating this design feature, invalid response protocols may be implemented and flag data for removal from the data set.

Including negatively or reverse-worded items on a scale is common practice, but this strategy is now known to be problematic. We have recently come to realize that negatively worded construct-related items may be associated with a confounding method effect and/or generate separate statistical factors that make interpretation of the scale values more ambiguous (Chen, Rendina-Gobioff, & Dedrick, 2010; DiStefano &

Motl, 2009; Podsakoff, MacKenzie, Lee, & Podsakoff, 2003; Schriesheim, Eisenbach, & Hill, 1991). If reverse-worded construct-related items are to be included, they should be carefully examined in the item evaluation step.

One possible way to guard against troublesome response sets but not cause methodological or statistical problems is to include reverse-worded *filler* (not-to-be-scored) items on the inventory. The key to success for this strategy is that the content of the filler items needs to be sufficiently similar to the scale content so that respondents do not recognize them as fillers. The responses on these filler items would not contribute to the scale or subscale score but would be used only to detect invalid profiles (and hopefully break an acquiescence bias).

Reviewing the Item Pool

With the initial item pool in hand, it is now time to consider having a panel of experts—a group of professional colleagues or experts in the field in general—evaluate the item content. Typically, experts are asked to evaluate each item in terms of *relevancy* to the target construct. Panel members can also evaluate each item's *clarity* as well as the possibility or potential for *bias* against any groups (e.g., inappropriate wording for a particular gender or ethnic group). Items presenting difficulties or concerns to the panel can be eliminated or rewritten. Panel members may also be able to suggest any facets of the construct that may have been overlooked, or a facet included in the item set that was interpreted incorrectly or incompletely by the item writers. Through the process of independent assessment of item relevancy, clarity, completeness, and correctness, evidence of *content validity* (the extent to which items measure a particular content domain) is enhanced (DeVellis, 2011).

Selecting Validation Scales

Whenever possible, scale developers should include additional measures in their data collection. DeVellis (2011) and Clark and Watson (1995) suggest at least two purposes to be served by these additional measures: bias evaluation and description of the relationship of the new scale to other measures.

It is possible to use some measures to detect potential *underlying problems or biases*. One particularly salient issue found throughout the behavioral and social sciences research literature deals with *social desirability* effects, where respondents may try to answer items with socially desirable answers that may not reflect their true opinions (Pauls & Stemmler, 2003; but for an alternative interpretation, see McCrae & Costa, 1983; Welte & Russell, 1993). As a consequence, many researchers employ a measure of social desirability (e.g., Crowne & Marlowe, 1960; Reynolds, 1982) administered with the new scale items. Lack of a substantial correlation between the social desirability scale and the scores of the new instrument can be considered as evidence that social desirability may not have contaminated the item responses of the sample (Paulus, 1991).

Scale developers also need to address the *construct validity* of the scale (Cronbach & Meehl, 1955). Construct validity addresses, in part, the relationship between scores on the new scale and scores on established measures of related constructs. To partly generate such construct validation evidence, respondents are asked to complete a set of inventories in addition to the pilot items of the scale that is under development. Most of these other measures should represent constructs that researchers believe are correlated (either positively or negatively) with the construct under study. Confirming these expectations provides evidence of *convergent* validity (evidence of shared variance between the scale and other constructs). For example, a measure designed to assess anxiety should correlate relatively strongly with measures of neuroticism and depression (represented by positive correlations) as well as with a measure of self-esteem (represented by a negative correlation).

It is also useful to include a measure or two that is believed to be unrelated to the construct for which the scale is being developed; confirming very weak relationships provides evidence of *divergent* validity (evidence of relative independence between the scale and other constructs). For example, a measure of social desirability is commonly used as one of these divergent measures. Together, convergent and divergent sources of evidence contribute toward providing evidence for the construct validity of the new scale.

Although most methodologists are supportive of using construct validation measures in scale construction, a few have argued that such efforts should be limited during the early stages of instrument development (Worthington & Whittaker, 2005). The reasoning for this is to reduce questionnaire length and respondent fatigue; reducing the number of additional scales also aids in minimizing potential bias introduced by additional measures.

Selecting the Sample

Composition of the Sample

With an initial item pool in place and construct-relevant additional scales also identified, scale developers can now focus on drawing a sample of respondents (Daniel, 2012). This sample should capture respondents who represent a wide range on the construct and who are representative of the population in which the new scale is expected to be implemented. Such representativeness can be based on standard demographic variables (e.g., sex, age, ethnicity) as well as specialized demographic considerations. As an example of the latter, a scale designed to assess satisfaction with primary care physicians, should draw this sample of patients from a variety of health care settings in proportion to what is descriptive of the population of patients.

Sample Size

Whether the individual items are scored in a binary (e.g., *yes-no*), summated response (e.g., 5-point graded response scale), or more continuous manner, an adequate sample size must be set as a goal so as to support the statistical analyses we use to evaluate both the individual items that constitute the scale and the efficacy of the composite score of scale itself. There are two not necessarily incompatible approaches to item and scale analysis, classical test theory (CTT) and item response theory (IRT), and these different approaches are associated with somewhat different sample size requirements; within each approach, the sample size requirements for the different item scoring rubrics are the same.

Sample size using CTT

The term *test* in CTT has the same meaning as the terms *scale* and *inventory* as we have used them in this chapter. At a very general level, CTT rests on the presumption articulated over a century ago by Charles Spearman (1904) that the observed scale score (X) of an individual is composed of two elements, a *true score* component (T) and an *error* component (E), which are interwoven in the single score we obtain for any test taker; thus, X = T + E.

Two related ideas follow from these presumptions. First, as suggested by Spearman (1907), the correlation computed between two measures results in an attenuated value of the correlation coefficient because of the presence of measurement error in the scores. Spearman argued that we should statistically correct for such attenuation in order to estimate the true correlation. Second, we can conceive of a statistic that came to be called a reliability coefficient representing, at least theoretically, the ratio of true score variance to observed score variance. Traub (1997) provides a relatively complete historical perspective of CTT.

From this general foundation of CTT, several statistical procedures relating to item and test analysis (covered later in this chapter) have been generated. For the results of these procedures to be stable requires a reasonably large sample size (DeVellis, 2011). It has been suggested that the sample should be a minimum of 300 respondents (Clark & Watson, 1995; Guadagnoli & Velicer, 1988; Nunnally & Bernstein, 1994). Such a sample size should eliminate any concerns about respondent variance and stands a better chance to have incorporated a diverse set of respondents.

CTT is still widely used today because it is simple and functional. It can meet the basic needs of many scale developers and does not require specialized software beyond the common statistical packages (e.g., IBM SPSS, SAS). However, there is a clear shift in the field toward the use of IRT when it is possible to do so. Although IRT does require special software, its impressive capability is attracting more users (Fan, 1998). Almost all of the major national educational testing programs, some of the intelligence testing programs, and increasingly more public health testing programs are based on IRT scale development and evaluation models.

Sample size using item response theory

According to the historical account of Hambleton and Jones (1993), Frederic Lord (1952, 1953) observed that respondents possess a certain amount of the characteristic or "ability" that is measured by the scale, and that their ability level thus mediates the score that they achieve on the measure. This may seem obvious, but certain consequences follow from it. For example, respondents with moderate levels of ability (e.g., people exhibiting moderate levels of knowledge) will exhibit relatively high scale scores on "easy" tests (e.g., measures testing for low levels of knowledge) and relatively low scale scores on "difficult" tests (e.g., measures testing for high levels of knowledge).

The implications of Lord's observation for the field of measurement were much less obvious but very far reaching, and led to the development IRT. It was originally called

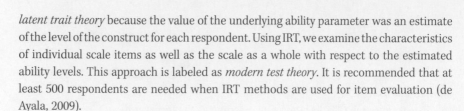

latent trait theory because the value of the underlying ability parameter was an estimate of the level of the construct for each respondent. Using IRT, we examine the characteristics of individual scale items as well as the scale as a whole with respect to the estimated ability levels. This approach is labeled as *modern test theory*. It is recommended that at least 500 respondents are needed when IRT methods are used for item evaluation (de Ayala, 2009).

Preliminary Statistical Evaluation of the Items

Recoding Reverse-Worded Items

Once the data have been collected from the sample of respondents and screened for coding violations (Meyers, Gamst, & Guarino, 2013a), any construct-related items that have been worded negatively must be reverse scored. For example, on a scale designed to assess the quality of physician care, the item "My physician is *not* attentive to my concerns" would need to be reverse scored. Assuming that a 5-point graded (ordered) response scale was used, the item should be recoded such that responses of 1 are transformed to 5, responses of 2 be transformed to 4, and so on. Thus, respondents with relatively high standing on the construct would have responded 1 or 2 to the original (reverse-worded) item but would have scores of 4 or 5 on the recoded item; it is this recoded item that is included in the data analysis rather than the original one.

Obtaining Item Means and Standard Deviations

Ideally, we wish to select items for the scale that exhibit a reasonable amount of variability (e.g., on a 5-point scale, standard deviations in the general range of 1.00 or higher). The variability of scores on an item is at least partly related to its mean. For example, if the mean for a given item assessed on a 5-point scale is 4.75, then the responses are concentrated at the upper end of the scale and the variability is therefore likely to be relatively low. It is also likely that the distribution of responses is highly skewed. Items with means toward the center of the scale are more likely to have acceptable variances and, all else equal, are preferred (DeVellis, 2011). Items with very limited variance (regardless of their means) are immediate candidates for removal, as the main statistical analyses will be based on the variance (how well the items differentiate respondents) and covariance (correlations) of the items.

Frequencies of Endorsement for the Response Alternatives

To supplement examining the item means and standard deviations, we also want to inspect the frequencies of endorsement for each response category to determine how many scale points were functionally being used by respondents. For example, it is possible that by infrequently selecting two of the five possible response categories a 5-point scale is functionally reduced down to a 3-point scale, and this loss of information will be reflected in the item variances.

Correlations of the Items

After reviewing the descriptive statistics and frequencies of endorsements for the response categories, it is important to examine the correlations of the items. This review should focus on two issues: the presence of negative correlations and the observation of very high correlation values. If two items are negatively correlated much beyond a zero value, then we infer that one is oriented positively and the other is oriented negatively on the construct. Had we properly identified all of the reverse-worded items and had we recoded them, we should not obtain negative correlations; the presence of such correlations suggests that one of the items was not recoded or is problematic, and that can be easily corrected at this point (e.g., deleting the item, recoding the item).

The other issue of interest in reviewing the correlation results is locating any relatively strong correlations among the item pairs, as the presence of such correlations could artificially generate a spurious factor in the structural analysis and may be a cause of local item dependence. Generally speaking, items correlated in the range of .70 or higher may be too strongly related for both to be appropriately retained as it is likely they are addressing very similar content. Ordinarily, the most expendable of these items (based on its content or its descriptive statistics) is removed at this point.

Performing a Structural Analysis

Measurement theory, whether CTT or IRT, presumes that there is a single underlying ability, characteristic, or dimension that is assessed by a scale (or subscale), thus allowing items to be combined in a meaningful way. The determination of whether it is appropriate to use a full scale score based on all of the items or separate subscale scores (and which items to combine if there are to be subscales) must be based on evidence of *internal structure* (AERA et al., 1999). Put simply, if the statistical analysis indicates that the items can all be combined together (the item set is unidimensional), then we may validly compute a full scale score; if the statistical analysis indicates that the items are more appropriately treated as subsets (the item set is multidimensional), then we may validly compute a set of subscale scores.

Identifying the Number of Underlying Dimensions

The next step of the scale development process is therefore to perform a structural analysis of the item data with the goal of identifying how many underlying latent dimensions are subsumed by the items (Briggs & Cheek, 1986; Clark & Watson, 1995; Comrey, 1988; Floyd & Widaman, 1995, Meyers et al., 2013a; Reise et al., 2000; Worthington & Whittaker, 2005). This can be accomplished by performing an exploratory factor analysis (EFA) for items that are not dichotomous, although EFA does not preclude conducting additional dimensional analyses in the context of IRT (M. C. Edwards, 2009; Wirth & Edwards, 2007). With dichotomous items, scale developers should go directly to an IRT nonlinear dimensional analysis (McLeod et al., 2001; Swygert, McLeod, & Thissen, 2001) or, if such an analysis is not feasible, at least use specialized software to factor analyze a matrix of tetrachoric correlations (see Panter, Swygert, Dahlstrom, & Tanaka, 1997).

All of the major software packages include several extraction (e.g., principal components, principal axis, unweighted and generalized least squares, maximum likelihood) and rotation methods (orthogonal strategies such as varimax and oblique strategies such as promax) within their EFA procedure. Most researchers use several extraction methods to ensure that the factor structure is stable across the methods and then select one to report; there is considerable evidence to indicate that these methods generally produce comparable results (e.g., Velicer & Jackson, 1990).

If the factor analysis indicates that there are multiple factors (facets of the construct), they are very likely to be correlated with each other because they derive from the larger construct. For the rotation phase, we therefore recommend starting with an oblique rotation strategy (e.g., promax) as such a strategy allows the factors to be correlated when they are rotated and will better represent the relationships between the variables than will an orthogonal rotation (Gorsuch, 1983, 1990, 2003; Meyers et al., 2013a; Thompson, 2004).

Examining the Relationships of the Items to the Factors

Most researchers adopt a pragmatic approach to achieving the final solution by examining two or three different rotated solutions, each with a different number of factors, and evaluating the strength of the coefficients relating each item to the factor with which it is most strongly correlated. Items should be associated with only one factor, an idea known as *simple structure* (Thurstone, 1947); items that correlate reasonably strongly with more than one factor (items that "cross-load" on the factors) should very likely be removed from the set at this point, as they are not adding to the clarity of the solution. Items exhibiting low correlations with all factors should also be eliminated. The factor analysis should be performed again without these problematic items, as it is possible that the factor structure can change somewhat with a reduced item set in the analysis.

Typically, scale items are deleted or retained depending on the magnitude of the structure/pattern coefficients (their "loadings" on the factors). Various suggestions have been offered regarding how high a coefficient value should be to recommend retention; these have ranged from a lenient value of .32 (Worthington & Whittaker, 2005) through a moderate value of .40 (Meyers et al., 2013a) to .50 when data reduction is a primary objective (Gamst et al., 2004).

Ultimately, by examining the content of those items most strongly associated with each factor, scale developers will reach the most reasonable and parsimonious interpretation of the factors with respect to existing theoretical models and empirical research. Factor interpretation is driven by the items that are most strongly correlated with it; that is, whatever content those items have in common (whatever ties them together conceptually) is the interpretation of the factor.

Working With the Items Retained From the Factor Analysis

Once the scale developers have settled on a rotated factor structure and have identified (named) their factor(s), they have an initial (tentative) list of items to consider bringing into the next step of scale development. Even after eliminating items that violate the criteria for simple structure, not all of the items are likely to survive to the next step, as some may not be sufficiently related to the factor to serve as indicators of it.

Of those items surviving this review, it is important to identify any that correlate inversely with respect to the other items (e.g., an item correlating negatively with its factor while all of the other items associated with that factor correlate positively). Such items will need to be recoded at this point, as the next step will be to combine all of the items within each factor, and they all need to be oriented in the same direction for the scale or subscale value to be properly interpreted.

If it has been determined that the scale appears to be multidimensional, a full-scale measure may not be completely out of the question. Researchers can use a technique known as (nonlinear) full-information *bifactor* analysis (within an IRT context). The issue addressed by such an analysis is whether the scale could be treated as being *essentially unidimensional* (Cai et al., 2011, Gibbons et al., 2007; Reise et al., 2007), thus permitting the subscales to be reabsorbed into a full-scale measure.

Assessing the Quality of Measurement

We now have a known factor structure (for discussion purposes we assume that the set of items is multidimensional) and we have identified the subsets of items that are related to each factor; in principle, we have our subscales, although some further trimming of more peripheral items should be expected. CTT analyses address the relationship of the items to the other items constituting the subscale and the amount of measurement error associated with each subscale. IRT analyses can then focus on item characteristics and test information/reliability. Both culminate in examining differential item functioning.

Assessing the Relationship of the Items to Their Respective Subscale

The score on each item constituting the subscale is expected to appropriately relate to that subscale value. Within CTT, this relationship is indexed by the *corrected item-total correlation*, which is the correlation between each subscale item and the total of the other subscale items. We compute this correlation for each item in each subscale and interpret the results as described in Table 13.3.

It should be noted that deleting items could affect the factor structure, and so the factor analysis should be performed on the reduced item set. Thus, factor analysis and item analysis represent iterative steps until a stable and workable set of high-quality items is achieved.

Measurement Error: Reliability as Indexed by Coefficient Alpha

Once the item set has been reduced, it is best practice to report the degree of measurement error associated with any developed scales (AERA et al., 1999). A commonly used index of measurement error is the reliability coefficient. Within CTT, an observed score is said to be composed of both true score and error variance, and a reliability coefficient can be conceived as representing the ratio of true score variance to total observed variance (Lord & Novick, 1986; Nunnally & Bernstein, 1994). Reliability theoretically ranges between 1.00 and .00, with 1.00 denoting that observed scores are composed only of true score variance (there is no measurement error) and .00 indicating that all of the observed variance is due to measurement error. The *coefficient alpha* developed by Cronbach (1951) is currently the most widely used reliability coefficient.

Coefficient alpha reflects the degree to which scale items are correlated and is said to represent the *internal consistency* of a scale; within CTT, it is the estimated lower boundary of the reliability for the population (McDonald, 1999). Generally recommended minimum alpha coefficients are .70 and preferably .80 or above when taking both item count and sample size into consideration (Clark & Watson, 1995; Nunnally & Bernstein, 1994; Ponterotto & Ruckdeschel, 2007).

There are two major limitations associated with coefficient alpha that are not necessarily recognized by casual users. First, coefficient alpha is very sensitive to the number of items on the scale; very generally, longer scales are associated with higher values of coefficient alpha. Because coefficient alpha can be artificially inflated by the number of items on the scale, the average item correlations should also be examined as a check on internal consistency (e.g., Clark & Watson, 1995; DeVellis, 2011; Meyers, Gamst, & Guarino, 2013b). The second major limitation associated with coefficient alpha is that high values of coefficient alpha do not guarantee that the items constitute a unidimensional item set. This is the case because sets of items each related to separate factors could correlate sufficiently strongly within their sets to yield a high value of coefficient alpha for the entire item array (Cortina, 1993).

Measurement Error: Standard Error

The reliability coefficient is a unit-free general index of the degree to which a scale is error-free, and we can use it to compare scales with each other. The standard error of measurement conveys the same information (the amount of measurement error) but does so in test score units; as such, it is specific to a particular scale.

We have known for more than half a century that the overall standard error of measurement is not constant across the range of test scores (Feldt, Steffen, & Gupta, 1985; Mollenkopf, 1949; Thorndike, 1951). If scale developers intend to address the error of measurement around any specific scale or subscale score, then they should compute the *conditional standard error of measurement*, that is, the value of the standard error of measurement around that particular score (e.g., using the procedure provided by Mollenkopf, 1949). The overall standard error of measurement is the average of the conditional standard errors of measurement across the score range.

IRT Models

For scales using ordered response categories, such as summated response formats, one of the more popular models (Edwards, 2009) that has been used to perform IRT analysis is the graded response model (GRM; Samejima, 1969, 1997), an

Table 13.3 Interpreting Corrected Item-Total Correlations for Scale Development

Valence	Magnitude	Interpretation
Positive	>.15	Desirable
		Higher scores on the item are associated with higher scale or subscale scores
		Item is a mini-indicator of scale or subscale
	.15 to .19	Acceptable
	.20 to .29	Good
	.30 to .39	Very good
	>.40	Excellent
Zero	.07 to −.07	Not desirable
		There is little or no relationship between scores on the item and scores on the scale or subscale
		Item is not an indicator to scale or subscale
		Item does not contribute to scale or subscale
		Item is a candidate for removal from scale or subscale
Negative	<−.07	Indicative of a problem with the item
		Higher scores on the item are associated with lower scores on scale or subscale
		Item is a counter-indicator of scale or subscale
		If missed in recoding any reverse worded items in scoring, then the item should be recoded and the reliability analysis should be performed again
		If it was not missed in recoding any reverse worded items, then it is likely that the item needs to be removed from scale or subscale and potentially replaced with one representing very similar content

extension of the more widely recognized two parameter logistic model (2PLM; Birnbaum, 1968) appropriate for dichotomously scored items. IRT analysis can model performance at both the item and the scale level. Evaluating both individual items and the scale as a whole using the same metrics allows scale developers to fine-tune the scale to meet the research or applied needs. For example, it would be possible to structure an inventory whose items in combination could maximally differentiate between patients who were on the brink of clinical depression versus those who were less severely depressed.

IRT Item Characteristics

IRT analyses fit S-shaped (e.g., logistic) functions with one, two, three, or (very rarely) four parameters to the item data. These functions, known as *item characteristic curves (ICCs)*, *item response functions*, or *trace lines*, depict for each item the relationship between theta (ability) on the horizontal axis and the probability of response on the vertical axis. Both the 2PLM and GRM estimate *discrimination* and *location* (*difficulty*) parameters. Discrimination (indexed by an *a* parameter) gauges how well items can differentiate respondents along the theta continuum; it represents the slope of the logistic function at its steepest point and is conceptually akin to loadings in factor analysis. All else equal, items with higher values on the discrimination parameter are more related to theta (they are more discriminating) and are stronger candidates for inclusion on the subscale; Baker (1985) suggests some criteria to evaluate the magnitude of this parameter.

Figure 13.1 illustrates ICCs for dichotomously scored items. The top graph depicts two relatively easier items, and the lower graph depicts two relatively more difficult items. Both are S-shaped, but the item with the steeper slope can do a better job of discriminating different ability levels of the respondents (within the range of steepness) than the item with the less steep slope.

Local Item Independence

Both CTT and IRT assume local item independence. In CTT, this is taken to mean that measurement errors are not correlated to the true scores of test takers (Yen, 1993). In IRT, the assumption of independence is met when, after fitting the IRT model to the data and removing the effects of ability as a common source of variance, little relationship between items remains (de Ayala, 2009; Yen, 1993).

Violations of local item independence can adversely affect the ordinary scoring and interpretation of scales (Steinberg & Thissen, 1996) and will produce overestimates of reliability and underestimates of the standard error of measurement (Sireci, Thissen, & Wainer, 1991; Thissen, Steinberg, & Mooney, 1989). Some of the new IRT software programs are designed to determine which pairs of items exhibit local dependence, allowing scale developers to either retain one of each pair in constructing the subscale or, if the situation warrants, score related (locally dependent) sets of items as testlets (Sireci et al., 1991; Steinberg & Thissen, 1996; Thissen et al., 1989; Yen, 1993).

Figure 13.1   Two Sets of Item Characteristic Curves (ICCs) Showing Differences in Discrimination for Relatively Easier Items and Relatively More Difficult Items

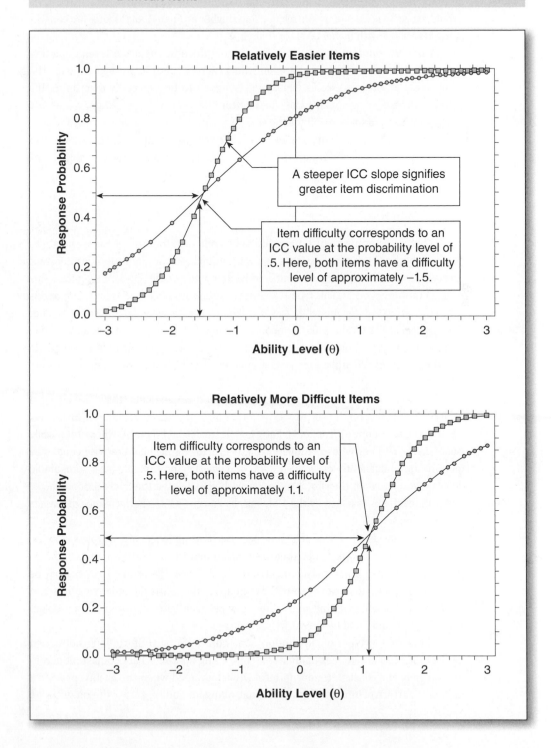

IRT Test Analysis

At the scale level, we can obtain from IRT a *test characteristic curve* that will inform us of the relationship between ability (theta) and the estimated total score. Generally, we would expect to see a monotonic relationship (higher estimated total scores are consistently associated with higher levels of ability).

A *test information function* can also be obtained at the scale level, depicting how well the scale can differentiate individuals across the ability range. Not surprisingly, most all-purpose scales (those not designed to be especially discriminating within only a narrow ability band) do a better job toward the middle of the ability range; however, it speaks well for the scale if it can provide a reasonable amount of information for most ability values. From the test information function, we also obtain a reliability (standard error of measurement) distribution across ability (see Embretson & Reise, 2000).

DIF Analysis

Once we determine which items are to be combined to form a scale or subscales and which items have characteristics that warrant inclusion on the scale, it is important that we perform an assessment of differential item functioning (DIF) on each item surviving the above process. This type of analysis has been available in a variety of iterations since the late 1950s (see Russell & Zickar, 2005) and can be carried out in the context of CTT as well as IRT (Oishi, 2006; Zumbo, 2007). For a DIF analysis to be performed, two or more groups based on relevant demographic variables (e.g., ethnicity, sex, geographic location, institutional affiliation, medical condition) within the respondent set must be identified.

DIF is said to occur when subsets of *equal ability* respondents (they have an equal estimated standing on the construct) perform differently on a given item (AERA et al., 1999; Hidalgo & López-Pina, 2004). For example, males and females whose total scale score (using CTT) or whose estimated ability level (using IRT) is otherwise equal may perform quite differently on a given item. Because they presumably have comparable ability levels based on their total scores or on their estimated theta levels, some factor other than what is assessed by the scale may be causing such a performance difference on that item.

DIF is considered to be problematic because, if the members of the groups have the same standing on the construct, then they should perform similarly on an item that is supposed to be part of its measurement. If DIF is obtained, then either the item may be *biased* with respect to one or more of those groups or the construct underlying that item may have a different meaning across those groups; in either case, it suggests a problem with the item and could be a basis for removing it.

There are two types of DIF: uniform and non-uniform. Uniform DIF is obtained when the group differences on an item (controlling for ability) are consistent across the range of the construct; non-uniform DIF is obtained when the groups provide a different pattern of item performance (controlling for ability) across the range of the construct.

Assembling Validation Evidence

At the time that the interim item pool was being pilot tested, respondents were also asked to complete a set of validation scales to establish the external validity of the to-be-developed scale. Now that the scale has been developed from the above steps, the scale or subscales may be computed and correlated with the other measures. Expectations about the relative strengths of these correlations have already been articulated in the process of their selection, and the correlation results will inform the scale developers about the convergent and divergent evidence to support use of the newly created scale.

Having developed a scale and provided validity evidence concerning its content, internal structure, and relationships with external measures may be sufficient for disseminating the scale in the professional literature or using it in applied settings, but the validation work is not complete. Subsequent research by the scale developers themselves and by other researchers in the field should be conducted (assuming that the scale has a wide enough appeal to be used in later research). Such later research is very likely to focus on additional applications of the scale and will likely involve examining its relationship with still other constructs to which it may eventually be linked.

An arena likely to be pursued in subsequent research is confirmatory factor analysis (CFA), one element of structural equation modeling (see Blunch, 2008; Cudeck & du Toit, 2009; Harrington, 2009; Raykov & Marcoulides, 2006; Thompson, 2004). Unlike EFA, a procedure that is intended to identify the initial factor structure of a scale, CFA is performed with the goal of assessing how well the proposed or hypothesized factor structure fits the data (Meyers et al., 2013a). This procedure allows for the new models to be directly compared to the original EFA (Worthington & Whittaker, 2005).

CFA may also be extended to a *multi-group analysis*. Here, the confirmatory model is applied to the data of two or more groups (e.g., males and females; African Americans, Latino/a Americans, and White Americans) to assess model *invariance*—the equivalency of the model across groups (Byrne, 2010). Should the groups differ in model fit, it is possible to determine where such differences may lie within the model, as there may be only one or two paths that are different across groups. Invariance analysis may also be conducted in the context of IRT; CFA and IRT analyses each have their advantages (Reise, Widaman, & Pugh, 1993).

Adopting a Multicultural Perspective

We live in a multinational world and in an increasingly multicultural environment. For example, in America the Latino/a and Asian populations are dramatically increasing (Dana & Allen, 2008). Further, nearly 30 million households speak Spanish at home, coupled with over 1 million people speaking languages other than English (APA, 2003). Historically, the social, behavioral, and health sciences have treated cultural variables in a historical progression from largely ignoring them or relegating them as extraneous factors or error variance to the more recent trend in research to incorporate multicultural phenomena as central contextual variables (Gamst, Liang, & Der-Karabetian, 2011; Hill, Pace, & Robbins, 2010).

With the increasing prominence of cultural and multicultural assessment, formulations, and considerations, it is useful for health-related scale developers to be cognizant of at least four cultural limitations embedded within much of the psychometric and methodological research literature:

- The focus has been on individual aspects of behavior, the capturing of individualistic appraisals, cognitions and values, with little concern for collectivistic and ecological behavioral determinants (Quintana, Troyano, & Taylor, 2001).
- Much of the research literature is built on convenience sampling (primarily college students), which may not be representative of the populations served in the arena of public health.
- Within-group racial/ethnic differences, often reflected in respondent social class, language preference, regional differences, tribal afflation, and so on (U.S. Department of Health and Human Services, 2001), are often ignored.
- Scale development can explicitly be designed to serve the communities it studies (LaFromboise & Jackson, 1996) and thus can be a collaborative process between the researchers and the community participants (Trimble & Fisher, 2006).

Scale developers would do well to become aware of the cultural limitations of the various standardized instruments, practices, and methods and how research participants with diverse characteristics interpret and respond to the scale items (Clarke, 2000; Helms, 2002; Ridley, Hills, & Li, 1998; Westermeyer & Janca, 1997).

EMERGING ISSUES AND FUTURE DIRECTIONS

The Institute of Medicine (2001) maintains that clinical protocols—the standards of care for a particular health condition developed by multidisciplinary groups that constitute best practices—need to be based on research evidence, which in turn is ultimately based on the measurement procedures underlying the research that generates such evidence. Although some of that measurement is focused on physical systems, much of that research addresses constructs that are appropriately assessed by scales. As the measurement field expands, refines our understanding of measurement, and enhances our measurement procedures, we can apply these advances in the domain of public health.

This chapter has outlined the steps to develop high-quality validated scales. The prescribed steps will undoubtedly increase the amount of time and cost to conduct research, but we believe the benefits of using valid measures in research to inform public health decisions is worth the additional resources. Some public health researchers may be met with resistance when attempting to obtain resources to develop and validate scales. However, if the need for these resources is articulated and the benefits for this investment demonstrated, then we may be able to build this often neglected pool of resources. Seeking input from colleagues outside the field of public health who routinely work on measurement refinement, such as those from psychology and education testing fields, may help us frame our argument for devoting more attention to measurement at the proposal writing stage. We can also increase expectation for the routine use of high-quality scales within the field of public health by including a set of validation scales in questionnaires to establish the external validity of new scales we are attempting to use and, importantly, report these findings at conferences and in journal articles. Over time these steps have potential to make standard the use of validated scales in public health research involving latent constructs.

ADDITIONAL RESOURCES

Clark, L. A., & Watson, D. (1995). Construction validity: Basic issues in objective scale development. *Psychological Assessment, 7,* 309–319.

DeVellis, R. F. (2011). *Scale development: Theory and applications* (3rd ed.). Thousand Oaks, CA: Sage.

Gamst, G., Liang, C. T. H., & Der-Karabetian, A. (2011). *Handbook of multicultural measures.* Thousand Oaks, CA: Sage.

Meyers, L. S., Gamst, G., & Guarino, A. J. (2013a). *Applied multivariate research: Design and interpretation* (2nd ed.). Thousand Oaks, CA: Sage.

Netemeyer, R. G., Bearden, W.O., & Sharma, S. (2003). *Scale development in the social sciences: Issues and applications.* Thousand Oaks, CA: Sage.

REFERENCES

Aiken, L. R. (1997). *Questionnaires and inventories: Surveying opinions and assessing personality.* New York, NY: Wiley.

American Educational Research Association, American Psychological Association, & National Council on Measurement in Education. (1999). *Standards for educational and psychological testing.* Washington, DC: American Psychological Association.

American Psychological Association. (2003). Guidelines on multicultural education, training, research, practice, and organizational change for psychologists. *American Psychologist, 58,* 377–402.

Baker, F. B. (1985). *The basics of item response theory.* Portsmouth, NH: Heinemann.

Birnbaum, A. (1968). Some latent trait models and their use in inferring an examinee's ability. In F. M. Lord & M. R. Novick (Eds.), *Statistical theories of mental test scores* (pp. 392–479). Reading, MA: Addison-Wesley.

Blunch, N. J. (2008). *Introduction to structural equation modeling using SPSS and AMOS.* Thousand Oaks. CA: Sage.

Briggs, S. R., & Cheek, J. M. (1986). The role of factor analysis in the development and evaluation of personality scales. *Journal of Personality, 54,* 106–148.

Brown, F. G. (1983). *Principles of educational and psychological testing* (3rd ed.). New York, NY: Holt, Rinehart & Winston.

Byrne, B. M. (2010). *Structural equation modeling with AMOS: Basic concepts, applications and programming* (2nd ed.). New York, NY: Routledge.

Cai, L, Yang, J. S., & Hansen, M. (2011). Generalized full-information item bifactor analysis. *Psychological Methods, 16,* 221–248.

Centers for Disease Control and Prevention. (2011). *CDC HRQOL-14 "healthy days measure."* Retrieved from http://www.cdc.gov/hrqol/hrqol14_measure.htm

Chen, Y.-H., Rendina-Gobioff, G., & Dedrick, R. F. (2010). Factorial invariance of a Chinese self-esteem scale for third and sixth grade students: Evaluating method effects associated with positively and negatively worded items. *International Journal of Educational and Psychological Assessment, 6,* 21–35.

Clark, L. A., & Watson, D. (1995). Construction validity: Basic issues in objective scale development. *Psychological Assessment, 7,* 309–319.

Clarke, I., III. (2000). Extreme response style in multicultural research: An empirical investigation. *Journal of Social Behavior and Personality, 15,* 291–311.

Comrey, A. L. (1988). Factor-analytic methods of scale development in personality and clinical psychology. *Journal of Consulting and Clinical Psychology, 56,* 754–761.

Cortina, J. M. (1993). What is coefficient alpha? An examination of theory and application. *Journal of Applied Psychology, 78,* 98–104.

Cronbach, L. J. (1951). Coefficient alpha and the internal structure of tests. *Psychometrika, 16,* 297–334.

Cronbach, L. J., & Meehl, P. E. (1955). Construct validity in psychological tests. *Psychological Bulletin, 52,* 281–302.

Crowne, D. P., & Marlowe, D. (1960). A new scale of social desirability independent of psychopathology. *Journal of Consulting Psychology, 24,* 349–354.

Cudeck, R., & du Toit, S. H. C. (2009). General structure equation models. In R. E. Millsap & A. Maydeu-Olivares (Eds.), *The SAGE handbook of quantitative methods in psychology* (pp. 515–539). Thousand Oaks, CA: Sage.

Dana, R. H., & Allen, J. (Eds.). (2008). *Cultural competency training in a global society.* New York, NY: Springer.

Daniel, J. (2012). *Sampling essentials: Practical guidelines for making sampling choices.* Thousand Oaks, CA: Sage.

Dawis, R. V. (1987). Scale construction. *Journal of Counseling Psychology, 34,* 481–489.

de Ayala, R. J. (2009). *The theory and practice of item response theory.* New York, NY: Guilford.

DeVellis, R. F. (2011). *Scale development: Theory and applications* (3rd ed.). Thousand Oaks, CA: Sage.

DiClemente, R. J., Boyer, C. B., & Morales, E. S. (1988). Minorities and AIDS: Knowledge, attitudes, and misconceptions among Black and Latino adolescents. *American Journal of Public Health, 78*(1), 55–57.

DiStefano, C., & Motl, R. W. (2009). Self-esteem and method effects associated with negatively worded items: Investigating factorial invariance by sex. *Structural Equation Modeling, 16,* 134–146.

Downing, S. M., & Haladyna, T. M. (Eds.). (2006). *Handbook of test development.* New York, NY: Routledge.

Edwards, A. (1970). *The measurement of personality traits by scales and inventories.* New York, NY: Holt, Rinehart & Winston.

Edwards, M. C. (2009). An introduction to item response theory using the Need for Cognition scale. *Social and Personality Compass, 3/4,* 507–529.

Embretson, S. E., & Reise, S. P. (2000). *Item response theory for psychologists.* Mahwah, NJ: Lawrence Erlbaum.

Fan, X. (1998). Item response theory and classical test theory: An empirical comparison of the item/person statistics. *Educational and Psychological Measurement, 58,* 357–381.

Feldt, L. S., Steffen, M., & Gupta, N. C. (1985). A comparison of five methods for estimating the standard error of measurement at specific score levels. *Applied Psychological Measurement, 9,* 351–361.

Fisher, T. D., Davis, C. M., Yarber, W. L., & Davis, S. L. (2011). Handbook of sexuality-related measures (3rd ed.). New York, NY: Routledge.

Floyd, F. J., & Widaman, K. F. (1995). Factor analysis in the development and refinement of clinical assessment instruments. *Psychology Assessment, 7,* 286–299.

Fowler, F. J., Jr. (1995). *Improving survey questions.* Thousand Oaks, CA: Sage.

Friedenberg, L. (1995). *Psychological testing: Design, analysis, and use.* Boston, MA: Allyn & Bacon.

Fry, E. (1977). Fry's readability graph: Clarification, validity, and extension to level 17. *Journal of Reading, 21,* 242–254.

Fry, E. (2002). Readability versus leveling. *The Reading Teacher, 56,* 286–292.

Gamst, G., Dana, R. H., Der-Karabetian, A., Aragon, M., Arellano, L., Morrow, G., & Martenson, L. (2004) Cultural competency revised: The California Brief Multicultural Competence Scale. *Measurement and Evaluation in Counseling and Development, 37,* 163–183.

Gamst, G., Liang, C. T. H., & Der-Karabetian, A. (2011). *Handbook of multicultural measures.* Thousand Oaks, CA: Sage.

Geary, C. W., Burke, H. M., & Wedderburn, M. (2006). Self-esteem and sexual health interventions: Development and use of a culturally-relevant "self-esteem" measure to evaluate the Vibes program in Jamaica. In A. P. Prescott (Ed.), *The concept of self in medicine and health care* (pp. 173–203). New York, NY: Nova Science.

Gibbons, R. D., Weiss, D. J., Segawa, E., Bhaumik, D. K., Kupfer, D. J., Frank, E., . . . Stover, A. (2007). Full-information bifactor analysis of graded response data. *Applied Psychological Measurement, 31,* 4–19.

Glanz, K., Rimer, B. K., & Viswanath, K. (2008). *Health behavior and health education: Theory, research, and practice* (4th ed.). San Francisco, CA: Jossey-Bass.

Gorsuch, R. L. (1983). *Factor analysis* (2nd ed.) Hillsdale, NJ: Lawrence Erlbaum.

Gorsuch, R. L. (1990). Common factor analysis versus component analysis: Some well and little known facts. *Multivariate Behavioral Research, 25,* 33–39.

Gorsuch, R. L. (2003). Factor analysis. In J. A. Schinka & W. F. Velicer (Eds.), Handbook of psychology: Vol. 2. Research methods in psychology (pp. 143–164). Hoboken, NJ: Wiley.

Green, D. P., Goldman, S. L., & Salovey, P. (1993). Measurement error masks bipolarity in affect ratings. *Journal of Personality and Social Psychology, 64,* 1029–1041.

Guadagnoli, E., & Velicer, W. F. (1988). Relation of sample size to the stability of component patterns. *Psychological Bulletin, 103,* 265–275.

Hambleton, R. K., & Jones, R. W. (1993). Comparison of classical test theory and item response theory and their applications to test development. *Educational Measurement: Issues and Practices, 12,* 38–47.

Harrington, D. (2009). *Confirmatory factor analysis.* New York, NY: Oxford University Press.

Heise, D. R. (2010). *Surveying cultures: Discovering shared conceptions and sentiments.* New York, NY: Wiley.

Helms, J. E. (2002). A remedy for the Black-White test-score disparity. *American Psychologist, 57,* 303–304.

Helweg-Larsen, M., & Collins, B. E. (1994). The UCLA Multidimensional Condom Attitudes Scale: Documenting the complex determinants of condom use in college students. *Health Psychology, 13,* 224–237.

Hidalgo, M. D., & López-Pina, J. A. (2004). Differential item functioning detection and effect size: A comparison between logistic regression and Mantel-Haenszel procedures. *Educational and Psychological Measurement, 64,* 903–915.

Hill, J. S., Pace, T. M., & Robbins, R. R. (2010). Decolonizing personality assessment and honoring indigenous voices: A critical examination of the MMPI-2. *Cultural Diversity and Ethnic Minority Psychology, 16*(1), 16–25.

Institute of Medicine. (2001). *Crossing the quality chasm: A new health system for the 21st century.* Washington, DC: National Academy of Sciences.

Kalichman, S. C., Simbayi, L. C., Jooste, S., Toefy, Y., Cain, D., Cherry, C., & Kagee, A. (2005). Development of a brief scale to measure AIDS-related stigma in South Africa. *AIDS Behavior, 9,* 135–143.

Kaplan, R. M., & Saccuzzo, D. P. (2012). *Psychological testing: Principles, applications, and issues* (8th ed). Belmont, CA: Thomson Wadsworth.

LaFromboise, T. D., & Jackson, M. (1996). MCT theory and Native-American populations. In D. W. Sue, A. E. Ivey, & P. B. Pedersen (Eds.), *A theory of multicultural counseling and therapy* (pp. 192–203). Pacific Grove, CA: Brooks/Cole.

Levenson, H. (1981). Differentiating among internality, powerful others, and chance. In H. Lefcourt (Ed.), *Research with the locus of control construct* (pp. 15–63). New York, NY: Academic Press.

Likert, R. (1932). A technique for the measurement of attitudes. *Archives of Psychology, 140,* 5–53.

Likert, R., Roslow, S., & Murphy, G. (1934). A simple and reliable method of scoring the Thurstone attitude scales. *Journal of Social Psychology, 5,* 228–238.

Loevinger, J. (1957). Objective tests as instruments of psychological theory. *Psychological Reports, 3,* 635–694.

Lord, F. M. (1952). A theory of test scores. *Psychometric Monographs, 7.*

Lord, F. M. (1953). The relation of test score to the trait underlying the test. *Educational and Psychological Measurement, 28,* 517–548.

Lord, F. M., & Novick, M. R. (1968). *Statistical theories of mental test scores.* Reading, MA: Addison-Wesley.

McCrae, R. R., & Costa, P. T. (1983). Social desirability scales: More substance than style. *Journal of Consulting and Clinical Psychology, 51,* 882–888.

McDowell, I. (2006). Measuring health: A guide to rating scales and questionnaires (3rd ed.). New York, NY: Oxford University Press.

McDonald, R. P. (1999). *Test theory: A unified approach.* Mahwah, NJ: Lawrence Erlbaum.

McLeod, L. D., Swygert, K. A., & Thissen, D. (2001). Factor analysis for items scored in two categories. In D. Thissen & H. Wainer (Eds.), *Test scoring* (pp. 189–216). New York, NY: Routledge.

Meyers, L. S., Gamst, G., & Guarino, A. J. (2013a). *Applied multivariate research: Design and interpretation* (2nd ed.). Thousand Oaks, CA: Sage.

Meyers. L. S., Gamst, G., & Guarino, A. J. (2013b). *Performing data analysis using IBM SPSS.* Hoboken, NJ: Wiley.

Mollenkopf, W. G. (1949). Variation of the standard error of measurement. *Psychometrika, 14,* 189–229.

Monette, D. R., Sullivan, T. J., & DeJong, C. R. (2011). *Applied social research: A tool for the human services* (8th ed.). Belmont, CA: Brooks/Cole.

Netemeyer, R. G., Bearden, W. O., & Sharma, S. (2003). *Scale development in the social sciences: Issues and applications.* Thousand Oaks, CA: Sage.

Nevo, B. (2005). Face validity revisited. *Journal of Educational Measurement, 22,* 287–293.

Nunnally, J. C., & Bernstein, I. H. (1994). *Psychometric theory* (3rd ed.). New York, NY: McGraw-Hill.

Oishi, S. (2006). The concept of life satisfaction across cultures: An IRT analysis. *Journal of Research in Personality, 40,* 411–423.

Osgood, C. E., May, W. H., & Miron, M. S. (1975). *Cross-cultural universals of affective meaning.* Urbana, IL: University of Illinois Press.

Osgood, C. E., Suci, G., & Tannenbaum, P. (1957). *The measurement of meaning.* Urbana, IL: University of Illinois Press.

Panter, A. T., Swygert, K. A., Dahlstrom, W. G., & Tanaka, J. S. (1997). Factor analytic approaches to personality item-level data. *Journal of Personality Assessment, 68,* 561–589.

Pauls, C. A., & Stemmler, G. (2003). Substance and bias in social desirability responding. *Personality and Individual Differences, 35,* 263–275.

Paulus, D. L. (1991). Measurement and control of response bias. In J. P. Robinson & P. R. Shaver (Eds.), *Measures of personality and social psychological attitudes* (pp. 17–59). San Diego, CA: Academic Press.

Pearlin, L. I., & Schooler, C. (1978). The structure of coping. *Journal of Health and Social Behavior, 19,* 2–21.

Podsakoff, P. M., MacKenzie, S. B., Lee, J.-Y., & Podsakoff, M. P. (2003). Common method biases in behavioral research: A critical review of the literature and recommended remedies. *Journal of Applied Psychology, 88,* 879–903.

Ponterotto, J. G., & Ruckdeschel, D. E. (2007). An overview of coefficient alpha and reliability matrix for estimating adequacy of internal consistency coefficient with psychological research measures. *Perceptual and Motor Skills, 105,* 997–1014.

Pulerwitz, J., & Barker, G. (2008). Measuring attitudes towards gender norms among young men in Brazil: Development and psychometric evaluation of the GEM scale. *Men and Masculinities, 10,* 322–338.

Quintana, S. M., Troyano, N., & Taylor, G. (2001). Cultural validity and inherent challenges in quantitative methods for multicultural research. In J. G. Ponterotto, J. M. Casas, L. A. Suzuki, & C. M. Alexander (Eds.), *Handbook of multicultural counseling* (2nd ed., pp. 604–630). Thousand Oaks, CA: Sage.

Raykov, T., & Marcoulides, G. A. (2006). A first course in structural equation modeling (2nd ed.). New York, NY: Routledge.

Reips, U. D., & Funke, F. (2008). Interval-level measurement with visual analogue scales in Internet-based research: VAS Generator. *Behavioral Research Methods, 40,* 699–704.

Reise, S. P., Morizot, J., & Hays, R. D. (2007). The role of the bifactor model in resolving dimensionality issues in health outcomes measures. *Quality of Life Research, 16,* 19–31.

Reise, S. P., Ventura, J., Keefe, R. S. E., Baade, L. E., Gold, J. M., Green, M. F., . . . Seidman, L. J. (2011). Bifactor and item response theory analysis of interviewer report scales of cognitive impairment in schizophrenia. *Psychological Assessment, 23,* 245–261.

Reise, S. P., Waller, N. G., & Comrey, A. L. (2000). Factor analysis and scale revision. *Psychological Assessment, 12,* 287–297.

Reise, S. P., Widaman, K. F., & Pugh, R. H. (1993). Confirmatory factor analysis and item response theory: Two approaches for exploring measurement invariance. *Psychological Bulletin, 114,* 552–566.

Reynolds, W. M. (1982). Development of reliable and valid short forms of the Marlowe-Crowne social desirability scale. *Journal of Clinical Psychology, 38,* 119–125.

Rhodes, S. D., McCoy, T. P., Vissman, A. T., DiClemente, R. J., Duck, S., & Hergenrather, K. C. (2011). A randomized controlled trial of a culturally congruent intervention to increase condom use and HIV testing among heterosexually active immigrant Latino men. *AIDS Behavior, 15,* 1764–1775.

Ridley, C. R., Hills, C., & Li, L. (1998). Revisiting and refining the multicultural assessment procedure. *Counseling Psychologist, 6,* 939–947.

Robinson, J. P., Shaver, P. R., & Wrightsman, L. S. (1991). *Measures of personality and social psychological attitudes.* San Diego, CA: Academic Press.

Rosenberg, M. (1965). *Society and the adolescent self-image.* Princeton, NJ: Princeton University Press.

Russell, S. S., & Zickar, M. J. (2005). An examination of differential item and test functioning across personality judgments. *Journal of Research in Personality, 39,* 354–368.

Samejima, F. (1969). Estimation of latent ability using a response pattern of graded scores. *Psychometric Monographs, 17.*

Samejima, F. (1997). Graded response model. In W. J. van der Linden & R. K. Hambleton (Eds.), *Handbook of modern item response theory* (pp. 85-100). New York, NY: Springer.

Schriesheim, C. A., Eisenbach, R. J., & Hill, K. D. (1991). The effect of negation and polar opposite item reversals on questionnaire reliability and validity: An experimental investigation. *Educational and Psychological Measurement, 51,* 67–78.

Singh, A. S., Vik, F. N., Chinapaw, M. J., Uijtdewilligen, L., Verloigne, M., Fernandez-Alvira, J. M., . . . Brug, J. (2011). Test-retest reliability and construct validity of the ENERGY-child questionnaire on energy balance-related behaviours and their potential determinants: The ENERGY-project. *International Journal of Nutrition and Physical Activity, 8,* 136.

Sireci, S. G., Thissen, D., & Wainer, H. (1991). On the reliability of testlet-based tests. *Journal of Educational Measurement, 28,* 237–247.

Spearman, C. (1904). The proof and measurement of association between two things. *American Journal of Psychology, 15,* 72–101.

Spearman, C. (1907). Demonstration of formulae for the true measurement of correlation. *American Journal of Psychology, 18,* 160–169.

Stamatakis, K. A., McQueen, A., Filler, C., Boland, E., Dreisinger, M., Brownson, R. C., & Luke, D. A. (2012). Measurement properties of a novel survey to assess stages of organizational readiness for evidence-based interventions in community chronic disease prevention settings. *Implementation Science, 7,* 65.

Steinberg, L., & Thissen, D. (1996). Uses of item response theory and the testlet concept in the measurement of psychopathology. *Psychological Methods, 1,* 81–92.

Stevens, S. S. (1946). On the theory of scales of measurement. *Science, 103,* 677–680.

Sudman, S., & Bradburn, N. M. (1982). *Asking questions: A practical guide to questionnaire design.* San Francisco, CA: Jossey-Bass.

Swygert, K. A., McLeod, L. D., & Thissen, D. (2001). Factor analysis for items or testlets scored in more than two categories. In D. Thissen & H. Wainer (Eds.), *Test scoring* (pp. 217–249). Mahwah, NJ: Lawrence Erlbaum.

Thissen, D., Steinberg, L., & Mooney, J. A. (1989). Trace lines for testlets: A use of multiple-categorical-response models. *Journal of Educational Measurement, 26,* 247–260.

Thompson, B. (2004). *Exploratory and confirmatory factor analysis: Understanding concepts and applications.* Washington, DC: American Psychological Association.

Thorndike, R. L. (1951). Reliability. In E. F. Lindquist (Ed.), *Educational measurement* (pp. 560–620). Washington, DC: E. F. Lindquist.

Thurstone, L. L. (1947). *Multiple-factor analysis.* Chicago, IL: University of Chicago Press.

Traub, R. E. (1997). Classical test theory in historical perspective. *Educational Measurement: Issues and Practice, 16,* 8–14.

Trimble, J. E., & Fisher, C. (2006). *Handbook of ethical considerations in conducting research with ethnocultural populations and communities.* Thousand Oaks, CA: Sage.

U.S. Department of Health and Human Services. (2001). *Mental health: Culture, race and ethnicity.* Rockville, MD: Author.

Velicer, W. F., & Jackson, D.N. (1990). Component analysis versus common factor analysis: Some issues in selecting an appropriate procedure. *Multivariate Behavioral Research, 25,* 1–28.

Wallston, B. S., Wallston, K. A., Kaplan, G. D., & Maides, S. A. (1976). Development and validation of the Health Locus of Control (HLC) Scale. *Journal of Consulting and Clinical Psychology, 44,* 580–585.

Wegmann, L., Bühler, A., Strunk, M., Lang, M., & Nowak, D. (2012). Smoking cessation with teenagers: The relationship between impulsivity, emotional problems, program retention and effectiveness. *Addiction Behavior, 37,* 463–464.

World Health Organization. (1993). *WHOQoL study protocol*. Geneva, Switzerland: World Health Organization.

Welte, J. W., & Russell, M. (1993). Influence of socially desirable responding in a study of stress and substance abuse. *Alcoholism: Clinical and Experimental Research, 17,* 758–761.

Westermeyer, J., & Janca, A. (1997). Language, culture and psychopathology: Conceptual and methodological issues. *Transcultural Psychiatry, 34,* 291–311.

Wirth, R. J., & Edwards, M. C. (2007). Item factor analysis: Current approaches and future directions. *Psychological Methods, 12,* 58–79.

Worthington, R. L., & Whittaker, T. A. (2005). Scale development research: A content analysis and recommendations for best practices. *Counseling Psychologist, 34,* 806–838.

Yen, W. M. (1993). Scaling performance assessments: Strategies for managing local item dependence. *Journal of Educational Measurement, 30,* 187–213.

Zumbo, B. D. (2007). Three generations of DIF analyses: Considering where it has been, where it is now, and where it is going. *Language Assessment Quarterly, 4,* 223–233.

14

Social Network Analysis[1]

Methods and Applications in Public Health

Elizabeth C. Costenbader and Thomas W. Valente

T he traditional epidemiologic approach considers attributes of a person as putting him- or herself at risk for a certain disease or health outcome. We see this focus on individual-level attributes and behaviors in the previous two chapters on survey design and scale development. Yet often demographic characteristics provide only a partial explanation for health outcomes. Similarly, some of the most popular and widely-used theories developed to understand health behaviors have focused on individual attributes such as individual levels of motivation (e.g., Theory of Planned Behavior) or individually-held health beliefs (e.g., Health Belief Model). In many instances, however, these theories have fallen short in their ability to explain why some people do things or are exposed to things, while others do not or are not. The limitations of theories and models focusing solely on individual attributes has contributed to the emergence over the last few decades of social network analysis (SNA) as a powerful investigative tool in public health. SNA is "the mapping and measuring of relationships and flows between people, groups, organizations, computers, URLs, and other connected information/knowledge entities" (Krebs, 2000–2013, para. 1).

In particular, the collection of tools, theories, and measures that constitute SNA are premised on the central insight that the social relationships within which an individual is embedded have a strong influence on behaviors and exposures. It is important to note that while all SNA shares this central insight or network perspective, SNA was developed from and often draws on multiple sociological theories. The term *network* is used to describe a set of relationships between people and between people and things. By studying relationships, network researchers add another dimension or set of factors that can explain human behavior.

THE RELEVANCE OF SOCIAL NETWORK ANALYSIS (SNA) TO PUBLIC HEALTH

The importance of network influences has been demonstrated in a wide variety of human health domains, including smoking initiation and cessation (Alexander, Piazza, Mekos, & Valente, 2001; Ennett & Bauman, 1993, 1994; Mercken, Snijders, Steglich, & de Vries, 2009; Steglich, Snijders, & Pearson, 2010), alcohol and other substance use (Friedman et al., 1997; Neaigus, Friedman, Kottiri, & Des Jarlais, 2001; Valente, Mouttapa, & Gallaher, 2004), family planning and reproductive health (Entwisle et al., 1996; Valente, Jato, Van der Straten, & Tsitol, 1997), sexually transmitted disease (STD) and HIV (Aral et al., 1999; Klovdahl, 1985; Kohler, 1997; Morris, 2004; Rothenberg et al., 1998), suicide (Bearman & Moody, 2004), physician behavior (Gross et al., 2002; Iyengar, Van den Bulte, & Valente, 2011), contraceptive use (Entwisle et al., 1996; Valente et al., 1997), obesity (Christakis & Fowler, 2007), and others.

Currently, studies of social support and its influence on mortality and morbidity probably represent the largest area of SNA application in the field (Albrecht & Adelman, 1987; Gottlieb, 1985; House, 1981; Knowlton, 2003; Sarason, Levine, Basham, & Sarason, 1983). In addition to studies of individual behaviors, community health projects have used network analysis to improve message dissemination and program implementation (Stoebenau & Valente, 2003), while interorganizational collaboration, cooperation, and exchange studies have been conducted to improve understanding of health service provision (Harris, Luke, Burke, & Mueller, 2008; Kwait, Valente, & Celentano, 2001; Provan, Nakama, Veazie, Teufel-Shone, & Huddleston, 2003; Thomas, Isler, Carter, & Torrone, 2007; Valente, Chou, & Pentz, 2007; Wickizer et al., 1993) and healthcare provider performance (Lomas et al., 1991; Soumerai et al., 1998). There are also numerous introductions and reviews of network methods and theory (Boissevain, 1974; Burt, 1980; Burt & Minor, 1983; Carrington, Scott, & Wasserman, 2005; Degenne & Forsé, 1999; Harary, Norman, & Cartwright, 1965; Knoke & Kuklinski, 1982; Knoke & Yang, 2008; Luke & Harris, 2007; Marsden, 1990; Marsden & Lin, 1982; Rogers & Kincaid, 1981; Scott, 2000; Valente, 2010; Wasserman & Faust, 1994; Wellman & Berkowitz, 1988). Table 14.1 provides additional illustrative examples of the ways social network analysis has been used in public health research and programs organized by both the type of network and the network mechanism being studied or utilized.

To cover all of the SNA approaches and methods available to public health practitioners is beyond the scope of a single chapter. We therefore aim in this chapter to provide an overview of network analysis—specifically, the set of assumptions, methods, and applications useful for addressing many social and behavioral issues in the field of public health—and to provide references for further exploration of the field.

THE METHODS OF SOCIAL NETWORK ANALYSIS

Types of Network Data

Network data are primarily collected and analyzed from one of two different vantage points: the level of the egocentric or personal network or the level of the

Table 14.1 Examples of Social Network Analysis Applications in Public Health

Network Types	Network Mechanism	Representative Outcomes	Example Citations
Social networks	Social support	Mortality and morbidity	House (1981)
	Social capital	Mortality	Kawachi, Kennedy, Lochner, & Prothrow-Stith (1997)
		Neighborhood violence	Sampson, Raudenbush, & Earls (1997)
		Mental health	Ziersch (2005)
	Social influence (selection)	Smoking	Ennett & Baumann (1993, 1994)
		Obesity	Christakis & Fowler (2007)
		Substance abuse and injection drug use	Friedman et al. (1997)
		Family planning	Stoebenau & Valente (2003)
		Diffusion of innovations	Valente (1995)
Two-mode networks	Affiliation	Smoking	Fujimoto, Wang, & Valente (in press)
Transmission networks	Sexual contact networks	HIV transmission	Morris & Kretzschmar (1997)
	Person-to-person networks	Tuberculosis	McElroy et al. (2003)
	Travel networks	Influenza	Apolloni, Poletto, & Colizza (2013)
Organizational or community networks	Community mobilization	Community engagement	Valente, Fujimoto, Palmer, & Tanjasiri (2010)
	Health service provision	Service improvement	Provan et al. (2003)

sociometric or complete network. Each of these vantage points yields a different type of data with unique management and analysis requirements and can provide the practitioner with different insights. It is important to understand the strengths and limitations of these vantage points in order to select the data collection and analysis approach most appropriate to your research or program objectives.

Data Collection Techniques

Egocentric

Egocentric (also referred to as local or personal) networks provide information uniquely from the respondent's (or ego's) perspective on his or her individual network contacts. Egocentric data are collected by asking individuals a name-generator question, which is a question specifically designed to elicit the names of network members (Campbell & Lee, 1991). The named individuals will not be interviewed, so the researcher need not record the full exact name (i.e., pseudonyms or initials are often sufficient). The name-generator question can either be open-ended as in "Who would you talk to if you needed x?" or bounded as in "Name up to five people you talk to about x." The named persons are referred to as alters. Once all of the alters have been named, additional information is collected about each alter's characteristics and his or her relationship to ego. The types of questions asked about each alter depend on the research question, but it is usually important to collect information on frequency of interaction and/or a subjective assessment of relationship importance or strength. These latter measures allow the researcher to distinguish ties that are strong (e.g., close relationships, relationships with frequent interactions) from weak ties (e.g., acquaintances, relationships with infrequent interaction). Additional characteristics that are typically asked about include all of the following:

1. Type of relation (e.g., family, friend, coworker, sex partner)

2. Demographic characteristics (e.g., age, residential location)

3. Socioeconomic characteristics (e.g., educational attainment, wealth, income)

4. Behavioral characteristics (e.g., smoke, practice safe sex, practice family planning)

5. Content of interaction (e.g., discuss health, have unprotected sex, share syringes)

Egocentric data provide measures of an individual's personal network in terms of the kind of people each respondent interacts with or is related to. The individual respondents surveyed about their personal networks can be selected through either random or purposive sampling techniques. In either case, since no exact names are elicited, there is no way to link specific individuals named with others that may be interviewed in the same study. These data, therefore, do not provide connected groups of respondents that can be mapped. The researcher can ask the respondent to indicate the degree of connectedness between the named alters to measure personal network density.

Sociometric

In order to assess links or ties in an entire community, sociometric or sociocentric network data are collected. Census sampling or interviewing all (or almost all) members of a community or population is the ideal approach to collecting information on all of the connections or ties existing within a sociometric network. Census sampling is preferred when the researcher can enumerate all members of the community, such as all organizations in an industry or all employees of an organization. Organizations, schools, and rural communities represent the most common sampling frames used in this type of data collection (Rogers & Kincaid, 1981; Valente, 1995, 1996). Increasingly, however, the advent of electronic communications provide census data for quite large communities.

Complete network data can be collected either with a name-generator question or by obtaining a roster of all the members of the community and asking the respondent to check those that he or she knows or interacts with. Roster census data usually result in many more nominations (limited only by the number of people on the roster), whereas nominations data typically limit the responding to naming five or seven close ties (Valente, 2010). The roster method is quite commonly used in organizations in which the size is fewer than 100 or so. Rosters are often distributed as an aid for the nomination question.

The main challenge to collection of complete network data, and census sample studies in general, is defining the boundary of the community (Laumann, Marsden, & Prensky, 1983). In school research, for instance, the network boundary can be the classroom, grade, or entire school depending on the research setting and school size. More typically however, the boundaries of a network are unknown or too big to allow for census sampling, yet we still want to understand something about the connections or relationships between individuals in the network. For instance, we may wish to track behavior or communications among network members or to recruit networks of related individuals into an intervention or study. In this case, snowball sampling can be used to generate partial network data.

There are two kinds of snowball samples that can be generated, one in which a subset of network members are randomly chosen as index respondents and then the interviewer attempts to contact and interview every one of the respondent's alters (all of their network). When the researcher starts with a set of randomly chosen index cases, then the network results provide a potentially valid parameter estimate of network structure. The second type of partial network entails interviewing some subset of alters based on a specific attribute of interest. For instance, the sample could be defined as alters with whom the respondents have the greatest frequency of interaction, thus capturing strong rather than weak ties. Alternately, the researcher might want to interview all the drug users in a community and so elects to have indexes provide the names of his or her friends who use drugs. This provides entrée into the drug-using community, and further interviews will yield a partial network from which the structure of the drug-using network can be assessed. When the alters are a randomly chosen subset, study results provide valid estimates of network properties attributable to the network.

Measures and Analysis

Egocentric

Egocentric data characterize people's immediate close social networks and allow researchers to determine whether the network characteristics are associated with substantive phenomenon. Analysis of egocentric data is usually done with standard attribute-based statistical programs such as SAS, SPSS, and STATA. Typically egocentric measures are of two types: compositional and variance. Compositional measures are those derived by counting or taking the average of egocentric network variables. For example, the number or proportion of males in the personal network is a compositional variable. For a behavioral example, the number of smokers in the personal network is a compositional variable. Variance measures are those derived by calculating the variance or standard deviation of the egocentric network variables. For example, the standard deviation of the age of the alters is a variance measure.

These personal network variables can be used to explain individual behavior. For example, it might be hypothesized that adolescents with network members who are older and more varied on age are at greater risk for substance use or other risky behaviors. Adolescents with older friends, and some much older friends, are probably exposed to more risk behavior in the form of friends who smoke or engage in unprotected sex. The measures and analyses mentioned thus far are derived from data that could be collected randomly; that is, the respondents are not connected in a preexisting social network. Statistical analysis of associations between these network variables and outcomes do not need to control for non-independence of observations other than what would normally apply to the data.

Egocentric data are often converted to dyadic format to facilitate statistical analysis. Dyadic data refer to observations comprising the respondent and one network alter. In other words, in dyadic data, each case is a relationship pair or dyad. Converting a regular attribute dataset to dyadic has certain advantages. Because each case is the respondent and the data on the alter he or she named, analysis can be conducted to test how relationship characteristics are associated with behavior. For example, one might ask survey respondents to name their five closest friends and then ask for their gender, age, religious beliefs, and smoking behavior. The researcher can test whether people report smoking more with same-gender friends versus non-same-gender friends.

If the data are converted to dyadic format, the observations are no longer independent but are clustered on the respondent. Some respondents may have provided information on one alter while others provided information on four or five alters. Consequently, the analysis needs to control for clustering on the respondent ID. This usually entails specifying a multilevel or hierarchal model to explicitly account for the clustering.

Sociometric

By virtue of collecting data from connected groups of respondents, sociometric (whether complete or partial) network data allow for several types of measurement and analysis not possible with egocentric data alone. It is wise to remember, however, that a sociometric network is composed of egocentric networks, and therefore the relational analyses possible with egocentric data are similarly possible with sociometric data. Connecting these egocentric networks allows us to visualize the network by creating graphs or sociograms (Figure 14.1) and to apply the many metrics and algorithms designed to describe the network's structure.

Figure 14.1   Sociogram Depicting Friendships in a Southern California Middle School Classroom

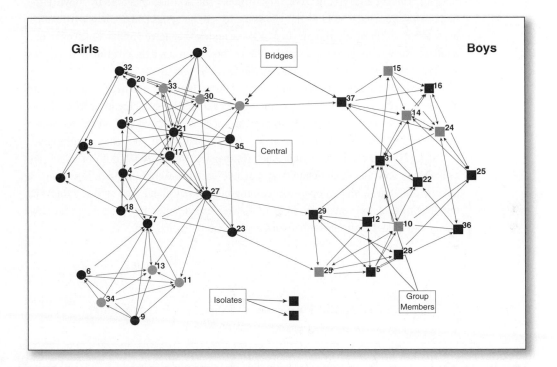

Graph made with Netdraw.

This figure shows the network of friendship choices among sixth-grade students who named their five closest friends in the class. Girls are depicted as circles and boys as squares. This sociogram identifies isolates, central members, group members, and bridges.

Network Visualization

The creation of a sociogram depicting relationships is one of the unique features of network data compared to other types of data. *Sociograms* display actors as *nodes* and the relational ties connecting actors as *lines*. Figure 14.1 shows a graph of the friendships between students in one classroom. Students were asked to name up to five of their closest friends in the class by writing their number from a class roster. Each circle or square is a node and the nodes in this network are the students in the classroom. The lines indicate friendship relationships or ties between students. The arrow heads indicate direction of relationship since some students named friends who did not name them in return; for example number 29 and 26 chose each other as friends, whereas 23 named 26 but 26 did not name 23. The lengths of the lines do not have meaning. People are placed on the graph based on how well connected they are; for example, those with many connections, such as number 21, are usually placed toward the center and then other nodes arrayed around them. Network graphing programs (here, we used Netdraw; Borgatti, Everett, & Freeman, 2002) try to make the pictures readable by moving the nodes away from each other so there is space to see the nodes and the labels (the numbers) while at the same time trying to keep nodes that have similar links near one another. There is no one correct way to draw a sociogram since the position of the nodes is somewhat arbitrary (Hennig, Brandes, Pfeffer, & Mergel, 2012).

Network diagrams are useful for showing the structure of a network, and there are a variety of techniques and computer programs available for graphing networks (Blythe, McGrath, & Krackhardt, 1996). Probably the most well-known and easily accessible visualization tools are Netdraw, which is the visualization tool that accompanies UCINET (Borgatti et al., 2002) and Pajek (Batagelj & Mrvar, 2007), both of which are available to download free online. Many people now use Gephi (Bastian, Heymann, & Jacomy, 2009), which is an open-source program also available free online. Table 14.2 provides more details on some of the most well-known computer programs that have been developed specifically for network analysis and visualization.

Table 14.2 Popular Social Network Analysis and Visualization Programs

Product	Description	License and Cost	Available at:
UCINET and Netdraw	A comprehensive package for the analysis of social network data Calculates centrality measures, subgroup identification, role analysis, elementary graph theory, and permutation-based statistical analysis Netdraw is the accompanying visualization tool	Commercial with free 60-day trial	https://sites .google.com/site/ ucinetsoftware/ downloads
StOCNET	Software package focusing on probabilistic (stochastic) models consists of five modules network analysis:	Free open-source software	www.gmw.rug .nl/~stocnet/ StOCNET.htm

Product	Description	License and Cost	Available at:
SIENA	Analysis of repeated measures on social networks		
BLOCKS	Stochastic blockmodeling of relational data		
p2	Analysis of binary network data with actor and/or dyadic covariates		
ULTRAS	Analysis of binary undirected network data using ultrametric measurement models		
ZO	Simulation and/or enumeration of graphs with given degrees		
statnet	A suite of R packages for social network analysis	Free open-source software	https://statnet .csde.washington .edu/trac/wiki/ Installation
sna	Performs sociometric analysis of networks		
ergm	A set of tools to analyze and simulate networks based on exponential random graph models		
network	Manipulates and displays network objects		
networksis	Provides tools for simulating bipartite networks with fixed marginal		
degreenet	Provides tools for statistical modeling of network degree distributions		
latentnet	Functions for network latent position and cluster models		
EgoNet	Program to assist in creating egocentric surveys, collecting the data, and providing general egocentric network measures and data matrixes	Commercial	www.mdlogix .com/solutions/ social-networks

(Continued)

(Continued)

Product	Description	License and Cost	Available at:
LinkAlyzer	Program to assist in linking of data records through matching of node attributes	Commercial	www.mdlogix .com/solutions/ social-networks
VisuaLyzer	Interactive tool for visualizing social network data Can create nodes and links directly or import data from Edgelist/Edgearray, Excel, or GraphML formats	Commercial with free 30 day trial	www.mdlogix .com/solutions/ social-networks
Social Networks Visualizer (SocNetV)	Computes basic network properties (i.e., density, diameter, shortest path lengths) as well as more advanced statistics such as centralities (i.e., closeness, betweenness, graph) and allows the researcher to draw social networks or plain graphs by clicking on a canvas	Free open-source software	http://socnetv .sourceforge.net/ index.html
Pajek	A visualization tool for large-scale networks that has some analytical capabilities such as calculating most centrality measures, identifying structural holes, and block-modeling	Free for noncommercial use	http://vlado.fmf .uni-lj.si/pub/ networks/pajek/
PNet	A program for the simulation and estimation of exponential random graph models (ERGMs) for social networks.	Free software	http://sna .unimelb.edu.au/ PNet
NetMiner 4	All-in-one software for network analysis and visualization Main features include analysis of large networks (+10,000,000 nodes), comprehensive network measures and models, exploratory and confirmatory analysis, interactive visual analytics	Commercial with free trial	www.netminer .com/index.php

Product	Description	License and Cost	Available at:
KrackPlot	A network visualization tool designed to be quick and easy to run Can read and write many graph formats and create output for Word or PowerPoint	Free software	www.isi.edu/~blythe/KP/
Gephi	An interactive visualization and exploration platform for all kinds of networks and complex systems, dynamic and hierarchical graphs	Free open-source software	https://gephi.org/
visone	Interactive graphical tool for manipulating, analyzing, and visualizing social networks Analysis methods include centrality indexes, clustering, cliques, components, and centralization	Free for noncommercial use	http://visone.info/

Once network data are collected, organizations, coalitions, and communities enjoy seeing their data reported back to them and viewing network diagrams because most people know their own personal networks, but no one can see the overall network structure unless the data are aggregated. Drawing network diagrams is one of the most attractive features of social network analysis as it provides a visual depiction of the overall structure of interactions (Freeman, 2000; McGrath, Krackhardt, & Blythe, 2002). However, network diagrams have their limitations. Large networks are hard to examine pictorially, and it is hard to compare different networks using only graphs.

Network-Level Measures

Although each person's connections may affect his or her behavior, the influence of these connections may vary depending on the overall pattern of relations in the complete network. The overall configuration or pattern of relationships in a network can also be important. The pattern of links in a complete network is referred to as the network structure—and structure matters. The network analysis field has created many metrics to use when describing the structure of a sociometric network.

Size is the most basic network measure and is a simple count of the number of people or things, referred to as nodes, in the network. **Network density** measures the proportion of ties in a network relative to the total number possible. In a dense network, there are lots of relationships between the nodes. **Mutuality**, or the extent to which ties are reciprocated, is also a network-level property and indicates whether there is a tendency for ties in the network to be reciprocated. While reciprocity compares the links between 2 nodes, the links between 3 nodes are referred to as **triads** and in a directed network there are 16 possible combinations of links connecting 3 nodes (Holland & Leinhardt, 1979; Wasserman & Faust; 1994). One measure of network structure, a **triad census,** describes the prevalence of these 16 types for the network. Of particular interest is transitivity in the network's triads. **Transitivity** in a network exists when there is the following combination of links among three nodes: if A → B, and B → C, then A → C. This triad is considered transitive because A and B both have the same relationship to C.

Transitivity forms the basis of much sociological thinking about how people function in groups. Balance theory (Heider, 1958) argues that people prefer a balanced social environment such that if A and B are friends (from A's perspective) and A likes C, then A would want B to also like C. In balance theory, C could be a person or an attitude or object, such as a political opinion, a new product on the market, a behavior, and so on. People struggle to keep their world in balance, and Festinger (1954) introduced the idea of cognitive dissonance, which is the discomfort one feels when one's environment is out of balance. Festinger argued that people will try to reduce their cognitive dissonance by trying to bring balance in their life—by trying to reduce intransitive triads.

Two other fundamental properties of a network are its **diameter**, the length of the longest path in the network, and the average distance between nodes, the **average path length**. Networks with the same number of nodes, and even the same density can have very different diameters since the diameter is the number of steps in the longest path in the network. Network diameter, then, is similar to a geographic diameter, the maximum distance from one peripheral spot to another. Unlike the diameter of the earth, however, the measurement is between the two most distal points in the network (as in a circle), not from a point back to itself. The average path length (APL) is the average of the distances between all the nodes in a network. APL is sometimes referred to as the characteristic path length. A small average path length indicates a cohesive network, while a large one indicates greater overall distances between nodes. APL is often used as a measure of network cohesion in which networks with low APL are considered cohesive. Networks with an APL greater than expected by chance are considered fragmented. APL and density often correlate.

Groups are aggregates of nodes who communicate or are connected to one another at a higher rate than others in the network. **Components** are the building blocks of group definitions and consist of all the nodes connected to each other through any number of steps in the network. Nodes that cannot reach each other are in different components. By definition, each **isolate** (i.e., node with no links to other nodes) is a separate component. This concept of the number of links defining a group can be generalized by creating K-cores.

A **K-core** is a subset of the network in which each node within the K-core is connected to at least K other people. Thus, a 2K-core is the set of people connected to at least two other nodes. All the nodes with zero or one link are dropped from the network.

Similarly, we can define a 3K-core as all the nodes with three or more links. As K is increased, successive pictures of who is left in the network will look increasingly dense. Once nodes are dropped from the network, the links from and to it are also dropped so the K criterion is calculated on the remaining nodes and links. The pattern of node removal as K is increased can be used to describe the network structure. For example, some networks have a core-periphery structure which is a network with a set of dense connections among a subset of nodes and another set residing on the periphery with fewer connections.

A **clique** is a subgroup of actors who are all directly connected to one another and no additional network member exists who is also connected to all members of the subgroup. The strict clique definition can be relaxed to define an n-clique which is the path length at which members of the clique are connected. For example, a 2n-clique is the set of people connected to each other by two steps. Two people are in the same clique if they are friends of the same friend. A second clique definition is a k-plex, defined as the set of points connected to all but k other nodes in the group. To find k-plexes the researcher sets both the k and n size of the groups. The minimum size for n, the size of the groups, is set to k-2 (because values of n close to k return trivial groups). For example, 2k-plexes with n = 7 will find all groups of size seven in which each person is connected to at least five others in the group. The k-cores, n-cliques, and k-plexes provide good measures of network structure, and as we study a network, these group identification methods provide insight into the pattern of affiliations such that we can characterize the network according to who is in which groups with whom.

As shown in Figure 14.2, network subgroups are often linked by structures known as **bridges**. Bridges can be either individual nodes or relationships. In Graph A, a relationship exists between two individuals that are part of separate subgroups, and this relationship serves as a bridging link. In contrast, in Graphs B and C, one node, node 10, connects two or more otherwise unconnected subgroups and thus serves as a bridging node. These bridges, whether individuals or relationships, reduce the overall distance in networks creating the well-known small world phenomenon.

The bridging node, node 10, in Graphs B and C in Figure 14.2 clearly occupies a critical or powerful position in this network. **Centrality** is an individual-level measure of the extent to which a node inhabits such a prestigious or critical position in the network. Centrality can be measured a variety of ways, each variation capturing a different dimension of network prominence (Borgatti & Everett, 2006). Most simply and intuitively, centrality can be measured as the number of nominations sent and received (i.e., measures of **centrality out-degree** and **in-degree**, respectively). Other centrality measures include **betweenness**, the extent to which a person lies on the shortest path connecting others in the network, and **closeness**, the average distance a person is from everyone else in the network (Freeman, 1979). **Centrality power** measures the degree to which an individual can exert control over the network (Bonacich, 1987), and **centrality flow** (Freeman, Borgatti, & White, 1991) and information (Stephenson & Zelen, 1989) measure the capacity of individuals to carry **information** within the network.

Figure 14.2   Three Variations of Subgroups Connected by Bridges

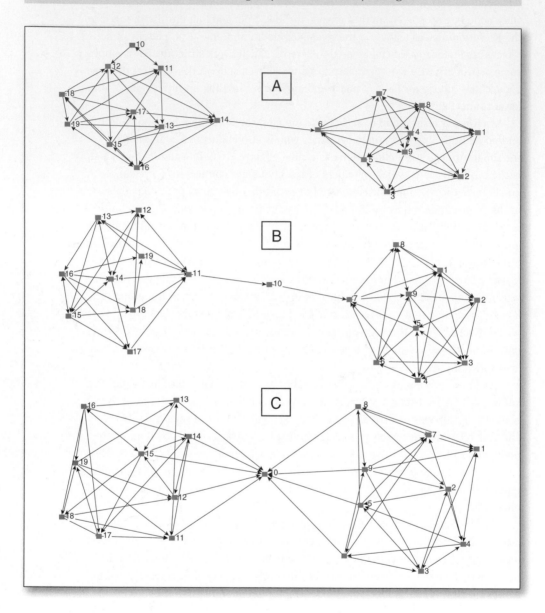

Centralization is the degree to which a network is focused on one or more central nodes. In centralized networks, one or a few nodes hold positions of power and control in the network, whereas decentralized networks have diffuse power and control structures. Centralization is calculated by determining the maximum individual centrality score in the network and subtracting it from all other individual scores in the network. These differences are summed and that total is divided by the maximum sum of differences theoretically possible in a network of that size. Similar calculations of centralization exist for centralization based on centrality closeness, betweenness, and others. Another way to calculate centralization is by simply calculating the standard deviation of the centrality scores for the network. A large standard deviation indicates a lot of variation in the individual centrality scores, whereas a small one indicates little variation and hence a decentralized structure. In Figure 14.3, two pairs of network sociograms show networks with different centralization scores yet the same densities, illustrating how density and centralization are not correlated and are independent structural measures.

Figure 14.3   A Comparison of Decentralized and Centralized Networks of the Same Densities

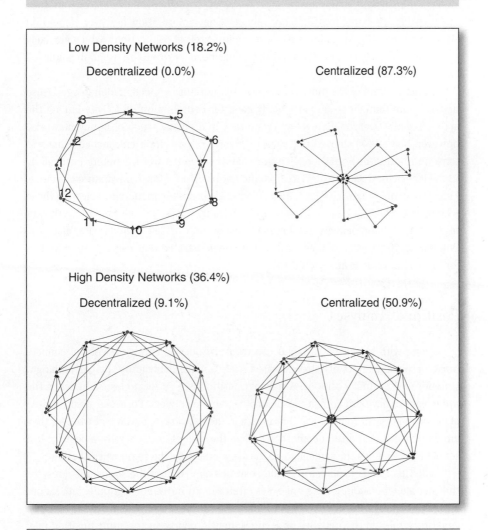

Graphs made with Netdraw.

Source: Borgatti (2002).

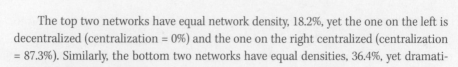

The top two networks have equal network density, 18.2%, yet the one on the left is decentralized (centralization = 0%) and the one on the right centralized (centralization = 87.3%). Similarly, the bottom two networks have equal densities, 36.4%, yet dramatically different centralizations.

Structural Analyses

Describing networks by these metrics is interesting, but these metrics are also useful in helping to inform understanding of—and ultimately to alter the distribution of—information, behaviors, and disease status in a network. For example, Granovetter's (1973, 1982) *strength of weak ties* theory proposes that information spreads rapidly through densely knit subgroups because actors are strongly connected to one another, and they directly share the information. Access to new information, however, comes into strongly connected groups through sources with external connections, which are likely to be weak. Identification of these weak ties has been shown to be useful in studies of diffusion and adoption.

Density is one of the most commonly used notions in social epidemiology. Dense networks are thought to be particularly good for coordination of activity among the actors because everyone knows everyone else. In a classic study of family networks, however, Bott (1957) showed that dense networks often exhibit entrenched value systems and norms, and that loose-knit or sparser networks were therefore particularly useful if an actor wanted to deviate from the norms of his or her immediate social circle. Finally, network opinion leaders can be identified with network data by selecting those who have the highest degree of centrality. At least 20 studies using social network data to identify opinion leaders for behavior change have been conducted (Valente & Pumpuang, 2007). Most of these studies have demonstrated that using opinion leaders for behavior change is an effective tactic.

Positional Analyses

Along with structural variables constructed from the entire network of connections, network analysts also have devised ways to analyze structure by partitioning a network into distinct positions. A network position is a set of nodes that occupy the same place or have similar relations with others in the network. Positions are composed of people who seem to be in the same space in the network, regardless of whether they are directly connected to one another, though they might be. Generally, a position is a set of nodes that has the same links to the same others, or the same types of others.

The theoretical basis for defining positions comes from the sociological insight that people who occupy the same roles often act similarly. For example, fathers are alike even though they are fathers to different children. Network-defined positions constitute roles in the network and, consequently, people in the same position may behave similarly. Positional analyses report the hierarchical structure of a network by partitioning individuals based on the degree of similarity in their network ties. Positional analyses do not provide individual measures, but rather provide indicators of equivalence (similarity) for all pairs of individuals in a network. The simplest positional measure computes the proportion of common ties for each pair of nodes in a network. This measure presents the percentage of links each pair of nodes has in common. The similarity criterion can then be used to form groups within the network based on their similarity scores.

Position analysis has been popular in social network analysis because it uncovers macro-level structure of the network from micro-level analysis of network relations. Position analysis can be conducted at both the individual and network levels. Individual-level position analysis is conducted by creating a measure of how equivalent two people are and then assigning a score for each pair of individuals based on that equivalence. Network-level position analysis is conducted by using mathematical algorithms to find positions in the network and then studying the relationships between these positions. Network-level position analysis consists of a set of positions and their interrelationships, whereas individual-level position analysis consists of a matrix of **positional equivalence** scores. Lorrain and White (1971) wrote an influential paper in which they proposed that the relations between people in a network can be reduced to a set of positions and the relations between these positions also treated as a network (a meta-level network). In some research, the network representing the relations between positions is referred to as the reduced-form network. Lorrain and White proposed that the network could be reduced to a set of blocks and the relations between blocks studied. This was called blockmodeling. Network researchers have developed different methods to identify the blocks (positions) and determine relations between positions (Doreian, Batagelj, & Ferligoj, 2005). The matrix or network that reports how the positions interact is referred to as the image matrix, the reduced form network, or matrix.

Finding positions in a network and assessing the degree of equivalence between actors is interesting from a research standpoint and can have substantive meaning when trying to understand networks. Yet from a disease perspective it is not immediately obvious how position equivalence affects one's likelihood of contracting a disease, since communicable diseases are spread by person-to-person contact. On the other hand, people in the same positions may be exposed to the same kinds of pathogens, so positional equivalence could be important to know.

For example, a positional analysis of sexual relations among a large network might reveal a set of positions such that one position is obviously a core group of sexually active individuals. Other positions that have contact with the core group may be at increased risk for sexually transmitted infections due to their contact with that group. All members of these positions may be at increased risk for disease. Although the risk factor is sexual contact, the positional analysis indicates why some people are at increased risk, even though their rate of sexual activity may be the same.

Glossary of Key Terms for Social Network Analysis

Average path length	Average distance connecting nodes in the network (AKA characteristic path length)
Bridge	The ability of an individual or a relationship to connect otherwise unconnected individuals or groups (Granovetter, 1973)
Centrality betweenness	The degree an individual lies on the shortest path connecting others in the network (Freeman, 1979)
Centrality closeness	The degree an individual is near others in the network (Freeman, 1979)
Centrality degree	The number of ties an individual sends (out-degree) or receives (in-degree; Freeman, 1979)
Centrality flow and information	Measures of the capacity of an individual to carry information within the network (Freeman et al., 1991; Stephenson & Zelen, 1989)
Centrality power	The degree an individual can exert control over other members of the network (Bonacich, 1987)
Centralization	The degree to which a network is focused on one or more central nodes.
Clique	A set of individuals who communicate more frequently with one another than with others in the community
Component	A set of individuals who are connected with another, but not with others in the community
Density	The number of ties in a network expressed as a proportion of the number possible (Scott, 2000)
Diameter	Length of the longest geodesic path; the distance between the two most distally connected nodes in the network
Dyad	Two nodes and their relationship
Egocentric	Network data collected from respondents about their contacts without interviewing those contacts (Burt & Minor, 1983)
Exponential random graph models	Used to test for structural properties of networks such as whether a network has a tendency for transitivity
Isolate	A node with no ties to other nodes
K-core	A subset of the network in which each node within the K-core is connected to at least K other people

Mutuality	The extent to which ties are reciprocated
Network	Set of relations between members of a community
Sociometric	Network data collected from the entire community (Wasserman & Faust, 1994)
Positional equivalence	The degree individuals have similar patterns of network ties in the community (status similarity; Burt, 1987); sometimes referred to as structural equivalence
Tie	Link between nodes
Triad	Configuration of links between three nodes
Transitivity	Tendency for two nodes linked to the same node to also be linked to each other
Triad census	The percentage of triads in a network that fall into 16 unique configurations

SNA APPLICATIONS AND RESEARCH FRONTS IN PUBLIC HEALTH

As network research has grown, several major areas of scholarly work have emerged. Those with the greatest applicability to public health issues and programs are described below.

Interventions

To date, evidence indicates that network data can be quite helpful in behavior change efforts (Valente, 2012; Valente & Fosados, 2006; Valente, Hoffman, Ritt-Olson, Lichtman, & Johnson, 2003; Valente et al., 2007). There are a number of approaches for applying network data to organizational or health promotion interventions (Valente & Fosados, 2006). The most common approach has been to identify opinion leaders using social network methodology and have these opinion leaders act as change agents (Lomas et al., 1991). Another approach is to identify subgroups in the network and approach them with behavior change promotions, or locate the leaders within the subgroups and enlist their assistance (Buller et al., 1999). Valente and Davis (1999) proposed identifying leaders first and forming groups around those leaders based on the social network nominations. Network data can also be used to identify groups and positional hierarchies and change efforts directed or tailored to these groups.

It is also possible to deliberately change networks so that bridges are created, strengthened, or removed. Network data in organizations or communities can be collected so that holes or gaps in the network can be spanned, or divisions that get revealed may be mended together via deliberate relationship building. Bridges represent potential bottlenecks to the flow of information within the community and in some cases may need to be strengthened to keep the community from fragmenting. It might also be the case that network analysis reveals one or a set of people who are central to disease spread or who are acting as bridges in the spread of disease between communities. Removing bridges in this latter case would slow the spread of a communicable disease such as HIV or STDs. These diagnostic tools provide many ways to inform interventions.

One of the challenges for network interventions is to incorporate network and behavioral data. It may not be sufficient to find opinion leaders; rather, it may be necessary to find opinion leaders who hold appropriate opinions about the behaviors being promoted. For example, getting employees to adopt a new treatment delivery system may require using network data to find the appropriate change agents in the organization, and it may be necessary that these change agents are both critical *and* supportive of the new system.

Social Capital

In addition to using network data to understand and alter behaviors, network data have been found to be informative in understanding the distribution of social resources. Traditionally, economic or material success was thought to be a product of one's intellect (known as human capital) and existing wealth (referred to as material capital; Borgatti, Jones, & Everett, 1998; Coleman, 1990). Lately, scholars have realized what every businessman knows: It is not what you know, but who you know. And further, not just who you know, but how well one uses his or her social resources. These social resources are referred to by some as social capital, which is the quality and quantity of resources available in a person's social network (Lin, 2001). Social capital provides access to job opportunities (Granovetter, 1973, 1974) and information on the job that provides an advantage. Social capital also can be used to provide access to health information or access to better or more appropriate health care. It has also been defined as the trust and/or the desire and ability to join civic groups. Putnam (2000), credited with popularizing the social capital concept, argued that social capital has been in decline in the United States because people are less inclined to join civic organizations, such as the Rotary Club, and more likely to spend their leisure time watching TV.

Many have measured social capital as the trust they have in their neighborhood (Moore, Shiell, Hawe, & Haines, 2005). This has led to research on how to define and identify social capital and considerations of its application to improving individual and community health. By trying to identify and strengthen available assets, social capital provides the opportunity to put a positive spin on the dire situation facing many underserved and deprived neighborhoods. Even the poorest have social capital manifested as knowledge about who has power and resources in the neighborhood. If this social capital can be mobilized, then perhaps some of the neighborhood's problems can be ameliorated. Conversely, focusing on social capital puts the burden on the community without acknowledging the institutional and historical causes that may have put communities in this disadvantaged position in the first place.

Exponential Random Graph Modeling

Perhaps the most significant development in the network field has been the advent of exponential random graph modeling (ERGM). ERGM is derived from the P* model which provided the basis for early statistical analysis of networks. The critical innovation in the P* model is the use of logistic regression analysis to determine the factors (individual characteristics and network metrics) associated with a link between two nodes. With ERGM, researchers generate simulated networks, which can then be compared to the observed network in order to statistically assess whether empirical networks exhibit certain structural properties (e.g., centrality, triadic transitivity). ERGM analysis can be used for (at least) three things:

1. Describe a network in terms of its structural properties

2. Determine if individual attributes (or node characteristics) are associated with network structural properties

3. Determine if individual attributes are associated with behaviors controlling for 1 and 2 (Robins, Pattison, Kalish, & Lusher, 2007)

For example, an ERGM model was used to test the probability that friendship ties existed (relative to no tie) among sixth-grade students as a function of network structural properties (e.g., density, reciprocity; Valente, Fujimoto, Chou, & Spruijt-Metz, 2009). Valente and others (2009) collected data from sixth-grade students in four schools in 15 classes. Students were asked to name their five closest friends in the class. Height and weight measurements were taken of all the students and their body mass index (BMI) calculated. BMI is typically used as an indicator of body composition, with adult BMI values greater than 30 signifying obesity. A common model was applied to all 15 classes and parameter estimates and their standard errors aggregated as in a meta-analysis to determine if the effects generalize across classes (Snijders & Baerveldt, 2003).

After controlling for structural effects, weight status similarity had a strong and statistically significant effect ($T^2 = 53.73$, $df = 15$, $p < .001$) with a mean effect size of 0.22 ($p < .001$), indicating that friendships were more likely to exist between students of the same rather than different weight statuses. The estimated between-classroom standard deviation of this effect size was 0.06 ($p = $ NS). The study also tested whether weight status was associated with naming more friends or being named as a friend. For naming friends, there was a significant main effect of weight status ($T^2 = 27.93$, $df = 15$, $p < .05$) with a mean effect size of .13 ($p < .05$), indicating that overweight adolescents named more friends than non-overweight adolescents. The estimated between-class standard deviation of this effect size was 0.13 ($p < .05$), indicating the estimated effect size was different between classes.

Note the ERGM results do not show the direction in which the association occurs. That is, there is an association between friendship and weight status which also means that non-obese students are also more likely to be friends with one another. The ERGM parameter estimate is not particularly informative as the researcher does not know how strong the association is. The ERGM analysis, however, does assure the researcher that the association between weight status and friendship is not a function of being connected to the same others in the class or other structural characteristics of the network. This study (Valente et al., 2009) also used regular random effects logistics regression to estimate the association between being at risk for obesity and having obese friends. The regression results indicated an approximate twofold increase in obesity for those with obese friends.

To this point, ERGM have been described as ways to determine whether an empirical network exhibits structural tendencies (e.g., amount of transitivity) and whether individual attributes may be associated with a link between two people. For example, do the actors tend to form reciprocal or transitive relationships, and are obese students more likely to be friends with other obese students? In addition to ERGM, statisticians have developed the underlying distributions of network properties well enough to create computer programs that also permit statistical testing of network dynamics and evolution (Banks & Carley, 1997; Doreian & Stokman, 1997).

Network Dynamics

In networks, change occurs at two levels: individual and network. Individuals add and lose relationships, and the nature of relationships can change, for example, from being close friends to acquaintances. At the network level, the overall network density, centralization, and transitivity (as well as other indicators) change over time. These dynamics create formidable analytic challenges because the set of people involved in the relationship may change. Given the inherent problem with comparing apples and oranges (changes in people), most social network dynamic research compares the same people or the same organizations over time. Researchers often need to choose whether they will study changes in individual indicators over time or study network evolution.

Identifying the evolution of social network preferences over time employs what have been called stochastic actor-oriented models (Burk, Steglich, & Snijders, 2007; Snijders 2001; Snijders, Steglich, Schweinberger, & Huisman, 2007). Instead of calculating frequencies of various types of social configurations as is done in ERGM, actor-oriented models simulate dynamic processes using what is essentially a form of agent-based modeling. The actor-oriented model follows similar logic to ERGMs except that rather than generating 500 simulated networks to compare against an empirical one, the researcher specifies the way the network at time 1 *evolves* to become the network at time 2. The estimation procedure allows researchers to identify whether behaviors are associated with the formation and/or dissolution of a tie between actors and whether network ties lead to changes in behaviors.

Currently there are two computer platforms used to test longitudinal network and behavior models, SIENA (Simulation Investigation of Empirical Network Analysis) and

PNET (see Table 14.2). These programs require the researcher to specify the parameters that are thought to govern how the network evolves from time 1 to time 2 and then generate a simulation of networks to determine whether imposing those rules will generate networks similar to the observed network at the later time point. The challenges for the researcher are to specify the structural and behavioral tendencies in the network. We encourage you to seek out more advanced materials and tutorials to learn how the analysis is conducted (Burk et al., 2007; Harrigan, 2009; Snijders, 2001; Snijders et al., 2007).

Diffusion/Contagion

The composition and evolution of networks have helped us understand what social networks look like. Network properties also have implications for how ideas, attitudes, and behaviors spread. As stated previously, a person's ideas, opinions, attitudes, beliefs, and behaviors are a function of his or her social networks' ideas, opinions, attitudes, beliefs, and behaviors. Diffusion of innovations is the process by which new ideas and practices spread within and between communities (Rogers, 2003). There is considerable evidence to suggest that a person's adoption of a new idea, attitude, opinion, or practice is strongly influenced by the behavior of his or her social network (Valente, 1995). Although this social influence may account for the spread of new ideas and practices, it is also true that the similarity of behaviors among people who are connected to one another arises because of selection.

Selection is the tendency for people to seek out friends whose behaviors are consistent with their own (Ennett & Bauman, 1993, 1994; Mercken et al., 2009; Valente, Fujimoto, Soto, Ritt-Olson, & Unger, 2013). A person who smokes is likely to seek out friends who smoke because this will reduce any cognitive dissonance that may emerge due to behavioral differences between the individual and his or her friends. Because smoking and perhaps other behaviors can be markers for cultural beliefs, a person might select friends based on these overt behaviors with the expectation the friends will hold the same beliefs and values as the focal person. Teasing out how social influence spreads—how an idea spreads through a network—can be complicated because of the way networks form (i.e., their homophily). Since people choose friends who are like themselves, it is hard to know whether networks influence behavior or whether people choose friends who engage in behaviors they want to emulate (Hoffman, Monge, Chou, & Valente, 2007).

There have been several notable studies of the diffusion of innovations through social networks. Three specific studies—on medical innovation (Coleman, Katz, & Menzel, 1966), Brazilian farmers (Rogers, Ascroft, & Röling, 1970), and Korean family planning (Rogers & Kincaid, 1981)—have become classics because they contain data specifically on when people adopted a new behavior and who in the community they were connected to via advice-seeking or discussion relationships. These three studies collected time-of-adoption data so the trajectory of diffusion could be plotted (see Figure 14.4). The network data in these studies permitted the investigation of how network characteristics were associated with adoption times (Valente, 1995).

The study of diffusion is further complicated by the long time span over which diffusion occurs. Very few new ideas and practices spread rapidly, and many adoption decisions are made by market forces beyond an individual's control. Still, networks matter, and whether by

Figure 14.4 Diffusion Curves for Three Studies: Medical Innovation, Brazilian Farmers, and Korean Family Planning

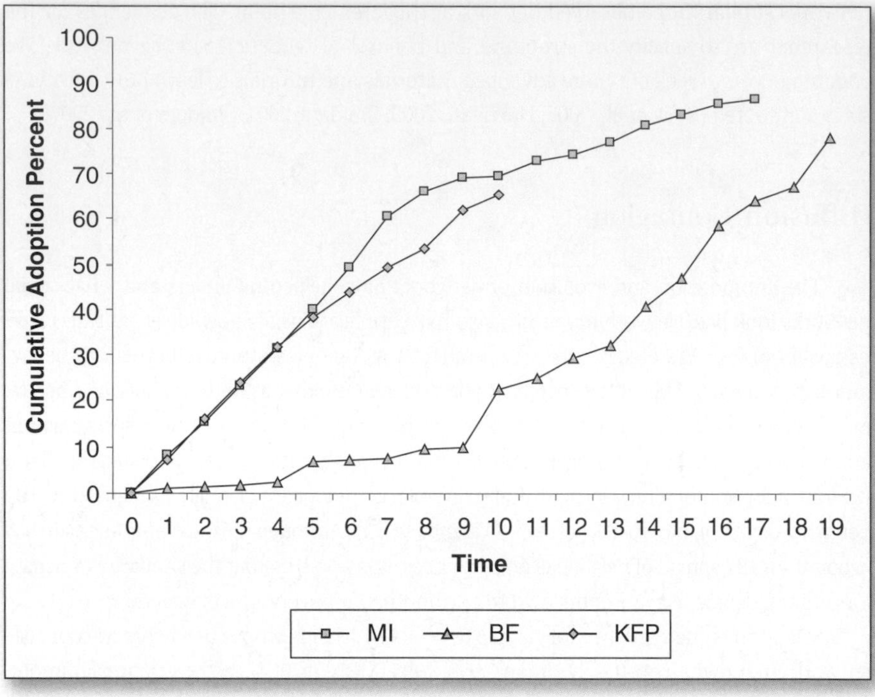

Each line represents the cumulative percentage of adopters over time in each study. Time in the medical innovation (MI) is months, for Brazilian Farmers (BF) and Korean Family Planning (KFP) it is years.

Source: Valente (2005).

selection or influence, the behavior of one's peers seems to have a strong effect on one's behavior, but there is considerable variation in how much. It seems that individuals have varying thresholds to adoption such that some people adopt an idea when no or few others have, while other people wait until a majority of others have adopted (see Figure A.10 in the Appendix to this volume). The distribution of thresholds governs how an idea or practice is adopted within a network (Valente, 1995, 1996). A population composed primarily of people with high thresholds will be resistant to diffusion, and hence diffusion will be slowed.

Another network factor shown to affect diffusion is one's position in the network (Becker, 1970). Several studies have found that people in the center of the network may be earlier adopters of certain ideas and behaviors (Alexander et al., 2001; Rogers & Kincaid, 1981; Valente, 2005). Being in a central position in the network provides an advantaged viewpoint of seeing what other people do and being exposed to ideas early (Christakis & Fowler, 2010). It also provides advantage in terms of influencing others, since opinion leaders, by definition, influence many others' opinions. Opinion leaders, often measured as central members in the network, both reflect and drive the diffusion process (Valente & Davis, 1999; Valente & Pumpuang, 2007).

In terms of behavior, the most significant area for future research is the collection of new data on the diffusion of innovation through a social (or other) network. Few studies have collected data on when individuals (or other nodes) adopt an innovation and the network contacts among the potential adopter units. New data that trace the diffusion of an idea or practice through multiple communities, complemented with social network data on who talks to whom or who is connected to whom, is needed to test diffusion models. Examples might be diffusion of a new process, procedure, or idea in organizations or branches of an organization; or adoption of policies or programs among teachers, administrators, or managers.

It may be that new diffusion data will become available within the course of research and application of network interventions. Building school- and community-based behavioral change programs that explicitly incorporate the power of social networks is a promising area of research and practice. Moreover, many groups are using network techniques to do community outreach and recruit community members into studies or interventions. Such interventions provide the opportunity to collect network data within the context of administering interventions that have the potential to improve individual and community health.

CURRENT ISSUES AND FUTURE DIRECTIONS

Much of the current work on diffusion consists of computer simulations or experiments using computer communications. These studies are extremely valuable for building theory and models to understand diffusion. Often they lack individual attributes and behaviors that can be used to more fully understand the behavior change process and test theories explicitly. Further, simulations are valuable to the extent they can mimic real-world issues and the assumptions are calibrated to empirical data. Thus, empirical data are urgently needed to build better agent-based models.

The growth in network applications has been fueled in part by the availability of sophisticated computer technology and programs that can simulate how networks function (Epstein, 2006). For instance, agent-based models can now simulate the simultaneous operations and interactions of multiple agents, in an attempt to recreate and predict the appearance of complex phenomena. As a result, scholars have been able to increase considerably the typologies of networks modeled, allowing for variation in network structures such as the reciprocity of ties or the amount of centrality. These models are also quite useful for contingency planning to explore "what if" scenarios. For example, bioterrorism and flu epidemic preparedness dictate that action plans be prepared for population-level threats such as virulent flu strains. Agent-based model programs can establish parameters on what level of flu virulence under what conditions of population connectivity will give rise to epidemic conditions. Other models can be run to determine who should be vaccinated first and the effects of vaccination sequences on epidemic spread.

Computer simulations may also be used to explore theoretical developments in hypothetical network analysis. For example, a network diffusion simulation was conducted comparing differences in diffusion in an empirical network to hypothetical diffusion in a random network. In the network condition it was assumed that 5% of the population adopted a new idea and that new adopters would adopt it when 15% of their personal network did so. The random condition was the same in size and density as the empirical one, but the network was generated randomly and ties distributed randomly. The simulation in the network condition showed unevenness in the diffusion process, with the adoption rate accelerating within pockets of interconnectivity in the network and leveling off as the innovation attempted to travel from one pocket of interconnectivity to another (Valente, 2005). The diffusion rate is smooth in the random condition, indicating that network structure does not affect the rate of diffusion.

The promise of social network research is that it will potentially provide a deeper understanding of human behavior on many different levels. For one, by modeling human relations, researchers can measure the strength of individual's relationships (e.g., strong and weak ties) or the differential social capital in different ties and show how these attributes influence behavior. At the network level, network analysis can be used to model explicitly the contact networks through which diseases are transmitted. Social network analysis can link macro- and micro-level structural influences by, for example, investigating whether personal network characteristics are differentially important based on network-level characteristics. Fourth, by understanding how ideas and behaviors spread or diffuse throughout networks, network interventions can be created to accelerate diffusion or curtail disease spread. Finally, important questions about how and with whom people interact and communicate can be posed and answered.

In sum, there are many different ways in which social network analysis can be added to the mix of methods used for public health research and programs. The avenues include the collection of empirical data and the use of modeling to understand and predict how networks influence the incidence and prevalence of many health behaviors and diseases, and to guide the development of network interventions to alter the diffusion or adoption of behaviors within networks. There is also ample opportunity to conduct research on methodological aspects of how best to collect network data and on algorithms to process it. At present, social networking technology has made the management and maintenance of social networks easier and more multidimensional than ever before. The increase in social networking platforms in combination with the increased availability of appropriate computational and statistical tools has meant that researchers interested in assessing and/or affecting changes in social networks are now limited only by their imaginations and perseverance.

ADDITIONAL RESOURCES

Carrington, P. J., Scott, J., & Wasserman, S. (2005). *Models and methods in social network analysis.* Cambridge, UK: Cambridge University Press.

Luke, D. A., & Harris, J. (2007). Network analysis in public health: History, methods, and applications. *Annual Review of Public Health, 28,* 69–93.

Scott, J. (2000). *Social network analysis: A handbook* (2nd ed.). Thousand Oaks, CA: Sage.

Valente, T. W. (2010). *Social networks and health: Models, methods, and applications.* New York, NY: Oxford University Press.

REFERENCES

Albrecht, T. L., & Adelman, M. B. (1987). *Communicating social support*. Newbury Park, CA: Sage.

Alexander, C., Piazza, M., Mekos, D., & Valente, T. W. (2001). Peer networks and adolescent cigarette smoking: An analysis of the national longitudinal study of adolescent health. *Journal of Adolescent Health, 29*, 22–30.

Apolloni, A., Poletto, C., & Colizza, V. (2013). Age-specific contacts and travel patterns in the spatial spread of 2009 H1N1 influenza pandemic. *BMC Infectious Diseases, 13,* 176.

Aral, S. O., Hughes, J. P., Stoner, B., Whittington, W., Handsfield, H. H., Anderson, R. M., & Holmes, K. K. (1999). Sexual mixing patterns in the spread of gonococcal and chlamydial infections. *American Journal of Public Health, 89,* 825–833.

Banks, D. L., & Carley, K. M. (1997). Models of network evolution. In P. Doreian & F. Stokman (Eds.), *Evolutions of social networks* (pp. 209–323). New York, NY: Routledge.

Bastian, M., Heymann, S., & Jacomy, M. (2009). Gephi: An open source software for exploring and manipulating networks. In *Proceedings of the Third International ICWSM Conference.* Palo Alto, CA: Association for the Advancement of Artificial Intelligence.

Batagelj, V., & Mrvar, A. (2007). *Pajek: Package for Large Network Analysis.* Ljubljana: University of Ljubljana, Slovenia.

Bearman, P. S., & Moody, J. (2004). Suicide and friendships among American adolescents. *American Journal of Public Health, 94,* 89–95.

Becker, M. H. (1970). Sociometric location and innovativeness: Reformulation and extension of the diffusion model. *American Sociological Review, 35,* 267–282.

Blythe, J., McGrath, C., & Krackhardt, D. (1996). The effect of graph layout on inference from social network data. *Graph Drawing, 1027,* 40–51.

Boissevain, J. (1974). *Friends of friends: Networks, manipulators and coalitions*. Oxford, UK: Blackwell.

Bonacich, P. (1987). Power and centrality: A family of measures. *American Journal of Sociology, 92,* 1170–1182.

Borgatti, S.P. (2002). *NetDraw software for network visualization.* Lexington, KY: Analytic Technologies.

Borgatti, S. P., & Everett, M. G. (2006). A graph-theoretic perspective on centrality. *Social Networks, 28,* 466–484.

Borgatti, S. P., Everett, M. G., & Freeman, L. C. (2002). *UCINET VI for Windows: Software for social network analysis.* Lexington, KY: Analytic Technologies.

Borgatti, S. P., Jones, C., & Everett, M. G. (1998). Network measures of social capital. *Connections, 21*(2), 27–36.

Bott, E. (1957). *Family and social network.* London, UK: Tavistock.

Buller, D. B., Morrill, C., Taren, D., Aickin, M., Sennott-Miller, L., Buller, M. K., . . . Wentzel, T. M. (1999). Randomized trial testing the effect of a peer education at increasing fruit and vegetable intake. *Journal of the National Cancer Institute, 91,* 1491–1500.

Burk, W. J., Steglich, C. E. G., & Snijders, T. A. B. (2007). Beyond dyadic interdependence: Actor-oriented models for co-evolving social networks and individual behaviors. *International Journal of Behavioral Development, 31,* 397–404.

Burt, R. S. (1980). Models of network structure. *Annual Review of Sociology, 6,* 79–141.

Burt, R. S. (1987). Social contagion and innovation: Cohesion versus structural equivalence. *American Journal of Sociology, 92,* 1287–1335.

Burt, R., & Minor, M. (Eds.). (1983). *Applied network analysis.* Newbury Park, CA: Sage.

Campbell, K. E., & Lee, B. A. (1991). Name generators in surveys of personal networks. *Social Networks, 13,* 203–221.

Carrington, P. J., Scott, J., & Wasserman, S. (2005). *Models and methods in social network analysis.* Cambridge, UK: Cambridge University Press.

Christakis, N. A., & Fowler, J. H. (2007). The spread of obesity in a large social network over 32 years. *New England Journal of Medicine, 357,* 370–379.

Christakis, N. A., & Fowler, J. H. (2010). Social network sensors for early detection of contagious outbreaks. *PLoS One, 5*(9), e12948.

Coleman, J. S. (1990). *Foundations of social theory.* Boston, MA: Harvard University Press.

Coleman, J. S., Katz, E., & Menzel, H. (1966). *Medical innovation: A diffusion study.* New York, NY: Bobbs Merrill.

Degenne, A., & Forsé, M. (1999). *Introducing social networks* (Trans. A. Borges). Thousand Oaks, CA: Sage.

Doreian, P., Batagelj, V., & Ferligoj, A. (2005). *Generalized blockmodeling,* New York, NY: Cambridge University Press.

Doreian, P., & Stokman, F. (Eds.). (1997). *Evolutions of social networks.* New York, NY: Routledge.

Ennett, S. T., & Bauman, K. E. (1993). Peer group structure and adolescent cigarette smoking: A social network analysis. *Journal of Health and Social Behavior, 34,* 226–236.

Ennett, S. T., & Bauman, K. E. (1994). The contribution of influence and selection to adolescent peer group homogeneity: The case of adolescent cigarette smoking. *Journal of Personality and Social Psychology, 67,* 653–663.

Entwisle, B., Rindfuss, R. D., Guilkey, D. K., Chamratrithirong, A., Curran, S. R., & Sawangdee, Y. (1996). Community and contraceptive choice in rural Thailand: A case study of Nang Rong. *Demography, 33,* 1–11.

Epstein, J. M. (2006). *Generative social science.* Princeton, NJ: Princeton University Press.

Festinger, L. (1954). A theory of social comparison processes. *Human Relations, 7,* 117–140.

Freeman, L. (1979). Centrality in social networks: Conceptual clarification. *Social Networks, 1,* 215–239.

Freeman, L. (2000). Visualizing social networks. *Journal of Social Structure, 1*(1).

Freeman, L. C., Borgatti, S. P., & White, D. R. (1991). Centrality in valued graphs: A measure of betweens based on network flow. *Social Networks, 13,* 141–154.

Friedman, S. R., Neaigus, A., Jose, B., Curtis, R., Goldstein, M., Ildefonso, G., . . . Des Jarlais, D. C. (1997). Sociometric risk networks and risk for HIV infection. *American Journal of Public Health, 87,* 1289–1296.

Fujimoto, K., Wang, P., & Valente, T. W. (in press). The decomposed affiliation exposure model: A network approach to segregating peer influences from crowds and organized sports. *Network Science.*

Gottlieb, B. H. (1985). Social support and the study of personal relationships. *Journal of Social Personality Relationships, 2,* 351–375.

Granovetter, M. (1973). The strength of weak ties. *American Journal of Sociology, 78,* 1360–1380.

Granovetter, M. (1974). *Getting a job: A study of contacts and careers.* Cambridge, MA: Harvard University Press.

Granovetter, M. (1982). The strength of weak ties: A network theory revisited. In P. V. Marsden & N. Lin (Eds.), *Social structure and network analysis* (pp. 105–130). Beverly Hills, CA: Sage.

Gross, C. P., Cruz-Correa, M., Canto, M. I., McNeil-Solis, C., Valente, T. W., & Powe, N. R. (2002). The adoption of ablation therapy for Barrett's esophagus: A cohort study of gastroenterologists. *American Journal of Gastroenterology, 97,* 279–286.

Harary, F., Norman, R., & Cartwright, D. (1965). *Structural models: An introduction to the theory of directed graphs.* New York, NY: Wiley.

Harrigan, N. (2009). *Exponential random graph (ERG) models and their application to the study of corporate elites.* Oxford, UK: Oxford University, Department of Politics and International Relations.

Harris, J. K., Luke, D. A., Burke, R. C., & Mueller, N. B. (2008). Seeing the forest and the trees: Using network analysis to develop an organizational blueprint of state tobacco control systems. *Social Science & Medicine, 67*, 1669–1678.

Heider, F. (1958). *The psychology of interpersonal relations.* New York, NY: Wiley.

Hennig, M., Brandes, U., Pfeffer, J., & Mergel, I. (2012). *Studying social networks: A guide to empirical research.* Frankfurt, NY: Campus.

Hoffman, B. R., Monge, P., Chou, C. P., & Valente, T. W. (2007). The roles of perceived peer influence and peer selection on adolescent smoking. *Addictive Behaviors, 32*, 1546–1554.

Holland, P. W., & Leinhardt, S. (1979). *Perspectives on social network research.* New York, NY: Academic Press.

House, J. S. (1981). *Work stress and social support.* Reading, MA: Addison-Wesley.

Iyengar, R., Van den Bulte, C., & Valente, T. W. (2011). Opinion leadership and contagion in new product diffusion. *Marketing Science, 30*, 195–212.

Kawachi, I., Kennedy, B. P., Lochner, K., & Prothrow-Stith, D. (1997). Social capital, income inequality, and mortality. *American Journal of Public Health, 100*, 1319–1325.

Klovdahl, A. S. (1985). Social networks and the spread of infectious diseases: The aids example. *Social Science Medicine, 21*, 1203–1216.

Knoke, D., & Kuklinski, J. H. (1982). *Network analysis.* Beverly Hills, CA: Sage.

Knoke, D., & Yang, S. (2008). *Social network analysis* (2nd ed.). Thousand Oaks, CA: Sage.

Knowlton, A. R. (2003). Informal HIV caregiving in a vulnerable population: Toward a network resource framework. *Social Science and Medicine, 56*, 1307–1320.

Kohler, H. P. (1997). Learning in social networks and contraceptive choice. *Demography, 34*, 369–383.

Krebs, V. (2000–2013). *Social network analysis, a brief introduction.* Retrieved from http://www.orgnet.com/sna.html

Kwait, J., Valente, T. W., & Celentano, D. D. (2001). Interorganizational relationships among HIV/AIDS service organizations in Baltimore: A network analysis. *Journal of Urban Health, 78*, 468–487.

Laumann, E., Marsden, P., & Prensky, D. (1983). The boundary specification problem in network analysis. In R. Burt & M. Minor (Eds.), *Applied network analysis.* Beverly Hills, CA: Sage.

Lin, N. (2001). *Social capital: A theory of social structure and action.* New York, NY: Cambridge University Press.

Lomas, J., Enkin, M., Anderson, G. M., Hanna, W. J., Vayda, E., & Singer, J. (1991). Opinion leaders vs. audit feedback to implement practice guidelines: Delivery after previous cesarean section. *Journal of the American Medical Association, 265*, 2202–2207.

Lorrain, F., & White, H. C. (1971). Structural equivalence of individuals in social networks. *Journal of Mathematical Sociology, 1*, 49–80.

Luke, D. A., & Harris, J. (2007). Network analysis in public health: History, methods, and applications. *Annual Review of Public Health, 28*, 69–93.

Marsden, P. V. (1990). Network data and measurement. *Annual Review of Sociology, 16*, 435–463.

Marsden, P. V., & Lin, N. (Eds.). (1982). *Social structure and network analysis.* Beverly Hills, CA: Sage.

McElroy, P. D., Rothenberg, R. B., Varghese, R., Woodruff, R., Minns, G. O., Muth, S. Q., . . . Ridzon, R. (2003). A network-informed approached to investigating a tuberculosis outbreak: Implications for enhancing contact investigations. *International Journal of Tuberculosis and Lung Disease, 7*(Suppl 3), S486–S493.

McGrath, C., Krackhardt, D., & Blythe, J. (2002). Visualizing complexity in networks: Seeing both the forest and the trees. *Connections, 25*(1), 30–34.

Mercken, L., Snijders, T. A., Steglich, C., & de Vries, H. (2009). Dynamics of adolescent friendship networks and smoking behavior: Social network analyses in six European countries. *Social Sciences & Medicine, 69*, 1506–1514.

Moore, S., Shiell, A., Hawe, P., & Haines, V. A. (2005). The privileging of communitarian ideas: Citation practices and the translation of social capital into public health research. *American Journal of Public Health, 95*, 1330–1337.

Morris, M. E. (Ed.). (2004). *Network epidemiology: A handbook for survey design and data collection.* New York, NY: Oxford University Press.

Morris, M., & Kretzschmar, M. (1997). Sexual networks and HIV. *AIDS, 11*, S209–S216.

Neaigus, A., Friedman, S. R., Kottiri, B. J., & Des Jarlais, D. C. (2001). HIV risk networks and HIV transmission among injecting drug users. *Evaluation and Program Planning, 24*, 221–226.

Provan, K. G., Nakama, L., Veazie, M. A., Teufel-Shone, N. I., & Huddleston, C. (2003). Building community capacity around chronic disease services through a collaborative interorganizational network. *Health Education and Behavior, 30*, 646–662.

Putnam, R. D. (2000). *Bowling alone: The collapse and revival of American community.* New York, NY: Simon & Schuster.

Robins, G., Pattison, P., Kalish, Y., & Lusher, D. (2007). An introduction to exponential random graph (p*) models for social networks. *Social Networks, 29*, 173–191.

Rogers, E. M. (2003). *Diffusion of innovations* (5th ed.). New York, NY: Free Press.

Rogers, E. M., Ascroft, J. R., & Röling, N. G. (1970). Diffusion of innovations in Brazil, Nigeria, and India. Unpublished manuscript, Michigan State University.

Rogers, E. M., & Kincaid, D. L. (1981). *Communication networks: A new paradigm for research.* New York, NY: Free Press.

Rothenberg, R., Sterk, C., Toomey, K. E., Potterat, J. J., Johnson, D., Schrader, M., & Hatch, S. (1998). Using social network and ethnographic tools to evaluate a syphilis transmission. *Sexually Transmitted Diseases, 25*, 154–160.

Sampson, R. J., Raudenbush, S. W., & Earls, F. (1997). Neighborhoods and violent crime: A multilevel study of collective efficacy. *Science, 277*, 918–924.

Sarason, I. G., Levine, H. M., Basham, R. B., & Sarason, B. R. (1983). Assessing social support: The social support questionnaire. *Journal of Personality and Social Psychology, 44*(1), 127–139.

Scott, J. (2000). *Network analysis: A handbook* (2nd ed.). Thousand Oaks, CA: Sage.

Snijders, T. A. B. (2001). The statistical evaluation of social network dynamics. *Sociological Methodology, 31*, 361–395.

Snijders, T. A. B., & Baerveldt, C. (2003). A multilevel network study of the effects of delinquent behavior on friendship evolution. *Journal of Mathematical Sociology, 27*, 123–151.

Snijders, T. A. B., Steglich, C. E. G., Schweinberger, M., & Huisman, M. (2007). *Manual for SIENA, version 3.* Groningen, Netherlands: University of Groningen.

Soumerai, S. B., McLaughlin, T. J., Gurwitz, J. H., Guadagnoli, E., Hauptman, P. J., Borbas, C., . . . Gobel, F. (1998). Effect of local medical opinion leaders on quality of care for acute myocardial infarction: A randomized controlled trial. *Journal of the American Medical Association, 279*, 1358–1363.

Steglich, C., Snijders, T. A. B., & Pearson, M. (2010), Dynamic networks and behavior: Separating selection from influence. *Sociological Methodology, 40*, 329–393.

Stephenson, K., & Zelen, M. (1989). Rethinking centrality: Methods and applications. *Social Networks, 11*, 1–37.

Stoebenau, K., & Valente, T. W. (2003). The role of network analysis in community-based program evaluation: A case study from Highland Madagascar. *International Family Planning Perspectives, 29*, 167–173.

Thomas, J. C., Isler, M. R., Carter, C., & Torrone, E. (2007). An interagency network perspective on HIV prevention. *Sexually Transmitted Diseases, 34*(2), 71–75.

Valente, T. W. (1995). Network models of the diffusion of innovations. Cresskill, NJ: Hampton Press.

Valente, T. W. (1996). Social network thresholds in the diffusion of innovations. *Social Networks, 18,* 69–89.

Valente, T. W. (2005). Models and methods for innovation diffusion. In P. Carrington, J. Scott, & S. Wasserman (Eds.), *Models and methods in social network analysis* (pp. 98–116). New York, NY: Cambridge University Press.

Valente, T. W. (2010). *Social networks and health: Models, methods, and applications.* New York, NY: Oxford University Press.

Valente, T. W. (2012). Network interventions. *Science, 337,* 49–53.

Valente, T. W., Chou, C. P., & Pentz, M. A. (2007). Community coalition networks as systems: Effects of network change on adoption of evidence-based prevention. *American Journal of Public Health, 97,* 880–886.

Valente, T. W., & Davis, R. L. (1999). Accelerating the diffusion of innovations using opinion leaders. *Annals of the American Academy of the Political and Social Sciences, 566,* 55–67.

Valente, T. W., & Fosados, R. (2006). Diffusion of innovations and network segmentation: The part played by people in the promotion of health. *Journal of Sexually Transmitted Diseases, 33,* S23–S31.

Valente, T. W., Fujimoto, K., Chou, C. P., & Spruijt-Metz, D. (2009). Friendship affiliations and adiposity: A social network analysis of adolescent friendships and weight status. *Journal of Adolescent Health, 45,* 202–204.

Valente, T. W., Fujimoto, K., Palmer, P., & Tanjasiri, S. P. (2010). A network assessment of community-based participatory research: Linking communities and universities to reduce cancer disparities. *American Journal of Public Health, 100,* 1319–1325.

Valente, T. W., Fujimoto, K., Soto, D., Ritt-Olson, A., & Unger, J. (2013). A comparison of peer influence measures as predictors of smoking among predominantly Hispanic/Latino high school adolescents. *Journal of Adolescent Health, 52,* 358–364.

Valente, T. W., Hoffman, B. R., Ritt-Olson, A., Lichtman, K., & Johnson, C. A. (2003). The effects of a social network method for group assignment strategies on peer led tobacco prevention programs in schools. *American Journal of Public Health, 93,* 1837–1843.

Valente, T. W., Jato, M. N., Van der Straten, A., & Tsitol, L. M. (1997). Social network influences on contraceptive use among Cameroonian women in voluntary associations. *Social Science and Medicine, 45,* 677–687.

Valente, T. W., Mouttapa, M., & Gallaher, M. (2004). Social network analysis for understanding substance abuse: A transdisciplinary perspective. *Substance Use & Misuse, 39,* 1685–1712.

Valente, T. W., & Pumpuang, P. (2007). Identifying opinion leaders to promote behavior change. *Health Education & Behavior, 34,* 881–896.

Wasserman, S., & Faust, K. (1994). *Social networks analysis: Methods and applications.* Cambridge, UK: Cambridge University Press.

Wellman, B., & Berkowitz, S. D. (Eds.). (1988). *Social structure: A network approach.* Cambridge, UK: Cambridge University Press.

Wickizer, T. M., Korff, M. V., Cheadle, A., Maeser, J., Wagner, E. H., Pearson, D., . . . Psaty, B. M. (1993). Activating communities for health promotion: A process evaluation method. *American Journal of Public Health, 83,* 561–567.

Ziersch, A. M. (2005). Health implications of access to social capital: Findings from an Australian study. *Social Sciences & Medicine, 61,* 2119–2131.

NOTE

1.   Adapted from Valente (2010).

15

Qualitative Research Methods

Emily E. Namey and Robert T. Trotter II

P ublic health researchers aim to address complex and multifaceted problems that often require empirical data on key behavioral, cultural, and environmental questions. The other methods covered in this section approach those questions by collecting and analyzing quantitative or number-based data. Qualitative research, by contrast, relies heavily on other forms of data—primarily text, narrative, direct observation, and images—to address issues in public health. Sometimes, we are interested in describing what people are doing, why they are doing it, and the context of their actions (when and where the activities take place) as a first step toward addressing a particular public health issue. For instance, what are the behaviors, motivations, and contexts related to adolescent drug use, or domestic violence, or prescription drug misuse? In other cases, epidemiological or quantitative survey data define the parameters of an issue, but we need to fill in the explanatory *why, where,* and *when* to help interpret or apply those data. This is the case when surveillance or secondary data (Chapters 5 and 9, respectively) reveal a trend that can't be explained by statistical correlation or the quantitative data alone. Qualitative research methods offer processes and techniques to help illuminate the relevant issues in both of these circumstances by examining the phenomena that underpin health beliefs, behaviors, or opinions.

THE QUALITATIVE-QUANTITATIVE COMPARISON

Attempts to discuss or define qualitative research often prompt stereotypical contrasts with quantitative research, summarized in the chart below.

	Qualitative	*Quantitative*
Data	Words, images, behaviors	Numbers
Purpose	Hypothesis generating, exploratory, validating	Hypothesis testing or confirmatory
Sampling	Nonprobabilistic sampling	Probabilistic sampling

These overly simplified comparisons may be helpful for demarcating points on the spectrum of scientific research methods; however, we would like to move away from this type of dichotomization because, like any broad generalization, it misses critical nuances. Qualitative research does frequently focus on nonnumeric or nominal-level data, including texts, images, behavioral descriptions, or sounds (Nkwi, Nyamongo, & Ryan, 2001). However, qualitative data collection and analysis activities also include ranking, grouping, and quantification processes, supported by a variety of univariate and multivariate statistical analyses. Similarly, while qualitative research is often exploratory and descriptive, so is a significant portion of quantitative research—and rigorous confirmatory qualitative research projects are increasingly common (Patton, 2002), particularly within mixed methods research designs (see Chapter 19).

Between 1990 and 2000, public health researchers engaged in a series of discussions, sometimes debates, on the consequences of the differences between quantitative and qualitative research design and methods (Baum, 1995; Johnson, 1990; Luborsky & Rubinstein, 1995). That debate focused on four critical issues: (1) theory in public health research, (2) sampling designs for public health research, (3) data collection techniques, and (4) analysis strategies relevant to public health policy and programs. The result of these discussions was validation of qualitative methods as highly important public health tools in research designs that include correctly targeted methods, defensible sampling plans, and theory-based analysis strategies (Creswell, Klassen, Plano Clark, & Clegg Smith, 2011; National Institutes of Health, 2000). We will touch on 2–4 here; a review of qualitative theory as linked to research designs is beyond the scope of this chapter, but there are several excellent baseline references on the topic (Bernard, 2013; Glaser & Strauss, 1967; Schensul & LeCompte, 2010; Trotter, 1997) as well as a review of common public health theories in the Appendix.

DEFINING QUALITATIVE RESEARCH

Like other research methods detailed in this book, qualitative research comprises a theoretical and methodological tool kit, and each tool in the kit has specific capabilities, applications, and limitations. We believe there are three characteristics that define qualitative research methods and help to set them apart from other approaches.

1. The ability to generate richly nuanced, personal- or public-level data through selection of knowledgeable informants, open-ended questioning about their attitudes and experiences, and inductive probing of their responses.

2. A sensitivity to context, the natural setting in which behaviors or beliefs occur or arise (Hammersley, 2008).

3. The capacity to meet the participant "where she or he is" by using local language and phrasing to ensure that the respondent has understood the question and has had the chance to explain her or his response.

Methodologically sound qualitative research also follows an iterative design that allows researchers to use preliminary discoveries to guide subsequent data collection and analysis, and may include the community in these efforts at all or some stages of research (see In Focus on community-based participatory research at the end of Chapter 4). Finally, as mentioned, much of the source data collected as part of qualitative research in the form of narrative, text, or images is itself qualitative. Figure 15.1 provides a general schematic of the research process, with typical qualitative research questions and data collection and analysis methods identified. Note that theory is used to varying degrees to inform each step of the process, from development of the research question and selecting appropriate methods, through to analysis and dissemination. (Chapter 2 covers the relationship between design and theory in more detail.)

Together, the qualities described above enable "qualitative methods [to] fill a gap in the public health toolbox; they help us understand underlying behaviors, attitudes, perceptions, and culture in a way that quantitative methods alone cannot" (Steckler, 2005, p. xiii). They help to explain the *why* and *how* of health issues and provide a more in-depth understanding of the *who*, *what*, and *when* (Bernard, 2011). Qualitative methods have contributed to the areas of nutrition, HIV prevention, diabetes treatment, maternal health, smoking cessation, vaccine avoidance, obesity, and most other current "hot topics" in public health. They provide efficient means for accessing, assessing, and capturing the context of *emerging* public health issues and are also often used in public health engagement and advocacy initiatives. In the subsequent sections, we offer an introduction to qualitative sampling, data collection, data management, and analysis and then provide illustrations of successful public health applications of these methods.

SAMPLING DESIGNS IN QUALITATIVE RESEARCH

Along with a credible research design, effective qualitative research hinges on proper selection of the sources of information that will address a given research question. The adage "garbage in, garbage out" applies: Collecting data from the wrong people leads to poor-quality or invalid data that cannot serve as the basis for evidence-based policies or programs. Consequently, sampling and the selection (from random to purposeful) of participants in qualitative public health research is a critical point of methodological discussion (Trotter, 2012; Trotter & Medina Mora, 2000).

Most qualitative research designs employ nonprobabilistic sampling strategies (Trotter & Medina Mora, 2000), some of which can lead to whole population descriptions and generalizability of findings (Frank & Snijders, 1994; Heckathorn, 1997), while

Figure 15.1 Basic Qualitative Research Design and Process

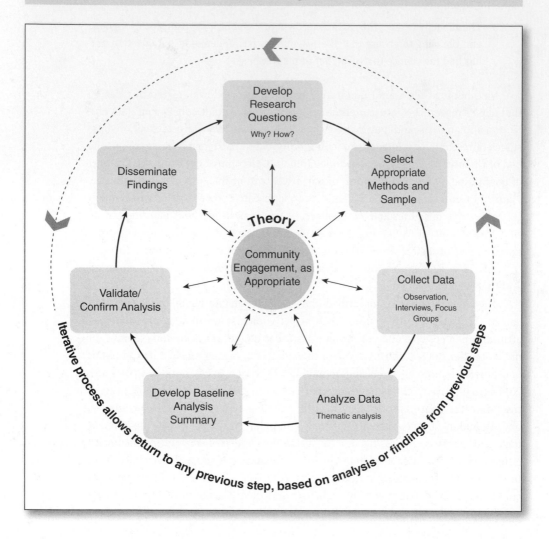

others are limited to describing much smaller populations. Probability (or random) samples are less frequently used in qualitative research for a few reasons:

- Much qualitative research is not intended or designed for statistical analysis or generalizability; it is designed for baseline description of people engaged in health behaviors and for theory and variable generation.
- There is little evidence of the normal distribution of the values, beliefs, attitudes, and perceptions across particular populations or topics (ACAPS, 2012).
- The potential for missing "experts" or specific individuals who have unique attributes (e.g., knowledge, experiences, social position) relative to the research question(s) is very high for most probabilistic samples, while qualitative sampling designs are specifically targeted at finding and engaging those cultural experts.

However, as Johnson (1990) shows in his seminal book on qualitative sampling, there are also qualitative research projects for which random or probabilistic sampling is feasible and absolutely appropriate (see Guest, Namey, & Mitchell, 2013, for examples).

The current state of the art for qualitative sampling includes four empirically tested techniques that produce scientifically defensible data relevant to public health (cf. Trotter, 2012): (1) nominated expert sampling, (2) intensive case finding through geographical sampling, (3) referral sampling, and (4) targeted sampling. Chapter 17 describes additional approaches to nonprobability sampling.

- **Nominated expert sampling** is a classic qualitative approach to exploring cultural and social meanings in various populations, communities, and cultural groups (Trotter, 2012; Trotter & Medina Mora, 2000). Defining the sample involves identifying consensus experts (those nominated by multiple other individuals in a community) to explore or confirm a specific area of knowledge or life experience. Since experts tend to agree about the majority of their subject area and also provide explanation of the variability in thought or experience, nominated expert samples produce a data set that is qualitatively valid, reliable, and culturally generalizable using a relatively small sample (Romney, Weller, & Batchelder, 1986).

- **Intensive case finding through geographical sampling** capitalizes on the condition that people with similar life experiences and views tend to congregate in identifiable locations. This allows researchers to characterize and target social settings that are ideal for drawing concentrated qualitative samples within subgroups of a larger population. The approach works particularly well for research on place-bound behaviors (such as those occurring in clinics, schools, bars, sporting venues, etc.). The researcher identifies a set of known (or discoverable) locations where the target behaviors occur on a regular basis and then recruits research participants from those locations using either a probabilistic or purposeful recruitment strategy (Curtis, Gesler, Smith, & Washburn, 2000).

- **Referral sampling** (snowball sampling and network-based sampling are the most common varieties) starts with an index individual who is identified as having the important characteristics, behaviors, or experiences relevant to the research objectives. This individual is then asked to refer others "like him or her" to participate in the research. The nominated individuals constitute a second wave of data collection, their nominees are the third wave, and so on until the required sample size is reached. One benefit of carefully designed nominated or referral samples is that they can provide a framework estimating the characteristics of whole populations (Frank & Snijders, 1994). Heckathorn's (1997) respondent-driven sampling is one of the most widely used variations on referral sampling. Another common referral sampling strategy is group identification and network sampling, which can be used to create defensible samples for studies of communities and bounded cultural groups (Schensul, Schensul, & LeCompte, 1999). Social network samples focus on mapping specific relationships (drug use, needle sharing, sexual partnerships) as well as their intensity, directionality, and frequency (see also Chapter 14). This type of sampling allows public health practitioners to make inferences about the type and quality of the relationships, core versus peripheral participation in the group, roles and statuses in the group, and dynamic interactions in the group (Salganik & Heckathorn, 2004).

- **Targeted sampling** is a well-substantiated sampling choice for mixed methods designs in hard-to-reach populations or where it is impossible to use an appropriate preexisting sampling frame. Targeted sampling (Robinson et al., 2006; Watters & Biernacki, 1989) consists of four steps: (1) initial mapping of county- and city-level indicators of behavior; (2) ethnographic mapping of candidate census tracts, neighborhoods, or other geopolitical entities; (3) development of initial recruitment plan for each site; and (4) ongoing revision of recruitment plans for each site (Bluthenthal & Watters, 1995). This strategy can be used as a reasonable substitute for strict probabilistic sampling designs in situations where qualitative and quantitative data are needed from the same population.

Often *theoretical saturation* is cited as a sampling parameter for qualitative research, meaning that you "interview to redundancy," or collect data until you are no longer learning something new about the topic. Most funders of public health research, however, require up-front estimates of sample size, which these sampling approaches can help to facilitate (see also Guest, Bunce, & Johnson, 2006; Guest et al. 2013). Qualitative sampling approaches do have limitations with regard to generalizing to large populations, especially highly diverse populations that are multimodal on beliefs, values, knowledge, and processes; however, this level of generalizability is typically not the aim of qualitative research or analysis.

OVERVIEW OF COMMON QUALITATIVE RESEARCH METHODS

The most common qualitative data collection methods are probably familiar, including **observation** (with a range of researcher involvement) and **interviewing** (including individual and group interview techniques). While there are various "camps" and approaches to qualitative research (see Creswell, 2006, for a description), qualitative researchers generally employ systematic, inductively oriented data collection processes, using in situ observation, open-ended questioning, and contextualized solicitation of ideas and opinions in people's own words. Analysis of the data generated through these methods is usually qualitative, using some form of thematic analysis (Charmaz, 2006; Corbin & Strauss, 2008; Guest, MacQueen, & Namey, 2012). We present a brief description of the main methods here; readers interested in more detailed coverage of the how-to of qualitative methods can find dedicated chapters on participant observation, in-depth interviews, and focus groups in *Collecting Qualitative Data* (Guest et al., 2013) and will also find references in the Additional Resources section at the end of this chapter.

Participant Observation

The term *participant observation* has two different referents. First, participant observation is a qualitative research paradigm that "puts you where the action is and lets you collect data" (Bernard, 2013, p. 310). A strong participant observation design is a systematic and integrated multi-method approach to field-based data collection (Schensul et al., 1999), developed to include specific methods, based on the project's guiding theory and research objectives. The basic methodological suite for participant observation includes the following:

1. Direct (in-context) observation of the environment and behaviors under study, including systematic—not impressionistic—recording of observational data. Observations can be guided by exploratory (inductive, grounded theory) approaches to highly quantified and operationally defined confirmatory or even hypothesis testing approaches, depending on the research question.

2. Participation by the primary researcher(s) in the experiential aspects of the behaviors under study, to the extent that is possible and ethical, in order to gain both an empirical and a humanistic understanding of those behaviors. This enhances both analysis and interpretation of the data.

3. Systematic collection of sociocultural narratives (through interviews, focus groups, natural environment conversations, dialogues, secondary data sources) that focus on "cultural expert" descriptions and explanations of the *what, why, who, where, when,* and context of the issues being studied.

4. A systematic approach to the management and analysis (and integration) of the complex data that a solidly designed participant observation study yields. The analysis can be based on emergent theory (grounded theory) and/or (simultaneously) existing theory to advance knowledge of public health conditions and issues (Trotter, Needle, Goosby, Bates, & Singer, 2001; Trotter, Needle, Goosby, Bates, & von Zinkernagel, 2000).

The second use of the term *participant observation* refers more narrowly to a technique combining elements 1 and 2 above: a process of in situ observation with some degree of interaction between the researcher and the environment/people being observed (DeWalt & DeWalt, 2011). The researcher may be an external *participant observer* seeking "to learn what life is like for an 'insider' while remaining, inevitably, an 'outsider'" (Mack, Woodsong, MacQueen, Guest, & Namey, 2005, p. 13) or an insider acting as an *observing participant*, noting and recording some aspect of life around her or him (Bernard, 2013). In either case, several types of data collection are possible in participant observation, as described in Table 15.1.

The strengths of observational activities are related to the embeddedness of the researcher and the ability to see and note what is happening in a given context. Within public health, observational methods are often used to do the following:

1. *Establish topics of inquiry for later, more structured data collection.* If knowledge of a social milieu is so minimal that research domains or questions cannot be formulated, participant observation is an excellent starting point.

Table 15.1 Types of Data Collection in Participant Observation

Data Type	Description	Pros and Cons
Observation notes, audio, video	The baseline for participant observation, notes and recordings are a written/transcribed/digital record of what the researcher saw or heard during the observation period	Very open to emergent data; little/no instrument bias. Can be difficult to capture in some venues, time-consuming to analyze, subject to the bias of the researcher regarding what to note or record.
Casual conversations, informal interviews	Notes or recordings of actual conversations	Capture data in the vernacular and in context. May not be relevant to research objectives; can be hard to accurately record in some settings. May be highly idiosyncratic and difficult to analyze.
Semistructured or structured interviews	Interviews conducted using an interview guide	Provide data relevant to the research objectives. Takes the encounter into a research mode that decreases some aspects of the natural context.
Counts of specific observations	Counts of the frequency/intensity/source of specific behaviors of interest; usually collected with the aid of a template listing the types of things to be counted	Provide data that can be used to identify norms or make comparisons between events, times, individuals, etc. Requires the development of a data collection instrument and the ability to accurately record the behavior of interest in the field setting.
Process flows	Visual or verbal records of common processes; often laid out in a flowchart or stepwise diagram	Excellent for understanding sequenced events (work flows, manufacturing processes, decision processes). Can be challenging to capture. Potential for capturing an idiosyncratic version.
Lists and categories	Lists of items, categories, and inclusion/exclusion rules	Provide both list content and cultural meaning. Can be tedious to collect and may be difficult to extract "rules."

Source: Guest et al. (2013).

2. *Avoid suspect self-reported data.* There are some topics for which people cannot or will not accurately report their own behavior (petty criminality, violations of social norms, etc.). Participant observation can lessen this form of self-report bias and yield a more valid understanding of these behaviors.

3. *Identify behaviors that might go unreported or be missed due to the limitations of procedural memory.* Highly routine or unconscious behaviors are notoriously easy to miss during interviews, focus groups, and surveys. Seeing these occur in a natural setting allows them to become part of the data.

4. *Lessen reporting biases.* Those without direct knowledge of a social scene may collect data that reflect their own points of view rather than the social reality of the people in it.

5. *Integrate the observed behavior into its physical context.* If the location and setting of the behavior of interest are critical to understanding, observation offers insights into how the setting and behavior interact.

6. *See the behavior you are interested in as it happens.* If your research questions are about observable behaviors, observation puts you in direct contact with the phenomena of interest in a way unrivaled by other data collection techniques (adapted from Guest et al., 2013).

A note of caution: The term *participant observation* is frequently misused in qualitatively oriented research proposals and publications. Too often, researchers use the term as an opaque catch-all, meaning, "Trust me, I know what I am doing, even though I don't want to tell you what that is, specifically." Be prepared to unpack the term if you use it, describing the research use of observation through a careful consideration of the areas, venues, times, and target populations to be included in the participant observation events, along with any other types of data collection involved. This technique should be systematic and grounded in the goals of research to keep it focused (Guest et al., 2013). Participant observers capture as much detail as possible in field notes or with recorders, sometimes using templates or guides to help focus observations or to keep them consistent across research team members. Patton (2002, p. 304) provides excellent examples of "good" and "bad" field notes that illustrate the difference between describing what is observed and making assumptions or interpretations about what is going on. Table 15.2 offers ideas of types of things to observe, though your project's aims will determine which types of observations are most relevant.

One classic example of a public health application of observation techniques comes from the 1990s, when researchers were interested in identifying how HIV transmission continued to spread among injecting drug users (IDUs), despite evidence that they were not sharing needles. To research the issue, Koester and Hoffer (1994) employed qualitative observation methods, joining IDUs in shooting galleries and other places where they went to inject drugs. There the researchers were close enough to the scene of the behavior to be able to observe each step in the process and ask on-the-spot questions about it. This allowed them to identify a crucial step that IDUs failed to consider when retelling their process of injecting: Drug injectors

Table 15.2 General Things to Observe

Category	Examples	Things to Note
Physical environment	Structural and geographical features	Map physical features of the environment as well as locations of particular behaviors and activities
Appearance of people	Demographics of individuals in the area, such as gender, estimated age and ethnicity, and any noteworthy physical appearance	Any trends and/or imbalances in demographic characteristics; range of types of individuals, including demographics, clothing, and unique appearance relative to others
Verbal behavior and interactions	Who speaks to whom and for how long, who initiates interaction; languages or dialects spoken	Any trends and/or imbalances in demographic characteristics in terms of interactions; range of languages/dialects spoken
Activities	Activities that occur in the area/venue; which people are engaged in which activities; duration of activities; temporal dimensions of activities	Range of activities; activity trends and associations of particular activities with certain types of individuals; temporal range and patterns of activities
Movement	Who enters and exits the area, and how many; time individuals spend in the area	When and where people enter and exit, where they come from, and how long they stay; demographic characteristics and whether they are alone or accompanied by others
Individuals who seem different from others in the area/group	Identifying people who dress or otherwise look different from others, or who are treated differently from others	Unique characteristics and what differentiates them from others; in many cases these individuals can be good key informants

shared other equipment, such as cottons and cookers used to filter and prepare drugs. Also, some users practiced "back-filling," opening the back of a syringe so that a friend could draw a specified amount of drugs from it. These sources of cross-contamination, dubbed *indirect sharing*, were potentially responsible for the continued transmission of HIV and hepatitis among the injecting drug user population.

Subsequent research confirmed the findings and offered more nuanced understanding of the intervention needs, which included education on the dangers of indirect sharing.

Page and Evans (2003) also employed the participant observation paradigm (and technique) to investigate a survey finding that tobacco use by African American youth was relatively low. The study team first observed adolescents smoking in public places and then conducted interviews with teens and their parents. "The field team's original intention for use of observational data was to gain a general picture of smoking behaviors among middle school age students, but in fact, several other kinds of information emerged" (p. 68). For instance, one of the main findings was that "Black & Milds," a cigarillo with 5 to 12 times the nicotine of cigarettes, was the tobacco product of choice among youth. The authors concluded that since users of these cigarillos "tend not to recognize them as tobacco and believe they contain no nicotine" (p. 64), the self-reported survey data was probably truthful, though an inaccurate representation of tobacco use among African American youth. Participant observation, including follow-up interviews, helped to refine and explain the survey findings and suggested intervention points—as well as potential changes to be made to items on tobacco use surveys for youth.

Individual and Group Interview Techniques

Virtually all qualitative researchers use interview techniques to some extent, and for many projects and researchers, interviews are the primary or sole source of data. This method is versatile across a range of study topics, adaptable to challenging field conditions, and excellent for not just providing information but generating understanding as well. We will discuss two types of interviews in detail here: one-on-one or in-depth interviews and focus group discussions. The basic processes for both are similar: A good interviewer or moderator will capitalize on interpersonal dynamics, using body language and verbal cues to encourage respondents to share their experiences and opinions (Green & Thorogood, 2009). The main difference between individual and group interviews relates to these dynamics and how they affect what people will say in a given context. Table 15.3 provides a comparison of in-depth interviews and focus groups and their uses.

In-Depth Interviews

An in-depth interview (IDI) is a guided conversation or narrative designed to elicit depth on a topic of interest. There are several features that characterize IDIs and that are essential to the power and utility of the technique. In general, IDIs

- are conducted one-on-one,
- use open-ended questioning,
- use inductive probing to get depth, and
- look and feel like a conversation.

Table 15.3 Individual In-Depth Interviews and Focus Group Comparison

Type of Interview	Strengths	Common Uses
Individual in-depth interviews	• Allow researchers to get "deep" answers to their questions from "experts" on the issue • Helpful for answering the *how* and *why* of processes, decision making, belief systems, mental models, interpretations, motivations, expectations, hopes, and fears • Can elucidate the meaning of norms, opinions, or experiences • Are more likely to capture individuals' personal opinions and values, rather than public or expected beliefs and values • Conversational, open-ended style is familiar to everyone • Easy to establish intimate setting and interpersonal rapport • Possible to have multiple, sequential conversations	• For narrower topics that require depth • If interested in personal narrative and individual experiences or opinions • To understand connections and relationships between particular events, phenomena, and beliefs • For sensitive or highly personal topics • When response independence is important
Focus group discussions	• Efficient for gathering a range of perspectives on a given topic • Group dynamics and cognitive triggers stimulate conversation • Can identify areas of consensus or disagreement • Provide an excellent window into "public discourse" and expected social norms and narratives • Can identify and discuss group norms	• For broader topics that require range • When studying social norms or seeking public-level narratives • If interested in group dynamics or process • To develop or pre-test campaigns or messages • To evaluate processes, programs, messages • As a way to "member check" findings from PO or IDI activities

IDIs can be used throughout the research process and at multiple points along the path of learning about a topic or issue. Weiss (1994) suggests that IDIs are useful for research that aims to develop detailed or holistic descriptions, integrate multiple perspectives, describe processes, learn how events are interpreted, and/or identify variables and frame hypotheses for quantitative research. This multiplex utility of IDIs is one of the reasons why they are so often one element of mixed method approaches in public health.

If we distill individual interviewing into the basic steps required, the process is (1) build rapport, (2) ask questions, (3) ask (probing) follow-up questions, and (4) repeat until the person has nothing new to add. The role of the interviewer is to *guide* the conversation. As Bernard (2013) puts it, "Get people on to a topic of interest and get out of the way. Let the informant provide information he or she thinks is important" (p. 185). During analysis you can look for consensus between participants and variability among them.

As noted in Table 15.3, in-depth interviews are typically the preferred approach for asking questions about polarizing, sensitive, confidential, or highly personal topics, since effective elicitation of information on these issues requires a space in which the interviewee can feel safe discussing matters that are usually kept private. For some sensitive or taboo topics, such as sexual activity, illicit behavior, or death, an interview serves as a forum where people can reflect on their own attitudes, opinions, and behaviors in a way they might not in a regular conversation. Similarly, because the setting is one-on-one, interviewees may be less concerned about offending someone else or answering in the "right" or socially acceptable way than if they were in a group setting (though potential for this kind of social desirability bias still exists). In some cases, discussing sensitive topics in a group or public setting could also put the interviewee at risks that range from social embarrassment to financial loss to actual physical harm.

One example of the productive use of IDIs in public health comes from work Lyerly and colleagues (2006) conducted on how women and couples think about what to do with "extra" frozen embryos. The objective was to explore the range of factors influencing couples' decision making in order to develop better counseling and policies surrounding frozen embryo disposition. Each of the four available options for handling the extra embryos was discussed: saving embryos for a future pregnancy attempt, thawing and discarding the embryos, donating them for stem cell research, or donating them to another infertile couple for adoption. The topic was sensitive in that it related to both infertility and morality (in terms of how people viewed their embryos). For many people, the interview was the first time they had to explicitly examine the beliefs and feelings guiding them about what to do with their frozen embryos.

The format of the interviews facilitated candid discussions about the meaning of the frozen embryos—for each individual, to the couple or family, and as a potential source of research material or adoption hope. One of the interesting findings from this research was that some women suggested there could be an alternative option to those presented—an option to return embryos to the woman's body at a time she was unlikely to get pregnant, allowing them to be reabsorbed instead of "discarded" in a lab somewhere. This idea was included in a subsequent national survey on the issue, and 19% of respondents said they would be likely or very likely to consider the option of transplanting the embryos to the woman's body at an infertile time (Lyerly et al., 2010). The findings from the in-depth interviews provided a response option for the survey that may never have been included—and one that nearly one-fifth of respondents agreed with.

Focus Group Discussions

Focus groups have the distinction of being the qualitative data collection technique with a name recognizable to the nonresearch public. The frequent use of the term, however, does not mean that everyone who says something about "focus groups" is talking about the same thing. From a research standpoint, it is important to define precisely what we mean by focus group discussion: a carefully planned conversation with a group of 8–12 people on a focused topic. Research focus groups generally have the following characteristics (Guest et al., 2013):

- A small group of people brought together explicitly to participate in a research discussion regarding a defined topic. This is substantially different from a debate, a cocktail party conversation, or a town hall meeting.
- Similarity among group members in terms of some aspect of their characteristics, experiences, or situation that causes them to feel they all have something in common (being female neurosurgeons or American men who were circumcised as adults, for example). This is key to building the rapport that makes a focus group successful.
- Lack of preexisting social relationships between the group members, so as to limit issues of hierarchy and to facilitate trust and openness during the discussion.
- Discussion guided by a skilled moderator or facilitator who controls the flow of questions and answers, and who explicitly uses group dynamics to uncover information and gain insights.

Focus group discussions rely on important elements of normal human conversation (sharing of experiences, opinions, perceptions, and reactions) and aspects of how we retrieve information stored in our memories (cognitive triggers) to enable the group to address the research objectives (Barbour, 2007). Just as human groups have certain characteristics and capabilities that are not just the sum of their individual members (a person can run in panic, but only a group can "stampede"), so too do focus groups yield data and insights that are more than just the sum of the perceptions, beliefs, and experiences of those taking part in the discussion (Patton, 2002).

Like IDIs, focus groups are a versatile technique that can be used for a wide variety of topics and research interests. Groups are an especially good method for collecting data on things that are inherently shared or that have a public aspect.

- *Group norms and normative expectations*—These can be at very broad levels (cultural norms) or much more specific (workplace routines, what happens during a visit to a doctor's office, what people do following a minor car accident, etc.).
- *Opinions and perspectives*—For topics on which a variety of viewpoints is known or expected to exist, groups can be a great way to explore the range of opinions. In these situations, the moderator stimulates mild debate among group members to discover how perspectives on the topic differ and how those holding different points of view support their positions.
- *Reactions and responses*—Focus groups are often used as a testing ground for reactions to social marketing campaigns, health product designs, public health interventions, service innovations, and so on. The focus group setting can capture both the direction and strength of the response, while ensuing discussion can critique or improve specific elements of the source material.

- *Problem solving and brainstorming*—The cognitive triggering in focus groups can often produce a team mentality in which the group members solve a problem, make suggestions, or brainstorm ideas for communications, products, or policies.
- *Group processes and group dynamics*—If your research topic is itself about a group process or about how people interact in groups, focus groups may enable you to observe these phenomena in action (Guest et al., 2013).

Successful conduct of a focus group requires training and skill. The moderator must carry a general idea of the topics to be covered, ask thoughtful questions, listen to answers with one ear toward how they relate to other topics on the list (to make smooth transitions) and the other ear toward the content of the response, pick up on and probe into interesting ideas or phrases, and at the same time skillfully make sure that everyone is engaged and is interacting with other members of the group (see also Seidman, 2006, pp. 78–79, for a description of the types of listening necessary for effective interviewing). In one-on-one interviews, too, the interviewer balances rapport and a conversation-like feel to the interview with an eye on the clock, the interview guide, and the research objectives to ensure that the "conversation" covers all of the necessary areas. In neither case should managing time be equated with administering Q1, Q2, Q3, Q4, getting a quick answer, and proceeding. One of the biggest advantages of the qualitative paradigm is the ability to probe into responses or observations as needed to obtain more detailed descriptions and explanations of experiences, behaviors, and beliefs, and it is up to the moderator (or interviewer for IDIs) to follow relevant leads.

Siddiqui and colleagues (n.d.) used focus groups to learn about norms around urinary incontinence among different ethnic groups in the southern United States. Epidemiological data show that urinary incontinence (UI) affects up to 45% of the female population of the United States, yet among women with UI, 70% of White compared to 16% Hispanic, 6% Black, and 5% Asian admitted to seeking care (Morrill et al., 2007). The goal of the study was to identify and compare normative beliefs about UI and to highlight potential intervention points for increasing treatment of UI in minority populations. Focus groups were convened with White, Hispanic, and Black women separately, stratified also by those who did and did not experience UI. All groups were asked the same questions about how UI was discussed among families and friends, within the larger ethnic community, and what they had learned from popular media. These questions were followed by questions about health seeking behaviors generally, and then more specifically for UI. A comparative thematic analysis of these data is underway, following an information-motivation-behavioral skill model.

How Do You Choose (or Know If Someone Has Chosen Wisely)?

Since focus groups and/or individual interviews are crucial to most projects, how do you choose between or mix and match them? Bernard (2000) usefully identifies "a continuum of interview situations based on the amount of control we try to exercise over people's responses" (p. 190). We refer to this level of control as the degree of

MODIFYING THE MEDIUM FOR CONDUCTING INTERVIEWS

While many of the examples presented in this chapter involved face-to-face interviewing of individuals or groups, there are several options for conducting interviews remotely. The table below summarizes a few of the more common options, along with some pros and cons to each. Note that you can also incorporate technology into data collection with things like videos or polling software (see www.polleverywhere.com). See the In Focus section at the end of Chapter 21 for more on mobile and digital data collection.

Medium	Pros	Cons
Phone or voice-over Internet	Enables cost-effective data collection with interviewees in geographically distant or highly dispersed locations. Can be useful when interviewees need to maintain a degree of anonymity.	Rapport can be harder to build without face-to-face contact. Data are less rich due to lack of body language. Requires both interviewer and interviewee to have access to reliable phone connections. In focus groups, it can be hard to tell when someone is ready to speak or would like to get in on the conversation.
Internet—written	Exchange of written question and answers can be done "live" in a single session or as a threaded discussion over days or weeks. Creates a full written record of responses. For some interviewees the process creates more thoughtful responses.	As with phone, rapport may be impaired and body language cues are absent from the data. Respondents who do not like to type may give shorter, less complete answers. Requires literate interviewees with Internet capability. Cross-typing (where more than one person types a response at a time) is frequent and can disrupt the flow of the conversation in "live" sessions.
Internet—video	Often a good approximation of face-to-face interviewing, cost-effective, and good for geographically distant or dispersed interviewees. Video capture enables a full record of the session.	Requires broadband Internet, webcam/speakers, and some degree of technical savvy on the part of both the interviewer and interviewee.

structure within the interview process. Three general terms used in this regard are unstructured, semistructured, and structured, but as Figure 15.2 illustrates, these are markers within a range (the x-axis). At one extreme are completely unscripted conversations, the type a researcher might have when doing participant observation or when almost nothing is known about a topic. At the other extreme fall highly structured interviews, in which the questions are asked verbatim and response categories are fixed (quantitative surveys). Most qualitative interviews are semistructured and fall somewhere in the middle, with more naturalistic interviews on the unstructured side and formal systematic qualitative techniques (freelists, pilesorts, social network interviews, decision modeling, cultural models interviews, etc.) on the more structured side.

Figure 15.2 General Interview Typology

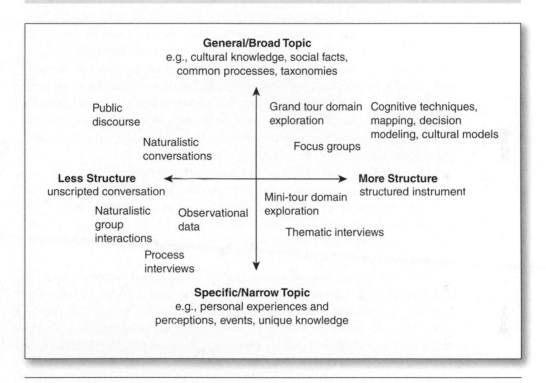

Source: Adapted from Guest et al. (2013, p. 115).

Figure 15.2 also includes, on the y-axis, a continuum of interview topics to consider. Topics that are more specific or narrow are better addressed in a one-on-one interview, where a respondent will have time to go in greater depth about a personal experience or specific knowledge. Broader or more general topics can be addressed by individual interviews as well, but group or focus group interviews may be more efficient, because a greater range of cultural knowledge can be generated quickly in a group setting.

Consider the following to choose between different interview methods:

- What are the main research questions that the interviews are intended to answer?
- What are the primary domains of content that should be covered in the interview?
- What types of data are needed to provide these answers (opinions, experiences, knowledge, attitudes—at a personal or public level)?

These questions, along with Table 15.3, provide some important considerations for identifying which type of interview goes with which type of data collection need. But theory, experience, and the need for flexibility factor in as well. For example, Namey and Lyerly (2010) collaborated on the Good Birth Project, a study investigating how U.S. women define a "good" birth experience, with an aim of improving maternity care (Lyerly, 2013). A senior consultant to the project insisted that focus groups would most efficiently and effectively address this topic, despite arguments that women's birth narratives were both extremely detailed (narrow) and highly personal (women were emotionally invested). The team agreed to conduct a pilot focus group, and Namey convened a group of women who were alike on two key dimensions of birth experience: All had delivered their babies vaginally and in a hospital setting. Though the group dynamic limited how much detail a woman could provide about her personal experiences, the discussion was open and productive—until the issue of epidural analgesia was raised. Some women in the group had requested and received epidurals, others had opted to "go natural."

The conversation then proceeded on eggshells, with women careful to couch their responses in socially acceptable ways. Those who had "gone natural" were lauded as brave or strong, which then caused those who had opted for an epidural to preface their remarks with slightly defensive comments about how or why an epidural was good or necessary. A veil of social correctness had fallen, and no amount of follow-up questioning could pull it away.

While this was extremely interesting data on the public-level narrative about birth (and provided good fodder for follow-up interviews), the group interview method was ill suited to the research objective of collecting rich, explanatory descriptions of the elements that made individual women's experiences good for them, regardless of what society had to say about their choices. It was hard for women to be honest about their experiences and opinions knowing that they may inadvertently offend another woman in the group who held precisely the opposite views or made different choices. In-depth interviews were used for the remainder of the data collection.

Additional Qualitative Research Methods That Enhance the Basic Set

While the core elements of participant observation and interviewing account for the bulk of qualitative research done in public health, there are a variety of additional, sometimes supplemental, methods that also rely on qualitative data collection techniques. These methods include free listing, ranking exercises, pile sorts, ethnographic

ENHANCING VALIDITY IN QUALITATIVE RESEARCH

Chapter 2 provides an introduction to some of the issues around validity in research. In qualitative research, validity is sometimes referred to as credibility, and it addresses the believability or accurateness of data on a particular issue within a particular population. The tips below provide "suggestions for enhancing rigor and transparency" to improve validity, but "procedures alone can never replace sound research or compensate for inadequate understanding of basic research principles" (Guest et al. 2013, p. 101).

Technique	What It Does
Research Design Stage	
Use multiple methods and/or data sources	• Collecting data via multiple methods and from a variety of sources provides the opportunity to compare findings in analysis for convergence or divergence (triangulation, constant comparative method).
Team-based instrument development (if using a guide) and pretest	• Involving the whole research team in steps of the instrument development processes increases validity by familiarizing the team with the connection between research objectives and questions on the guide at an early stage. • Brainstorming specific questions to include may increase validity of the questions, since multiple perspectives will be considered (reduces bias from any one person). • Pretesting facilitates validity by ensuring questions make sense to participants.
Data Collection Stage	
Train field team in collection techniques	• Training data collectors on the purpose behind the questions and probing techniques improves the relevance of data collected (that is, interviewers are more likely to ask follow-up questions directly related to the study objectives).
Monitor data as they come in	• Providing data collectors with immediate feedback (or receiving feedback on your own data) improves data quality and consistency. Debriefing on a regular basis is an important element in qualitative reliability and validity checks.

(Continued)

(Continued)

Technique	What It Does
Elicit feedback from participants after summarizing their interview	• Having participants review what they said improves validity and provides the researcher with an opportunity to clarify anything that was unclear or ambiguous.
Data Analysis Stage	
Transcribe data using a transcription protocol	• Transcription provides a verbatim account of the data collection event, thereby enhancing validity. • Using a transcription protocol ensures that transcription is done consistently and is of the appropriate type for the analytic aims.
Establish translation expectations from the start	• Translation techniques and styles vary greatly. Establishing your translation approach up front increases the likelihood that your data will be useful for the analysis planned. Improper translation protocols result in highly questionable data, analysis, and interpretation.
Develop and use a precise codebook	• The vast majority of coding reliability problems are due to differing interpretations of code meanings. The more descriptive and precise a codebook, the better inter-coder reliability will result. • Good codebooks also facilitate data comparison if using the same codes in a different study. • This provides easy access to code meanings for internal reviews.
Use multiple coders and inter-coder agreement checks	• Coding agreement comparisons facilitate coding reliability by providing checks on individual biases and variance in interpretation of code definitions. • Coding comparisons generate iterative revisions to the codebook, improving the precision of code definitions. • Intercoder agreement exercises can provide a metric for assessing progress in consistency of code application (if using percent agreement or Kappa statistic).
External and/or peer review of coding and summaries	• Outside review facilitates coding validity by providing checks on individual biases and variance in interpretation of code definition (a reliability issue as well).

Technique	What It Does
Create an audit trail	• Such a trail makes the analysis process more transparent for other researchers to review. • It also facilitates internal review of processes and the ability to accurately replicate procedures if desired.
Triangulate, combine, or cross-reference data sources	• If analyzed properly, convergent data from different methods/sources validate findings. • Divergence of data indicates a need to adapt explanatory models and provide potential reasons for the discordance.
Negative case analysis	• Consciously including negative cases in an analysis mitigates analyst biases by forcing analysts to look for and report any evidence contrary to prevailing patterns identified in the data.
Support themes and interpretations with quotes	• Using verbatim quotes increases validity of findings by directly connecting the researcher's interpretations with what participants actually said.

Source: Adapted from Guest et al. (2013, pp. 99–101).

decision modeling, visual elicitation techniques, and others. We have provided a brief description of many of these techniques, along with common applications and key references, in Table 15.4.

QUALITATIVE DATA MANAGEMENT AND ANALYSIS

Qualitative Data Management

Data management includes "all the processes necessary for systematically and consistently collecting, tracking, preparing, processing, organizing, storing, securing, retrieving, verifying, and sharing qualitative data so that it can be used to (a) inform subsequent data collection and (b) perform data analysis" (McLellan-Lemal, 2008, p. 168). As such, there is no single data management "step" to be performed on qualitative data; it is an ongoing, dynamic series of activities that is interwoven with recruitment, data collection, coding, and analysis in an attempt to organize interrelated data and make them accessible for full analysis. Table 15.5 identifies specific data management tasks that run for the life of a project.

Table 15.4 Overview of Additional Qualitative Data Collection Techniques

Technique	Description
Free listing	Elicitation of an exhaustive list of elements or items in a particular domain. Usually phrased as, "What are all of the X in Y," followed by probes of "Can you think of anything else?" Example: *What are all of the health problems in your community?*
Potential uses	• When you have limited information about your research topic • When you want to identify the range and parameters of a domain • When you want to create the primary items for other techniques such as surveys or domain classification techniques • To get people brainstorming about a topic as a warm-up
References	Bernard (2000); Bernard & Ryan (2010); Borgatti (1999); Weller & Romney (1988)
Context	Group or one-on-one
Rating or ranking exercises	Research participants rate or rank a series of items, either provided by the researcher or generated within the interview (e.g., during free listing). May be done orally, visually (using stickers), or in writing. Example: *Which health problems in your community are the most important to you?*
Potential uses	• To establish priorities • To reach consensus on most relevant issues • To identify important sequences of events
References	Bernard (2011); Weller & Romney (1988)
Context	Group or one-on-one
Pile sorting	Research participants put items (words, pictures, objects, sometimes generated through free listing) in piles that make sense to them. Example: *Ask participants to place free-listed health problems together in groups that make sense to them. Participants might make a pile for chronic disease, infectious disease, pediatric issues, geriatric issues, structural issues, etc.*
Potential uses	• To construct a taxonomy for a given domain • To elicit judgments of similarity among items in a cultural domain

Technique	Description
	• To identify attributes people use to distinguish items • To identify underlying dimensions in complex domains
References	Borgatti (1999); Weller & Romney (1988)
Context	Group or one-on-one
Mapping	Research participants are asked to create a map of a particular area or behavior, with a specific objective in mind. Example: *Draw a map of all of the areas around your school where teenagers smoke.*
Potential uses	• To address research questions with a spatial dimension • To identify spatial sequences of behavior • To collect stacked information—qualitative, quantitative, social, behavioral, and geographic—in one sitting • To see the participant's geographic view of the issue • To create concept maps
References	Perkins (2007); Kuznar & Werner (2001)
Context	Group or one-on-one
Visual elicitation techniques	The use of video, photographs, drawings, or maps—created by the research participants or the researcher—as stimuli to generate discussion or reveal elusive concepts. As a general rule of thumb, less ambiguous stimuli will tend to elicit more factual and tangible responses. More ambiguous stimuli are presumed to better reveal inner values, emotions, and beliefs. Example: *Tell me a story about these three photographs of the community that I have here. [Ask follow-up questions about the topic of interest: How do the factories here affect your daily life?]*
Potential uses	• To reveal underlying values or cognitive and emotive processes that verbal questioning might not reach • To collect information on symbolic elements within a culture (e.g., graffiti, religious symbols, gang markers) that relate to the research topic • To document environmental context (both social and physical) • To get feedback on a visual campaign item
References	Banks (2001, 2007); Pink (2007); Soley & Smith (2008)

(Continued)

(Continued)

Technique	Description
Context	Group or one-on-one
Photovoice	Research participants are asked to take photographs over a prescribed period of time, after developing a theme to guide the topics of the photos. They are then asked to come back and discuss their pictures and create a display or story to share with policymakers or community leaders. Example: *Take photographs to show how malaria affects your life.*
Potential uses	• To allow research participants to present a visual view of their world and then explain it • To collect compelling firsthand accounts for advocacy or community health efforts
References	Blackman (2007); Wang (1999); Wang, Yi, Tao, & Carovano (1998)
Context	Group or one-on-one, particularly effective with adolescents
Drawings and collages	Research participants are asked to draw something or create a collage as a way of representing their thoughts, feelings, or opinions about a particular topic. Example: *Draw a picture or make a collage to represent how drinking alcohol affects your life.*
Potential uses	• To explore ideas or opinions that may be better communicated visually • To allow research participants to present a visual view of their world and then explain it • To conduct a thematic apperception substudy
References	Bagnoli (2009)
Context	Group or one-on-one, particularly effective with children
Laddering	An interviewing technique used to reveal core values regarding a particular belief or behavior. Example: *Asking a series of* why *questions to uncover attributes, consequences, and ultimately underlying values related to choices of unhealthy foods.*
Potential uses	• To develop effective communications or education campaigns • To identify deeply held values that affect motivations to act
References	Guest et al. (2013); Reynolds & Gutman (1988)

Technique	Description
Context	One-on-one
Ethnographic decision modeling	A method to model aggregate decision-making processes across a group, community, or culture. *Example: How do mothers in your community decide whether to take a sick child to the doctor?*
Potential uses	• To identify, document, and predict behavioral decision points • To strategize interventions (one to match each decision point)
References	Gladwin (1989); Ryan & Bernard (2006)
Context	One-on-one

Table 15.5   Data Management Activities for Qualitative Research

Keeping a record of events	When were data collected? By whom? When were data transcribed/translated? By whom? When were data coded? Using what version of the codebook? By whom? What summaries, matrices, or queries were created using data? When and by whom?
Maintaining standard labeling, organization, and storage procedures	What will study files be called? How will they be organized? (by date, number, subpopulation) Where will they be kept?
Monitoring data quality and study progress	Are data reflecting information that respond to research objectives? Are data of good quality? (appropriate probing, moderation, sufficient detail of field notes, etc.) Is recruitment on schedule with the study timeline? Are coding and analysis?

Additional details on qualitative data management are available in Schensul and LeCompte (2010), Bernard (2013), Guest et al. (2013), and McLellan-Lemal (2008). Public health–oriented data management processes and action plans are described in detail in the Centers for Disease Control and Prevention–supported RARE (Rapid Assessment, Response, and Evaluation) and I-RARE (International RARE) manuals and publications (Trotter et al., 2000; Trotter et al., 2001; Trotter & Singer, 2005).

Qualitative Data Analysis

Qualitative analysis typically includes the systematic analysis of qualitative data (what, how, who, when, where) based either on an emergent (grounded) theory framework or on an existing culture theory framework (Bernard, 2012; Schensul, Schensul, & LeCompte, 2013). It also typically includes an exposition of the qualitative *why* factors in the data by providing a dual interpretation of the data from the perspective of the people who provided it and from the perspective of the researchers who analyzed it (Wolcott, 1994). A number of consistent, defensible approaches to qualitative analysis are tied to the various theoretical frameworks used to collect the data. Some researchers feel that an interpretivist perspective is more closely aligned with a grounded theory approach to qualitative data analysis. Grounded theory is a set of inductive and iterative techniques designed to identify categories and concepts within text that are then linked into formal theoretical models (Corbin & Strauss, 2008; Glaser & Strauss, 1967). A postpositivist approach may draw on the same type of thematic analysis, but will be more focused on supplying evidence (sometimes in the form of theme frequencies or advanced data visualizations) for any interpretations generated. Applied thematic analysis (Guest et al., 2012) borrows useful techniques from varied theoretical and methodological perspectives and adapts them to an applied research context—a context where ensuring the credibility of findings to an external audience is necessary, and achieving this goal is facilitated by systematic methods and procedures.

In most cases, the basic steps of a thematic analysis of qualitative data include the following:

- reading/reviewing data with research/analysis objectives in mind
- identifying key concepts, ideas, and themes in data
- defining and codifying important ideas and themes in a codebook
- coding data, preferably with two independent coders
- summarizing coded data by
  - looking for patterns and relationships among themes
  - identifying theme frequencies to help identify the most salient ideas across data
  - using quantitative data reduction techniques as appropriate
  - referring back to qualitative data, using quotes to emphasize findings

Figure 15.3 illustrates the general flow of the qualitative analysis process.

Qualitative Data Analysis Software

Qualitative data management and analysis can be facilitated by qualitative analysis software. There are several commercial varieties and a few free programs. Most share a core set of functions:

- facilitated application of a complex coding scheme that links segments of narrative to a theme, concept, or issue (a qualitative code)

Figure 15.3   The Qualitative Analysis Process

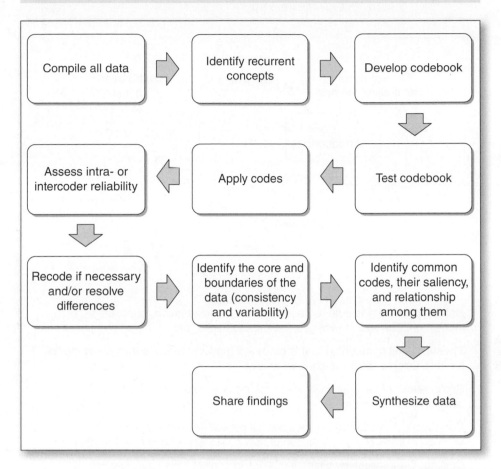

- retrieval of key segments of textual data from large databases
- linkage of concepts and themes within and between interviews or other textual data
- linkage of external variables/data to each narrative (such as the demographic characteristics of the informants, or contextual variables that might have a bearing on the content of the interview)
- strong Boolean and proximity search capabilities that, if carefully and appropriately used, can accommodate highly quantitative content analysis processes

Note that qualitative data analysis software cannot *do* analysis for you. It helps you work with large amounts of data and the codes you create to tag and organize those data. Figure 15.4 illustrates how qualitative data and metadata (the codes and notes we add to data) are related, and it defines common terms.

Figure 15.4 Definitions of and Relationships Among Data and Metadata Items in Qualitative Analysis

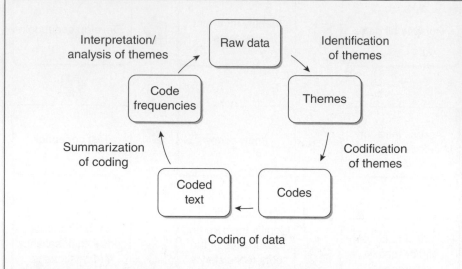

Data: Typically the textual representation of a conversation, observation, or interaction. Can also be images, lists, photographs, etc.

Theme: A unit of meaning that is observed (noticed) in the data by a reader of the text. Often a recurrent concept or idea.

Code: A textual description of the semantic boundaries of a theme or a component of a theme.

Codebook: A structured compendium of codes that includes a definition of each code and often a description of how codes are related to each other.

Coding: The process by which a qualitative analyst links specific codes to specific data segments as a way of tagging examples of themes.

Source: Adapted from Guest et al. (2012, pp. 50, 139).

APPLICATIONS OF QUALITATIVE RESEARCH METHODS TO PUBLIC HEALTH

To this point, we have provided a basic overview of qualitative research methods, focusing on the rationale and implementation of systematic qualitative research. Public health practitioners employ qualitative methods in various contexts, including study of health behaviors and behavior change; health communications; needs assessments; environmental scans; and monitoring and evaluation, to name a few. Table 15.6 links the rationale for and common usage of qualitative methods within these approaches, while the sections below provide examples of recent applications in public health. Note that qualitative research is also often a component of community-based and participatory action research, with mapping, interview, and focus group activities used to assess community resources, strengths, and challenges. This application of qualitative methods is covered in the In Focus section at the end of Chapter 4.

Table 15.6   Strengths of Qualitative Research Methods for Common Public Health Approaches

Public Health Area	Strengths of Qualitative Methods	Method(s) of Choice
Behavior and behavior change	• Identification of routines, motivations, behavioral triggers, and decision points • Ability to distinguish between public and nonpublic levels of personal narrative	In-depth interviews for personal, individual-level; focus groups for public-level narrative; participant observation of current behavior where possible
Health communications	• Identification of health beliefs, knowledge, and attitudes • Exploration of how and why current beliefs, knowledge, and attitudes came to be • Ability to involve target audience in message development and testing	In-depth interviews for design and development; focus groups for testing messages
Needs assessments and environmental scans	• Systematic overview of current context and activities • Open-ended identification of what is needed and why • Ability to describe range of facilitators and barriers • Inclusion of end users and stakeholders in discussion of how to best meet need(s)	Observations for scanning; focus groups with end-users; in-depth interviews with key stakeholders

(Continued)

(Continued)

Public Health Area	Strengths of Qualitative Methods	Method(s) of Choice
Monitoring and evaluation	• Documentation of what occurred during a program, campaign, or intervention • Examination of how participants or recipients experience(d) the project • Qualitative rapid assessment provides timely feedback	Observation to collect data on ongoing activities; in-depth interviews or focus groups to ascertain progress during and after the project (from participants' view)

Behavior and Behavior Change Research

Public health research into behavior and behavior change often focuses on questions of *how* (how do people wash their hands, how do mothers treat their newborns, how do aging adults keep track of their medications) and *why* (why don't people use condoms, why do teens take up smoking, why do people avoid annual check-ups), with an eye toward changing behavior or improving practice for a better public health result.

For example, Torres, Meetze, and Smithwick-Leone (2013) used Photovoice to engage Latina mothers in South Carolina in a conversation about increasing physical activity for their children. The purpose of the study was to have these mothers identify the barriers and opportunities for physical activity for Latino children in their community, reflect on their consensus findings, and then draft policy recommendations. The research team conducted 12 in-depth interviews with Latina mothers, who also took pictures of their families and communities for discussion, and 8 interviews with community stakeholders and school staff. In subsequent focus groups, the Latina mothers identified barriers to physical activity, such as lack of transportation, poor English skills, lack of knowledge about school-based opportunities, and anti-immigrant discrimination. They then developed solutions to address or mitigate these issues and presented their plans using their photos on flipcharts (Torres et al., 2013).

In another example, Lyerly, Namey, Gray, Swamy, and Faden (2012) used in-depth interviews with pregnant women who had received H1N1 vaccine in the context of a clinical trial during the height of the 2009 epidemic to better understand women's reasons for participating in research during pregnancy. They found "that women participated in order to obtain early access to vaccines, to do so in a situation where they would be closely monitored, and to do so in a way that would produce knowledge that might help other pregnant women" (p. 5). These data provide evidence that some pregnant women see research participation as a benefit, and argue against the de facto exclusion of pregnant women from medical research.

Health Communications Research

Qualitative research methods that allow respondents to answer questions using their own words, values, and behaviors can be particularly useful to public health practitioners trying to develop messages or campaigns to influence behaviors or motivate actions. Individual and group interview techniques provide a chance to understand *how* local communities express their understanding of an issue, *what* the important issues or topics are for a given subpopulation, along with information on *why* they are important. All of this feeds into culturally and socially relevant models of how best to package or disseminate information. The text box below highlights some common uses of qualitative methods in the development of effective health communications programs or podcasts.

A study undertaken by Wray and colleagues (2008) used focus groups and cognitive interviews to identify challenges in communicating with the public about emergent health threats. They were interested in assessing the public's baseline knowledge of nonconventional weapons and the health threats they posed. They also wanted to

---

Making Health Communication Programs Work: Common Uses of Qualitative Research Methods

Developing a communication strategy
  o Learning about feelings, motivators, and past experiences related to a health topic
  o Exploring the feasibility of various potential actions (from the intended audience's viewpoint)
  o Identifying barriers to those actions
  o Exploring what benefits the intended audience members find compelling and what results they expect from taking a particular action
  o Learning about the intended audience's use of settings, channels, and activities
  o Capturing the language used by the intended audience to discuss issues

Exploring reactions to message concepts (concept testing)
  o Identifying concepts that do or do not resonate and understanding why
  o Identifying concepts that have a different meaning for participants than those anticipated (cognitive debriefing processes)
  o Triggering the creative thinking of communication professionals
  o Illustrating to others how the intended audience thinks and talks about a health issue

---

Source: Adapted from National Cancer Institute (2001).

understand the types of information that the public would want, expect, and react to in case of an emergency and the sources they would turn to for information. The research team found

> limited public understanding of emerging biological, chemical, and radioactive materials threats and of the differences between them; demand for concrete, accurate, and consistent information about actions needed for protection of self and family; active information seeking from media, local authorities, and selected national sources; and areas in which current emergency messaging [could] be improved. (p. 2214)

These findings help public health officials plan and prepare for a threat situation by highlighting the types of content and delivery routes needed for future messages. Since qualitative data are usually collected in the way "real" people talk *in context*, we then also have information on key words or phrases to include in public health messaging.

The National Institute on Drug Abuse's Cultural Epidemiology Working Group, concerned with both the emergence of new drugs and street uses of existing drugs, has consistently employed qualitative research methods to monitor epidemiological changes in drug use across the nation. As highlighted in their proceedings, "Qualitative information from ethnographic studies or local key informants is also used to describe drug use patterns and trends, and it may be particularly informative in the early identification of new issues or substances being misused or abused" (U.S. Department of Health and Human Services, 2012, p. 7). One key communication element of that monitoring is the constantly changing street names of drugs. Ongoing qualitative research provides street-level updates on naming conventions so that epidemiologists have critical linguistic equivalents that drug abuse respondents will recognize. Epidemiologists can then quantitatively monitor trends and changes in drug use regionally and nationwide by surveying respondents on a regular basis using the latest terms.

Needs Assessment Research

One of the aims of public health practitioners is to make any new public health program or service relevant, significant, and sustainable (Centers for Disease Control and Prevention, 2009). Toward this end, needs assessments are conducted to document the needs of a community or population prior to implementing a new program. The use of qualitative methods during needs assessment activities helps ensure that those needs are not just enumerated, but explained and contextualized. For this reason, there is a growing trend among public and private funding sources to require mixed methods community needs assessment programs to elaborate both the perceived and evidence-based needs for communities. These approaches identify not only the level of need, but also the individuals in need (who), the kinds of needs they have (what), the distribution of those needs (where and when), and the local understanding of those needs (why). In many cases, public health practitioners will conduct a series of in-depth interviews with a range of local stakeholders—politicians, health care providers, clinic administrators, religious leaders, first-responders—to develop a broader- and higher-level view of the issues to consider. These can happen prior to or concurrent with focus groups that bring together members of the end-user community, perhaps mothers, teenagers, teachers, or a specific cultural subpopulation.

Peragallo Urrutia and colleagues (2012) conducted a needs assessment in 2009, in Leogane, Haiti, as plans for a new donor-funded health clinic were being developed. Using a survey of existing health services in Leogane as a basis, the researchers conducted a series of focus groups to ask women from the community to identify their most pressing health needs, barriers to meeting those needs, and how they thought the community and outside organizations should be involved in addressing them. The Haiti earthquake of 2010 disrupted planning for this new clinic and necessitated a reprioritization of resources, though the health needs identified by the community—nutritious food and drink, access to affordable and available medical care, potable water, education/training, and improved sanitation—likely remained similar, if exacerbated. As one woman told the researchers, "We have not eaten anything since this morning . . . some parents do not have anything to give their children. They leave for school in the morning and come back home without eating anything" (p. 95).

The use of qualitative methods in this type of research helps to better match policy and programs to specific populations' needs by soliciting the unconstrained opinions of those populations. Quotes like the one above can help to emotionally underscore the importance of the findings. The RARE method developed by Trotter and colleagues (2000, 2001), provides additional guidance for incorporating assessment activities into a wider framework of intervention development and program evaluation.

Monitoring and Evaluation Research

Funding agencies often require high-quality evaluation of public health programs, initiatives, interventions, and education efforts. Qualitative methods are crucial for

- identifying and defining key stages of development, critical mileposts, and complex accomplishments;
- identifying the logical processes and connections implicit in the program; and
- creating feedback loops within the program for mid-course correction rather than after-the-fact criticism of program challenges and failures. "Quantitative measures can parsimoniously capture snapshots of pre- and post-states, even some interim steps, but qualitative methods are more appropriate for capturing evolutionary and transformational developmental dynamics" (Patton, 2002, p. 168).

Most state-of-the-art evaluation models incorporate both qualitative assessments and quantitative metrics to meet the standards for evaluation design. One example of a complex mixed methods evaluation design is the model developed for the Native American Cancer Prevention (NACP) Program, through a collaborative agreement between the University of Arizona Comprehensive Cancer Center and Northern Arizona

University (NCI U54). The basic design is a technological transfer from industry to public health (cancer prevention) called a *logic model plus* design (Trotter & Singer, 2005). As those familiar with public health monitoring and evaluation will note, an evaluation logic model is a required element of most program evaluations. The "plus" part of the design is the inclusion of qualitative research methods and a query-based approach that uses qualitative questions to monitor progress and identify the achievement of milestones. This approach allows evaluators to capture the initiative as a whole (short-, medium-, and long-term outcomes, plus impact) and also provides a way to target the unique evaluation needs of each specific NACP core, or specific project.

As mentioned in Chapter 1, the distinction between monitoring and evaluation (M&E) activities and research is sometimes a blurry one. Here we've only skimmed the surface of M&E to point out how qualitative methods can fit into the process. For additional information on monitoring and evaluation, see Wholey, Hatry, and Newcomer (2010), which includes chapters on the use of qualitative methods for evaluation.

QUALITATIVE APPROACHES AND GLOBAL HEALTH ISSUES

Moving public health research across borders or between cultures presents additional considerations for planning and conducting qualitative research. As with other research methods, using qualitative research methods in an international or multi-site setting typically increases timelines and budgets and requires consideration of local context in areas such as informed consent and autonomy. The considerations for global health research that are specific to qualitative methods relate to translation, literally—because of the text-based nature of many of the data collection and analysis tasks—and more figuratively, in terms of translating the strengths of the methods presented in this chapter to appropriately reflect the cultural and social norms of the participant population.

In terms of research design, global health research contexts can guide or constrain your use of specific qualitative methods. If, for example, the political or social context is one of big brother–style surveillance, observation activities won't be the best choice for collecting public health data—even if they would most efficiently provide the data necessary to meet study objectives. Similarly, the topic of interviewer-interviewee matching (having researcher and respondent be the same on some key characteristic like gender, age, or ethnic group) can take on increased importance in places where social norms prevent men and women from being in mixed company or where it would be impertinent to have a 20-something asking personal questions of an elder. In research we conducted in West Africa, for instance, we found during pretesting that female sex workers were actually more comfortable speaking to male interviewers than females. They provided two reasons for this: They dealt with men more regularly, as part of their business, and felt that men would be less judgmental about their profession than women would be. We therefore had the men on the research team conduct the interviews.

Contracting with local research agencies can help to overcome some of the translation and implementation challenges related to culture and language. Field teams trained in the research objectives will likely be able to provide a better translation of consent forms, data collection instruments, and eventually the data themselves. Engagement of local researchers also provides an opportunity for capacity building, as training on specific research methods may be required.

CURRENT ISSUES AND FUTURE DIRECTIONS

Qualitative research methodologies have evolved extensively in the last few decades, producing useful, empirically tested mid-range theories, scientifically justified sampling protocols, and analytical strategies that are useful and appropriate for public health practitioners. Using qualitative research methods, we can elicit a range and depth of opinions without having to predefine all of the potential options. We can also explore the context of those opinions and whether they translate to behaviors with public health consequences. Observation and interviewing techniques offer different ways of exploring health behaviors and opinions, but each focuses on selecting appropriate participants and letting them be the "experts" who show or tell us the important (or mundane) details and context of their experiences and beliefs. Qualitative research methods—whether stand-alone or part of a mixed methods design—facilitate explanations and understandings of issues important to the public's health, by allowing us to explore global issues on a local (action) level.

At the same time, qualitative research faces some challenges that will need to be resolved through a continuing evolution of theory, methods, and analytical strategies. One of the continuing challenges for qualitative research is the issue of appropriately protecting both individuals and communities from unintended harm. Qualitative research is frequently "high touch," up close and personal. Anonymity is normally impossible for any meaningful, longer-term qualitative data collection and community explorations, especially among vulnerable populations where the stakes are particularly high, and confidentiality must be maintained at the highest level possible. The continual evolution of human subject protections is an area for both current and future development of research practices and protections (see Whiteford & Trotter, 2008, for discussions of cross-cultural qualitative research ethics and vulnerable populations).

There are several emerging directions in qualitative research that are relevant to public health research. One that is particularly germane for this chapter is the growing utilization of technology in both the dissemination and the testing of public health prevention and intervention programs. There will be significant qualitative contributions to this rapidly changing field, including (1) formative research with end-user communities, populations, and individuals to construct socially and culturally congruent applications; (2) qualitative content explorations of existing websites and social media interactions to form baseline information on what is out there and what it means; and (3) direct contact qualitative research through electronic media and social media that parallels community-based research on similar topics. There are significant theoretical, methodological, and epistemological issues at play in this context. In addition, the need for field-based (ethnographic, participant observational, etc.) research on the use of technology (from medical telemetry, to Internet-based intervention programs, etc.) in "real life" is increasingly apparent. Many technology-based public health programs are treating technology as a potential panacea for face-to-face contact, without investigating the context of use or the barriers to use in specific groups or communities. The interface between technology and people is a highly productive area for qualitative research in the public health context and will remain so as long as technology continues to change at its current pace (see also Chapter 21).

ADDITIONAL RESOURCES

Qualitative Methods for Public Health (general)

Green, J., & Thorogood, N. (2009). *Qualitative methods for health research* (2nd ed.). Thousand Oaks, CA: Sage.

Lindlof, T. R., & Taylor, B. C. (2010). *Qualitative methods for health communication* (3rd ed.). Thousand Oaks, CA: Sage.

Patton, M. Q. (2001). *Qualitative research and evaluation methods*. Thousand Oaks, CA: Sage.

Trotter, R. T., II, & Singer, M. (2005). Rapid assessment strategies for public health: Promise and problems. In E. Trickett & W. Pequeqnat (Eds.), *Community Intervention and AIDS*. Oxford, UK: Oxford University Press.

Qualitative Research Sampling

Guest, G. (in press) Sampling and selecting participants in field research. In H. Bernard & C. Gravlee (Eds.), *Handbook of methods in cultural anthropology* (2nd ed.). Lanham, MD: Altamira.

Guest, G., Namey, E., & Mitchell, M. (2013). *Collecting qualitative data: A field manual* (Chapter 2). Thousand Oaks, CA: Sage.

Trotter, R. T., II (2012). Qualitative research sample design and sample size: Resolving and unresolved issues and inferential imperatives. *Preventative Medicine, 55,* 398–400.

Qualitative Data Collection

Angrosino, M. (2008). *Doing ethnographic and observational research*. Thousand Oaks, CA: Sage.

Guest, G., Namey, E., & Mitchell, M. (2013). *Collecting qualitative data: A field manual*. Thousand Oaks, CA: Sage.

Kreuger, R. A., & Casey, M. A. (2009). *Focus groups: A practical guide for applied research*. Thousand Oaks, CA: Sage.

Rubin, H. J., & Rubin, I. S. (2012). *Qualitative interviewing: The art of hearing data*. Thousand Oaks, CA: Sage.

Qualitative Data Analysis

Charmaz, K. (2006). *Constructing grounded theory: A practical guide through qualitative analysis*. Thousand Oaks, CA: Sage.

Corbin, J., & Strauss, A. (2008). *Basics of qualitative research: Techniques and procedures for developing grounded theory*. Thousand Oaks, CA: Sage.

Guest, G., MacQueen, K. M., & Namey, E. (2012). *Applied thematic analysis*. Thousand Oaks, CA: Sage.

Web Resources

Qualitative Research Consultants Association, http://www.qrca.org/

Social Research Solutions, http://www.socialresearchsolutions.com

Qualitative Health Research, http://qhr.sagepub.com/

The Qualitative Report, http://www.nova.edu/ssss/QR/qualres.html

Qualitative Research Resources - University of Georgia, http://www.qualitativeresearch.uga.edu/QualPage/

Qualitative Research Resources - University of Manchester, http://www.socialsciences.manchester.ac.uk/morgancentre/realities/teaching/

Qualitative Research and Resource Center - York University, http://www.yorku.ca/laps/soci/qrrc/

REFERENCES

ACAPS. (2012). *Qualitative and Quantitative research techniques for humanitarian needs assessment: An introductory brief.* Geneva, Switzerland: Author. Retrieved from http://www.parkdatabase.org/documents/download/qualitative_and_quantitative_research_techniques.pdf.

Bagnoli, A. (2009). Beyond the standard interview: The use of graphic elicitation and arts-based methods. *Qualitative Research, 9,* 547–570.

Banks, M. (2001). *Visual methods in social research.* Thousand Oaks, CA: Sage.

Banks, M. (2007). *Using visual data in qualitative research.* Thousand Oaks, CA: Sage.

Barbour, R. (2007). *Doing focus groups.* London, UK: Sage.

Baum, F. (1995). Researching public health: Behind the qualitative-quantitative methodological debate. *Social Science & Medicine, 40,* 459–468.

Bernard, H. R. (2000). *Social research methods: Qualitative and quantitative approaches.* Thousand Oaks. CA: Sage.

Bernard, H. R. (2011). *Research methods in anthropology: Qualitative and quantitative approaches* (5th ed.). Lanham, MD: Altamira.

Bernard, H. R. (2013). *Social research methods: Qualitative and quantitative approaches* (2nd ed.). Thousand Oaks, CA: Sage.

Bernard, H. R., & Ryan, G. (2010). *Qualitative data analysis: Systematic approaches.* Thousand Oaks, CA: Sage.

Blackman, A. (2007). *The PhotoVoice manual: A guide to designing and running participatory photography projects.* London, UK: PhotoVoice.

Bluthenthal, R. N., & Watters, J. K. (1995). Multimethod research from targeted sampling to HIV risk. *NIDA Research Monograph, 157,* 212–230.

Borgatti, S. (1999). Elicitation techniques for cultural domain analysis. In J. Schensul & M. LeCompte (Eds.), *The ethnographer's toolkit: Vol. 3* (pp. 115–151). Walnut Creek, CA: Altamira Press.

Centers for Disease Control and Prevention, Healthy Communities Program. (2009). *A sustainability planning guide for healthy communities.* Atlanta, GA: Author. Retrieved from http://www.cdc.gov/healthycommunitiesprogram/pdf/sustainability_guide.pdf

Charmaz, K. (2006). *Constructing grounded theory: A practical guide through qualitative analysis.* Thousand Oaks, CA: Sage.

Corbin, J., & Strauss, A. (2008). *Basics of qualitative research: Techniques and procedures for developing grounded theory*. Thousand Oaks, CA: Sage.

Creswell, J. W. (2006). *Qualitative inquiry and research design: Choosing among five approaches.* Thousand Oaks, CA: Sage.

Creswell, J. W., Klassen, A. C., Plano Clark, V. I., & Clegg Smith, K. (2011). *Best practices for mixed methods research in health sciences.* Washington, DC: U.S. Department of Health and Human Services, Office of Behavioral and Social Sciences Research.

Curtis, S., Gesler, W., Smith, G., & Washburn, S. (2000). Approaches to sampling and case selection in qualitative research: Examples in the geography of health. *Social Science & Medicine, 50,* 1001–1014.

DeWalt, K. M., & DeWalt, B. R. (2011). *Participant observation: A guide for fieldworkers* (2nd ed.). Lanham, MD: AltaMira.

Frank, O., & Snijders, T. (1994). Estimating the size of hidden populations using snowball sampling. *Journal of Official Statistics, 10,* 53–67.

Gladwin, C. (1989). *Ethnographic decision tree modeling.* Newbury Park, CA: Sage.

Glaser, B., & Strauss, A. (1967). *The discovery of grounded theory: Strategies for qualitative research.* New York, NY: Aldine.

Green, J., & Thorogood, N. (2009). *Qualitative methods for health research* (2nd ed.). Thousand Oaks, CA: Sage.

Guest, G., Bunce, A., & Johnson, L. (2006). How many interviews are enough? An experiment with data saturation and variability. *Field Methods, 18,* 59–82.

Guest, G., MacQueen, K. M., & Namey, E. (2012). *Applied thematic analysis.* Thousand Oaks, CA: Sage.

Guest, G., Namey, E., & Mitchell, M. (2013). Sampling. In *Collecting qualitative data: A field manual for applied research* (pp. 41–74). Thousand Oaks, CA: Sage.

Hammersley, M. (2008). Context and contextuality. In L. Given (Ed.), *The SAGE encyclopedia of qualitative research methods* (pp. 122–123). Thousand Oaks, CA: Sage.

Heckathorn, D. D. (1997). Respondent driven sampling: A new approach to the study of hidden populations. *Social Problems, 44*(2),174–199.

Johnson, J. C. (1990). *Selecting ethnographic informants.* Thousand Oaks, CA: Sage.

Koester, S., & Hoffer, L. (1994). Indirect sharing: Additional risks associated with drug injection. *AIDS and Public Policy, 9*(2), 100–105.

Kuznar, L. A., & Werner, O. (2001). Ethnographic mapmaking: Part 1. Principles. *Field Methods, 13,* 204–213.

Luborsky, M. R., & Rubinstein, R. L. (1995). Sampling in qualitative research: Rationale, issues, and methods. *Research on Aging, 17*(1), 89–114.

Lyerly, A. D. (2013). *A good birth: Finding the positive and profound in your childbirth experience.* New York, NY: Avery.

Lyerly, A. D., Namey, E., Gray, B., Swamy, G., & Faden, R. R. (2012) Women's views about participating in research while pregnant. *IRB Ethics and Human Research, 34*(4), 1–8.

Lyerly, A. D., Steinhauser, K., Namey, E., Tulsky, J. Cook-Deegan, R., Sugarman, J., . . . Wallach, E. (2006). Factors that affect decision making about frozen embryo disposition: Infertility patient perspectives. *Fertility and Sterility, 85,* 1620–1630.

Lyerly, A. D., Steinhauser, K., Voils, C., Namey, E., Alexander, C., Bankowski, B., . . . Wallach, E. (2010). Fertility patients' views about frozen embryo disposition: Results of a multi-institutional U.S. survey. *Fertility and Sterility, 93,* 499–509.

Mack, N. Woodsong, MacQueen, Guest, & Namey. (2005). *Qualitative research methods: A data collector's field guide.* Research Triangle Park, NC: Family Health International.

McLellan-Lemal, E. (2008). Qualitative data management. In G. Guest & K. M. MacQueen (Eds.), *Handbook for team-based qualitative research* (pp. 165–188). Lanham, MD: AltaMira.

Morrill, M., Lukacz, E. S., Lawrence, J. M., Nager, C. W., Contreras, R., & Luber, K. M. (2007). Seeking healthcare for pelvic floor disorders: A population-based study. *American Journal of Obstetrics and Gynecology, 197*(1), e81–86.

Namey, E., & Lyerly, A. D. (2010). The meaning of "control" for childbearing women in the US. *Social Science and Medicine, 71*, 769–776.

National Cancer Institute. (2001). *Making health communication programs work: A planner's guide* (Rev. ed.). Bethesda, MD: Author. Retrieved from http://www.cancer.gov/cancertopics/cancerlibrary/pinkbook

National Institutes of Health. (2000). *Qualitative methods in health research: Opportunities and considerations in application and review.* Washington, DC: National Institutes of Health, Office of Behavioral and Social Sciences Research. Retrieved from http://obssr.od.nih.gov/pdf/qualitative.pdf

Nkwi, P., Nyamongo, I., & Ryan, G. (2001). *Field research into socio-cultural issues: Methodological guidelines.* Yaounde, Cameroon: International Center for Applied Social Sciences, Research, and Training/UNFPA.

Page, J. B., & Evans, S. (2003). Cigars, cigarillos, and youth. *Journal of Ethnicity in Substance Abuse, 2*(4), 63–76.

Patton, M. Q. (2002). *Qualitative research and evaluation methods* (3rd ed.). Thousand Oaks, CA: Sage.

Peragallo Urrutia, R., Merisier, D., Small, M., Urrutia, E., Tinfo, N., & Walmer, D. (2012). Unmet health needs identified by Haitian women as priorities for attention: A qualitative study. *Reproductive Health Matters, 20*(39), 93–103.

Perkins, C. (2007). Community mapping. *Cartographic Journal, 44*(2), 127–137.

Pink, S. (2007). *Doing visual ethnography* (2nd ed.). Thousand Oaks, CA: Sage.

Reynolds, T., & Gutman, J. (1988). Laddering theory, method, analysis, and interpretation. *Journal of Advertising Research, 28*, 11–31.

Robinson, W. T., Risser, J. M. H., McGoy, S., Becker, A. B., Rehman, H., Jefferson, M., . . . Tortu, S. (2006). Recruiting injection drug users: A three-site comparison of results and experiences with respondent-driven and targeted sampling procedures. *Journal of Urban Health, 83*(1), 29–38.

Romney, A. K., Weller, S. C., & Batchelder, W. H. (1986). Culture as consensus: A theory of culture and informant accuracy. *American Anthropologist, 88*, 313–338.

Ryan, G., & Bernard, H. (2006). Testing an ethnographic decision tree model on a national sample: Recycling beverage cans. *Human Organization, 65*, 103–114.

Salganik, M. J., & Heckathorn, D. D. (2004). Sampling and estimation in hidden populations using respondent-driven sampling. *Sociological Methodology, 34*, 193–239.

Schensul, J. J., & LeCompte, M. D. (2010). *Designing and conducting ethnographic research: An introduction.* Walnut Creek, CA: Altamira Press.

Schensul, S. L., Schensul, J. J., & LeCompte, M. D. (1999). Essential ethnographic methods: Observations, interviews, and questionnaires. *Book 3: The Ethnographers Tool Kit.* Walnut Creek, CA: Altamira Press.

Schensul, S. L., Schensul, J. J., & LeCompte, M. D. (2013). *Initiating ethnographic research: A mixed methods approach.* Plymouth, UK. AltaMira Press.

Seidman, I. (2006). *Interviewing as qualitative research.* New York, NY: Teachers College Press.

Siddiqui, N., Ammarell, N., Namey, E., Wu, J. M., Sandoval, J. S., & Bosworth, H. B. (n.d.). *Urinary incontinence and health seeking behavior among White, Black, and Latina women.* Manuscript in preparation.

Soley, L., & Smith, A. (2008). *Projective techniques for social science and business research.* Milwaukee, WI: Southshore Press.

Steckler, A. (2005). Foreword. In P. R. Ulin, E. T. Robinson, & E. E. Tolley, *Qualitative methods in public health* (p. xiii). San Francisco, CA: Jossey-Bass.

Torres, M. E., Meetze, E. G., & Smithwick-Leone, J. (2013). Latina voices in childhood obesity: A pilot study using photovoice in South Carolina. *American Journal of Preventive Medicine, 44,* S225–S231.

Trotter, R. T., II. (1997). Anthropological midrange theories in mental health research: Selected theory, methods, and systematic approaches to at-risk populations. *Ethos, 25,* 259–274.

Trotter, R. T., II. (2012). Qualitative research sample design and sample size: Resolving and unresolved issues and inferential imperatives. *Preventative Medicine, 55,* 398–400.

Trotter, R. T., II, & Medina Mora, M. A. (2000). Qualitative methods. In *Guide to drug abuse epidemiology* (pp. 93–123). Geneva, Switzerland: World Health Organization, Non-communicable Disease and Mental Health Cluster.

Trotter, R. T., II, Needle, R. H., Goosby, E., Bates, C., & Singer, M. (2001). A methodological model for rapid assessment, response, and evaluation: The RARE program in public health. *Field Methods, 13*(2), 137–159.

Trotter, R. T., II, Needle, R. H., Goosby, E., Bates, C., & von Zinkernagel, D. (2000). *RARE evaluation protocols manual.* Washington, DC: U.S. Department of Health and Human Services, Office of Public Health and Science, Office of HIV/AIDS Policy.

Trotter, R. T., II, & Singer, M. (2005). Rapid assessment strategies for public health: Promise and problems. In E. Trickett & W. Pequeqnat (Eds.), *Community intervention and AIDS* (pp. 130–152). Oxford, UK: Oxford University Press.

U.S. Department of Health and Human Services, National Institutes of Health, National Institute on Drug Abuse. (2012). *Epidemiologic trends in drug abuse: Proceedings of the community epidemiology work group.* Bethesda, MD: Author. Retrieved from http://www.drugabuse.gov/sites/default/files/cewg_january_2012_tagged_v2.pdf

Wang, C. (1999). Photovoice: A participatory action research strategy applied to women's health. *Journal of Women's Health, 8,* 185–192.

Wang, C., Yi, W., Tao, Z., & Carovano, K. (1998). Photovoice as a participatory health promotion strategy. *Health Promotion International, 13,* 75–86.

Watters, J. K., & Biernacki, P. (1989). Targeted sampling: Options for the study of hidden populations. *Social Problems, 36,* 416–430.

Weiss, R. S. (1994). *Learning from strangers: The art and method of qualitative interview studies.* New York, NY: Free Press.

Weller, S., & Romney, A. (1988). *Systematic data collection.* Thousand Oaks, CA: Sage.

Werner, O. & Kuznar, L.A. (2001). Ethnographic mapmaking: Part 2 practical concerns and triangulation. *Field Methods, 13:* 291–296.

Whiteford, L. M., & Trotter, R. T., II. (2008). *Ethics for anthropological research and practice.* Boston, MA: Wadsworth.

Wholey, J., Hatry, H., & Newcomer, K. (2010). *Handbook of practical program evaluation* (3rd ed.). San Francisco, CA: Jossey-Bass.

Wolcott, H. F. (1994). *Transforming qualitative data: Description, analysis, and interpretation.* Thousand Oaks, CA, Sage.

Wray, R. J., Becker, S. M., Henderson, N., Glik, D., Jupka, K., Middleton, S., . . . Mitchell, E. W. (2008). Communicating with the public about emerging health threats: Lessons from the pre-event message development project. *American Journal of Public Health, 98,* 2214–2222.

16

Randomized Controlled Trials for Psychosocial Interventions

Phyllis Solomon and Mary Cavanaugh

As detailed in Chapter 8, randomized controlled trials (RCTs) have been primarily employed in biomedical research, but they have more recently moved into the arena of psychosocial interventions. In the public health arena, these psychosocial RCTs are directed at examining the effectiveness of health promotion, health education, and disease prevention and management interventions in order to improve the health and social and emotional well-being of a designated population. Frequently, these psychosocial service interventions are delivered in health clinic settings, but may also be delivered in one's home, school setting, or work site as well.

The kinds of topics that can be addressed by psychosocial RCTs include determining whether public health education and promotion interventions are effective for things like promoting the use of condoms to prevent the spread of HIV, educating youth in the risks and consequences of tobacco use to reduce the uptake of smoking, educating obese individuals on healthy eating habits toward the goal of increasing weight loss, or educating persons with various diseases to more effectively manage the symptoms of their illness. RCTs use experimental strategies to assess whether these innovative psychosocial interventions are more effective approaches to achieving knowledge gains and changes in attitude, beliefs, and behavior than what is usually offered.

PSYCHOSOCIAL RANDOMIZED CONTROLLED TRIALS (RCTs) IN CONTEXT

Effectiveness Versus Efficacy RCTs

Despite the accumulating evidence of effective interventions both for health promotion and disease management, there is growing concern regarding the lack of translation of research into the public health practice arena. This gap has resulted in the inability to achieve many of the recommendations of Healthy People 2000, a situation likely to continue with Healthy People 2020, as it has even more ambitious goals (Centers for Disease Control and Prevention, 2013; Glasgow, Lichtenstein, & Marcus, 2003).

The gap between research evidence and practice is in part attributable to the fact that these efficacious interventions do not translate well into the real world of everyday practice of public health. This, in turn, is related to the difference between efficacy and effectiveness. **Efficacy studies** are conducted under ideal circumstances with highly trained providers and stringent inclusion criteria. An efficacy trial is considered an explanatory trial in that its purpose is to determine whether the intervention produces the expected beneficial (and no harm) outcome under the most ideal circumstances. An **effectiveness study**, by contrast, takes place in a routine practice setting with real-world providers and a broadening of the range of eligible recipients. The effectiveness trial is viewed as a pragmatic trial that is evaluating the degree of benefit derived from the intervention in the usual service setting (Garthehner, Hansen, Nissman, Lohr, & Carey, 2006; see Chapter 11 for more on the rationale for this). Thus, the two trial types address different questions. This psychosocial model of RCTs is referred to as an effectiveness trial, as opposed to the traditional RCTs discussed in Chapter 8, which are designated as efficacy trials.

Another factor that distinguishes the two types of RCTs is that the internal validity of an efficacy study is much stronger given that confounds from provider delivery and recipients are controlled for, including the employment of double blinding, which is usually not feasible in effectiveness trials. However, these constraints that increase internal validity in efficacy trials result in far less external validity than in effectiveness trials (see Table 16.1). The inclusion criteria are often so narrowly defined that the results are applicable to only a limited number of settings and to small subpopulations of those served in routine practice settings. For instance, one of the major shortcomings of efficacy studies in the United States is that they are frequently limited to middle-class, White populations rather than to low-income, ethnically diverse populations who are more often served in public or private nonprofit settings in which routine practice occurs. In contrast, effectiveness studies often focus on the latter population who are primarily served in these settings.

General Qualities of Psychosocial RCTs

As you may have gathered from the comparison above, RCTs for psychosocial interventions are most often effectiveness studies that generally take place in community

Table 16.1   Effectiveness and Efficacy RCTs

	Effectiveness	*Efficacy*
Type of setting	– Real-world, routine practice – Community settings (e.g., agencies, schools, institutions)	– Ideal circumstances – Laboratory – Academic health settings
Purpose	Pragmatic	Explanatory
Sample	Broad inclusion criteria, including comorbid disorders, minority and low-income populations	Highly restrictive inclusion criteria (i.e., often limited to "majority" populations)
Blinding	Usually no blinding, possibly data collectors blinded to participants' assigned condition	Frequently double blinding (neither participants nor providers know participants' assigned condition) or triple blinding (researcher also does not know assignment)
Interventionists	– Trained usual care providers – Experimental intervention is only one of their responsibilities	– Trained, highly qualified research staff – Dedicated to experimental intervention
Intervention	According to a standardized intervention protocol, but with flexibility for adaptation	Strictly adheres to a standardized intervention protocol
Validity	Higher in external than internal validity	Higher in internal than external validity

settings (e.g., schools, mental health clinics, substance abuse agencies) rather than in a laboratory or academic research setting. This is the "real-world" quality of an effectiveness study that is necessary for testing the practicality or feasibility of a health promotion or education intervention. Despite differences with biomedical or efficacy RCTs, psychosocial RCTs retain the primary feature of randomly allocating individuals into their assigned group condition. This chance allocation procedure is used with the expectation that the groups will have equal distributions of both measured and unmeasured characteristics. Therefore, with a large enough sample, possible confounding factors that may produce a difference in group outcomes are controlled with strong internal validity afforded by an experimental design. This enables investigators to more confidently make causal statements about their findings due to the isolation of the manipulated interventions as the primary influence on the outcomes.

This chapter concentrates on effectiveness RCTs for psychosocial interventions that are focused on selected and indicated preventive interventions rather than universal interventions, using the Institute of Medicine's (Mrazek & Haggerty, 1994) classification system for psychosocial interventions. Indicated preventive interventions are targeted at an issue, challenge, or disorder of specific individuals and will emphasize individual random allocation rather than cluster or place-based random assignment by groups such as schools, medical practices, and work sites (see Chapters 8 and 17 for more on RCT and general sampling strategies, respectively). Thus, this chapter is primarily concerned with presenting methods and issues of importance to effectiveness trials, in contrast to the primarily biomedical efficacy and safety RCTs featured in Chapter 8. Many of the basic methods of efficacy RCT designs are relevant to these designs as well, such as randomization procedures and control groups, and will be discussed only with regard to how they relate to psychosocial RCTs.

IMPORTANCE OF QUALITATIVE METHODS TO RCTS

RCT study designs like those described in Chapter 8 are challenging to use with complex and multifactorial psychosocial interventions, and they are limited in their ability to capture the social and behavioral processes involved in producing the outcomes of these interventions. There are several challenges with using strict RCT designs in psychosocial research:

- Frequently in psychosocial public health research, the experimental intervention is not standardized, but is designed to be individualized and flexible to meet the varying needs of a diversity of individuals.
- Given that these RCT take place in real-world settings, the environmental context in which the study is set may influence the intervention in unknown ways to affect the outcomes.
- Provider characteristics, expertise, and experience, and recipients' characteristics, preferences, and beliefs may interact with the intervention and study design to affect outcomes.
- RCTs are designed to answer the question of whether the experimental intervention works, but not why it works or for whom it works (Lewin, Glenton, & Oxman, 2009; Oakley et al., 2006; Verhoef, Casebeer, & Hilsden, 2002).

Given these limitations, incorporating qualitative methods (see Chapter 15) into quantitative RCT designs has been found to enhance understanding of measured outcomes, compared to looking at RCT study findings alone. A recent review of studies employing qualitative methods in conjunction with randomized controlled trials found that it was relatively uncommon to include qualitative methods in RCTs (Lewin et al., 2009; see text box). Table 16.2 lists various purposes for incorporating a qualitative component into an RCT. Many of these approaches will be elaborated on throughout the rest of the chapter.

Table 16.2   Purposes for Inclusion of Qualitative Methods in RCTs

Prior to an RCT

- To explore issues related to question of interest
- To explore environmental context for the RCT
- To generate hypotheses for examination in RCT
- To develop and refine experimental intervention
- To define and specify standard of care, potential comparison condition
- To develop or select appropriate outcome measures

During an RCT

- To examine whether experimental intervention delivered as intended, including describing experimental intervention as delivered
- To assess processes of implementation and change
- To examine the social context in which RCT is delivered and contextual factors that impact intervention
- To examine interactions between provider and recipients
- To examine providers' and recipients' responses to and meanings of the intervention, possibly by subgroups

After an RCT

- To explore reasons for outcomes of RCT
- To explain variation in effectiveness for various subgroups
- To examine the appropriateness of underlying conceptualization of RCT
- To generate further questions or hypotheses

Source: Adapted from Lewin et al. (2009); incorporates information from Verhoef et al. (2002) and Oakley et al. (2006).

DESIGNING AND CONDUCTING RCTS FOR PSYCHOSOCIAL INTERVENTIONS

In this section we discuss the methods to be employed in designing RCTs for effectiveness studies of psychosocial interventions. The section begins with ethical considerations as they underlie the entire design and conduct of the study, including whether one should go forward to execute an RCT. From there we move through planning, theoretical considerations, and issues relating to design, sampling, and implementing the RCT.

EXAMPLE OF PSYCHOSOCIAL RCT WITH QUALITATIVE COMPONENT: ENCOURAGING CONTRACEPTIVE UPTAKE—THE MALAWI MALE MOTIVATOR PROJECT

Objective: To examine effectiveness of Malawi Motivator intervention on couples' uptake of contraception.

Methods: RCT with a sample comprising 400 men recruited from 257 villages in Mangochi district of Malawi. Only 1 man from each village was assigned to the experimental intervention. To be eligible men were at least 18 years old, married or living with a female sexual partner younger than 25 (not currently pregnant or breastfeeding a child younger than 6 months). Participants were not sterilized or using modern contraceptives for the past 3 months.

Outcomes included contraceptive uptake, and researchers used the information-motivation-behavioral skills model to evaluate changes in family planning knowledge, attitudes, and self-efficacy; gender norms; and communication regarding family planning.

Intervention: Male motivators, 30-year-old married men who enthusiastically used modern contraception, had five visits with participants in which they initially shared family planning information, then discussed motivating factors to using family planning including using own experiences. They subsequently employed role-playing and skill teaching to communicate about family planning and benefits of contraceptive use.

Results: At posttest, contraceptive use increased in both conditions, but more so in the experimental intervention.

Qualitative Assessment: 10% of participants in the intervention condition who completed postintervention surveys were randomly selected to participate in an in-depth interview. Open-ended questions assessed perceptions of the study, whether men were using contraception and the rationale for using, opinions of information shared during the intervention, and comfort with discussing family planning.

Qualitative Findings: Qualitative findings supported and enhanced quantitative results. Participants noted that their overall communication with wife/girlfriend was improved by being able to comfortably discuss family planning. Some even attributed this openness to improving their relationships. Some also looked forward to visits with the motivator as it provided them with skills that they previously did not have.

Source: Shattuck et al. (2011).

Ethical Considerations

Chapter 3 covered the basics of research ethics; here we provide specific issues related to psychosocial RCTs and safeguards necessary to prevent harming participants as a result of a RCT intervention. One of the main differences with psychosocial RCTs is that they combine the ethics of both *practice* and *research*. *Practice* is defined in the Belmont Report (National Commission for the Protection of Human Subjects of Biomedical and Behavioral Research, 1979) as "interventions that are designed solely to enhance the well-being of an individual, patient, or client and that have a reasonable expectation of success"; whereas, *research* is defined as activities "designed to test a hypothesis, permit conclusions to be drawn, and thereby to develop or contribute to generalizable knowledge" (p. 3). In RCTs the experimental intervention is theoretically expected to produce more effective outcomes than the control condition. However, for ethical purposes, if the intervention addresses disease management, it needs to be at least as effective as routine practice. The RCT must meet the principle of equipoise, mentioned in Chapter 8, which means there is some degree of uncertainty about effectiveness—otherwise there is no ethical justification for the study. In other words, if existing empirical evidence has already established that the experimental intervention is more effective than routine practice for the targeted population, there is no ethical reason to conduct the RCT.

Unlike many efficacy RCTs, a placebo is not usually ethically justified in psychosocial RCTs if the population requires services in the management of their illness, as it may be unethical to deny services. Therefore, routine practice or standard of care is commonly used as the control condition rather than a placebo. If, normally, participants would need to wait for service, a waitlist condition may be justified. (Although if, due to the study, they need to wait longer than they would otherwise, then it would not be ethically justified.) For health promotion or preventative RCTs, which are often educational interventions, where the participants would not be receiving any intervention if it was not for the RCT, then a placebo, a waitlist, or an "inert" control condition would be ethically justified.

Informed Consent

Informed consent must be obtained prior to randomization to a condition. It is not ethical to have a study participant sign a consent form that indicates that the condition to which he or she will be assigned is unknown, if the assignment is already known to the investigator. This type of research requires two separate consent forms, one for each condition, and the individual needs to be asked to sign the consent for the condition to which he or she has been assigned. Moreover, assigning a participant in advance of obtaining consent may result in biased attrition (dropout from the study), as individuals who have a strong preference for a particular condition may not agree to join the study. This occurrence makes for a less valid design and thus a less ethical study. Consent forms need to contain a clear description of both the experimental intervention and the control condition if it is, for example, routine care. Merely stating that it is routine care is not clearly informing the potential participant, thus more detail is warranted.

In some RCTs multiple consent forms may be needed for each individual. For example, if extensive prescreening is necessary to determine one's eligibility for study inclusion, and those screening questions ask for detailed personal information, such as a psychiatric diagnostic assessment, a consent form for determining eligibility would be required. It would not be justified to include this screening as part of the RCT consent form, as the individual may not be eligible to be included in the study.

Consent forms may be needed for providers as well. Providers who are being asked to engage in activities that are outside of their scope of service provision responsibilities become research subjects or become research personnel, as discussed below. For example, the first author was involved in a prevention intervention for HIV for persons with severe mental illness where agency-based case managers were randomly assigned to deliver the experimental prevention intervention to consenting clients or not. Although the agency agreed to this random assignment procedure, the agency cannot agree on behalf of its workers to engage in such a procedure. Consequently, only those case managers who consented were randomly assigned. In addition, these same case managers were asked their personal opinions about their alliance with their clients. They had to consent to this as well. If information collected were data routinely included in the client's case record, then the case manager would not need to be consented as this information pertains to the client and the client would therefore need to consent. However, if providers are being asked about their personal beliefs, opinions, attitudes, and knowledge, they are considered research subjects.

Ethical Responsibility at RCT Termination

RCTs have a set time frame for the intervention, but for RCTs testing disease management approaches, it does not mean that participants do not require continued care upon termination of the RCT—even if the intervention is highly successful. Ethically, it is the responsibility of the intervention providers to ensure that appropriate referrals are made and receipt of services is obtained for participants. Furthermore, at termination of the intervention providers need to deal with issues of closure for participants. This is where the ethics of practice and research clearly intersect.

Ethics of Internet RCTs

Currently, a number of psychosocial RCTs are being conducted via the Internet. Special considerations for these must be kept in mind in order to protect the safety and confidentiality of the subjects. For example, with consent forms it is important to warn about risks of revealing personal information and being sure to disable standard signatures when corresponding with others in the study. The first author is currently involved in a parenting educational RCT for mothers with severe mental illness that has a Listserv component. Although this intervention is not a treatment study, clinical issues of concern arise given the nature of the target population. For instance, one participant posted an entry that suggested she was suicidal. However, in order to maintain confidentiality, study personnel were unable to determine the participant's identity as her postings were anonymous. After this incident, the study team decided that determining who sent specific emails was an important aspect to include in the study protocol and changes were instituted accordingly. For example, the consent form was revised to indicate that the investigators could break confidentiality when the situation warranted.

Administrative Arrangements for Human Subject Protections

Beyond Institutional Review Board (IRB) approval from the home institution of the primary investigator, RCTs may have additional administrative requirements for protections of human subjects from the agency or facility setting. This may occur when the intervention is being conducted in an agency and the agency personnel are carrying out the intervention. These employees are engaged in research and therefore become research personnel. Additionally, agency research providers may be required to take human subjects research training so they are knowledgeable regarding protection of human subjects. If the research is funded by the federal government and requires IRB oversight, the agency needs to apply for a Federal-Wide Assurance (FWA) from the National Institutes of Health's Office of Research Protection. Should the agency or facility merely be offering their site for recruitment and delivery of intervention by the study's own research personnel, then an FWA is not necessary, as the principal investigator's IRB approved the study and is overseeing it.

In addition, agencies and facilities may have their own IRBs or research review committees that need to review and approve the research. If the RCT is conducted in a medical or mental health facility or agency, the research must meet the requirements of the Health Insurance Portability and Accountability Act privacy rule. Furthermore, as with efficacy RCTs, effectiveness RCTs that are funded from the federal government require a Data Safety and Monitoring Board be put in place to oversee and monitor the study. The members of the committee must have relevant expertise and the degree to which they monitor the RCT is commensurate with the potential risk. For most psychosocial RCTs, the committee comprises three or four members who are provided with summary materials of the status of the study, are apprised of any adverse events, and meet in person or via conference call about quarterly.

Planning Psychosocial Effectiveness

When planning a psychosocial RCT, a few elements are essential. First, the research question needs to be significant to the field of public health and to be ethically and conceptually sound. Based on theory and empirical research, there has to be a well-developed justification for considering that the experimental intervention is more effective than the control condition. Second, the experimental intervention must be well defined and able to be implemented in an appropriate setting—which will need to be selected and negotiated.

Selecting and Negotiating a Setting

As in many kinds of research, a site assessment is an important step in the planning of research. When selecting a site, the researcher has to assess whether the site is not only willing to participate in the RCT, but also sufficiently motivated to sustain the study to completion. Often, the site will need to implement the intervention, assist in recruitment of participants, and maintain them in the intervention, which will require qualified staff, resources, and eligible and willing participants. And funds must be available for implementing the intervention out of either research funds or agency resources. For example, might this experimental intervention be a billable service? If not, are there ways to adapt the intervention so that it could be a reimbursable service? Without these necessary prerequisites in place, there is no reason to move forward in designing the protocol.

Negotiating site issues can be a delicate matter, because a commitment needs to be secured from the head administrator as well as from those who will be implementing the research, such as assisting in recruitment and conducting the intervention. Failure to obtain buy-in from setting personnel may well lead to implementation failure. Often the process is both a bottom-up and a top-down process. To design the protocol one must work at the organizational level where the RCT will actually be carried out. The designing of an RCT should be a collaborative process between the researcher and the provider, or it may not be feasibly implemented at the site. Clearly, roles and expectations of both researchers and providers need to be developed in advance. Trust between parties is essential. Table 16.3 outlines the principles for working with providers and clients in designing and conducting RCTs (Solomon, Cavanaugh, & Draine, 2009).

Pilot Studies

Before designing an RCT, researchers frequently conduct a pilot or small-scale study to determine the feasibility and importance of a full-scale RCT. Pilot studies that are well conceptualized with clear objectives are likely to lead to higher quality RCTs (Lancaster, Dodd, & Williamson, 2004). External pilot studies are stand-alone research studies that

---

Table 16.3 Principles for Working With Providers in Designing and Implementing RCTs—REAL SCORE

Respect for providers

Establish credibility

Acknowledge strengths

Low burden

Shared ownership-reciprocity

Collaborative relationship

Offer incentives—be responsive and appreciative of providers

Recognize environmental constraints—be flexible

Ensure trust—be sure providers feel heard

Source: Randomized Controlled Trials: Design and Implementation for Community-Based Psychosocial Interventions by Phyllis Solomon et al (2009) Table 3.1 from p. 52. By permission of Oxford University Press, USA.

are carried out prior to the design of the RCT. In contrast, internal pilot studies are a part of the RCT, often a first phase (Torgerson & Torgerson, 2008). Pilot studies serve to assess "the worthiness, practicality, feasibility, and acceptability of the intervention, recruitment, retention, and data collection procedures" (Solomon et al., 2009, p. 52).

There are, therefore, several reasons to conduct a pilot study prior to designing the RCT (see Table 16.4). One primary reason for conducting a pilot study is to obtain data in order to calculate a well-powered RCT. There are some statisticians and researchers that caution against using an underpowered study (which is often the case for pilots as they are small-scale studies) to estimate an effect size (Kraemer, Mintz, Noda, Tinklinberg, & Yesavage, 2006), but many others believe some data are better than no data.

All too often investigators overestimate the available number of eligible participants for their RCT. Consequently, a pipeline study may be important to conduct prior to designing the RCT. Boruch (1997) suggests conducting "scouting research" as means to become familiar with the recruitment site and determine where and how potentially eligible individuals can be recruited. Such an assessment "directs attention to how, why, and when individuals may be included in the experiment or excluded and the number of individuals who may enter or exit the study at any given point" (p. 88). Here is where qualitative methods of participant observation can be particularly helpful. With these data the researcher can make a determination as to whether it is feasible to conduct the RCT at this site and/or add other sites. Trying to recruit some eligible participants to determine their willingness to participate and, if they are not willing, to assess why not is equally important. In-depth interviews may provide additional insights. In these ways, a pilot study can help the researcher estimate how many eligible and willing participates there are likely to be.

Since the target populations of psychosocial effectiveness RCTs are often ethnic and minority groups, there is a need for specific recruitment strategies. Witte and her colleagues (2004) conducted a review of the literature regarding strategies for successful recruitment of an ethnically diverse target population. They found four categories of recruitment strategies:

- **Individual** strategies that include incorporating appropriate cultural beliefs, practices, and lifestyles in promotional material; providing compensation; and offering child care and transportation
- **Researcher-driven** strategies, which involve demonstrating the usefulness of the project and concern for safety, along with employing ethnically and racially matched recruitment staff
- **Site** strategies, which include site staff in the development of the study design and procedures defining their roles
- **Community** strategies that involve community members and organizations in the development of recruitment procedures and protocols, and in demonstrating study benefits to the larger community (Solomon et al., 2009)

A recent systematic review of community-based participatory research (CBPR, see Chapter 4) found that this approach enhanced RCTs in the recruitment and retention of racial and ethnic minority groups. The authors concluded that RCTs investigating health care issues like health promotion or screening for diseases may well benefit from the CBPR paradigm (De Las Nueces, Hacker, DiGiralamo, & Hicks, 2012).

Pilot work is also essential for the retention of participants in both the intervention and measurement portions of the study (Davis, Broome, & Cox, 2002), particularly given that the target populations of these types of RCTs are often low income, living in unstable housing, and/or employed in inflexible jobs. These and other issues contribute to attrition in RCTs, which can frequently be lengthy. Some feedback on the receptivity of both the experimental and control conditions is therefore helpful in designing the protocol. Participant perception of the interventions as desirable and beneficial is fundamental to retention (Good & Schuler, 1997). Site staff involvement in intervention development results in their greater buy-in and in encouraging participant retention as well (Solomon et al., 2009; see Table 16.4).

Table 16.4 Primary Purposes of Pilot RCTs

Determine general feasibility of RCT

Conduct pipeline assessment for recruitment of needed sample

Obtain data to calculate sample size

Determine retention strategies

Determine practicality, feasibility, and acceptability of interventions

Finding and Developing Intervention Manuals

A major assumption of RCTs is that the intervention is delivered in a standardized manner, with each interventionist engaged in the same processes and practices with each participant (Solomon et al., 2009). To achieve standardization in efficacy trials, treatment manuals are used. A treatment manual specifies the intervention, provides standards for evaluating adherence in the intervention, offers guidance for training, provides quality assurance standards, facilitates replication, and stimulates dissemination and transfer of effective interventions. These manuals often include a brief literature review, general guidelines for establishing a therapeutic relationship, descriptions of specific techniques and content, suggestions for structurally sequencing activities, and strategies for dealing with special problems, implementation issues, and termination (Solomon et al., 2009, p. 194).

However, community-based psychosocial interventions dealing with management of diseases or conditions are difficult to put into standard operating procedures as they occur in multiple sites with diverse practitioners and participants and involve a myriad of activities that are flexible interventions (Bond, Evans, Salyers, Williams, & Kim, 2000). These may be more program/operation manuals that contain instructions for structural elements of the program, such as caseload size, types and numbers of staff and their qualifications, and requirements of site location. Health promotion interventions involving educational curricula are easier to standardize, as they are more highly focused and follow curriculum development procedures.

Regardless of which type of intervention, the expectation today is that effectiveness RCTs will have some type of manual or curriculum, which will have to be developed, located, or adapted. The development of a manual or a curriculum is an iterative process that requires expert input and pilot testing prior to the intervention being used in a fully developed RCT. There are a number of ways to locate existing manuals or curricula, such as Internet search engines, literature searches, particular websites, and federal agencies. Also, the Substance Abuse Mental Health Services Administration has downloadable toolkits of evidence-based interventions for substance abuse and mental health. Finally, the text *Randomized Controlled Trials* (Solomon et al., 2009) offers some guidance on the development of interventions based on the work of Carroll and associates (Carroll & Nuro, 1997, 2002; Carroll & Rounsaville, 2008).

There are various models for adapting existing interventions so they may be utilized for new settings and new target populations. Ethnographic approaches are effective for adapting existing manuals (Wingood & DiClemente, 2008). Focus groups and elicitation interviews may assist in reviewing existing interventions, pretesting the intervention, and/or drafting a new intervention. Focus groups and in-depth interviews with providers, supervisors, administrators, service recipients, and their families may be conducted to adapt existing standardized interventions.

Other more structured procedures may be employed to define and refine an existing intervention such as the Delphi method or concept mapping. The Delphi method is a means to generate ideas from a group of individuals who eventually come to a consensus on a topic. This method may be used to generate the components, activities, and processes of an intervention, as Flander and Burns (2000) utilized to categorize the work of intensive case managers. Similarly, concept mapping is a group process of brainstorming about a topic and is a way to sort and rate emerging items, and cluster the items with the output being a visual display of the relationship of the clusters to each other. This procedure has been employed to delineate program activities and their sequence in addition to the contextual factors that affect a program (Trochim, Cook, & Setze, 1994). Often programs are implemented and called by the same name, but no one to date has developed a manual or specified the exact structure, processes, or procedures that are involved. Consequently, a good deal of preliminary work needs to be carried out prior to conducting an RCT of the effectiveness of such an intervention.

Developing Fidelity and Leakage Assessments

Once the intervention is well specified and a manual has been developed, the next step is to develop a fidelity assessment (which is usually included in the final manual). The elements in the manual are the basis for evaluating the fidelity of the intervention. **Fidelity** indicates the extent to which the intervention is implemented as delineated in the manual; this is essential to determine whether the RCT is testing the effectiveness of the proposed experimental intervention. Lack of fidelity may result in an incorrect conclusion from the RCT; that is, that the intervention was ineffective in producing the intended outcomes, when in reality the intended intervention was not carried out

(Orwin, 2000). A **fidelity measure** is a scale or tool that assesses the adequacy of an intervention and is a quantifiable means to determining the extent to which an intervention was implemented (Bond, Evans, et al., 2000).

To fully evaluate implementation, the assessment needs to answer not only whether the intervention was delivered as intended but also whether it was received by recipients as well. Thus, multiple measures are needed, which may also include extraction of data from charts or service billing forms, service logs, observations, or use of videotaping. If interventions employ an educational curriculum, a checklist may be created for use on an observational or self-report form. The construction of these measures is similar to developing any scale (see Chapter 13). Bond, Williams, and colleagues (2000) have a manual on the development of fidelity measures for psychiatric rehabilitation programs that can serve for other types of programs as well. Solomon and colleagues (2009) present examples of how to develop fidelity measures. One example is in the study of HIV prevention with persons with severe mental illness and co-occurring substance abuse. The educational curriculum was provided to case managers on cards with assigned numbers for each card. When submitting billing forms for an incentive, case managers listed the card numbers that they reviewed with each client. In this way, the researchers could monitor the extent to which the intervention was delivered.

Also, it is important to ensure that the specific intervention differs from other interventions, in some cases from what is implemented in routine practice. Therefore, elements of this other intervention may be incorporated into the fidelity measure as well (Bellig et al., 2004). To assess the extent of contamination between conditions, a leakage scale is used. Such a scale captures the extent to which those in a control condition may have received portions of the intervention intended only for experimental participants. In some situations, the fidelity measure completed by those in the control condition may serve this purpose. In order to develop methodologically sound fidelity and leakage measures, the psychosocial intervention needs to be extremely well specified in terms of structural and behavioral elements, and in such a manner that they can be measured. This is not an easy task given the complexity and multiple aspects of many of these interventions (Burns, Burchard, Suter, Leventz-Brady, & Force, 2004).

Theoretical Basis of Psychosocial RCTs

As with any research study, an RCT requires a theoretical justification as to why the intervention is expected to produce the behavioral changes in the outcome. There are a number of commonly employed theories for psychosocial interventions for health promotion and disease management, including social learning theory, social support, the theory of planned behavior, the theory of reasoned action, and the transtheoretical model of change (Solomon et al., 2009; see the Appendix for more on theory). These theories are generally coupled with empirical research to justify the RCT. And more than one of these theoretical frameworks may be used, depending on the research objective. For example, the first author conducted an RCT of an educational intervention for families of relatives with a severe mental illness and the theoretical justification included stress coping and adaptation, as well as social support and social learning theory. The family education intervention focused on teaching how to cope with and adapt to the severe illness of the relative, taught behavioral skills, and offered support through other group participants.

Stronger theoretical models are those that include mediators and moderators based on Baron and Kenny's (1986) conceptualization that has become commonly used in RCTs. Mediators offer explanations as to what produces the change in the outcomes of the RCT. Mediator models help to understand the processes of change or the mechanisms by which change occurs in specified outcomes. The mediator is the conceptual link that comes between the cause-and-effect relationship; in other words it follows the intervention, but comes before the outcome. For example, in the family education intervention mentioned earlier, the mediators were the degree of coping ability and social supports, which were proposed to lead to decreases in stress and burden of family members (rather than severity of illness having merely a direct effect on the outcomes).

Moderators generally alter the effect or the strength of the relationship of the intervention with the outcome. The moderator interacts with the intervention to produce a different outcome or different degree of the outcome. For example, a particular intervention for youth may be more effective in the behavioral outcomes for high-risk youth than for low-risk youth. Thus, moderators are often characteristics that participants bring to the RCT. Moderator assessment enables one to more effectively determine for whom the intervention was most effective.

Considerations in Designing a Psychosocial RCT

After the necessary pilot work and conceptualization is completed, the researcher is ready to design the study. The randomization procedure enables a scientific comparison to be made between conditions. The comparisons to be made have been determined based on the pilot work conducted up to this point. There may be more than one experimental condition and more than one control condition, such as comparisons of routine practice with a benign intervention in order to control for attention bias or a practice condition. Thus, in each case the RCT builds on the classic experimental design of random assignment to the experimental versus the control condition, and the outcomes are measured before the intervention is manipulated and then after the intervention is complete. In some instances, it is not feasible to obtain a pre-measure. In others, the nature of the pretest may be expected to interact with the intervention, so the pretest is excluded on two conditions (one experimental and one control), and two conditions (experimental and control) are added with pretests in the design to test for this interaction affect. This design is referred to as the Solomon Four Group Design (no relation to the first author).

Many psychosocial RCTs test very complex programs with a number of interlocking services. Again, great care is required in the RCT design to identify what exactly is producing the change in outcomes. For example, Cosden and his colleagues (Cosden, Ellens, Schnell, & Yamini-Diouf, 2005; Cosden, Ellens, Schnell, Yamini-Diouf, & Wolfe, 2003) designed a study where those facing criminal charges were randomly assigned to a mental health court or the usual court. Mental health courts are specialized courts that are designed to be less adversarial than the usual court for persons with mental illness who come in contact with the legal system and are referred for mental health services in lieu of jail time. Those assigned to the mental health court also received assertive community treatment (ACT; a comprehensive self-contained program of mental health treatment and rehabilitation services delivered by a team of professionals) and supportive housing services (where supports are provided to individuals in independent housing) or the usual routine mental health services available in the community. Although this study has provided some of the most positive evidence for mental health courts to date, it is unclear what produced the positive effect. Was it the mental health court, ACT plus supportive housing, or the interaction of the mental health court and ACT plus supportive housing? It is unknown from this design. These service components should have been separated into three experimental conditions plus a control condition design to be able to answer the question of the effectiveness of mental health courts versus usual court.

Threats to Internal Validity

There are a number of confounds that threaten the internal validity of an RCT. The usual culprits will not be reviewed, as a discussion of them can be found in most basic research methods books (and Chapter 2), but rather the focus will be on those that need particular attention in regard to psychosocial RCTs. For instance, in psychosocial RCTs, certain differences between the control and experimental conditions may result in instrument problems. Instrumentation refers to measurement differences that are not inherent to the measure per se but are changes in the calibration of the measure due to differing circumstances and procedures between administrations. For example, the data collectors for the experimental and control conditions may not be the same individuals. If they are trained the same and are equally qualified and have similar amounts of time, interest, and motivation, it may not be a problem. However, the two may be at different locations, intentionally to control for potential contamination (discussed below), that may have different commitments or interest in the RCT, resulting in data collectors being more or less committed to the RCT. This commitment differential may result in changes in the reliability of the measure being different by site location. To mitigate these issues, the same data collectors should be used for all conditions whenever possible.

Contamination between conditions is another potential threat to the internal validity of a psychosocial RCT. Contamination is also referred to as drift, blurring of conditions, or treatment dilution or diffusion. This threat occurs when the control condition receives some of the beneficial elements intended only for the experimental condition. This can occur if

- control condition providers learn about the experimental condition and inadvertently or intentionally utilize these service elements with control condition recipients;
- control service recipients learn about experimental services or educational elements from experimental service recipients;
- experimental providers over time drift more toward the way in which they implemented service provision prior to the RCT, which is the control condition for the study; or

- the social environment around the RCT changes, as when a new policy mandate requires all providers to engage in certain practices, which may be exactly the practices of the experimental condition.

Seemingly innocent events or activities can result in contamination. In some cases, service recipients sitting in the same waiting room may discuss the benefits of their service, leading control recipients to ask for elements intended for the experimental group only. Table 16.5 summarizes strategies to reduce and assess contamination in a psychosocial RCT.

Table 16.5   Methods to Minimize and Assess Contamination

To minimize the potential for contamination . . .
- Employ cluster/place randomized designs
- Use different providers for experimental and control conditions
- Limit interaction of experimental and control providers and participants

To assess whether contamination has occurred . . .
- Conduct leakage measures
- Observe implementation of RCT (use qualitative methods)

Changes in the environmental context of the RCT may threaten the internal validity of the design. In the usual parlance of research methodology this threat is referred to as *history*, which is an event that occurs in the environment including the agency, community, or system level that may serve as a competing explanation for a change in the outcome other than the experimental intervention. Since it is sometimes difficult to anticipate events in advance (for example, there are often policy changes that occur during an RCT), one of the best means to capture potential threats is to build a qualitative component into the study, such as participant observations and periodic interviews with key informants.

Attrition is a common problem with psychosocial RCTs as they take place in the community, with individuals who are characteristically difficult to find and to engage in service, and they occur over an extended period of time. One method that has been employed is to have introductory sessions prior to recruitment of participants so that those not really interested or motivated will likely not consent to the study. However, some researchers are concerned that this compromises external validity of the study. Another method to reduce attrition is incentive payments, such as providing a bonus for completing all data points in the study. Should participants drop out of the intervention, it does not mean that they have to drop out from the data collection aspect of the RCT. There are statistical procedures for handling missing data, but one has to anticipate issues regarding attrition and collect the minimal data required to conduct the analytic procedures.

Randomization Procedures

The standard approaches to randomization in RCTs were introduced in Chapter 8, so here we provide only examples from psychosocial RCTs. **Cluster randomization** is sometimes employed, where randomization occurs at the group or cluster level rather than the individual level, to control for contamination. For example, the first author was involved in an RCT where case managers were randomly assigned to either deliver an HIV prevention intervention or not to clients with a severe mental illness and a co-morbid substance abuse problem. Case managers who were assigned the educational intervention delivered it to all their consenting clients, while those case managers assigned to the control condition did nothing different.

Cluster randomized designs, or place-based randomized designs, have also been used in community-wide health promotion programs. For example, a hand washing program in Jerusalem randomly assigned 40 preschools to receive a hygiene intervention or serve as a waitlist control school. All children attending the schools assigned to the hygiene program received the intervention (Rosen, Manor, Engelhard, & Zucker, 2006). Later, control schools also received the hygiene intervention. Sikkema (2005) reports on a community level RCT where nine demographically matched pairs of low-income housing developments in five U.S cities were assigned either to the experimental HIV prevention intervention or to the control condition. To control for contamination, the housing developments in a given city were at least 2 miles apart. There are a number of issues specific to these cluster randomized designs, including informed consent, misidentifying the unit level of analysis, and others. For more detail see Donner and Klar (2004).

Random assignment in some instances needs to be implemented in blocks in order to better maintain control of how many subjects enter particular conditions within a set period of time. The **block** is a specified number of units, such as a block of 4, 8, or 10, and balances the number of individuals who enter each condition at the end of each block. In the first author's RCT of family education, there was a group educational workshop, an individual consultation, and a waitlist condition. The providers were unable to handle too many cases at one time and enough individuals needed to begin a group, so block randomization was necessary to meet these stipulations. This enabled a manageable flow of participants to the three conditions.

Blinding of providers and participants to the assigned condition is included in many traditional RCTs to control for potential bias. With psychosocial RCTs, particularly in health promotion or disease management, it is impossible for providers and participants to not know whether they are receiving or delivering the experimental or control condition. It is possible, however, for data collectors to be blind to the assigned condition of the study participant on whom they are collecting data (Gellis, McGinty, Horowitz, Bruce, & Misener, 2007), though sometimes participants inadvertently tell the data collector to which condition they were assigned.

Sampling Procedures

Samples for psychosocial RCTs are frequently convenience or consecutive samples of individuals who meet the study criteria and consent to participate. As with any study, the criteria for inclusion and exclusion of participants need to be clearly operationalized. For example, merely delineating specific diagnoses for inclusion criteria does not indicate how the recruiter will know that a specific individual has one of these diagnoses. Diagnoses can be operationalized as reported by the participant, extracted from the medical chart of the participant, or determined by using a specific diagnostic measurement tool. Psychosocial RCTs typically have few exclusion criteria as samples are far less restrictive than in traditional RCTs. Inclusion criteria might comprise a specific diagnosis with or without comorbidities. Again, a power analysis will need to be conducted to determine the required sample size to show an effect. The predesign work done during the planning stage will help to develop the case that the proposed sample size can be obtained, taking into account incligibles, refusers, and attrition. The sample size needs to compensate for these factors so that sufficient sample size is available for the final data analysis.

Outcome Measures

Specific outcomes for a psychosocial RCT will depend on the objectives and theoretical framework for the RCT, but the researcher needs to consider how reasonable it is to expect a change in behavior within the time frame of the RCT. For example, it may be unrealistic to assume that an intervention designed to change the functioning level of persons with severe mental illness will effect a measurable change in only 6 months. Once realistic outcomes are determined based on theory and time period, the next step is to find reliable and valid measures for the outcomes within the target population, keeping in mind that often these populations are ethnically diverse. Outcomes may be obtained at a number of points during the intervention to assess the impact of the process of the intervention on the participants; how this is done will depend on whether data will be obtained directly from participants, providers, or existing data sources such as case records. More than one source of data is usually recommended, with the expectation that an intent-to-treat analysis will be conducted. Intent-to-treat analysis examines outcomes based on participants' assigned groups, regardless of whether they attended the intervention, and is based on the assumption that in the real world of practice this is how participants are likely to function. However, in order to conduct such an analysis the outcome data need to be available. If the expectation is that a number of the sample participants will be difficult to locate, then the use of administrative data may result in less missing data.

Implementing RCTs

Preparing the Site

Before implementing the RCT, the investigator needs to prepare the setting for the RCT. Remember that researchers need the setting more than the setting needs the RCT, so there must be real buy-in at the site. Understanding the perspective of the agency, organization, and/or providers (as learned during the planning stage) will help. The actual implementation, then, must be collaborative, typically with regularly scheduled meetings between the research team and providers, including administrators who are responsible for decision making. If the project team is hiring interventionists, researchers have some control over selecting the most qualified providers. However, if agency personnel are to deliver the interventions, researchers will have to accommodate this. On-site personnel may not have the motivation or possess the level of qualifications essential to implement the intervention. Recent focus in the field on training agency personnel in the implementation of evidence-based practices provides a guide; efforts to train personnel to implement interventions are essentially the same. Research has found that stand-alone didactic training on an intervention is insufficient, because there needs to be ongoing monitoring and coaching for providers to gain confidence in delivering an intervention (Fixsen, Blase, Naoom, & Wallace, 2009). Supervisors too require training in the intervention, even if they are not delivering it, so they can appropriately oversee implementation. In addition, the control condition providers will likely have to be trained in data collection and in human subject protections.

Monitoring Fidelity and Process

Implementation of an intervention is a developmental process; until there is a full complement of participants, the intervention is not fully implemented. Full implementation will depend in part on the rate of recruitment, which will also influence when fidelity assessments should be conducted. Monitoring and employing fidelity assessments of the intervention are incorporated at regular and/or strategic intervals to ensure the intervention is being implemented according to the manual; otherwise a lack of fidelity remains a source of error in the study (McGrew, Bond, Dietzen, & Salyers, 1994).

The amount of the intervention that participants receive, termed dosage, is also an important data point. These data may be obtained from billing records, administrative data, or service logs kept by providers. The investigator may also need to know whether participants are receiving services from other entities. Furthermore, documentation of the actual process of implementation and the environmental context are essential to understanding the RCT. Glisson, Dukes, and Green (2006) found that organizational climate and culture have an impact on interventions. Both qualitative and quantitative methods can be employed to help systematically measure these factors (see description of a process monitoring system in Chapter 15).

Enrollment Tracking

Another ongoing and essential feature of RCT implementation is the tracking of recruitment and retention of participants through completion. This requires the development of a computerized system that can monitor the enrollment of participants on a continuous basis. Enrollment logs can help avert the need for last-ditch recruitment drives to meet sample size and can facilitate participant follow-up. A tracking form needs to be developed at the beginning of the study to complete with each participant at baseline data collection and to review at all follow-up data collection points. Tracking data might include not just basic information like current address, but also names and contact information of individuals who are likely to know where the participants are and places they are likely to go should their financial or housing situation change. Solomon and colleagues (2009) provide a comprehensive listing of retention and tracking information and techniques.

RANDOMIZED CONTROLLED TRIALS AND GLOBAL HEALTH

As mentioned in Chapter 1, the utilization of RCTs has both its supporters and detractors, particularly within the global health arena. Supporters believe that RCTs provide rigorous evidence on the effectiveness of interventions addressing individual- and community-level problems. Detractors assert that, particularly from an international perspective, there are significant translational challenges in the design and implementation of RCTs. Contextual issues can indeed affect the external validity of a randomized trial. What may be demonstrated as an effective intervention in one sociopolitical and economic environment may not show similar effects in another. Factors such as culture, race, class, gender, and/or sociopolitical environment can significantly affect the development and implementation of an RCT.

There are also ethical concerns regarding the application of RCTs across populations (Victora, Habicht, & Bryce, 2004). Vulnerable socioeconomic groups may be more prone to the adverse consequences of RCT participation: Individuals and social groups from poor and disadvantaged countries have shown to be at higher risk for exploitation in the name of rigorous science (Council on Foreign Relations, 2012). However, with awareness of contextual issues, thorough IRB review, and ethical safeguards in place, RCTs can provide rich information to aid in the development and application of interventions that may reduce personal and social issues and challenges globally (see text box). The Cochrane Collaboration's call for larger efforts to include global health topics in systematic reviews is viewed by many as a positive sign in a movement toward this goal (Richards, 2004). With increased emphasis on evidence-based interventions globally, it is essential to conduct effectiveness RCTs in each new setting, especially after any adaptation, as the effectiveness of an intervention in one setting may not apply to another.

EXAMPLE OF PLACED-BASED RCT AND GLOBAL HEALTH—REDUCING HIV-RELATED STIGMA IN HEALTH CARE SETTINGS: A RANDOMIZED CONTROLLED TRIAL IN CHINA

Objective: To examine the effectiveness of White Coat, Warm Heart Intervention in reducing health providers' stigmatizing attitudes and behaviors toward people living with HIV.

Methods:

Sample: Forty county-level hospitals in two provinces in China were randomized to an intervention or control condition. Systematic sampling was employed to select the provider participants who had regular contact with

(Continued)

(Continued)

patients. Forty-four service providers were selected from each hospital, resulting in a sample size of 1,760.

Outcomes: Primary outcomes were prejudicial attitudes, avoidance intent toward people living with HIV, and perceived institutional support related to protection from infections and HIV care in the hospital.

Intervention: Popular opinion leaders (POLs) were identified through hospital coworkers, gatekeepers, and department heads. Twenty to 25 POLs were trained in each intervention hospital, for a total of 450. They were trained in employing universal precautions, fighting stigma and improving patient relationships, and improving patient care. POLs were to function as behavior changers, and prescribed messages were to be delivered by POLs. POLs were given opportunities for practicing and refining skills to deliver messages. Control and intervention hospitals received standard information packages and the same amount of universal precaution supplies.

Results: Intervention hospitals had significant reduction in prejudicial attitudes, reduction in avoidance intent toward people living with HIV, and perceived increase in institutional support at 6 months; results were sustained for 12 months.

Source: Li et al. (2013).

CURRENT ISSUES AND FUTURE DIRECTIONS

Public health and medicine have been transformed by the evidence provided by RCTs. Bukens, Keusch, Belizan, and Bhutta (2004) identify a need, however, for more trials of behavioral interventions at the global level. The need is perhaps greatest where populations are heavily affected by macro-level factors, such as poverty and institutionalized racism, yet there are issues that affect the development and implementation of RCTs in these areas. For instance, access to samples, feasibility issues, and the cost-effectiveness of trials in an era of depleting resources pose particular challenges when attempting to conduct RCTs with vulnerable populations. Psychosocial RCTs require a close collaboration between the research team and agency personnel/community members, which can be difficult given the complex realities of community settings. For this reason community-based participatory research has been proposed by some researchers to be conducted in conjunction with RCTs (Jones, Koegel, & Wells, 2008; see Chapter 4). Nevertheless, the need is great for evidence-based strategies to address the varied and complex problems faced by those most in need. With collaboration and teamwork, researchers and community members can carefully plan to address problems that may affect intervention outcomes and work together to close the gap between research evidence and the real-world needs of community settings.

ADDITIONAL RESOURCES

Newman, J., Rawlings, L., & Gertler, P. (1994). Using randomized control designs in evaluating social sector programs in developing countries. *World Bank Research Observer, 9,* 181–201.

Plantadosi, S. (2005). *Clinical trials: Methodological perspective.* New York, NY: Wiley.

Shadish, W., Cook, T., & Campbell, D. (2002). Experimental and quasi-experimental designs for generalized causal inference. Boston, MA: Houghton Mifflin.

REFERENCES

Baron, R., & Kenny, D. (1986). The moderator-mediator variable distinction in social psychological research: Conceptual, strategic, and statistical considerations. *Journal of Personality & Social Psychology, 5,* 1173–1182.

Bellig, A., Borrelli, B., Resnick, B., Hecht, J., Minicucci, D., Ory, M., . . . Czajkowski, S. (2004). Enhancing treatment fidelity in health behavior change studies: Best practices and recommendations from the NIH Behavior Change Consortium. *Health Psychology, 23,* 443–451.

Bond, G., Evans, L., Salyers, M., Williams, J., & Kim, H. (2000). Measurement of fidelity in psychiatric rehabilitation. *Mental Health Services Research, 2,* 75–87.

Bond, G., Williams, J., Evans, L., Salyers, M., Kim, H., Sharpe, H., & Leff, S. (2000). *Psychiatric rehabilitation fidelity toolkit.* Cambridge, MA: Human Service Research Institute.

Boruch, R. (1997). *Randomized field experiments for planning and evaluation.* Thousand Oaks, CA: Sage.

Bukens, P., Keusch, G., Belizan, J., & Bhutta, Z. A. (2004). Evidence-based global health. *Journal of the American Medical Association, 291,* 2639–2641.

Burns, E., Burchard, J., Suter, J., Leventz-Brady, K., & Force, M. (2004). Assessing fidelity to a community-based treatment for youth: The Wraparound Fidelity Index. *Journal of Emotional and Behavioral Disorders, 12,* 79–89.

Carroll, K., & Nuro, K. (1997). The use and development of treatment manuals. In K. Carroll (Ed.), *Improving compliance with alcoholism treatment* (pp. 53–72). Bethesda, MD: National Institute of Alcohol Abuse and Alcoholism.

Carroll, K., & Nuro, K. (2002). One size cannot fit all: A stage model for psychotherapy manual development. *Clinical Psychology: Science and Practice, 9,* 396–406.

Carroll, K., & Rounsaville, B. (2008). Efficacy and effectiveness in developing treatment manuals. In A. Nezu & C. Nezu (Eds.), *Evidence-based outcome research* (pp. 219–243). New York, NY: Oxford University Press.

Centers for Disease Control and Prevention. (2013). *Healthy People 2020 final review.* Retrieved from http://www.cdc.gov/nchs/healthy_people/hp2010/hp2010_final_review.htm

Cosden, M., Ellens, J., Schnell, J., & Yamini-Diouf, Y. (2005). Efficacy of a mental health treatment court with assertive community treatment. *Behavioral Sciences and the Law, 23,* 199–214.

Cosden, M., Ellens, J., Schnell, J., Yamini-Diouf, Y., & Wolfe, M. (2003). Evaluation of a mental health treatment court with assertive community treatment. *Behavioral Sciences and the Law, 21,* 415–427.

Council on Foreign Relations. (2012). *Are randomized controlled trials a good way to evaluate development projects?* Washington, DC: Author.

Davis, L., Broome, M., & Cox, R. (2002). Maximizing retention in community-based clinical trials. *Journal of Nursing Scholarship, 334,* 47–53.

De Las Nueces, D., Hacker, K., DiGiralamo, A., & Hicks, L. (2012). A systematic review of community-based participatory research to enhance clinical trials in racial and ethnic minority groups. *Health Services Research, 47,* 1363–1386.

Donner, A., & Klar, N. (2004). Pitfalls of and controversies in cluster randomization trials. *American Journal of Public Health, 94,* 418–422.

Fixsen, D., Blase, K., Naoom, S., & Wallace, F. (2009). Core implementation components. *Research on Social Work Practice, 19,* 531–540.

Flander, M., & Burns, T. (2000). A Delphi approach to describing service models of community mental health practice. *Psychiatric Services, 51,* 656–658.

Gartlehner, G., Hansen, R. A., Nissman, D., Lohr, K. N., & Carey, T. S. (2006). *Criteria for distinguishing effectiveness from efficacy trials in systematic reviews* (AHRQ Publication No. 060046). Rockville, MD: Agency for Healthcare Research and Quality.

Gellis, Z., McGinty, J., Horowitz, A., Bruce, M., & Misener, E. (2007). Problem-solving therapy for late life depression in home care: A randomized field trial. *American Journal of Geriatric Psychiatry, 15,* 968–978.

Glasgow, R., Lichtenstein, E., & Marcus, A. (2003). Why don't we see more translation of health promotion research to practice? Rethinking the efficacy-to-effectiveness transition. *American Journal of Public Health, 93,* 1261–1267.

Glisson, C., Dukes, D., & Green, P. (2006). The effects of ARC: Organizational intervention on case-worker turnover, climate, and culture in children's service system. *Child Abuse & Neglect, 30,* 855–880.

Good, M., & Schuler, L. (1997). Subject retention in a controlled clinical trial. *Journal of Advanced Nursing, 26,* 351–355.

Jones, L., Koegel, P., & Wells, K. (2008). Bridging experimental design to community-partnered participatory research. In M. Minkler & N. Wallerstein (Eds.), *Community-based participatory research in health from process to outcomes* (pp. 67–84). San Francisco, CA: Jossey-Bass.

Kraemer, H., Mintz, J., Noda, A., Tinklinberg, J., & Yesavage, J. (2006). Caution regarding the use of pilot studies to guide power calculations for study proposals. *Archives of General Psychiatry, 63,* 484–489.

Lancaster, G., Dodd, S., & Williamson, P. (2004). Design and analysis of pilot studies: Recommendations for good practice. *Journal of Evaluation in Clinical Practice, 10,* 307–312.

Lewin, S., Glenton, C., & Oxman, A. (2009). Use of qualitative methods alongside randomized controlled trials of complex healthcare interventions: Methodological study. *BMJ, 339,* b3496.

Li, L., Wu, Z., Llang, L., Lin, C., Guan, J., Jia, M., . . . Yan, Z. (2013). Reducing HIV-related stigma in health care settings: A randomized controlled trial in China. *American Journal of Public Health, 103,* 286–292.

McGrew, J., Bond, G., Dietzen, L., & Salyers, M. (1994). Measuring fidelity of implementation of a mental health program model. *Journal of Consulting and Clinical Psychology, 62,* 670–678.

Mrazek, P., & Haggerty, R. (Eds.). (1994). *Reducing risks for mental disorders: Frontiers for preventive intervention research.* Washington, DC: National Academy Press.

National Commission for the Protection of Human Subjects of Biomedical and Behavioral Research. (1978). *The Belmont Report: Ethical principles and guidelines for the protection of human subjects of research.* Washington, DC: U.S. Government Printing Office.

Oakley, A., Strange, V., Bonell, C., Allen, E., Stephenson, J., & RIPPLE Study Team. (2006). Process evaluation in randomized controlled trials of complex interventions. *BMJ, 332,* 413–416.

Orwin, R. (2000). Methodological challenges in study design and implementation: Assessing program fidelity in substance abuse health services research. *Addiction, 95,* S309–S327.

Richards, T. (2004). Poor countries lack relevant health information. *BMJ, 328,* 310.

Rosen, L., Manor, O., Engelhard, D., & Zucker, D. (2006). In defense of the randomized controlled trial for health promotion research. *American Journal of Public Health, 96,* 1181–1188.

Shattuck, D., Kemer, B., Gilles, K., Hartman, M., Ng'ombe, T., & Guest, G. (2011). Encouraging contraceptive uptake by motivating men to communicate about family planning: The Malawi Male Motivator Project. *American Journal of Public Health, 101,* 1089–1095.

Sikkema, K. (2005). HIV prevention among women in low-income housing developments: Issues and intervention outcomes in a place-based randomized controlled trial. *Annals of the American Academy of Political and Social Science, 599,* 52–70.

Solomon, P., Cavanaugh, M., & Draine, J. (2009). *Randomized controlled trials: Design and implementation for community-based psychosocial interventions.* New York, NY: Oxford University Press.

Torgerson, D., & Torgerson, C. (2008). *Designing randomized trials in health, education and social sciences.* New York, NY: Palgrave Macmillan.

Trochim, W., Cook, J., & Setze, P. (1994). Using concept mapping to develop a conceptual framework of staff's views of supported employment program for individuals with severe mental illness. *Journal of Consulting and Clinical Psychology, 62,* 766–775.

Verhoef, M., Casebeer, A., & Hilsden, R. (2002). Assessing efficacy of complementary medicine: Adding qualitative research methods to the "gold standard." *Journal of Alternative and Complementary Medicine, 8,* 275–281.

Victora, C. G., Habicht, J. P., & Bryce, J. (2004). Evidence-based public health: Moving beyond randomized trials. *American Journal of Public Health, 94,* 400–405.

Wingood, G., & DiClemente, R. (2008). The ADAPT-ITT model: A novel method of adapting evidence-based HIV interventions. *Journal of Acquired Immune Deficiency Syndrome, 47,* S40–S46.

Witte, S., Bassel, N., Gilbert, L., Wiu, E., Chang, M., & Steinglass, P. (2004). Recruitment of minority women and their main sexual partner in an HIV/STI prevention trial. *Journal of Women's Health, 13,* 1137–1147.

PART V

Cross-Cutting Methods and Approaches

17

Sampling

The Foundation of Good Research

Johnnie Daniel

The previous three sections in this book reviewed specific research methods employed in public health. This section uses a wider lens to look at research design components that cut across all types of public health research, beginning in this chapter with a discussion of sampling. **Sampling** is a set of procedures for selecting study elements from, or about, which data are collected. The sampling procedures used in a study determine the size of its data collection effort, the amount of resources and skills necessary to conduct the study, the characteristics of the elements selected, and the appropriateness of different data collection instruments and data analysis procedures. Sampling also determines whether, and how much, we can generalize from the elements included in the study to those elements not included in the study. Ultimately, the procedures used to select study elements affect the extent to which the objectives of a study are met. To simplify the process of choosing an appropriate sampling strategy and sample size for your study, the sampling process in this chapter is divided into six fundamental steps listed in Figure 17.1.

Figure 17.1 The Six Steps of the Sampling Process

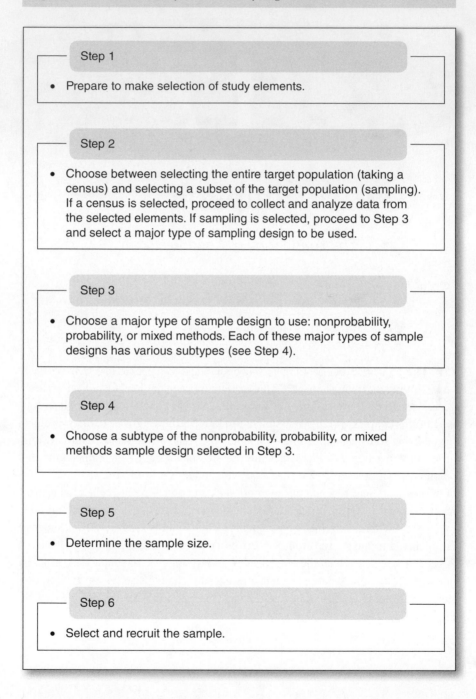

Step 1

- Prepare to make selection of study elements.

Step 2

- Choose between selecting the entire target population (taking a census) and selecting a subset of the target population (sampling). If a census is selected, proceed to collect and analyze data from the selected elements. If sampling is selected, proceed to Step 3 and select a major type of sampling design to be used.

Step 3

- Choose a major type of sample design to use: nonprobability, probability, or mixed methods. Each of these major types of sample designs has various subtypes (see Step 4).

Step 4

- Choose a subtype of the nonprobability, probability, or mixed methods sample design selected in Step 3.

Step 5

- Determine the sample size.

Step 6

- Select and recruit the sample.

This chapter has also been organized to introduce each of these steps in detail, to identify the choices you'll have to make along the way, and to highlight advantages and disadvantages of different sampling choices.

KEY CONCEPTS AND DEFINITIONS

Target population is the set of elements to which a researcher desires to apply the findings of a study. The target population of a study may be persons experiencing a particular medical problem, physicians working in a specific hospital, or residents of a specific community.

Census is a total enumeration of a target population. All members of the target population of a study are selected for inclusion in the study. A census of employees of a hospital would select all employees of the hospital for inclusion in the study.

Sampling is the selection of a subset of the members of a population for inclusion in a study. A sample of employees of a hospital would include only a selected subset of the employees of the hospital.

Sampling element is the item (person, location, event, etc.) from, or about, which data are collected.

Sampling frame is a listing of the entire target population. A good frame would include every member of the target population once and only once, and no other elements.

Probability sampling is a sampling procedure that gives every element in the target population a known and nonzero probability of being selected.

Nonprobability sampling is a sampling procedure that does not give every element in the target population a known and nonzero chance of being selected. Some members of the target population would have an opportunity to be selected for the study, and others would not have a chance to be selected.

Mixed methods sampling involves the combination of different types of sample designs. Within-methods designs combine different types of probability sample designs or different types of nonprobability sample designs. Cross-methods designs combine probability sample designs and nonprobability sample designs.

PREPARE TO SELECT STUDY ELEMENTS

The selection of study elements begins with thoughtful preparation. Such preparation must be sufficient to fully answer the following questions:

- What are the objectives of the study?
- What is the target population?
- What is the nature of the target population?

- What resources are available to conduct the study?
- What research design issues should be considered?

The answers to these questions drive the choices that are made in the subsequent steps. Answering these questions may involve an extensive literature review and/or formative research.

What Are the Objectives of the Study?

The elements for a given study should have a good fit with the objectives of the study. Broadly, the objectives of a research project may fall in the categories of exploration, description, prediction, evaluation, explanation, or a combination of these categories (explained in Chapter 2). Research that has an exploratory purpose might require a less rigorous procedure for selecting study elements; nonprobability sampling and/or a sample with a small sample size may suffice. At the other end of the spectrum, research aiming to provide information for biomedical decision making will require more rigorous procedures for selecting study elements, including probability sampling and a relatively large sample size. Of course, a study may have multiple objectives and require a combination of sampling approaches.

What Is the Target Population?

Before selecting the elements for a study, identify the target population by defining clear inclusion and exclusion criteria for selecting the elements to be studied. **Inclusion criteria** are a set of conditions that must be met in order to participate in a study, and **exclusion criteria** are a set of conditions that disqualify elements from participation. We also need to decide whether the objectives of a study require focus on a single target population, multiple target populations, or various segments of a target population. A health survey may have multiple target populations, with more detailed analyses of some of the populations than for others.

As Gales, Maxwell, and Norris (2008) note, defining the target population in public health research can be rather challenging:

> Let us take a situation where a town is hit by a hurricane. Researchers may be interested in assessing all those who were affected by this event. But who are those persons? Are all persons in the town through which the hurricane passed "affected"? Or would the affected be only persons who saw the hurricane? Or those who had property damage as a result of the hurricane? If the latter is the desired group, how much property damage is sufficient for a person to be considered to be part of the sampling frame? (pp. S21–S22)

Clear definitions are therefore crucial to delimiting the target population for a particular study.

What Is the Nature of the Target Population?

Along with a clear definition of the target population, we should have a good understanding of the nature of the target population, in terms of content, size, heterogeneity, accessibility, and spatial distribution. In public health research the target population may be people (e.g., patients, health care workers), locations (e.g., hospitals, health departments, cities, restaurants), things (e.g., illegal drugs, cigarettes, medications), events (e.g., tornados, floods, doctor's visits), or time (e.g., time of day, day of week). All may require different contingencies for selecting the elements for a study. Moreover, the size of the target population is critical in determining how to select the elements for a study. It will affect the funds, time, and number of personnel necessary to conduct the study: A nationwide survey will take more resources than a community survey. Relatedly, the spatial distribution of the target population affects the resources necessary to conduct a study. In conducting personal interview health surveys, the travel time of interviewers covering sparsely populated rural areas is likely to be significantly greater than the travel time of interviewers covering densely populated urban areas.

Target populations that are diverse may also require different sampling procedures than relatively homogeneous populations; the more homogeneous a population, the fewer the number of elements necessary to represent the population. A health survey of a community whose residents are of the same ethnic group would likely require a smaller sample size than a health survey of a widely ethnically diverse community. Accessibility is another consideration: We may end up with a biased sample if members of the target population who are accessible are very different from its members who are not accessible. Persons with a particular medical problem sitting in the admission room of a clinic or hospital are more accessible than persons with the same medical problems who are not in the admission room; however, there may be significant differences in these two categories of patients with regard to socioeconomic status, severity of condition, and other key variables.

MORE KEY CONCEPTS AND DEFINITIONS

Over-coverage bias occurs if a sampling frame or sampling procedures include elements that are not members of the target population of a study. An example is a sampling frame of employees of a hospital that includes persons who are not employees. They may be former employees or persons whose names are listed due to errors.

Under-coverage bias is due to the use of a sampling frame that excludes members of the target population of a study. An example is a sampling frame of employees of a hospital that does not include all employees. It may exclude newly hired employees and part-time employees.

(Continued)

(Continued)

Clustered-frame bias is due to the use of a sampling frame that includes units with more than one element of the target population. An example is a sampling frame of the names of the primary insurer of a family health insurance plan. Some of the names in the list represent households that include a spouse, while others include a spouse and children.

Multiple-coverage bias is due to the use of a sampling frame that includes elements more than once. An example is a sampling frame of employees of a hospital that includes the names of some employees more than once, potentially because they work in more than one department.

What Resources Are Available to Conduct the Study?

With information on the nature of the target population in hand, we can assess the availability of resources (e.g., money, time, personnel, authority, facilities, information sources, equipment, sampling frame) to conduct the study. This assessment will affect our decisions about how to select the elements of a study. One important resource to consider is a **sampling frame**, a listing of the target population. A good sampling frame is free of over-coverage bias, under-coverage bias, multiple-coverage bias, and clustered-frame bias (see More Key Concepts and Definitions text box). It also includes accurate, reliable, and up-to-date information on each element. Whether a frame is available—and if available, the extent to which it has coverage bias—will affect the selection of different types of sample designs.

What Research Design Issues Should Be Considered?

Along with the research objectives, the research design and data collection and analysis techniques will influence the choice of sampling approaches. Much of qualitative research is based on nonnumeric data and seeks to interpret meanings, perspectives, and understandings. Quantitative research, by contrast, typically uses numerical data to estimate population parameters and analyze the statistical relationships among variables. Generally speaking, nonprobability sampling tends to be a better fit with qualitative research designs, and probability sampling tends to be a better fit with quantitative research designs. Mixed methods research designs often use mixed methods sample designs. Experimental and quasi-experimental research designs typically use nonprobability sample designs (e.g., availability sampling, purposive sampling, quota sampling) in selecting and allocating subjects to different treatment modalities. Due to attrition, mortality, and loss of contact, longitudinal research designs generally require larger sample sizes than cross-sectional research designs.

CHOOSE BETWEEN SAMPLING OR TAKING A CENSUS

In deciding whether to take a **census** (select all members of the target population for inclusion in the study) or to **sample** (select only some of the members of the target population for inclusion in the study), one should relate the results of Step 1 to the advantages and disadvantages of taking a census and sampling outlined below. A census technically is not a sampling method since no selective process is involved; everyone in the population is selected for inclusion in the study. Logistical constraints typically prevent employing censuses in field research. Most study populations are large, and including everyone from a population in a research study—even if you have a sampling frame—is usually prohibitively time-consuming and costly.

Advantages and Disadvantage of Taking a Census and Sampling	
Census	
Advantages of taking a census	Since sampling is not done, there is no sampling error.
	Information may be collected on all members of the target population, including small subgroups.
	Depending on the amount of nonresponse, true representation of the target population may be obtained
Disadvantages of taking a census	Data collection, processing, and analysis may be too time-consuming.
	It may be too costly in terms of personnel and money.
Sampling	
Advantages of sampling	Data collection, processing, and analysis are not as time-consuming as taking a census.
	It requires fewer personnel and less money.
	Depending on sample design, one may be able to accurately estimate population parameters.
	It may be possible to spend more resources on quality control, minimizing bias.
Disadvantages of sampling	Sampling error will exist; how much depends on the sample design.
	Small subgroups may not be represented in the sample in sufficient numbers for small-group analyses.
	Sampling may not be feasible, ethical, or legal.
	Members of the target population not selected may feel their opinions are not valued.

That said, a census will not have sampling error, and depending on the extent of nonresponse, it is likely to be better for addressing important objectives by providing information that represents the whole of the target population (rather than estimating from some sample of that population). Characteristics of the target population can also influence your choice to use a census. The heterogeneity of a population may warrant a census in order to represent all segments of a population. Similarly, a census would, if complete, include small or hidden subgroups in the study population.

Sampling, on the other hand, is best employed in the following cases:

- *The research has an exploratory purpose.* Generally, an exploratory study does not require a large number of elements.
- *You need to make a quick decision.* Studies utilizing sampling take less time than studies taking a census.
- *You need to regularly collect up-to-date information.* It takes more time to take a census than to sample. By the time the findings of the census are reported, the data might not be relevant to current situations.
- *You are interested in a homogeneous population.* The more homogeneous the population, the fewer the number of elements necessary to represent the population. Sampling will often suffice for homogeneous populations.
- *You need to target specific elements of the population.* Only those elements specifically targeted should be selected.
- *The target population size is large.* The larger the population, the more resources are necessary to take a census. With limited resources and a large population, sampling is often the only choice.
- *The population is highly scattered.* Collecting data from a highly scattered population could be expensive, making sampling the better choice.
- *You have limited available resources (time, money, personnel, etc.).* Sampling requires fewer resources than taking a census.

Based on the factors described, you can decide whether to take a census or to sample. If you decide to take a census, the task of determining how to select study elements is completed, and you proceed to collecting and analyzing the data from the elements. If you decide to sample, the next task is to determine which type of sampling procedure is most appropriate. These choices are made in Step 3.

CHOOSE BETWEEN NONPROBABILITY SAMPLING, PROBABILITY SAMPLING, AND MIXED METHODS SAMPLING

Non-probability sampling refers to any method of sampling that does not use random procedures in selecting sampling elements. As such, it does not give every item/person in the target population a known, nonzero chance to be selected. Nonprobability sampling does not allow the researcher to determine the odds of each sample member being selected. Conversely, **probability sampling** employs some form of random selection and therefore gives every element in the target population a known, nonzero chance to be selected. Probability sampling allows the researcher to determine the odds of each sample unit being selected. A **mixed methods** sample is a combination of multiple types of sample designs, which can be either nonprobability or probability based. Table 17.1 summarizes some of the factors that favor the selection of one approach over another; each is also discussed in greater detail below.

Table 17.1 Factors Affecting Choice of Sampling Approach

Factors Favoring Nonprobability Sampling	Factors Favoring Probability Sampling	Factors Favoring Mixed Methods Sampling
Research has an exploratory purpose	Purpose of research is to provide information useful in reaching conclusions or decisions	Research has multiple purposes
Need for quick decisions	Not a need for quick decisions	Not a need for quick decisions
Need to target specific elements of the population and/or illustrative examples	Not a need to target specific elements of the population	Need for a representative sample and to make statistical inferences; but also, target specific elements of the population
Homogeneous population	Heterogeneous population	Heterogeneous population
Difficult to gain access or locate population elements	Accessible population	Difficult to gain access or locate segments of the population
Population is highly scattered	Population not highly scattered	Population is highly scattered
Limited available resources	Sufficient resources are available	Sufficient resources are available
Appropriate sampling frame is not available	Appropriate sampling frame is available	Appropriate sampling frame is available
Qualitative research design is used	Quantitative research design is used	Mixed methods research design is used
Not important to make statistical generalizations	Important to make statistical generalizations	Important to make statistical generalizations
Important to use easy operational procedures	Not important to use easy operational procedures	Not important to use easy operational procedures
Very small sample is targeted	Need to minimize selection bias	Need to minimize selection bias

Source: Daniel (2012).

Factors Favoring the Use of Nonprobability Sampling

Generally, nonprobability sampling requires fewer resources than probability sampling. It can be done quicker, cheaper, and with less information and skill than required for probability sampling. On the other hand, it tends to have greater selection bias, does not provide a basis for estimating sampling error, and limits the use of inferential statistics (first column of Table 17.1). As Guest (in press) summarizes, "Non-probabilistic sampling is the norm when using qualitative data collection methods. The primary reason for this is qualitative inquiry is generally not intended or designed for statistical generalizability."

Highlighting another reason for the use of nonprobability sampling, Stueve, O'Donnell, Duran, San Doval, and Blome (2001) noted the problems in using probability sampling in studying HIV prevention among men who have sex with men:

> Probability-based sampling has many advantages, but can be difficult and costly to implement in HIV prevention research. This is especially the case for risk groups whose relatively small size, residential dispersion, and experiences with stigma make them difficult to reach with traditional probability methods such as random-digit dialing and household sampling. Minority young men who have sex with men (MSM) are a notable example. Despite elevated prevalence of diagnosed AIDS cases, HIV infection, and related risk behaviors, minority young MSM have been virtually invisible in general population surveys, and surveys that target specific population segments such as racial/ethnic groups. To increase sample sizes, some researchers use random-digit dialing or household sampling in areas known to have large gay populations and screen for MSM. Although these studies yield larger numbers of MSM than do general population surveys, they are likely to represent more affluent, gay-identified men. (p. 922)

In this example we see the potential for missing "experts" or specific individuals who have unique attributes (e.g., knowledge, experiences, social position) relative to the research question(s) when using probabilistic samples, making nonprobabilistic sampling the appropriate choice for many qualitative research questions asked of key informants or stakeholders.

Factors Favoring the Use of Probability Sampling

Generally, probability sampling requires more time, money, people, and skills than nonprobability sampling does. In return for this investment, researchers gain a sample that is more likely to represent the target population, with a statistical basis for making inferences to a target population. Depending on sample design, it may also be possible to accurately estimate sampling errors. However, probability sampling may miss small subgroups, and probability sampling may not be possible without an adequate sampling frame. Factors favoring the use of probability sampling are listed in the middle column of Table 17.1. Generally speaking, probability sampling is warranted when

- the statistical methods you plan to use for data analysis require a probabilistic sample (the case for most statistics), or

- study objectives require you to statistically generalize results from a sample to the larger study population. Statistical generalization includes probability estimates such as sampling error, standard error, and confidence intervals.

Based on these criteria, it makes sense to use probability sampling for many studies that involve quantitatively oriented data collection and analyses, such as structured surveys, structured observation techniques, and confirmatory content analysis of text.

Factors Favoring the Use of Mixed Methods Sampling

Mixed methods sample designs combine different types of sample designs in conducting a study, giving them the flexibility to accommodate studies with multiple purposes, targeting different populations, or using complex research designs—at the cost of increased resource needs. Multiphase sampling is common practice in larger, more complex field studies. The factors that favor the use of such sample designs are summarized in the right-hand column of Table 17.1. Consider your target population(s) and how you want to connect data from your samples, theoretically and analytically, and then combine methods to best meet your research objectives and study context.

CHOOSE THE SAMPLING SUBTYPE

After deciding among the main types of sample designs, you next must choose which subtype to employ. In this section we review several options for each type of sample design, identifying what is involved, advantages and disadvantages, and factors favoring their use (see Table 17.2 at the end of this section).

Subtypes of Nonprobability Sampling

Availability Sampling

Availability sampling is a subtype of nonprobability sampling that includes a number of related sampling procedures. The commonality of these procedures is that elements are selected from the target population on the basis of their availability or convenience and those of the researcher; data are collected from whatever cases present themselves. A number of different kinds of nonprobability sampling fall within the category of availability sampling, including convenience sampling, haphazard sampling, accidental sampling, chunk sampling, grab sampling, opportunistic sampling, fortuitous sampling, incidental sampling, straw polling, volunteer sampling, nonprobability systematic sampling, and nonprobability web-based sampling. These approaches, typically termed convenience sampling, have the lowest credibility of all sampling approaches, so should be viewed as a last resort. You will have to explicitly justify use of this technique when writing research proposals or disseminating findings. Conducting research in conflict zones, for example, may permit only convenience samples due to security issues.

Or in ethnographic research, initial interviews may be convenience based, until the researcher becomes more familiar with the study community.

Availability sampling has four basic steps:

1. Define the target population.

2. Identify convenient ways to recruit and select available elements in the target population.

3. Determine the sample size.

4. Select the targeted number of population elements.

Advantages and Disadvantages of Availability Sampling	
Advantages	*Disadvantages*
• Least resources (time, money, personnel) required • Simple operational procedures • Least effort requirements • Least skills required	• Sample is not likely to be representative of the target population • Sampling error cannot be estimated • Elements of the population that are difficult to locate may be excluded from the study • Selection of individual elements is subjective • Researcher has little control over sample characteristics • Potential volunteerism bias • Least reliable sampling procedure

Purposive Sampling

Purposive sampling is a nonprobability sampling procedure in which elements are selected from the target population on the basis of their fit with a specific set of inclusion/exclusion criteria. This is the most commonly employed nonprobabilistic sampling approach (also sometimes called judgment sampling). Perhaps the most intuitive way to think of purposive sampling is that you choose study participants based on the purpose of their involvement in the study. In Bernard's (2000) words, "you decide the purpose you want your informants (or communities) to serve, and you go out and find some" (p. 176). Daniel (2012) has proposed a framework to classify four major categories of purposive sampling on the basis of the nature of the inclusion/exclusion criteria employed. These categories include sampling procedures using selection criteria based on the following:

1. Consistency or inconsistency with central tendency

2. The amount of variability

3. Theory/model development

4. Judgment or reputation

Purposive sampling procedures that use selection criteria based on central tendency seek to select elements either because they are typical or because they are not typical. These sampling procedures include typical case sampling, modal instance sampling, deviant case sampling, rare element sampling, extreme case sampling, intensity case sampling, and outlier sampling.

Purposive sampling that uses selection criteria based on variability seek to create either a homogeneous or heterogeneous sample. These sampling procedures include homogeneous sampling, maximum variation sampling, heterogeneity sampling, and diversity sampling.

Purposive sampling procedures that employ selection criteria based on the judgment, reputation, or specialized knowledge include the following types of sampling: judgment sampling, subjective sampling, bellwether case sampling, reputational sampling, politically important sampling, expert sampling, and informant sampling.

Table 17.2   Major Subtypes of Purposive Sampling

Selection criteria	Subtypes	Description	Example: Study of visitors to hospital waiting room
Central tendency: Selection based on whether elements are considered to be average members of the target population	Typical case sampling, modal instance sampling	Elements selected because they are considered to be average	Selection of visitors in the waiting room considered to be typical or average
	Rare element sampling, extreme case sampling, deviant case sampling, outlier sampling	Elements selected because they are considered to be different from average	Selection of visitors in the waiting room considered to be very different from average visitors
Variability: Selection based on whether elements would create a homogeneous sample or a heterogeneous sample	Homogeneous sampling	Elements selected on the basis of their common characteristics	Selection of visitors in the waiting room who are similar to average visitors
	Maximum variation sampling, heterogeneity sampling, diversity sampling	Elements selected on the basis of their differences	Selection of visitors in the waiting room considered to be very different from average visitors

(Continued)

(Continued)

Selection criteria	Subtypes	Description	Example: Study of visitors to hospital waiting room
Theoretical model: Selection based on whether elements are consistent or inconsistent with theoretical model, hypothesis, or comparison group	Confirmatory sampling, theoretical sampling	Elements selected because they should confirm a theory or hypothesis	Selection of visitors in the waiting room who are likely to confirm one's hypothesis
	Disconfirming sampling, negative case sampling	Elements selected because they should disconfirm a theory or hypothesis	Selection of visitors in the waiting room who are likely to disconfirm one's hypothesis
	Matched sampling	Elements selected because their characteristics match a comparison group	Selection of visitors in the waiting room to create comparison groups with similar characteristics
Judgment: Selection based on judgment, reputation, intense characteristics, or past experiences	Judgment sampling, expert sampling, informant sampling, subjective sampling	Elements selected on the basis of subjective judgment and/or to provide their judgment	Selection of visitors in the waiting room based on judgment of who will best fit the purposes of the study and/or to be used as informants
	Politically important cases, intensity case sampling, critical case sampling, reputational sampling, bellwether case sampling	Elements selected because of their reputations or because they are considered to have rich information relating to the topic of the study	Selection of visitors in the waiting room on the basis of reputation, the richness of their past experiences, and/or their political importance

Source: Daniel (2012).

The following steps are used to select a purposive sample:

1. Define the target population.

2. Identify the inclusion/exclusion criteria to be used.

3. Create a plan to recruit and select population elements that satisfy the inclusion/exclusion criteria.

4. Determine the sample size.

5. Select the targeted number of population elements.

Inclusion criteria can be broad, such as being an adult male (which, by default, excludes children and women). A criterion can also be very specific (and/or rare), such as having been the victim of a serious surgical error in the past 3 months. Typically, multiple criteria are specified for a given study and can be demographic, behavioral, and/or biological.

Advantages and Disadvantages of Purposive Sampling	
Advantages	*Disadvantages*
• Permits the targeting of specific elements of the population • Takes advantage of the researcher's knowledge of the population	• Researcher must have adequate information and knowledge about the population, the sites, and the conditions of the research • Selection of individual elements is subjective • Sampling error cannot be estimated

Quota Sampling

Like purposive sampling, **quota sampling** is a nonprobability sampling procedure in which elements are selected from the target population on the basis of their fit with a specific set of inclusion/exclusion criteria. However, quota sampling has a few additional features. Categories of the target population are created, and data collectors are assigned targeted numbers of elements within each category to be selected and included in the sample (quota controls).

There are two major subtypes of quota sampling: proportional and nonproportional. In **proportional quota sampling**, the quotas given to the data collectors are set so that the proportions of the categories in the sample are consistent with their proportions in the target population. On the other hand, in **nonproportional quota sampling**, the quotas given to the data collectors are not necessarily set so that the categories would be proportional to their representation in the target population. They may be set to have an equal number of elements. Nonproportional quota sampling tends to be used when the proportions of categories in the population are not known, when it is desired to compare categories to each other, and when it is necessary to oversample a certain segment of the target population.

The following steps are used to select a purposive sample:

1. Define the target population.

2. Identify inclusion/exclusion criteria for the sample.

3. Create a plan to recruit and select population elements that satisfy the inclusion/exclusion criteria.

4. Determine the total sample size.

5. Determine the number of elements each data collector should select from categories of the inclusion/exclusion criteria.

6. Select the targeted number of population elements per the quota controls.

As an example, imagine that your study population is injection drug users in city X and the population comprises approximately 95% men and 5% women. You want to sample 100 individuals from this population. If you are interested in getting a representative cross-section of the population, as is, you would use proportional quota sampling and would select about 95 men and 5 women for your sample. If, however, you wanted to do a comparison between men and women within your population, such a strategy would render too small of a female subsample to say anything meaningful. In this latter case, you would use a nonproportional quota sample and select approximately 50 men and 50 women from your population.

Advantages and Disadvantages of Quota Sampling	
Advantages	*Disadvantages*
• Makes possible the inclusion of specific numbers of different segments of the target population in the sample • Facilitates the study of within-group and between-group subgroup differences within a population	• Greater resources are necessary to train and manage field workers • Researcher needs up-to-date information and knowledge about the population, the sites, and the conditions of the research • Sampling error cannot be estimated • Elements of the population that are difficult to locate may be excluded from the study • Selection of individual elements is subjective • Sample may not be representative of the target population

Respondent-Assisted Sampling

Respondent-assisted sampling is a nonprobability sampling procedure in which elements are selected from a target population with the assistance of elements previously selected. Initial participants are recruited using a particular form of sampling and then are subsequently asked to refer other members of the target population to the research project. Those referred are asked in turn to refer other members, and so on until the targeted sample size is reached or no new members of the target population are referred.

Subtypes of this form of sampling include snowball sampling, chain-referral sampling, referral sampling, network sampling, and respondent-driven sampling (RDS). RDS is a relatively new sampling procedure that makes fundamental modifications to the other forms of respondent-assisted sampling (Heckathorn, 1997). In this approach, respondents, instead of the researcher, make the contact with those referred, and special statistical modeling procedures are used in analyzing the data collected. As part of the analysis, a mathematical model of the recruitment process weights the data to compensate for nonrandom sample selection process. It is argued that these procedures yield unbiased estimates of population parameters (Heckathorn, 2007; Salganik, 2006; Salganik & Heckathorn, 2004; Semaan, 2010).

RDS is now widely used in public health research and has been adopted by the Centers for Disease Control and Prevention and other public health organizations throughout the world (Lansky et al., 2007). However, claims that its statistical modeling procedures produce unbiased estimates of population parameters are still under review (see Gales et al., 2008; Gile & Handcock, 2010; Goel & Salganik, 2010; Johnston, Malekinejad, Kendall, Iuppa, & Rutherford, 2008; Lansky et al., 2012; McCreesh et al., 2012).

Respondent-assisted sampling has the following basic steps:

1. Define the target population.

2. Identify inclusion/exclusion criteria for the sample.

3. Recruit and select initial "seeds."

4. Collect data from those selected.

5. Ask those selected for referrals.

6. Contact those referred.

7. Repeat Steps 4 through 6 with new referrals until targeted sample size or saturation (no new referrals are forthcoming) is achieved.

These basic steps are modified somewhat when using respondent-driven sampling (see Distinguishing [and Required] Features of RDS text box).

As mentioned below, RDS, and respondent referral techniques in general, are excellent techniques for sampling hard-to-reach, or "hidden," populations such as those engaged in illicit or socially condemned behavior. Malekinejad and colleagues (2008), for example, used respondent-driven sampling in collecting behavioral surveillance data on injection drug users in San Francisco. They found RDS to be effective in including many individuals who would otherwise be missed if sampling from drug treatment and HIV prevention service facilities. Further demonstrating the effectiveness of RDS in terms of inclusivity is a study by Wei,

DISTINGUISHING (AND REQUIRED) FEATURES OF RDS

- Information is collected on the size and nature of the respondents' personal networks (acquaintances, friends, and relatives who fall within the target population). These data are used to later weight and map the data.
- Instead of the researcher contacting those referred and asking them to participate in the research, the participants make the contact and invite others to participate in the research.
- Coupons are used to track who recruited whom and to map the respondents' networks. Once an initial seed completes the data collection process, he or she is given coupons (typically three) with unique ID numbers and instructions to give the coupons to other members of the target population and invite them to participate in the study.
- Multiple waves are carried out to minimize the effect of the selection process of the initial seed. The recruitment process continues until the targeted sample size is reached or until subsequent selections of waves do not differ in participant characteristics of concern.
- Using the data collected, statistical models are used to estimate parameters of the target population.

McFarland, Colfax, Fuqua, and Raymond (2012). They compared the results of two independent studies of Black men who have sex with men. One study used RDS and the other study used time-location sampling. The RDS sample was socioeconomically more diverse, indicating it better captured the existing heterogeneity within the target population.

Advantages and Disadvantages of Respondent-Assisted Sampling	
Advantages	*Disadvantages*
<ul><li>Procedures are in place to include rare and hard-to-reach populations</li><li>Facilitates the study of social networks</li></ul>	<ul><li>Selection of individual elements is subjective</li><li>Sample may not be representative of the target population</li><li>Potential bias produced by the initial seeds</li><li>Potential volunteerism bias</li><li>Size of network may influence selection</li><li>Respondents are not likely to refer persons they do not like, persons they have personal conflicts with, persons they fear, etc.</li><li>Researcher has little control over the sampling procedures</li></ul>

Table 17.3   Factors Favoring Different Types of Nonprobability Sampling

Factors Favoring Availability Sampling	Factors Favoring Purposive Sampling	Factors Favoring Quota Sampling	Factors Favoring Respondent-Assisted Sampling
Least resources (time, money, personnel) available	Need to target specific elements of the population	Need to guarantee the inclusion of members of different subpopulations	Need to sample rare and hard-to-reach populations
Need for the simplest operational procedures	Researcher has up-to-date information and knowledge about the population, the sites, and the conditions of the research	Purpose of study to compare subgroups	Members of the target population know each other, and are willing to request others to participate in the research
Least effort and skills required	Need to take advantage of the researcher's knowledge of the population and the research sites	Need for the proportion of subgroups in the sample to be a certain number	Very little information is known about the target population
Study consists of a pilot test of questionnaire, exploratory research		Resources available to manage fieldwork	
Not necessary to select a representative sample		Researcher has up-to-date information and knowledge about the population, the sites, and conditions of the research	

Source: Daniel (2012).

Subtypes of Probability Sampling

If a decision is made to select probability sampling, you must decide which subtype to use. There are four major subtypes of probability sample designs: simple random, stratified, systematic, and cluster. In this section we describe these forms of sampling, steps in carrying out the designs, their advantages and disadvantages, and factors favoring their use.

Simple Random Sample

Simple random sampling is a probability sampling procedure that gives every element in the target population, and each possible sample of a given size, an equal and independent chance of being selected.

The following steps are used to select a simple random sample:

1. Define the target population.

2. Identify an existing sampling frame of the target population, or develop a new one.

3. Evaluate the sampling frame for under-coverage, over-coverage, multiple coverage, and clustering of elements, and make adjustments where necessary.

4. Assign a unique number to each element in the frame.

5. Determine the sample size.

6. Randomly select the targeted number of population elements using the lottery method, a table of random numbers, or a random number generator.

Simple random sampling is extremely common in public health research. If a sampling frame exists, or can be easily constructed, a simple random sample is an ideal option. In one example (among thousands), Kantor, Bilker, Glasser, and Margolis (2002) employed simple random sampling in their study of erectile dysfunction and depression. They selected a simple random sample from a list of patients aggregated across 73 general medical practices affiliated with a referral center in Pennsylvania. In another example, Chan et al. (2006) utilized listings on the Hong Kong Doctors Homepage, a website developed and maintained by the Hong Kong Medical Association, as a sampling frame. From this list they selected a simple random sample of Hong Kong doctors for inclusion in their study.

Advantages and Disadvantages of Simple Random Sampling	
Advantages	*Disadvantages*
• Not necessary for sampling frame to include auxiliary information on the elements in the population • Every possible combination of sampling units has an equal and independent chance of being selected	• Adequate sampling frame is required • Members of subgroups of the population may not be included in the sample in sufficient numbers, if at all

Advantages	Disadvantages
• Possible to estimate sampling error • Easy to communicate procedures to others • Estimates are easy to calculate; advanced statistical software is not necessary • Not necessary to weight the data during the data analysis phase of a study as every element has an equal and independent chance of selection	• Resulting sample may not be representative of the target population • Data collection could be time consuming and costly if the target population is widely dispersed geographically • Does not make use of auxiliary information on the elements of the population

Systematic Sampling

Systematic sampling is a probability sampling procedure in which a random selection is made of the first element for the sample, and then subsequent elements are selected at a fixed interval.

Typically, the following steps are used to select a systematic sample:

1. Define the target population.

2. Determine the desired sample size (n).

3. Identify an existing sampling frame, or develop a sampling frame of the target population.

4. Evaluate the sampling frame for under-coverage, over-coverage, multiple coverage, clustering, and periodicity, and make adjustments where necessary. Ideally, the list will be in a random order.

5. Determine the number of elements in the sampling frame (N).

6. Calculate the sampling interval (i) by dividing the number of elements in the sampling frame (N) by the targeted sample size (n).

7. Randomly select a number (r) from 1 through i.

8. Select for the sample (r), r + i, r + 2i, r + 3i, and so forth, until the frame is exhausted.

Systematic sampling is an appropriate and useful sampling option when a sampling frame cannot be obtained or generated. As with simple random sampling, one could find thousands of examples of its use in public health research. To cite one, Hendry, Beattie, and Heaney (2005) used systematic sampling in their study of children with minor illness or injury who came to pediatric accident and emergency departments. Every third child who registered as a patient was included in their sample. Systematic sampling procedures are also often used when intercept interviewing (in health facilities or elsewhere) or doing household surveys if the community/town has not been enumerated.

Advantages and Disadvantages of Systematic Sampling	
Advantages	*Disadvantages*
• Spreads the sample across the target population • Easier to draw and implement than simple random sampling • If a randomized sampling frame is used, the results may be similar to those of simple random sampling	• If a sampling frame is used that includes periodicities that are correlated with the interval that is used, the resulting sample may not be representative of the population • If a sampling frame is not used, one must be able to accurately estimate the population size for the determination of the sampling interval

Stratified Sampling

Stratified sampling is a probability sampling procedure in which the target population is first separated into mutually exclusive, homogeneous categories (strata), and then a simple random sample is selected from each category (stratum). There are two major subtypes of stratified sampling: proportionate stratified sampling (PSS) and disproportionate stratified sampling (DSS). In PSS, the number of elements allocated to the various strata is proportional to their representation in the target population. On the other hand, in DSS the number of elements allocated to the various strata is not proportional to their representation in the target population. PSS is often used when the objective of the study is to estimate population parameters. DSS is often used when the objectives of the study require detailed analyses of certain categories, comparison of categories of different sizes, and the use of different data collection procedures within the different categories.

The following steps are used to select a stratified sample:

1. Define the target population.

2. Identify the stratification variable(s) and determine the number of strata to be used. Ideally, these will be variables that are correlated with one's study variables.

3. Identify an existing sampling frame, or develop a sampling frame that includes information on the stratification variable(s) for each element in the target population. Variability within strata should be minimized, and variability between strata should be maximized.

4. Evaluate the sampling frame for under-coverage, over-coverage, multiple coverage, and clustering, and make adjustments where necessary.

5. Divide the sampling frame into strata. Within-stratum differences should be minimized, and between-strata differences should be maximized. The strata must not be overlapping, and every element of the target population must be in one, and only one, stratum. Assign a unique number to each element.

6. Determine the sample size for each stratum.

7. Randomly select the targeted number of elements from each stratum.

As noted above, stratified sampling is typically used when (a) estimating population parameters is a study objective or (b) a need to oversample an under-represented subpopulation exists. An example of the former is a study by Keane, Marx, and Ricci (2001). The researchers used a proportionate stratified sampling approach in their nationwide study of local health departments. They stratified the population by size of jurisdiction served by the local health department and then selected a simple random sample from each stratum. In another example, Linnan et al. (2008) used a disproportionate stratified sampling design in their nationwide study of work site health promotion programs throughout the United States. Due to the preponderance of work sites with fewer than 50 employees, sites with more than 50 employees were oversampled to ensure that estimates would be appropriate for all sites of all sizes.

Advantages and Disadvantages of Stratified Sampling	
Advantages	*Disadvantages*
• Possible to make inferences to the target population, within a stratum, and comparisons across strata facilitating the study of within-group and between-group subgroup differences within a population • Less sampling error than simple random sampling • May ensure representation of specific subpopulations in the sample • Different data collection procedures may be used in different strata	• Requires a sampling frame with relevant auxiliary information • Requires knowledge of the population • Requires more effort than simple random sampling • Calculation of population estimates may be complicated • More time consuming than simple random sampling • If disproportionate stratified sampling is used, the data collected must be weighted in order to accurately estimate population parameters

Cluster Sampling

Cluster sampling is a probability sampling procedure in which naturally occurring aggregates or clusters of elements of the population are randomly selected. Subtypes of cluster sampling may be classified on the basis of the number of sampling events (single-stage cluster sampling, two-stage cluster sampling, and multistage cluster sampling) and on the basis of the proportional representation of the clusters in the sample (probability proportional to size and probability disproportional to size). In single-stage cluster sampling, once an aggregate or cluster is selected, all the elements in the selected cluster are included in the sample. In two-stage cluster sampling and multistage cluster sampling, additional sampling is done after the first stage. In probability-proportional-to-size cluster sampling, the number of elements selected from a cluster is proportional to the size of the cluster in the total population, and in probability-disproportional-to-size cluster sampling, the number of elements selected is not proportional to the size of the cluster in the total population.

The following steps are used to select a cluster sample:

1. Define the target population.

2. Determine the desired sample size.

3. Identify an existing sampling frame, or develop a new sampling frame of clusters of the target population.

4. Evaluate the sampling frame for under-coverage, over-coverage, multiple coverage, and clustering, and make adjustments where necessary. Ideally, the clusters would be as heterogeneous as the population, mutually exclusive, and collectively exhaustive.

5. Determine the number of clusters to be selected. This may be done by dividing the sample size by estimated average number of population elements in each cluster.

6. Randomly select the targeted number of clusters.

7. If two-stage or multistage cluster sampling is done, either randomly select individual elements from the selected clusters (two-stage cluster sampling) or randomly select additional clusters from the selected clusters and then randomly select individual elements (multistage cluster sampling).

Multistage cluster sampling is common when sampling in geographically large and populous areas. And, in many cases, other sampling strategies are included in these more complex sampling designs. Lippert, Fendrich, and Johnson (2008), for example, used a multistage sampling design in their study of the impact of the 9/11 attacks on substance use in Chicago, Illinois. Their target population was English-speaking residents between the ages of 18 and 40 years. In their first stage, census tracts in Chicago (i.e., first-stage clusters) were selected randomly. In the second stage, one block (i.e., second-stage cluster) was selected randomly from within each sampled tract. In the third stage, every household on the sampled block was screened for eligibility (census). In the final stage one adult was randomly selected from within each eligible household (systematic).

Subtypes of Mixed Methods Sampling

Mixed methods sample designs may be categorized into different subtypes, described below (for more detailed descriptions of mixed methods sampling, see Collins, Onwuegbuzie, & Jiao, 2006, 2007; Daniel, 2012).

Advantages and Disadvantages of Cluster Sampling	
Advantages	*Disadvantages*
• Does not require a sampling frame of the target population • May minimize data collection costs and efforts • Less administrative time required	• Higher sampling error than simple random sampling • Sampling errors may be extremely large if clusters differ significantly from each other • Researcher must be able to clearly delineate boundaries to the clusters • Calculation of population estimates may be complicated

Table 17.4   Factors Favoring Different Types of Probability Sampling

Favors Favoring Simple Random Sampling	*Favors Favoring Systematic Sampling*	*Favors Favoring Stratified Sampling*	*Favors Favoring Cluster Sampling*
• When it is necessary to give every element of the population an equal chance to be selected • When an adequate sampling frame of the target population is available • When comparing subgroups is not critical to study objectives • Works best for small, homogeneous populations that are not widely dispersed	• Easy to use • Can use without a sampling frame • Useful when the distribution of the target population is not an order that corresponds to the sampling interval that is used	• An adequate sampling frame that includes information to allow subgrouping (i.e., stratification) of individuals • Appropriate when it is important that elements in certain subcategories are represented in the sample • Used when it is necessary to compare and/or use different procedures for different segments of the population	• When an appropriate sampling frame of individual elements of the target population is not available • If it is necessary to minimize data collection costs and target population is dispersed across a large geographical area • Distribution of the elements of the population occur in distinguishable clusters • When it is necessary to estimate characteristics of clusters as well as the target population

First, they may be classified into two categories: within-methods designs and cross-methods designs. A within-method design combines either multiple nonprobability sample designs or multiple probability sample designs. A cross-method design combines one or more nonprobability sample designs with one or more probability sample designs. Next, the sample designs may be classified according to the time order in which they are implemented. They may be implemented concurrently, at the same time (concurrent designs), or sequentially, one after another (sequential designs).

The relationship that the sample designs have with each other may also be used in characterizing additional subtypes. The sample designs may have any one of three types of relationships with each other: equivalent status, nested, and multilevel. Sample designs that have an equivalent status with each other have the same level of dominance. Neither design is subordinate to the other(s). Nested designs are methods composed of one or more dominant sample design and one or more subordinate sample designs. Multilevel designs are methods that sample components of a target that are at different levels of generality.

Sampling Based on the Nature of the Sampling Unit

Often population-based sampling is not practical due to the lack of a good sampling frame of the population or lack of fit with the purposes of the study. The sampling procedures described above may be applied to alternative sampling units such as spaces, locations, time, venues, telephone numbers, email addresses, website visitors, and postal addresses.

Cross-tabulating the dimensions described above, 18 subtypes of mixed methods sampling may be identified. An outline of these subtypes, with brief examples, is presented in Table 17.5. Chapter 19 provides a description of the numerous variations of mixed methods designs.

Additional Sampling Approaches

Time-Space Sampling

Time-space sampling is a set of sampling procedures that utilize space as a sampling unit. This type of sampling is also referred to as area sampling and spatial sampling and is particularly useful for sampling individuals who tend to congregate, live, or work in known geographic areas. The spaces may be geographical units (typical sampling units used in multistage cluster sampling described above), the floor space of a shopping mall, grids on a map, and so on. It may also be referred to as location-based sampling. Time-based sampling consists of a set of sampling procedures that use units of time as sampling units. Time units may be hours, days, weeks, months, or years depending on the subject matter of the research. Venue-based sampling may be viewed as a combination of space-based sampling, location-based sampling, and time-based sampling. First, formative research is conducted to determine locations and time periods in which members of the target population tend to be present. A sampling frame of these space/location/time units is created, and a sample of these units is then randomly selected. Data collectors then go to the selected location/time periods and select members of the target population using systematic sampling.

Table 17.5 Subtypes of Mixed Methods Sample Design

Within-methods designs: Probability	Concurrent designs	Parallel	In a study of the attitudes of nurses toward a health policy, one may simultaneously select a simple random sample of nurses at one hospital and a cluster sample of nurses at another hospital.
		Nested	In a study of the attitudes of nurses toward a health policy, one may simultaneously select a stratified sample of nurses, and from those selected, using simple random sampling, select a subsample of the nurses for more detailed data collection.
		Multilevel	In a study of the attitudes of nurses toward a health policy, one may simultaneously select a simple random sample of hospital administrators and a stratified sample of nurses.
	Sequential designs	Parallel	In a study of the attitudes of nurses toward a health policy, one may first select a simple random sample of nurses at one hospital and later select a cluster sample of nurses at another hospital.
		Nested	In a study of the attitudes of nurses toward a health policy, one may first select a stratified sample of nurses, and using the information collected, later select a simple random sample of nurses previously selected for more detailed data collection.
		Multilevel	In a study of the attitudes of hospital employees toward a health policy, one may first select a simple random sample of hospital administrators and later select a stratified sample of nurses.

(Continued)

(Continued)

Cross-methods designs: Nonprobability and probability combinations	Concurrent designs	Parallel	In a study of the attitudes of nurses toward a health policy, one may simultaneously select an availability sample of nurses at one hospital and a simple random sample of nurses at another hospital.
		Nested	In a study of the attitudes of nurses toward a health policy, one may simultaneously select an availability sample of nurses, and from those selected, using simple random sampling, select a subsample of the nurses for more detailed data collection.
		Multilevel	In a study of the attitudes of nurses toward a health policy, one may simultaneously select a purposive sample of hospital administrators and a stratified sample of nurses.
	Sequential designs	Parallel	In a study of the attitudes of nurses toward a health policy, one may first select a simple random sample of nurses at one hospital and later select an availability sample of nurses at another hospital.
		Nested	In a study of the attitudes of nurses toward a health policy, one may first select a stratified sample of nurses, and using the information collected, later select a purposive sample of nurses previously selected for more detailed data collection.
		Multilevel	In a study of the attitudes of hospital employees toward a health policy, one may first select a purposive sample of hospital administrators and later select a stratified sample of nurses.

Source: Daniel (2012); Onwuegbuzie and Collins (2007).

Weinbaum et al. (2008) used venue-based sampling in their study of the prevalence of hepatitis B virus (HBV) immunization and HBV infection among men aged 23 to 29 years who have sex with men. First, they identified venues for enrollment from advertisements, individual and group interviews, and field observations. They then constructed sampling frames of venues and time periods of the day during which a minimum of seven eligible men might be encountered during a 4-hour sampling effort. Each month, they randomly selected 12 or more venues and their associated times. During sampling events, recruiters then approached men who appeared to be under age 30 years and asked them to participate in the study.

Telephone-Based Sampling

Telephone-based sampling utilizes telephone numbers as sampling units. Three major types of telephone-based sampling have been used: list-based sampling, basic random digit dialing (RDD), and list-assisted random digit dialing. List-based sampling involves selecting a sample from a list of telephone numbers using simple random sampling, systematic sampling, or an add-a-digit procedure whereby one randomly selects a telephone number from a list and then adds a number to it before dialing. The add-a-digit procedure is used to cover telephone numbers that are unlisted. Basic RDD involves randomly generating the complete telephone numbers. List-assisted RDD involves using listed telephone numbers in assisting the random generation of telephone numbers so as to make the process more efficient.

A study by Crawford, McGraw, Smith, McKinlay, and Pierson (1994) offers a good example of telephone-based sampling. They used random digit dialing in their study of differences between Black and White adults in patterns of coronary heart disease–related care. They chose to employ RDD rather than sampling from hospital discharge records in order to include persons not in regular contact with the health care system. The same number of dialings was made in each exchange in the targeted communities to ensure that all households with telephones in the area had the same probability of being contacted. All eligible adults, persons 44 to 75 years of age at the time of the interview, in a household were asked to complete a telephone interview approximately 20 minutes in length.

Web-Based Sampling

Web-based sampling involves either the probability or nonprobability selection of email addresses, website visits, and/or recruited users of the Internet. Hirshfield et al.'s (2012) study provides an illustrative example in the context of public health. The researchers conducted an online randomized controlled trial assessing the impact of two HIV prevention videos and an HIV prevention webpage. They placed a banner ad on four gay-oriented sexual networking websites for U.S. men. One of the websites further agreed to send emails through its internal system to all of its U.S. members (i.e., a list-based sampling frame of emails). During the study, a total of 609,960 emails were sent nationwide. While Internet and email-based sampling techniques are fraught with nonresponse problems, they can reach a lot of people in a short amount of time.

Address-Based Sampling

Address-based sampling (ABS) is a set of sampling procedures that utilizes postal addresses as sampling units. As the number of cell phone–only households increased, the use of telephone surveys decreased and the use of mail surveys increased. The increase in mail surveys is in part due to the availability of addresses via the Delivery Sequence File of the U.S. Postal Service. This file contains addresses that the Postal Service uses for mail delivery throughout the United States. The list is used as a sampling frame for mail surveys (see Daniel 2012; Link, Battaglia, Frankel, Osborn, & Mokdad, 2006). The CDC has also recently incorporated ABS in its REACH U.S. Risk Factor Survey, which monitors racial/ethnic health disparities (Liao et al., 2011).

DETERMINE THE SAMPLE SIZE

The size of a sample may be too small, or it may be too large. A study that uses a sample size that is larger than required (an oversized study) is a misuse of resources and unethically involves more elements in the study than necessary. A study that uses a sample size that is too small (an undersized study) is likely to have inconclusive findings and therefore be a waste of resources. Listed below are factors that favor small sample sizes and factors that favor large sample sizes.

The decision about how many elements to be sampled should be made via a systematic process, and not simply via the application of a gut feeling or the use of a statistical formula. This process begins with a consideration of factors reviewed in Step 1, selecting a sample.

1. *Consider the objectives of the study.* Typically, studies with exploratory objectives do not require large sample sizes. On the other hand, conclusive research and research for important decision making tend to require larger sample sizes. One should have a clear understanding of the objectives of the study.

2. *Consider ethical considerations.* Given the burden research places on participants, a sample size that is too small (e.g., to detect a significant effect) is unethical, and a sample size that is too large (e.g., one that indicates that a very small difference is statistically significant even though the difference may be meaningless from a practical or clinical perspective) is unethical.

3. *Consider the nature of the population.* Aspects relating to the nature of the population that should be taken into account in determining one's sample size are the number of target populations, the size of the target population, the homogeneity/heterogeneity of the population, and the spatial distribution of the population. Health surveys that have multiple target populations, large, heterogeneous populations that are widely, geographically distributed, require larger sample sizes than those that target a single, small homogeneous population that is not widely, geographically distributed.

4. *Consider available resources.* One of the most critical factors in determining sample size is the amount of available resources (money, time, facilities, personnel, etc.) one has to conduct a study. Generally, the more limited one's resources, the more consideration should be given to choosing a smaller sample rather than a larger sample.

5. *Consider the type of research design.* One should take into consideration that quantitative research designs tend to require larger sample sizes than qualitative research designs, nonexperimental designs tend to require larger sample sizes than experimental research designs, and longitudinal research designs tend to have larger sample sizes than cross-sectional research designs.

6. *Consider the data analysis design.* Several factors relating to the procedures that researchers plan to use in analyzing the data of a study should be taken into consideration in determining sample size. This is especially the case for quantitative research in which inferential statistics will be used. It is important that researchers consider the sample size assumptions of the statistical procedures, the number of variables included in the analyses, the amount of detail the data analysis design requires, the strength of the expected relationship of relationships studies, and the size of the differences between categories for comparative studies.

7. *Consider the type of sample design employed.* Nonprobability sample designs tend to have smaller sample sizes than probability sample designs. Although often the sample size of a study is arbitrarily set, for both of these types of sample designs two basic approaches are used in determining sample size: a fixed approach and a sequential, or inductive, approach. A **fixed approach** involves setting a fixed number of elements to be selected from the population targeted prior to data collection. In a **sequential approach**, participants are added to the study until saturation is obtained, or the point at which data are no longer adding to the understanding of the topic being investigated, and redundancy sets in (Birks & Mills, 2011; Charmaz, 2006). A sequential approach is commonly used in ethnographic inquiry (Chapter 15) in which a researcher is embedded in the study community for long periods of time. One can also use a sequential approach in a probability sampling context. In this case researchers would preselect a set of decision rules or stopping rules to govern when sampling will stop, such as a specific margin of error.

Francis et al. (2010) proposed four principles be used in specifying data saturation. The first principle includes selecting 10 cases as an initial analysis sample. The second principle relates to the stopping criterion. It proposes that three additional cases be selected to determine if any new themes emerge. Additional cases will be added until an additional set of three cases does not suggest new themes. The third principle proposes that two independent coders be used. And the fourth principle proposes that the methodology employed be clearly reported so as to permit an evaluation of the evidence.

Notwithstanding, most applied public health research requires fixed, predetermined sampling procedures for probability and nonprobability samples alike. This is because sample size specification is typically required by those who review research proposals, such as funders, scientific review committees, and Institutional Review Boards (Chapter 3). So how are adequate sample sizes estimated prior to collecting data? The methods differ between the two major types of sampling approaches: probability and nonprobability.

Estimating Probability Sample Sizes

Fixed approaches to probability sampling involve the calculation of sample sizes based on such factors as one's desired level of confidence (how sure one desires to be that the results are true), level of significance (probability of a Type I error), power level (probability of a Type II error), and margin of error (how close an estimate is to the true figure). A sample size is selected so as to balance these factors. Larger sample sizes are associated with higher levels of confidence, lower probabilities of Type 1 and Type II errors, and smaller margins of error. Using statistical formulas, one calculates the sample size taking these factors and the variability of the population into account.

> **Type I error:** Concluding that a difference exists between two groups when, in fact, there is no difference.
>
> **Type II error:** Concluding that a difference does not exist between two groups when, in fact, there is a difference between the groups.

A detailed discussion of the determination of sample size is beyond the scope of this chapter. For a description of statistical calculations of sample sizes for different types of research designs, including power calculations, see Cohen (1988), Walters (2004), Carlin and Doyle (2002), Kelly, Webster, and Craig (2010), and Suresh and Chandrashekara (2012). It is always a good idea to consult a sampling statistician for large, complex sample designs. For simpler studies, one can choose from a number of online services that provide assistance in calculating sample size:

Creative Research Systems: www.surveysystem.com/sscalc.htm

Raosoft: www.raosoft.com/samplesize.html

National Statistical Service:

    www.nss.gov.au/nss/home.nsf/pages/Sample+size+calculator

Pivotal Research: www.pivotalresearch.ca/resources-sample-calc.php

Estimating Nonprobability Sample Sizes

Although power calculations can be (and sometimes are), in practice, used to estimate nonprobability sample sizes for quantitative studies, doing so violates many of the assumptions underlying statistical power analysis (that is, most quantitative data collection procedures assume a probability sample and a normal distribution within a population).

For smaller, particularly qualitative, studies, the most cited determining factor in selecting sample size is saturation (Guest, Bunce, & Johnson, 2006), a concept relevant only to sequential and inductive sampling contexts. So for fixed sampling contexts, how does one go about estimating when saturation will occur *before* data are collected? An empirical study conducted by Guest et al. (2006) showed that, from a sample of 60 in-depth interviews (across two countries), the dataset was relatively "thematically saturated" after only 12 interviews. After analyzing 12 of the 60 interviews, 100 of the 114 (88%) total codes applied to the entire dataset had been identified and developed. Seventy percent of all codes were identified within the first six interviews (Figure 17.2).

Figure 17.2   Code Creation Over the Course of Data Analysis

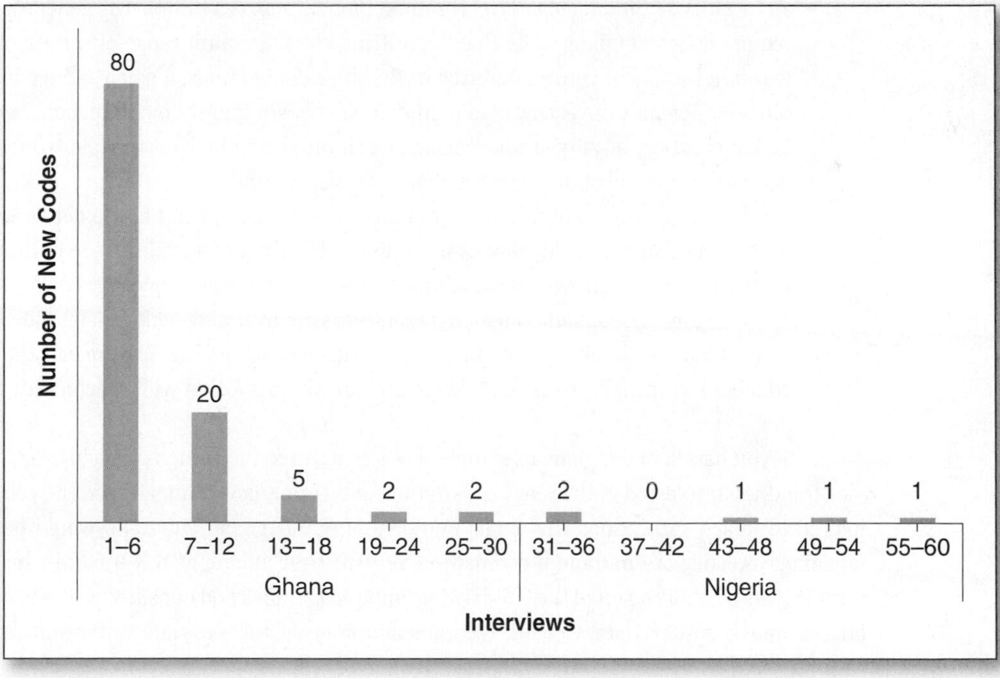

Source: Guest et al. (2006).

The magic number of six interviews is consistent with one other empirically based study (Morgan, Fischoff, Bostrom, & Atman, 2002) and Morse's (1994) recommendation for phenomenological studies. While helpful, be aware that the numbers above come with two important caveats.

Caveat 1: All Studies Are Different

The studies from which the saturation data above were derived have three important factors in common. Each of these studies (a) involved a fairly homogenous sample, (b) used a semistructured data collection approach, and (c) was interested in finding patterns across the sample. Not every qualitative study exhibits any one, let alone all, of these characteristics. In general, the rapidity at which saturation is reached is related to five factors.

- *The degree of instrument structure:* The more structure embodied in the instrument, the sooner saturation will be reached. Note that for studies using an unstructured instrument, or no instrument at all, saturation may never be reached.
- *The degree of sample homogeneity:* The more homogeneous the sample, the quicker saturation is achieved. Groups that are alike on various dimensions are more likely to think in similar ways and have similar experiences.
- *The complexity and focus of the study topic:* For more complex and intricate topics, it will take longer to reach saturation than for simpler and more targeted topics.
- *Study purpose:* Finding high-level common themes across a sample will generally require fewer sampling units than identifying the maximum range of variation within a sample. If you're interested in finding the big issues, a small sample is often sufficient. Conversely, if your study objectives require the comprehensive documentation of all the idiosyncrasies exhibited within your sample, you'll need to sample substantially more than 6 or even 12 units.
- *Analyst categorization style:* Some folks are "splitters"; they tend to see detail in everything and create codebooks accordingly. On the other end of the continuum are "lumpers"; these individuals like to group things into a few large conceptual categories. Codebooks created by splitters will invariably include a lot more codes than codebooks created by analysts with a lumper bent. The smaller the codebook being used to code the data, the quicker saturation will be achieved.

So if you have a heterogeneous sample, a less structured instrument, a highly complex topic, are interested in the range of variation, and your analysts are all splitters, you may never reach saturation. The magic numbers of 6 and 12 per subgroup would be meaningless. They are minimum estimates. Use your best judgment to estimate your sample sizes by building off of the few existing empirical studies and considering the five factors above, rather than viewing recommendations as the ultimate authoritative source.

Caveat 2: Your Audience May Have Different Standards

While data suggest that a sample size of 6–12 individuals per group is sufficient for many (but not all!) types of qualitative studies, for many audiences (e.g., journals, funders, clients) this number is perceived as too small, regardless of the empirical or anecdotal evidence.

8. *Make final adjustments:* Once a targeted sample size has been determined taking into account the above considerations, one should make adjustments taking into account such factors as the potential ineligibility rate, nonresponse rate, and attrition rate. Table 17.6 summarizes factors to consider when choosing or estimating sample sizes.

Ineligibility rate: The percentage of elements selected to be part of the sample but later found out not to be members of the target population.

Nonresponse rate: The percentage of individuals selected who fail to take part in the study.

Attrition rate: Persons who began participating in a longitudinal study but drop out before completing the study.

Table 17.6 Factors to Consider When Choosing or Estimating Sample Sizes

Factors Favoring Small Samples	*Factors Favoring Large Samples*
• The research has an exploratory research objective • The population is homogeneous • The population is scattered, making data collection difficult and expensive • There are limited resources • A high eligibility rate and high response rate are anticipated • A qualitative research design is employed • The study involves a small number of variables • The data analysis design does not require a large sample size	• The research has a nonexploratory research objective • The research has multiple objectives • It is important to make inferences to the target population with a small margin of error • The population is heterogeneous • Resources are sufficient to accommodate a large sample • Low eligibility rates are anticipated • Low response rates are anticipated • The study involves a large number of variables • A complex quantitative research design is employed • The data analysis design requires a large sample size

SELECT AND RECRUIT THE SAMPLE

Recruiting methods are related to sampling strategies, but they are not the same thing. Recruitment of study participants refers to the process by which participants are first informed about and, if eligible, asked to join a study. Recruitment is the means used to obtain a desired sample. As with every other dimension in research design, your method of recruitment will be determined by a combination of research objectives, logistical constraints, contextual parameters, and ethical considerations. Table 17.7 provides a summary of the various recruitment methods used in public health research.

Table 17.7   Recruitment Techniques and Characteristics

Type	Technique	Advantages	Disadvantages
Media-based (indirect and passive)	Posters/flyers	• Inexpensive • Targeted coverage • In many cases the choice of venues acts as a prescreen for qualified interviewees	• Dependent on visibility of the recruiting message • May miss many qualified interviewees
	Newspaper/magazine	• Relatively wide coverage	• Expensive
	Radio/TV	• Wide coverage	• Expensive • Coverage not highly targeted
	Internet	• Inexpensive	• Little control over coverage • Dependent on visibility of the recruiting message • May miss many qualified interviewees
Investigator-initiated	Door-to-door	• Higher response rates (than approaches that are not face-to-face)	• Labor intensive
	Facility-based	• Good response rates	• Generalizability limited to facility patrons
	Intercept	• If done at a venue relevant to the study topic or target interview population, can be an efficient way to locate qualified participants who might be hard to find through other methods • May be linked to time/space sampling	• Involves approaching individuals in public places • Subject to bias created by lack of representativeness of the intercept location(s) or by approach bias from the recruiter doing the intercepts

Type	Technique	Advantages	Disadvantages
	Email	• Inexpensive • In many cases the choice of email addresses acts as a prescreen for qualified interviewees	• Limits sample to Internet users • Potentially low response rate (dependent on population and topic) • Subject to self-selection bias
	Phone	• If randomly selected, useful for getting unbiased representation of residents of a particular area	• Limits sample to those with phones • Obtaining sampling frame may be difficult • Can be time consuming, especially if the screening criteria disqualify many from participation
	Mail	• Inexpensive	• Lower response rates
Socially based	Chain referral (participants refer other participants)	• Good for hard-to-reach populations	• Participants must have substantial social ties • Social connections between the interviewees may create bias in the research findings
	External referral (nonparticipants refer participants)	• Can be effective, depending on who is referring (e.g., community leaders)	• Possible ethical issues relating to participant volition
	National panel	• Prescreened lists, usually balanced to provide a nationally representative source of market research participants, can be easily screened to provide participants matching almost any set of demographic,	• Expensive • Depending on how the panel is developed and maintained, panels may contain people who participate in studies simply to get the incentive money or who

(Continued)

(Continued)

Type	Technique	Advantages	Disadvantages
		behavioral, attitudinal, or other characteristics	take on the personae of "professional respondents," causing skewed data • May miss particularly well-qualified interviewees who are not part of the database
Panel/list-based	Research facility or professional/ affiliation based panel	• Range in cost from free to expensive • Range in quality, depending on how the lists are developed and maintained	
		• Assuming the lists closely match the screening criteria, makes for fast, efficient recruiting of highly qualified interviewees • Useful for tough-to-locate categories of interviewees	• Dependent on the quality/ representativeness of the lists • Use of some lists may raise issues of privacy if those on the list have not preapproved being contacted by researchers

Source: Guest, Namey, and Mitchell (2013).

SAMPLING IN INTERNATIONAL CONTEXTS

Theoretically, political borders and cultural practices have no bearing on sampling strategies. Sampling methods should be chosen, first and foremost, based on their appropriateness with respect to the proposed data analysis, their ability to achieve the desired research objectives, and ethical considerations. But geography and culture can affect the logistics of implementing a particular sampling approach. In many developing countries, physical access to the study population can be impeded due to poor roads (whose conditions can be highly seasonal) or lack of transportation routes altogether. Resources, such as recruiting companies or reliable data to construct sampling frames, are less likely to exist in developing countries.

To compensate for these challenges, researchers are advised to involve local collaborators before designing sampling strategies. As noted in Chapters 4 and 22, community engagement is always a good idea before initiating a research study. It is especially critical, however, when doing research in international settings. Not only is community and stakeholder cooperation necessary for the successful implementation of a study, but local experts can tell you which recruitment techniques are most appropriate—and more important, which ones are inappropriate—for your study population. Even experienced ethnographers, who may be very familiar with a particular community, rely on local community members to provide guidance for research processes and to gain entry into local communities. These same tenets hold true if conducting research among subpopulations in your own country, such as immigrant communities or socially isolated or deviant subpopulations.

FUTURE DIRECTIONS

Developing an appropriate sampling strategy can be a complicated endeavor involving the conceptual (and sometimes mathematical) integration of numerous competing factors. And if your study involves multiple data collection methods, these steps will need to be applied to each different data collection method you employ. Adding to the complexity is an ever-evolving technological landscape in the research world (see the In Focus at the end of Chapter 21).

It is expected that technological changes will continue to have a significant impact on research methodology, including sampling techniques. The increasing use of cell phones and other mobile devices, for example, has made telephone surveys more difficult. On the other hand, researchers can now more easily sample individuals from geographically dispersed areas, through the Internet and mobile devices. New sampling and recruitment approaches are likely to develop in adjusting to these ongoing changes.

Another emerging area in the field of sampling is the operationalization of the concept of saturation. Only a few empirical studies have been conducted on this topic, leaving numerous knowledge gaps left to explore. The few data saturation studies carried out on in-depth interviews, for example, employed relatively homogenous samples and semistructured instruments. A key question remains: How does the saturation point change if these parameters are altered? Empirical data are also absent regarding the number of focus groups required to research saturation. These and many other important questions pertaining to nonprobability sampling are in need of investigation.

ADDITIONAL RESOURCES

Cohen, J. (1988). *Statistical power analysis for the behavioral sciences* (2nd ed.). New York, NY: Psychology Press.

Daniel, J. (2012). *Sampling essentials: Practical guidelines for making sampling choices.* Thousand Oaks, CA: Sage.

Guest, G. (in press). Selecting and recruiting participants for field research. In H. Bernard & L. Gravlee (Eds.), *Handbook for methods in cultural anthropology* (2nd ed.). Lanham, MD: AltaMira Press.

Magnani, R. Sabin, K., Saidel, T., & Heckathorn, D. (2005). Review of sampling hard-to-reach and hidden populations for HIV surveillance. *AIDS*, 19, S67–S72.

Onwuegbuzie, A., & Collins, K. (2007). A typology of mixed methods sampling designs in social science research. *The Qualitative Report*, 12, 281–316.

REFERENCES

Bernard, H. R. (2000). *Social research methods: Qualitative and quantitative* approaches. Thousand Oaks, CA: Sage.

Birks, M., & Mills, J. (2011). *Grounded theory: A practical guide.* Thousand Oaks, CA: Sage.

Carlin, J. B., & Doyle. L. W. (2002). Statistics for clinicians, 7: Sample size. *Journal of Paediatrics & Child Health, 38,* 300–304.

Chan, W. K., Chung, T. S., Lau, B. S., Law, H. T., Yeung, A. K., & Wong, C. H. (2006). Management of hypertension by private doctors in Hong Kong. *Hong Kong Medical Journal, 2,* 115–118.

Charmaz, K. (2006). *Constructing grounded theory: A practical guide through qualitative analysis.* Thousand Oaks, CA: Pine Forge Press.

Cohen, J. (1988). *Statistical power analysis for the behavioral sciences* (2nd ed.). Mahwah, NJ: Lawrence Erlbaum.

Collins, K. M. T., Onwuegbuzie, A. J., & Jiao, Q. G. (2006). Prevalence of mixed-methods sampling designs in social science research. *Evaluation and Research in Education, 19:* 83–101.

Collins, K. M. T., Onwuegbuzie, A. J., & Jiao, Q. G. (2007). A mixed-methods investigation of mixed methods sampling designs in social and health science research. *Journal of Mixed Methods Research, 1:* 267–294.

Crawford, S. L., McGraw, S. A., Smith, K. W., McKinlay, J. B., & Pierson, J. E. (1994). Do Blacks and Whites differ in their use of health care for symptoms of coronary heart disease? *American Journal of Public Health, 84,* 957–964.

Daniel, J. (2012). *Sampling essentials: Practical guidelines for making sampling choices.* Thousands Oak, CA: Sage.

Francis, J. J., Johnston, M., Robertson, C., Glidewell, L., Entwistle, V., Eccles, M. P., & Grimshaw, J. M. (2010). What is an adequate sample size? Operationalising data saturation for theory-based interview studies. *Psychology and Health, 25,* 1229–1245.

Gales, S., Maxwell, A. R., & Norris, F. (2008). Sampling and design challenges in studying the mental health consequences of disasters. *International Journal of Methods in Psychiatric Research, 17,* S21–S28.

Gile, K. J., & Handcock, M. S. (2010). Respondent-driven sampling: An assessment of current methodology. *Sociological Methodology, 40*(1), 285–327.

Goel, S., & Salganik, M. J. (2010). Assessing respondent-driven sampling. *Proceedings of the National Academy of Sciences of the United States of America, 107,* 6743–6747.

Guest, G. (in press). Selecting and recruiting participants for field research. In H. Bernard & L. Gravlee (Eds.), *Handbook for methods in cultural anthropology* (2nd ed.). Lanham, MD: AltaMira Press.

Guest, G., Bunce, A., & Johnson, L. (2006). How many interviews are enough? An experiment with data saturation and variability. *Field Methods,* 18, 59–82.

Guest, G., Namey, E., & Mitchell, M. (2013). *Collecting qualitative data: A field manual for applied research.* Thousand Oaks, CA: Sage.

Heckathorn, D. D. (1997). Respondent driven sampling: A new approach to the study of hidden populations. *Social Problems,* 44 174–199.

Heckathorn, D. D. (2007). Extensions of respondent-driven sampling: Analyzing continuous variables and controlling for differential recruitment. *Sociological Methodology, 37:* 151–208.

Hirshfield, S., Chiasson, M. A., Joseph, H., Schneinmann, R., Johnson, W. D., Remien, R. H., . . . Margolis, A. D. (2012). An online randomized controlled trial evaluating HIV prevention digital media interventions for men who have sex with men. *PLoS One, 7*(10), e46252.

Hendry, S. J., Beattie, T., & Heaney, D. (2005). Minor illness and injury: Factors influencing attendance at a paediatric accident and emergency department. *Archives of Disease in Childhood, 90,* 629–633.

Johnston, L. G., Malekinejad, M., Kendall, C., Iuppa, I. M., & Rutherford, G. W. (2008). Implementation challenges to using respondent-driven sampling methodology for HIV biological and behavioral surveillance: Field experiences in international settings. *AIDS and Behavior, 12,* S131–S141.

Kantor, J., Bilker, W. B., Glasser, D. B., & Margolis, D. J. (2002). Prevalence of erectile dysfunction and active depression: An analytic cross-sectional study of general medical patients. *American Journal of Epidemiology, 156,* 1035–1042.

Keane, C., Marx, J., & Ricci, E. (2001). Privatization and the scope of public health: A national survey of local health department directors. *American Journal of Public Health, 91,* 611–617.

Kelly, P. J., Webster, A. C., & Craig, J. C. (2010). How many patients do we need for a clinical trial? Demystifying sample size calculations. *Nephrology, 15,* 725–731.

Lansky, A, Drake, A., Wejnert, C., Pham, H., Cribbin, M., & Heckathorn, D. D. (2012). Assessing the assumptions of respondent-driven sampling in the National HIV Behavioral Surveillance System among injecting drug users. *Open AIDS Journal, 6,* 77–82.

Lansky, A. Abdul-Quader, A. S., Cribbin, M., Hall, T., Finlayson, T. J., Garfein, R. S., . . . Sullivan, P. S. (2007). Developing an HIV behavioral surveillance system for injecting drug users: The National HIV Behavioral Surveillance System. *Public Health Reports, 122,* 48–55.

Liao, Y., Bang, D., Cosgrove, S., Dulin, R., Harris, Z., Stewart, A., . . . Giles, W. (2011). Surveillance of health status in minority communities—Racial and Ethnic Approaches to Community Health Across the U.S. (REACH U.S.) Risk Factor Survey, United States, 2009. *Morbidity and Mortality Weekly Report, 60*(6), 1–44.

Link, M. K., Battaglia, M. P., Frankel, M. R., Osborn, L., & Mokdad, A. H. (2006). Address-based versus random-digit-dial surveys: Comparison of key health and risk indicators. *American Journal of Epidemiology, 164,* 1019–1025.

Linnan, L., Bowling, M., Childress, J., Lindsay, G., Blakey, C., Pronk, S., . . . Royall, P. (2008). Results of the 2004 National Worksite Health Promotion Survey. *American Journal of Public Health, 98,* 1503–1509.

Lippert, A. M., Fendrich, M., & Johnson, T. P. (2008). Vicarious exposure to terrorist attacks and substance use: Results from an Urban Household Survey. *Journal of Urban Health, 85,* 411–427.

Malekinejad, M., Johnston, L. G., Kendall, C., Kerr, L. R., Rifkin, M. R., & Rutherford, G. W. (2008). Using respondent-driven sampling methodology for HIV biological and behavioral surveillance in international settings: A systematic review. *AIDS and Behavior, 12,* S105–S130.

McCreesh, N., Frost, S. D., Seeley, J., Katongole, J., Tarsh, M. N., Ndunguse, R., . . . White, R. G. (2012). Evaluation of respondent-driven sampling. *Epidemiology, 23,* 138–147.

Morgan, M., Fischoff, B., Bostrom, A., & Atman, C. (2002). *Risk communication: A mental models approach.* New York, NY: Cambridge University Press.

Morse, J. (1994). Designing funded qualitative research. In N. Denzin & Y. Lincoln (Eds.), *Handbook for qualitative research* (pp. 220–235). Thousand Oaks, CA: Sage.

Onwuegbuzie, A., & Collins, K. (2007). A typology of mixed methods sampling designs in social science research. *The Qualitative Report, 12,* 281–316.

Salganik, M. J. (2006). Variance estimation, design effects, and sample size calculations for respondent-driven sampling. *Journal of Urban Health, 83*(Suppl 1), 98–112.

Salganik, M. J., & Heckathorn, D. D. (2004). Sampling and estimation in hidden populations using respondent-driven sampling. *Sociological Methodology, 34,* 193–239.

Sandelowski, M. (1995). Sample-size in qualitative research. *Research in Nursing & Health, 18,* 179–183.

Semaan, S. (2010). Time-space sampling and respondent-driven sampling with hard-to-reach populations. *Methodological Innovations Online, 5,* 60–75.

Stueve, A., O'Donnell, L. N., Duran, R., San Doval, A., & Blome, J. (2001). Time-space sampling in minority communities: Results with young Latino men who have sex with men. *American Journal of Public Health, 91,* 922–926.

Suresh, K. P., & Chandrashekara, S. (2012). Sample size estimation and power analysis for clinical research studies. *Journal of Human Reproductive Sciences, 5*(1), 7–13.

Walters, S. J. (2004). Sample size and power estimation for studies with health related quality of life outcomes: A comparison of four methods using the SF-36. *Health & Quality of Life Outcomes, 2*, 26.

Wei, C., McFarland, W., Colfax, G. N., Fuqua, V., & Raymond, H. F. (2012). Reaching black men who have sex with men: A comparison between respondent-driven sampling and time-location sampling. *Sexually Transmitted Infections, 88*, 622–626.

Weinbaum, C. M., Lyerla, R., MacKellar, D. A., Valleroy, L. A., Secura, G. M., Behel, S. K., . . . Torian, L. V. (2008). The Young Men's Survey Phase II: Hepatitis B immunization and infection among young men who have sex with men. *American Journal of Public Health, 98*, 839–845.

18

Statistical Methods in Public Health Research

Mark A. Weaver

This chapter presents an overview of statistical analysis methods commonly applied in public health research. The material is presented conceptually, with very few mathematical formulas, and is intended to be accessible to readers with no prior exposure to statistics. My primary goal is not to teach readers how to do statistics but, rather, to enable readers to better understand and critically evaluate methods applied in the literature. For the motivated reader, there are many textbooks from which to learn the fundamentals of applied statistics; Norman and Streiner (2008) provide one comprehensive (and amusing) introduction to the field.

Statistics is an ever-broadening field, so the scope here is necessarily limited. Chapter 1 provided a very brief history of the development of statistical methods, and I expand on this only slightly. For an entertaining account of the development of statistics throughout the 20th century, see Salsburg's (2001) *The Lady Tasting Tea*. Unavoidably, some current exciting frontiers in public health statistics fall outside the scope of this chapter, including "high-dimensional problems" in genetics and medical imaging as well as the study of environmental interactions that lead to changes in gene expression, so-called epigenetics. However, the material I present should provide a suitable foundation upon which you can start to build knowledge in these advanced areas.

Typically, any statistical analysis would begin with a descriptive summary of the data, either by tabulating some meaningful values (e.g., means, standard deviations, medians, and ranges for ordinal variables, frequencies and percent distributions for categorical variables) or by generating informative visual displays. Although this is the preferred first step in every analysis, I postpone further discussion of descriptive statistics until the final section of this chapter. Instead, I begin by introducing some inferential basics that are integral to most modern statistical methods. I then provide examples from the global health literature of commonly applied statistical methods. I conclude with a section on current issues and future directions for statistics in public health research.

THE BASICS OF STATISTICAL INFERENCE

Imagine that we wanted to know the proportion of all males between the ages of 18 and 65 living in Botswana who would test HIV-positive at some moment in time. Theoretically, we could know the true proportion exactly, if only we were able to quickly screen every member of the population. Realistically, however, financial and time limitations prevent us from ever doing that. How, then, could we get a reasonable estimate of this proportion?

Or suppose we wished to know if a new cancer treatment was better than a standard treatment. If we can only treat any individual patient once, how can we learn whether a group of patients as a whole would have fared better with one drug or the other?

Questions such as these can be addressed using **inferential statistics**, methods for drawing conclusions about some well-defined *population* based on data from a *sample* of that population. But what allows us to make valid inferences about an entire population based only on a relatively small sample? The answer is *probability*, generated as the result of some random process. Shortly, I will describe two such random processes used extensively in public health research that were already mentioned in preceding chapters: random sampling and randomization. But first I need to define precisely what I mean by probability.

Probability as a Basis for Statistical Inference

As mentioned in Chapter 1, the modern conception of probability dates back to a series of letters written between Blaise Pascal and Pierre de Fermat in 1654 (Devlin, 2008). The pair's correspondence started after a gambler requested Pascal's help in determining the proper way to split the pot from a game of chance that was abruptly interrupted. This idea of probability, stemming from games of chance, was further developed by Jakob and Nikolaus Bernoulli, Abraham de Moivre, John Venn, and, in the 20th century, notable statisticians and philosophers such as Sir Ronald Fisher, Jerzy Neyman, and Karl Popper, among others.

This notion of probability has been called **frequentist probability**, defined as the long-run relative frequency of a (hypothetically) *repeatable* event. The most familiar example features a fairly balanced coin flipped repeatedly many times: The relative frequency with which the coin lands heads will rapidly converge to 50% as the number of flips increases. Similarly, when rolling a well-balanced six-sided die many times, the die will land showing either a one or two about a third of the time, for a probability of 33.3%.

Finally, the probability is 0.00001% that my ticket will win in a fair lottery if one ticket is to be drawn out of 10,000,000 tickets sold. It's because of examples such as the latter that the word *hypothetically* has been inserted into the definition; although the actual lottery will occur only once, I *know* the relative frequency with which my ticket would be drawn if the *same* fair lottery were to be repeated indefinitely.

There is an alternative conception of probability, called **subjective probability**, typically defined as a personal degree of belief in a proposition or hypothesis. For example, I might indicate that I'm 95% certain that I turned the oven off before leaving home this morning. This form of probability is often encountered in Bayesian methods of statistical inference, which I will revisit briefly in the last section of this chapter. Until then, I consider only frequentist methods of statistical inference.

Random Sampling From a Finite Population

Consider a large, but finite, population of size N (e.g., N could be 1,000, 100,000, or 900,000,000), and assume that the population is sufficiently well defined such that we could, theoretically at least, list every member. Suppose we wish to determine something about that population, but taking a census of every member would be prohibitively expensive. As described in Chapter 17, in public health research we typically approach such problems by taking a random sample of size n from this population, where n is usually much smaller than N. In theory, we could list all possible distinct samples of size n that we could obtain from this population. Thus, we could compute the selection probability for any individual in the population simply by counting the number of samples in which she was included and dividing by the total number of possible samples. As a very basic example, consider a bag containing four equally sized marbles ($N = 4$), numbered 1 through 4. Suppose we decided to randomly select two marbles from the bag ($n = 2$). The following are the six possible samples of size two: {1, 2}, {1, 3}, {1, 4}, {2, 3}, {2, 4}, and {3, 4}. Notice that each marble is contained in half of the possible samples, meaning that the selection probability is 50% for each marble.

Given a random sample, it is straightforward to estimate the number of units in the population that have some characteristic in common. Using each sampled individual's selection probability, which can generally be calculated, or at least approximated, whenever the population size N is known, we simply "up-weight" their contribution to the sample to estimate the number of similar individuals in the population. For example, imagine an urn containing 1,000 balls, some of which are red and the rest black. You reach into the urn and randomly pull out 10 balls; thus, the selection probability for any ball in the urn is simply 10/1,000 or 1%. Suppose you observe one red ball in your sample. Then your estimate for the number of red balls in the urn would simply be 1/0.01 or 100. Replace those balls, mix the urn again, and repeat. This time, you observe 2 red balls, so your new estimate would be 200 red balls in the urn. Suppose, unbeknownst to you, there were really 150 red balls in the urn. If you were to continue repeating this sampling process, each time pulling out 10 balls, counting the number of reds, throwing them back in and remixing, note that your estimate from any single sample could never possibly equal this true value. However, probability theory assures us that the average over all of your many samples would be very close to 150. This is what is meant by an **unbiased estimate**.

It should be clear in the above example that our inference about the number of red balls can only directly apply to the actual urn from which we sampled. We can say nothing about other urns full of balls, no matter how "similar to" or "representative of" our urn they might appear. Thus, we say that our **inference space** is the urn from which our samples were drawn. Similarly, when our goal is to estimate something about a population of people, our statistical inference space should typically be confined to the specific population from which our random sample was actually drawn.

Randomization

Suppose we conducted an experiment to compare a new weight loss drug, FitFad, to placebo. We enrolled some number of people, N, into our study and randomized half to FitFad and half to placebo, fully blinded of course, as described in Chapter 8. Contrary to the above discussion, our study population (these N people) would represent a sample of convenience. They are people who both met our inclusion criteria and consented to join our study, and, as such, do not represent a random sample from any easily definable larger population. Can any statistical inferences that we make based on the results of our study be meaningful? They certainly can, but with limitations that possibly aren't well understood, even by many researchers.

Consider the following simplified example. Suppose we enrolled just four people ($N = 4$) and randomly assigned 2 each to FitFad and placebo. Numbering these people 1 through 4 (their study ID), we note that there are six possible allocations (Table 18.1). For example, in allocation 1, participants 1 and 2 would be assigned to FitFad while 3 and 4 would receive placebo. Randomization essentially consists of randomly selecting one allocation from the list of possible allocations, revealing a connection with random sampling as described in the previous section.[1] Suppose in our study we randomly selected the third allocation, so that participants 1 and 4 received FitFad while participants 2 and 3 received placebo.

Table 18.1 Ways to Allocate Four Participants to Two Groups With Two in Each

Allocation	FitFad	Placebo
1	1, 2	3, 4
2	1, 3	2, 4
3	1, 4	2, 3
4	3, 4	1, 2
5	2, 4	1, 3
6	2, 3	1, 4

Suppose we observed the results presented in Table 18.2. Both participants assigned to FitFad lost more weight than those assigned to placebo. Is this sufficient evidence to declare FitFad effective for weight loss? One reasonable summary comparison, or **test statistic**, would be to calculate the mean weight lost for each group and take the difference. For this example, an average of 8 pounds was lost on FitFad, compared with an average of 2 pounds on placebo, for a mean difference of 6 pounds.

Table 18.2 Weight Loss for Each Hypothetical Participant

Participant	Group	Weight Lost
1	FitFad	10 lbs.
2	Placebo	4 lbs.
3	Placebo	0 lbs.
4	FitFad	6 lbs.

How can we assess whether this weight loss was caused by FitFad as opposed to simply being a product of chance (perhaps the participants most inclined to lose weight just happened to end up in the FitFad group)? To answer this question, we begin by assuming that FitFad provides no benefit over placebo for weight loss; that is, in the terminology of the next subsection, we will assume that the **null hypothesis** is true. Since assignment was random, this assumption implies that each participant would have lost exactly the same amount of weight regardless of which drug he or she received. That is, under the null hypothesis, we assume that participant 1 would have lost 10 pounds whether she received FitFad, as she actually did, or whether she had, counterfactually, received placebo. Table 18.3 shows these hypothetical results for each possible allocation. Recall that our observed results correspond to allocation 3.

Table 18.3 Hypothetical Results for Each Random Allocation Assuming no Difference Between FitFad and Placebo

	Participants		Observed Weight Loss		Difference in
Allocation	FitFad	Placebo	FitFad	Placebo	Means
1	1, 2	3, 4	10, 4	0, 6	4
2	1, 3	2, 4	10, 0	4, 6	0
3	1, 4	2, 3	10, 6	4, 0	6
4	3, 4	1, 2	0, 6	10, 4	−4
5	2, 4	1, 3	4, 6	10, 0	0
6	2, 3	1, 4	4, 0	10, 6	−6

In statistical hypothesis testing, a **p-value** is defined as the probability of observing a test statistic as or more extreme (that is, further away from the null hypothesis) than the one observed, assuming that the null hypothesis is true. We will discuss the logic behind hypothesis testing below, but for now we can use this definition and the results in Table 18.3 to calculate an *exact* (one-sided[2]) p-value. Notice that our observed mean difference of 6 pounds is the most extreme test statistic favoring FitFad over placebo. Since each possible random allocation had an equal selection probability, we can calculate an exact p-value as 1/6, or about 0.17. As we will see below, we typically require $p < 0.05$ before declaring sufficient evidence to reject the null hypothesis. We would thus conclude that our small experiment provided insufficient evidence to support the claim that FitFad actually caused the observed weight loss.

As with random sampling, it is important to consider our statistical inference space, that is, the population to which results directly apply. I noted above that the study population for randomized trials is typically not a random sample from any larger population. However, as we saw in Table 18.3, our observed results can be thought of as a random sample from some population, namely the finite population of all admissible randomizations among our enrolled participants. Thus, the primary inference from a randomized trial should typically relate to this finite population (Stewart, 2002).

In this section, we used a randomization-based *permutation test* to analyze our hypothetical data. In reality, such methods are rarely used. Typically, methods based in one way or another on the *normal*, or Gaussian, *distribution*, such as those that I describe in the next section, are used instead because they are more familiar or accessible. However, even when these alternative methods are applied, it is imperative to remember that randomization provides the validity (Cook & DeMets, 2008; Fisher, 1966).

Random Sampling From an Ambiguous Population or Use of Nonrandom Samples

Occasionally, studies are conducted in which the participants truly are randomly selected from a large or ambiguous population where the total population size is unknown. For example, consider a study intending to measure the continued use of hormonal contraceptives in which health clinics are first randomly selected from a country's population of clinics. Then, within each selected clinic, study participants are randomly sampled from all female clients who present within some specified time frame. In such cases, it would seem intuitively reasonable that statistical inferences should apply to the population of women who presented to any of the country's clinics during the study period, even if selection probabilities can only be roughly estimated.

More often, however, participants in public health studies represent nonrandom samples of convenience. To apply the inferential approaches emphasized in this chapter to epidemiologic observational data or when generalizing inferences from a randomized trial to a broader patient population, one must implicitly assume (or imagine) that study participants represent a random sample from some larger, perhaps infinite, hypothetical population. How reasonable are such assumptions? The answer most likely varies across studies, but Kempthorne (1979) provided a very clear demarcation: "I have never met random samples except when sampling has been under human control and choice as in random sampling from a finite population or in experimental randomization" (p. 123). Greenland (1990) also addressed this question: "In most epidemiologic studies, randomization and random sampling play little or no role. . . . I therefore conclude that probabilistic interpretations of conventional statistics are rarely justified" (p. 421). Greenland proposed several alternative approaches for analyzing nonrandom data, which we will revisit in the final section of this chapter.

The Logic of Hypothesis Testing

Fisher (1925) first formalized the principles for testing statistical hypotheses using the chi-squared statistic previously developed by Karl Pearson and the t-statistic developed by William "Student" Gosset. Using Fisher's method of **significance testing**, one specifies only a null hypothesis, collects sample data, and computes a test statistic to determine how incompatible the observed data are with what would have been expected under the null. In Fisher's approach, there was no need to specify an alternative hypothesis. Jerzy Neyman and Egon Pearson, Karl's son, extended Fisher's approach, despite Fisher's objections, to the familiar modern conception of **hypothesis testing** in which both the null and alternative hypotheses are specified prior to testing. In this section, I describe the logic underlying the Neyman-Pearson approach.

As previously mentioned, the statistical hypothesis to be tested is typically called the **null hypothesis**, expressed as H_0. The null often, but not always,[3] includes the hypothesis of no difference or no association. The null hypothesis for the weight loss example would be that the average weight loss using FitFad is less than *or equal to* that using placebo.

The investigator's research hypothesis (i.e., what the investigator would hope to conclude) is generally part of the **alternative hypothesis**. For the example, the alternative hypothesis would be that average weight loss with FitFad is greater than with placebo. Typically, the null and alternative hypotheses are specified such that they are mutually exclusive and exhaustive.[4] The goal of hypothesis testing is almost always to reject the null hypothesis, which would allow one to conclude that the alternative must be true.[5]

Based on observed data, we decide whether to reject H_0 or not. If the data are consistent with H_0, we decide to not reject; but if they are sufficiently inconsistent, we reject H_0 and conclude the alternative. But how should we decide whether the data are sufficiently inconsistent with H_0? Typically, we use the data to compute a **test statistic** (e.g., chi-squared or t-statistic), such that larger values of this statistic correspond with more evidence against H_0. To standardize interpretation, we then use either tabulated values or, more frequently nowadays, a computer to convert the test statistic to a p-value. Recall that the p-value is defined as the probability of obtaining a test statistic as or more extreme than the one that was observed, assuming that H_0 is true. If this probability is suitably small, we conclude that either H_0 is false or a very unlikely event has occurred. We generally prespecify a decision rule such that if the p-value is less than a certain threshold α, referred to as the **significance level**, then we reject H_0; otherwise, we do not reject.

Now, in truth, H_0 is either true or false, but we rarely get to know the actual truth within the entire population of interest. Based only on our observed sample data, we decide to either reject H_0 or not. In making this decision, there is a potential for two types of errors: A type I error occurs when we incorrectly reject a true null; a type II error occurs when we decide against rejecting a false null (Table 18.4). Although we can never rule out such errors, we can employ procedures such that the probabilities of these errors are controlled or minimized. In the Neyman-Pearson approach, the type I error probability (i.e., the significance level α) is typically controlled at a prespecified level, conventionally 5% although other values are sometimes used. The type II error probability, denoted as β, depends on the selected α, the specific value of the alternative hypothesis (i.e., the true magnitude of effect), and the sample size. The probability of correctly rejecting H_0, $1 - \beta$, is called **power**. This relationship between power and sample size is very important when designing a public health study. Although the details of sample size calculations are beyond the scope of this introductory chapter, they can be found in many texts (e.g., Cook & DeMets, 2008; Hulley, Cummings, Browner, Grady & Newman, 2007).

Table 18.4   Statistical Error Probabilities

		Truth	
		H_0 is true	H_0 is false
Decision	Do not reject H_0	Correct decision *Probability: (1 − α)*	Type II error *Probability: β*
	Reject H_0	Type I error *Probability: α = significance level*	Correct decision *Probability: (1 − β) = power*

Note that the emphasis in hypothesis testing is on rejecting H_0 or not; we typically do not "accept" H_0. P-values quantify the evidence in the data against H_0, but failing to reject does not provide evidence that the null is true.[6] Thus, in public health research, it is best to avoid conclusions such as "no difference between groups" or "no association between X and Y"; rather, it is preferable to conclude that "the data provide insufficient evidence" of a difference or an association. One should also bear in mind that p-values are calculated assuming that H_0 is true, and so should avoid interpreting p-values as though they conversely represent the probability that the null is true.

Key Points

- Hypothesis tests are used to decide to reject (or not) the null hypothesis.
- It is always possible that decisions based on observed data might result in errors.
- The error probabilities can be controlled.

Genesis of a Confidence Interval

Researchers calculate point estimates and confidence intervals to estimate population parameters using sample data. Such parameters could include proportions or means from a single population or, when comparing populations, differences in proportions or means, odds ratios, incidence rate ratios, or really almost any quantity that might be estimated using standard statistical methods. The nature of the parameter to be estimated is almost irrelevant to the following discussion,[7] so I focus on estimating a simple population mean.

Suppose we wanted to estimate the mean age at first childbirth among Mexican women and that, unbeknownst to us, the true mean was 21.3 years. We could estimate the population mean, for example, by calculating the sample mean among a random sampling of 100 Mexican women. Naturally, we shouldn't expect our singular sample mean to exactly equal the population mean, and if we were to repeat our sample multiple times we would get different estimates each time: The first estimate might be 21.0 years, the next 21.9, the next 20.5, and so on. This variation of sample means around the true mean is called the **sampling distribution**. Thanks to a well-known statistical result called the Central Limit Theorem,[8] we know that the sampling distribution will follow a normal (i.e., bell-shaped, or Gaussian) distribution, centered at the true mean (Figure 18.1). For larger sample sizes, say 200 or 1,000, the sampling distribution will remain normal, only less dispersed around the true mean with increasing sample size.

Figure 18.1   Hypothetical Sample Means and Sampling Distributions

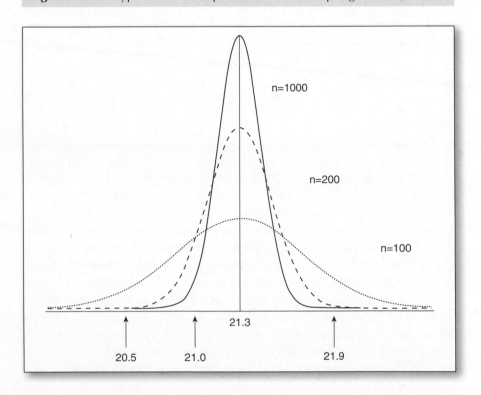

How do we benefit from knowing that the sampling distribution is Gaussian? Although we know neither the true population mean (the reason for sampling in the first place) nor the true **standard error** of the sampling distribution (a measure of dispersion which, for the sample mean, is equal to the standard deviation divided by the square root of the sample size), we know with absolute certainty that approximately 68% and 95% of all sample means would fall within one or two standard errors, respectively, of the true mean (Figure 18.2). Therefore, if we could only cast a net that was about two standard errors wide on either side of our observed *sample* mean, we would capture the *true* mean somewhere in that net 95% of the time. This is the essence of a **confidence interval**.

Figure 18.2   Properties of the Normal Distribution

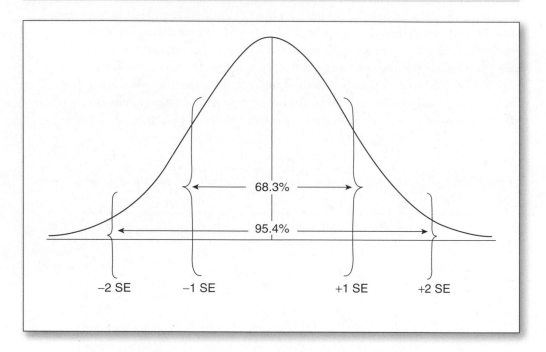

In public health studies, we typically take only one sample, not multiple. Suppose we observed a mean of 20.5 years and a standard deviation of 6 years in our sample of size 100. Although unknown to us, suppose that the true standard deviation is 5 years, implying that the true standard error is 0.5, but we would estimate it to be 0.6. We then calculate a 95% confidence interval by taking the sample mean plus and minus (approximately[9]) two times the estimated standard error, or 19.3 to 21.7. At the study's conclusion, all we really see is our point estimate along with the 95% confidence interval (Figure 18.3). In particular, note from Figure 18.3 that there is no normal distribution of values within the confidence interval itself; this is a common misconception regarding the role of the normal distribution in confidence intervals. We should not necessarily assume that the true value is likely to be near the center of the interval. Recall from Figure 18.2 that approximately 32% of all sample means will fall more than one standard error from the population mean. This implies that in nearly one third of all samples, one end of a 95% confidence interval (which end we cannot possibly know) will be closer to the true value than is the sample mean!

Figure 18.3   Hypothetical Point Estimate and Confidence Interval

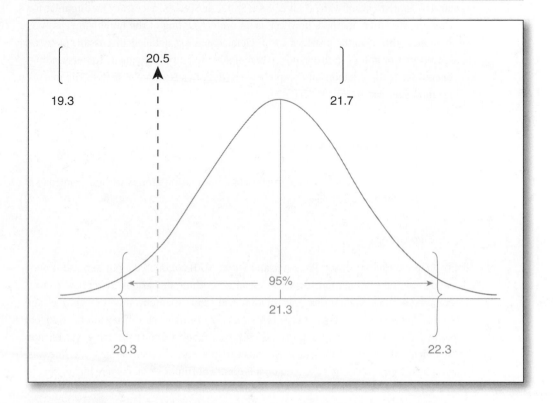

Key Points

- Confidence intervals provide a range of plausible values for a population parameter.
- In a single observed confidence interval, one should have no more confidence that the true value is near the center of the interval (i.e., the point estimate) than near one of the endpoints.

BASIC COMPARISONS AND ADVANCED MODELS: APPLICATIONS IN PUBLIC HEALTH

This section presents examples of some statistical methods commonly applied in public health research. The five studies that serve as the examples employed a broad range of study designs (individual- and cluster-randomized trials, probability sampling, cross-sectional convenience sampling, and longitudinal service statistics) with populations from four countries. Furthermore, the studies span various public health domains, from disparities-based community participatory research through health services research.

I provide broad overviews of statistical methods and avoid mathematical details to the extent possible. Given the data, most results can be easily computed using any standard statistical software, such as SAS, Stata, or SPSS. A necessary requirement for using any statistical method, however, is an understanding of the underlying assumptions; alas, this chapter provides insufficient space for detailed discussion of these assumptions or appropriate diagnostic techniques. To gain the requisite understanding, I encourage readers to consult comprehensive statistics textbooks, such as the marvelous modeling text by Freedman (2009).

Unadjusted Comparisons

First, we discuss some simple methods for comparing groups without controlling or adjusting for other variables.

Two Groups

O'Brien, Halbert, Bixby, Pimentel, and Shea (2010) conducted a randomized trial of an educational intervention to reduce racial and ethnic disparities in cervical cancer screening in the United States. They randomized 120 Hispanic women to receive either the intervention, consisting of two short workshops, or usual care. They intended to follow participants for 6 months postrandomization. Their primary outcome was receipt of cervical cancer screening, a dichotomous variable, and a key secondary outcome was self-efficacy for screening, measured on a 5-point continuous scale where higher scores indicate greater self-efficacy.

The results for the screening outcome appear in Table 18.5; issues related to the diminished sample sizes are discussed below. The observed screening rate was higher in the intervention compared to the control group (65% vs. 36%). We desire to test whether this discrepancy is higher than might be expected by chance if the intervention really provided no benefit over usual care; that is, we desire a p-value. For a comparison with a dichotomous outcome, a chi-squared test (either the conventional test due to Pearson or an "exact" randomization-based test due to Fisher) would be appropriate. The calculated p-values were 0.02 and 0.03 for the Pearson and Fisher tests, respectively, both of which were lower than the prespecified 5% significance level. (Generally, Fisher's test, which is more computer-intensive, is preferred for randomized comparisons or small sample sizes, but the two tests will converge for larger sample sizes.) These authors concluded that their intervention successfully increased screening rates.

For self-efficacy, the observed means (and standard deviations) were 4.7 (0.7) and 4.0 (0.8) in the intervention and control groups, respectively. Recall that higher scores are better on this continuous variable, so we might ask whether an observed mean difference of 0.7 on this 5-point scale provides evidence of an intervention benefit. The authors applied "Student's" two-sample t-test, which is appropriate regardless of sample size if the data are

Table 18.5   Cervical Cancer Screening, Frequency (Percentage)

	Screened	Not screened	Total
Intervention	22 (65%)	12 (35%)	34
Control	13 (36%)	23 (64%)	36

Source: O'Brien, et al. (2010).

at least approximately normally distributed or with large sample sizes (e.g., $n > 30$ in each group). The authors reported a p-value of 0.002 and concluded that the intervention was also beneficial for raising screening self-efficacy. For small sample sizes with distinctly non-normal data, a nonparametric (or distribution-free) test, such as the Wilcoxon rank sum test, might be preferable. Alternatively, a test based on the randomization permutation distribution, as described previously, could have been applied.

Assuming that the data were reported accurately, the conclusions made by O'Brien et al. (2010) would be warranted from a fair randomized comparison. However, as alluded to in Chapters 8 and 16, one key assumption required for valid interpretation of a randomized trial is that any postrandomization loss or withdrawal of participants is nondifferential between groups (i.e., reasons for exclusion are not related to either group or the outcomes). Note that only 70 of 120 randomized women were included in the analysis. The authors reported that 17 participants randomized to the intervention group were excluded from analyses because they did not receive the intervention and 9 others were lost to follow-up. Twenty-four of the control participants were reportedly lost. Although some loss is typically unavoidable, postrandomization exclusions are never advisable as they create potential for selection bias.[10] In this case, it is conceivable that only the most motivated intervention participants provided complete data. Thus, it would seem sensible to view the results of this study with some skepticism until they can be replicated in a more effectively controlled trial.

Multiple Groups

Vadiakas, Oulis, Tsinidou, Mamai-Homata, and Polychronopoulou (2011) reported on a national probability sample to assess periodontal health among Greek adolescents. The survey design consisted of a stratified cluster sample; geographic areas (the strata) were designated as urban or rural, and schools (the clusters) were randomly selected from within each area. Finally, 12- and 15-year-old students were randomly sampled from within the selected schools. In all, 1,216 12-year-olds and 1,249 15-year-olds contributed data to the analysis. Dental examinations determined counts of decayed, missing, and filled teeth surfaces (DMFS) as well as the presence of untreated dental caries.

One question of interest concerned whether children's self-assessments of their oral health agreed with results of their dental exams. The observed average DMFS counts, by age and self-assessment, are shown in Figure 18.4. Analysis of variance (ANOVA) is an appropriate statistical test for comparing more than two groups. The authors conducted one-way ANOVAs (i.e., only one grouping variable, self-assessment) separately for each age group and reported p-values < 0.001 for each test, clearly indicating that self-assessments were related to actual oral health within this population. Alternatively, the authors could have combined the 12- and 15-year-olds and conducted a single two-way ANOVA, which would have allowed for direct comparisons between the age groups.

Figure 18.4   Average Oral Health by Age and Self-Assessment Groups

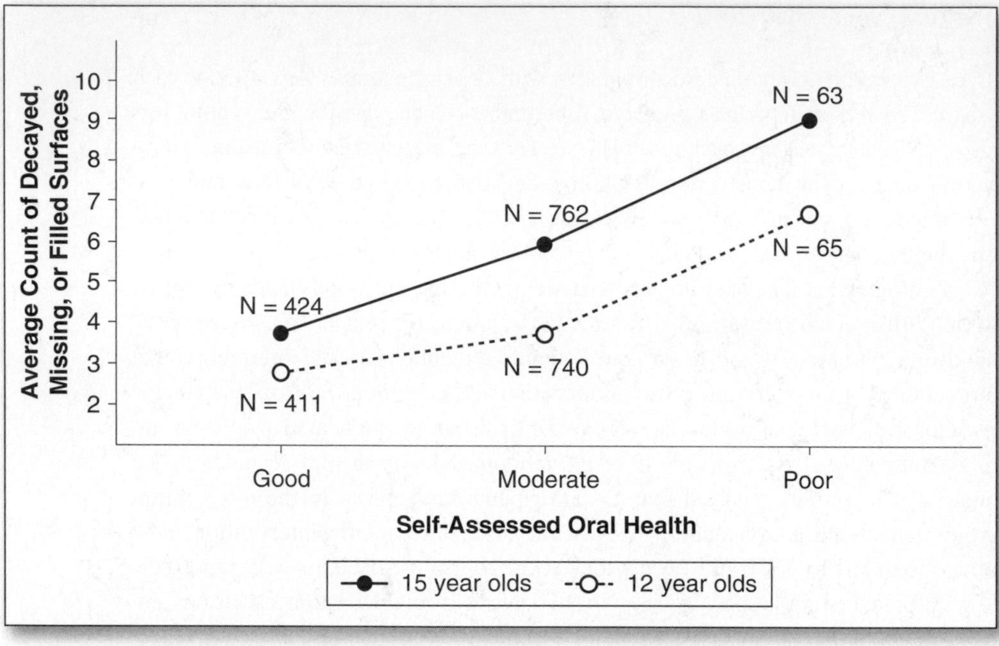

Source: Vadiakas et al. (2011).

Vadiakas et al. (2011) also tested whether child self-assessment was related to the presence of untreated caries (Table 18.6). A chi-squared test (either Pearson's or Fisher's) provides an appropriate test for categorical outcomes and easily generalizes to multiple groups. For each age group, either test would result in a p-value < 0.001, again indicating that the self-assessment was related to actual dental health in this population.

Because the results reported by Vadiakas et al. (2011) stem from a national probability sample, it seems reasonable to assume that they are valid for comparing respective subsets of the Greek adolescent population. However, the authors did not account for the sampling design (stratification and clustering) in their analyses, nor did they appropriately weight their analyses using selection probabilities. Ignoring clustering during analysis leads to underestimating standard errors, confidence intervals that are too narrow, and p-values that are too small; conversely, ignoring stratification can lead to counteractive effects. Thus, the supported inferences are somewhat unclear in this case.

Table 18.6 Untreated Dental Caries, Frequency (Percent)

Self-assessed oral health	12-year-olds		15-year-olds	
	Caries	No caries	Caries	No caries
Good	144 (35%)	267 (65%)	162 (38%)	262 (62%)
Moderate	355 (48%)	385 (52%)	443 (58%)	319 (42%)
Poor	45 (69%)	20 (31%)	46 (73%)	17 (27%)

Source: Vadiakas et al. (2011).

Adjustment via Regression Models

Regression models are frequently used to obtain estimates and comparisons adjusted for other important variables that might also influence the outcome. Controlling for these other variables within a model allows researchers to reduce their influences when estimating the effect(s) of the main variable(s) of interest (i.e., to compare like with like). For example, in estimating the relationship between smoking and lung cancer, researchers might decide to control for participant gender, allowing them, in effect, to compare nonsmoking and smoking males and females, separately; the model then mathematically combines results across genders into a single, adjusted estimate. Depending on the type of outcome, regression analysis comes in many varieties, including linear regression for continuous outcomes, logistic regression for dichotomous or categorical outcomes, and proportional hazards regression for survival or time-to-event outcomes. I introduce logistic and linear regression in the following two subsections, but will delay the discussion of proportional hazards until the survival analysis discussion later in the chapter.

Logistic Regression

As described previously, the primary comparisons reported by O'Brien et al. (2010) were unadjusted for any baseline variables. However, when estimating treatment effects, public health researchers frequently prefer to report estimates adjusted for baseline variables thought to be related to the outcome. O'Brien et al. used logistic regression to estimate the effect of their educational intervention, relative to usual care, adjusted for such variables as age, education, and parity, along with several others.

Let q represent the probability of a "success" for a dichotomous outcome. For the example, q is the probability that a woman gets screened for cervical cancer. Then $q/(1 - q)$ represents the *odds* of being screened. Logistic regression models the logarithm of the odds, or the *logit*:

$$\text{Log } q/(1 - q) = \text{Logit}(q) = \alpha + \beta^*X + \boldsymbol{\theta}^*\mathbf{Z},$$

where α is an intercept, X equals 1 for intervention and 0 for usual care, β is the intervention effect, and $\boldsymbol{\theta}^*\mathbf{Z}$ represents terms for the adjustment or control variables. It is straightforward to show that $\exp(\beta)$ provides the adjusted odds ratio for comparing intervention to usual care.

O'Brien et al. (2010) estimated an adjusted odds ratio of 6.7 with a 95% confidence interval from 1.8 to 25.7. Thus, the estimated odds for getting screened were almost seven times higher among intervention participants than among controls. Note that the confidence interval excludes the value 1, which would be the value of the odds ratio if q were the same for the two groups. Thus, this result is consistent with the unadjusted hypothesis test described previously. Note also that the confidence interval is very wide due to the small sample size. Thus, these data are consistent with both a doubling and a 25-fold increase in the screening odds!

Linear Regression

Linear regression is used to model the mean of a continuous outcome as a function of selected covariates or independent variables. In their study, Vadiakas et al. (2011) used linear regression to compare mean DMFS counts[11] between male and female respondents, simultaneously controlling for location (urban/rural), parents' educational status, brushing frequency, and dental visit history. Among 12-year-old Greek adolescents, they found sufficient evidence ($p = 0.006$) to reject the null hypothesis that males and females have the same mean number of dental problems. In particular, they estimated that males have, on average, about 0.9 more tooth surface problems than females, with a 95% confidence interval from 0.25 to 1.54. However, among 15-year-olds, they found insufficient evidence to reject the null at the traditional 5% significance level ($p = 0.099$); they estimated that males have, on average, 0.7 more tooth surface problems, but with a 95% confidence interval from −0.05 to 1.53, which spans zero, consistent with the test result. Based on these comparisons alone, should we infer that the gender difference decreases, or even vanishes, as Greek children age? Absolutely not! Recall that a nonsignificant comparison does not provide evidence for the null, which implies that significant and nonsignificant results do not necessarily contradict one another. If we desired to test for such an effect, we could model the data for the two age groups together and include an age-by-gender interaction term in the model, a test of which would provide a comparison of the gender difference across age groups. Although the authors do not report the results of such an interaction test, we can surmise that had they done so they would have obtained a nonsignificant result because the two confidence intervals virtually overlay one another.

Correlated Outcomes

In the previous sections, we discussed analysis methods appropriate for independent outcomes (i.e., each unit contributes only one observation to an analysis). In this section, I briefly introduce methods for correlated outcomes. When analyzing paired observations from the same unit or *cluster* (e.g., two eyes from the same individual, studies involving identical twins), the two-sample t-test described previously won't do; a paired t-test is required. In the following subsections, I describe two study designs that naturally lead to correlated outcomes—longitudinal studies measuring the same individuals over time and cluster-randomized trials—and briefly introduce two modern advanced methods for handling correlated outcomes: mixed effects regression models and generalized estimating equations.

Longitudinal Data

To evaluate an intervention designed to increase access to antiretroviral therapy (ART) by shifting certain healthcare tasks from doctors to nurses, Shumbusho et al. (2009) reported on health outcomes among 435 HIV patients initiating ART at three selected rural health centers in Rwanda. The authors extracted data from the health records of enrolled patients for up to two years after they first started taking ART. Data included CD4 cell count and patient weight at each follow-up visit as well as patient characteristics at the time of ART initiation, such as WHO HIV stage classification (a value from 1 to 4, with higher numbers indicating sicker patients). Most patients contributed multiple CD4 measurements to the analysis, and it would seem reasonable to expect repeated measurements from any single patient to be positively correlated.

To model change in CD4 count over time, the authors applied a linear mixed regression model, that is, an advanced version of linear regression that simultaneously models both the mean outcome and the correlation structure between outcomes.[12] The authors chose to model mean CD4 count as a quadratic function of time, controlling for WHO stage, health center, age, gender, weight, and ART regimen. One often-noted benefit of using mixed models is that they allow for different patients to have differently timed, or even some missing, outcome assessments. The resulting model-estimated mean CD4 cell counts, all of which dramatically increased over time, are presented in Figure 18.5.

Figure 18.5   Mean CD4 Cell Counts by Initial WHO HIV Stage

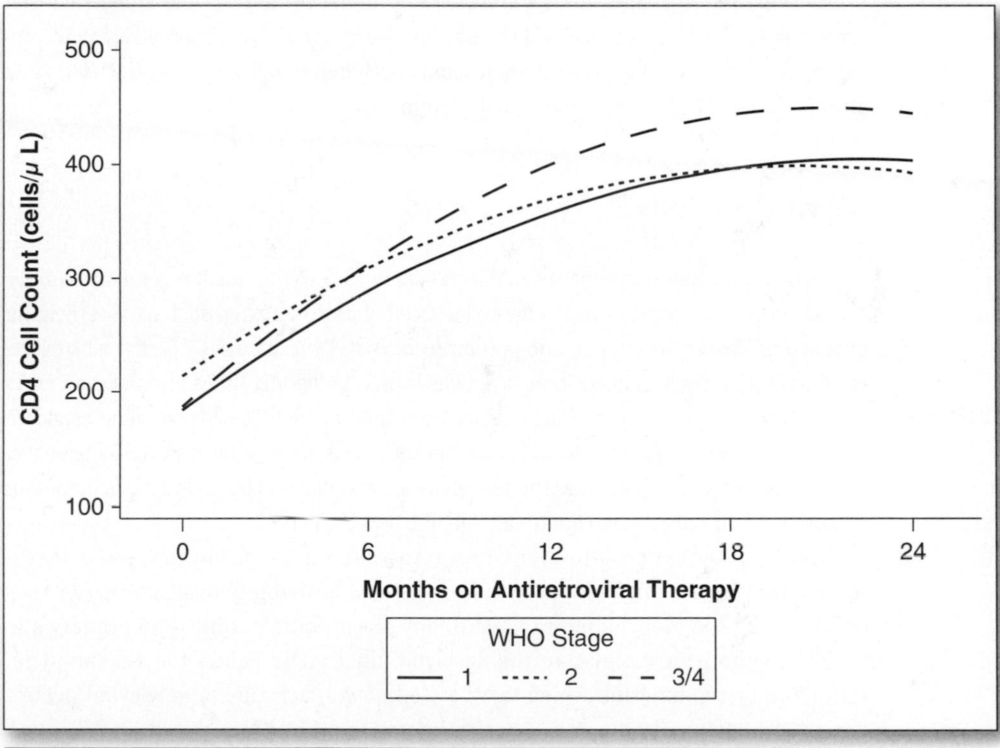

Source: Shumbusho et al. (2009).

Shumbusho et al. (2009) emphasized the descriptive nature of their analyses and appropriately noted the inferential limitations: "The fact that neither the sites nor the patients were randomly selected implies that our findings cannot necessarily be generalized to other sites or even to other patients at these particular sites" (p. 8).

Cluster-Randomized Trials

Cluster-randomized trials, in which intact groups of individuals, rather than individuals themselves, are randomized to treatment group, represent another design resulting in correlated outcomes. Individuals from the same cluster tend to be more similar, in some sense, than individuals from different clusters. This similarity induces an *intra-cluster correlation* among outcomes contributed by individuals from the same cluster. As with longitudinal data, appropriate analysis methods account for this correlation. Generalized estimating equations (GEE) provide a very flexible mechanism for modeling correlated outcomes of many different types, whether continuous, dichotomous, or counts. Similar to mixed models, GEE also allows for certain types of missing outcome data.

Reynolds, Toroitich-Ruto, Nasution, Beaston-Blaakman, and Janowitz (2008) conducted a cluster-randomized health services research study to evaluate a training intervention for improving the quality of reproductive health care among facilities in Kenya. They randomized supervisors from 60 facilities to either receive the training or not (30 each), and they measured many different outcomes at the facility, provider, and client levels. One key set of outcomes of interest involved steps that providers in these facilities took to prevent infections, particularly hand-washing before and after client examinations. The authors applied a logistic regression model using GEE and concluded that providers in facilities that received the training were significantly more likely than providers in control facilities to wash their hands both before (38% vs. 13%, $p = 0.001$) and after (48% vs. 13%, $p < 0.001$) individual examinations.

Survival Analysis

Survival analysis encompasses a collection of tools useful for analyzing the time until a specific **event** (a transition from one well-defined state to another, such as alive/dead or disease-free/disease) occurs. One important feature of survival analysis is that all subjects must have a precisely defined "time 0" at which their individual times at risk for an event begin. Another is that survival analysis includes built-in methods for handling **censored** observations, or data from subjects for whom event time is not directly observed for whatever reason (e.g., dropout). This makes survival analysis a valuable tool for analyzing dichotomous outcomes when subjects contribute varying time to the dataset.

With survival or time-to-event data, researchers are typically interested in estimating the **survivor function**, which provides the probability of surviving (without experiencing the event of interest) up to any given point in time. The primary statistical method for estimating the survivor function is called the Kaplan-Meier estimator, a step function which takes a step down each time a new event occurs. Figure 18.6 shows the Kaplan-Meier estimates for time from initiating ART until death, by CD4 cell count at the time of initiation, for the data reported by

Shumbusho et al. (2009). We note from Figure 18.6 that an HIV patient who initiated ART with a very low CD4 cell count had almost 25% chance of dying within the first 6 months, whereas a patient who initiated with a higher CD4 count had better than 90% chance of surviving at least two years.

Figure 18.6   Kaplan-Meier Estimates of Survivor Functions by CD4 Cell Count

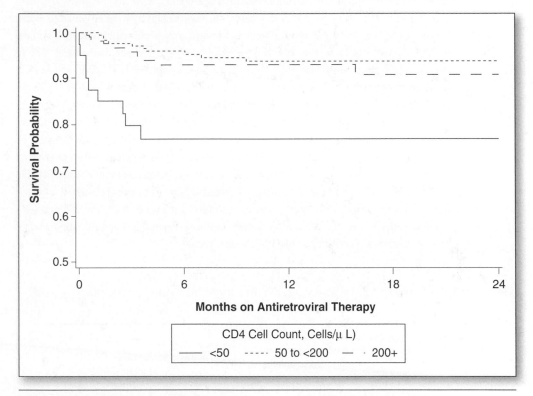

Source: Shumbusho et al. (2009).

Survival analysis also provides a method, called the **log-rank test**, for testing the null hypothesis that the survivor functions of several groups are exactly the same. The log-rank p-value for the data presented in Figure 18.6 was < 0.001, indicating that the survivor functions were significantly different, although we should bear in mind the previously mentioned inferential limitations when interpreting this result because the patients were not randomly sampled.

The survival analysis toolbox also includes a regression method for making adjusted comparisons, called Cox proportional hazards regression in honor of its originator, Sir David Cox. Just as logistic regression estimates odds ratios, proportional hazards regression estimates **hazard ratios**, measures of how much more likely certain individuals are than others to experience an event at any given point in time. For the Shumbusho et al. (2009) example, patients who initiated ART with CD4 count less than 50 were about 2.4 (95% confidence interval 1.0 to 5.4) times more likely to die at any point in time than were those who initiated with higher CD4 counts, controlling for weight and WHO stage (results not presented in the original paper).

Structural Equation Models

Structural equation models (SEM) represent a very broad class of models, capable of simultaneously modeling complex relationships between many variables, including both **manifest** (directly observed) and **latent** (unobserved and possibly unobservable) variables. Although initially developed primarily in the social sciences, SEM are finding more and varied applications in public health research.

Rao et al. (2012) applied SEM to investigate the relationships between HIV-related social stigma, depression, and medication adherence among a cross-sectional convenience sample of 720 HIV patients in Seattle, Washington. Figure 18.7 shows their final model, which includes three latent variables—HIV stigma, depressive symptoms, and adherence to HIV medication—each of which is measured by a number of manifest variables. An SEM can be broken down into two components: a **structural model** that specifies relationships between latent constructs and a **measurement model** that specifies relationships between latent constructs and manifest indicator variables. In Figure 18.7, the structural model consists of the paths connecting HIV stigma, depressive symptoms, and adherence, as well as the control variables age, sex, and race. The model also contains three measurement models, one for each latent construct. For example, the concept of overall adherence to one's prescribed medication (which is not easily directly measured) was indirectly measured using five different self-reported indexes covering various time frames. Depressive symptoms and HIV stigma were both measured using previously validated cognitive scales.

Figure 18.7 Structural Equation Model With Estimated Path Coefficients

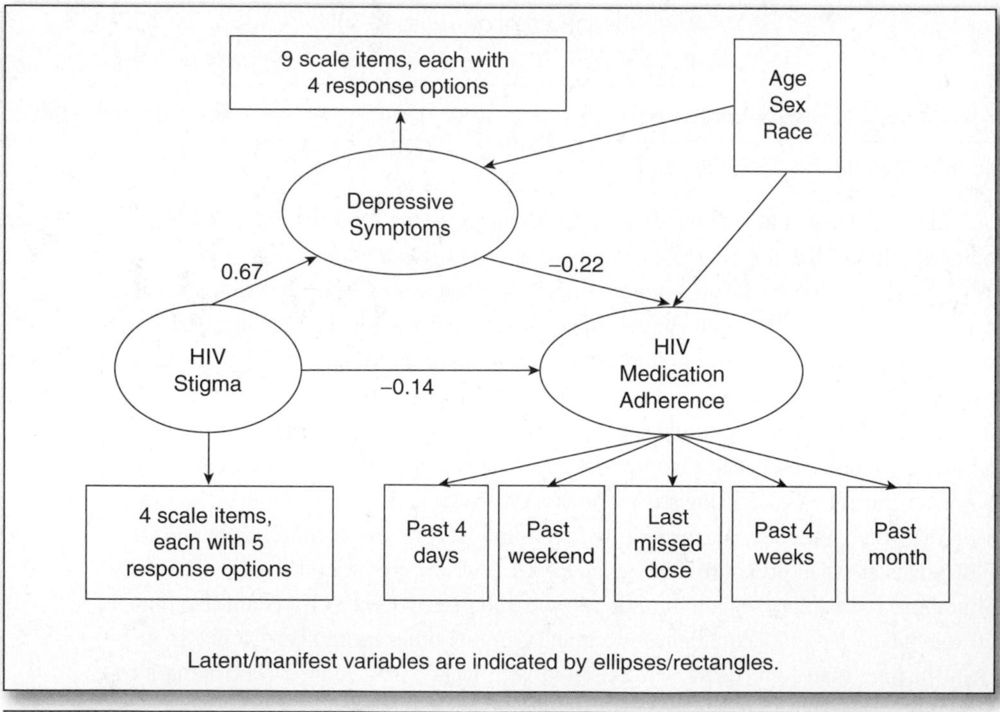

Latent/manifest variables are indicated by ellipses/rectangles.

Source: Rao et al. (2012).

Note that the structural part of this model depicts two simultaneous regression relationships, one for depressive symptoms regressed on HIV stigma and another for HIV medication adherence regressed on both depressive symptoms and HIV stigma. Both models control for age, sex, and race. This exemplifies one of the key benefits of SEM: the ability to simultaneously fit multiple regression models. The estimated path coefficients for these models, shown in Figure 18.7, indicate a positive relationship between stigma and depressive symptoms (i.e., greater stigma is associated with worse depressive symptoms) but negative relationships between medication adherence and both stigma and depressive symptoms. The authors concluded that depressive symptoms partially **mediated** (were intermediary in) the relationship between stigma and adherence.

As with other modeling approaches, SEM assume that the fitted model is the "correct" model, and many different **fit indexes** have been proposed to evaluate this assumption. One commonly used index, the root mean-square error of approximation (RMSEA), is typically interpreted such that values less than 0.05 indicate a model that fits the observed data well, values between 0.05 and 0.10 indicate reasonable fit, while values greater than this indicate poor fit. The authors reported an RMSEA of 0.07, indicating that their model provides one reasonable approximation to the relationships present in their observed data. Of course, it's never possible to completely rule out the potential for even better fitting alternative models within these, or any, data.

Table 18.7   Overview of Statistical Methods Described in This Section

Method	Typical use[13]
Chi-squared test	Compares the occurrence of a binary (yes/no) event between two or more groups
Two-sample t-test	Compares the means of a continuous outcome between two independent groups
Paired t-test	Compares the means of a continuous outcome between pairs of correlated measurements
Analysis of variance	Compares the means of a continuous outcome across multiple groups
Logistic regression models	Model probability of a binary event as a function of one or more predictor variables
Linear regression models	Model the mean of a continuous outcome as a function of one or more predictor variables

(Continued)

(Continued)

Method	Typical use[13]
Mixed effects regression models or generalized estimating equations	Model correlated outcomes (e.g., repeated measurements from the same person, such as longitudinal measurements or one measurement from each eye, or otherwise clustered responses) as a function of one or more predictor variables
Survival analysis Kaplan-Meier estimates of survival curves Log-rank test for comparing survival curves Cox proportional hazards regression model	Describe, compare, or model incidence of binary events when subjects contribute varying time to the analysis
Structural equation models	Simultaneously estimate multiple regression models specifying relationships between latent (unobserved) and manifest (observed) variables

CURRENT ISSUES AND FUTURE DIRECTIONS

Alternative Approaches for Nonrandom Samples

I noted previously that Greenland (1990) discussed several alternative approaches to analyzing data from nonrandom samples. Here, I briefly discuss three approaches: descriptive statistics, Bayesian statistics, and causal inference.

Descriptive Statistics

The vast realm of descriptive statistics includes any method that one might use to organize and summarize data in a clear and concise manner. This often involves tabulating summary statistics, but the great utility of informative graphical displays should not be overlooked or underemphasized. Perhaps the best repository for creative descriptive analysis remains Tukey's (1977) *Exploratory Data Analysis*. Presentation of descriptive statistics should generally be the first analytical step and, in many instances, may be the only analysis that can be readily justified. Unfortunately, editors of public health journals may be reluctant to publish results of purely descriptive analyses even in these latter cases.

Bayesian Statistics

Bayesian statistical methods, named for the Reverend Thomas Bayes, model uncertainties regarding unknown parameters using two complementary probability distributions. The *prior probability* represents an analyst's subjective beliefs about the model parameters before the data have been observed, while the *posterior probability* is conditioned on (or "updated by") the evidence provided in the observed data. These probabilities are related by the following formula (Greenland, 2006):

$$P(\text{parameters} \mid \text{data}) = P(\text{parameters})\,P(\text{data} \mid \text{parameters})\,/\,P(\text{data})$$

Here, P(parameters | data) represents the posterior probability of the parameters conditional on the observed data, P(parameters) represents the prior probability, and P(data | parameters) is called the *likelihood*. Acceptability of these methods is growing in public health research due to the perception that they provide a straightforward way to update old knowledge with emerging evidence.

With data from nonrandom samples, Bayesian methods attempt to avoid the interpretational problems associated with standard frequentist methods by explicitly modeling as many potential sources of bias as possible. Often, the resulting models have many layers of complexity. One obvious limitation to this approach is that the validity of conclusions rests on the correctness of the model assumptions, a limitation shared with frequentist likelihood-based methods (Freedman, 2009). Another, perhaps more serious, limitation is that two analysts who model the same data using different priors often reach conflicting conclusions. As emphasized by Greenland (2006), Bayesian inference is strongly dependent on the selected prior, the assumed model, and the observed data. Thus, although clearly useful in the context of personal decision making, it is less clear what role Bayesian statistics should play when it comes to making far-reaching public health recommendations.

Causal Inference With Nonrandomized Data

Public health research is often conducted to investigate the potential for cause-effect relationships between exposures (e.g., smoking) and diseases (e.g., lung cancer). However, as discussed in Chapter 7, establishing such causal relationships in nonrandomized studies is complicated by the ubiquitous presence of confounding effects (i.e., common causes of both the exposure and outcome). Failure to control adequately for confounding has led many researchers to misinterpret associations as evidence of causality. For example, through observation one might be tempted to conclude that carrying a cigarette lighter causes lung cancer when, in fact, both the exposure and the outcome are responses to smoking cigarettes.

Many statistical approaches have been proposed as attempts to isolate causal effects in the presence of confounding. The most frequently applied is to simply adjust for all "known" and measured potential confounders using one of the regression models described previously. More advanced methods include graphical techniques such as directed acyclic graphs, propensity score or risk set matching, and marginal structural models (Hernán & Robins, 2012). However, these increasingly innovative approaches all share a common serious limitation, namely, the utter inability to control for unmeasured or, perhaps more likely and definitely more insidious, *unknown* confounders. Importantly, because confounding, like any bias, can go in either a positive or negative direction, even adjusting for all known confounders does not necessarily lead to a decrease in the net confounding bias (Greenland & Robins, 1986). Further, Greenland and Robins (1986) emphasize that "the property of being a confounder is not directly verifiable from data" (p. 418). Moreover, systematic biases, such as confounding, cannot be reduced by increasing the sample size. Randomization provides the only sure means to control for confounding,[14] although incomplete follow-up can cause bias even in properly randomized studies.

Meta-Analysis

Multiple independent trials of varying sizes, from small to very large, are often conducted to assess the effects of a particular intervention or treatment on a clinical outcome. Meta-analyses are systematic overviews that use statistical methods to synthesize results across these trials, weighting each trial according to its sample size. For example, Peto, Collins, and Gray (1995) presented the results of a meta-analysis of 11 randomized trials, each of which enrolled between 80 and 5,000 patients, all designed to test the beneficial effects of antiplatelet therapy following myocardial infarction on subsequent stroke or vascular death. Although sometimes used for nonrandomized studies, Peto (1987) emphasized that meta-analyses should generally be restricted to properly randomized trials to avoid the many biases associated with nonrandomized studies that might swamp small to moderate treatment effects. As mentioned in Chapter 1, the Cochrane Collaboration maintains a large database of meta-analyses, primarily of randomized trials.

Broadly speaking, there are essentially two statistical approaches to meta-analyses, typically termed *fixed-effect* and *random-effects models*. It is often implied that fixed-effect methods assume that the treatment effect remains constant across all trials, whereas random-effects models allow for a more realistic assumption that the effect may vary across trials. However, Peto and colleagues (1995) pointed out that neither implication is entirely accurate. They showed that a simple fixed-effect approach "provides a valid, efficient, and assumption-free test of the [null] hypothesis that treatment does nothing in any trial" (p. 36), regardless of the extent of heterogeneity across trials. Furthermore, they explained that random-effects models, which purport to estimate an "average treatment effect", require a strong, somewhat unrealistic, assumption that the varying treatment effects were randomly sampled from a larger population of effects.

The primary limitation associated with meta-analyses is the potential for publication bias, which results when some relevant trials, particularly those with disappointing results, have not been published. Bias can also be introduced if meta-analysts selectively choose which trials to include or exclude. Potential for these biases can be mitigated somewhat by requiring that all clinical trials be preregistered in a trial database (such as ClinicalTrials.gov) and that a protocol for the meta-analysis, including trial selection criteria, be developed in advance. Nevertheless, meta-analysis is not a substitute for conducting large, properly randomized trials (Peto et al. 1995).

Moving Forward, Looking Back

Here at the beginning of the 21st century, statistics has become the mathematical language that pervades almost all of science. New statistical methods have been developed at an amazing clip in efforts to keep pace with complex scientific problems. However, the classical methods developed in the early parts of the 20th century, methods based on the frequentist interpretation of probability, continue to be the most applied and provide the foundations for many of the new methods. In particular, it is rare to find a quantitative public health research paper that does not include at least one (and often scores more!) p-value or confidence interval. Fisher (1966), who developed the logical foundation for significance tests, warned that "the physical act of randomization . . . is necessary for the validity of any test of significance" (p. 45). Nonetheless, this fact seems to have "escaped recognition," to use Fisher's words, as these statistics appear in publication after publication, irrespective of how the data actually came to be observed.

According to two recent reviews (Ioannidis, 2005; Young & Karr, 2011), a surprisingly high proportion (more than 80%) of associations identified as statistically significant in large and frequently cited nonrandomized studies failed to replicate when subsequently tested in randomized trials. One notable case was the seemingly beneficial effect (subsequently found, in two large randomized trials, to actually be harmful) of postmenopausal hormone replacement therapy for preventing coronary artery disease observed in a large cohort of almost 50,000 women (Ioannidis, 2005). Young and Karr (2011) discussed two primary reasons for such spurious associations. The first relates to confounding and other biases discussed previously. The second relates to multiple testing, sometimes pejoratively referred to as "data dredging" or "fishing." As noted in the section on hypothesis testing, a single test conducted at the 5% significance level has a 5% chance of identifying an association when in fact none exists. However, when multiple tests are conducted using a single dataset, the chance of making at least one false claim rises exponentially (Figure 18.8). Conducting 14 independent tests leads to greater than 50% chance of making at least one false claim, while conducting more than 60 tests makes a false claim almost a certainty. Many public health articles report (either explicitly or implicitly) more than 14 tests, and a fair number report more than 60!

Given the limitations acknowledged in this section, what can be done moving forward to improve applications of statistical methods in public health research? First, we would do well to recall the definition of frequentist probability and to carefully consider whether it could reasonably apply to any particular study or situation. Second, for nonrandomized studies, we can follow Greenland's (1990) recommendations, such as to "deemphasize inferential statistics in favor of pure data descriptors" (p. 428). Finally, and perhaps above all, we should maintain "respect for the origins of the data" (Rothman, 1990, p. 418); data generated from a well-controlled randomized trial or random sample should be analyzed and interpreted accordingly. In the absence of actual randomization or random sampling, researchers should take care to explicate the random process, either real or assumed, that underlies their intended statistical inferences.

Figure 18.8   Multiple Testing and the Probability of Making False Claims

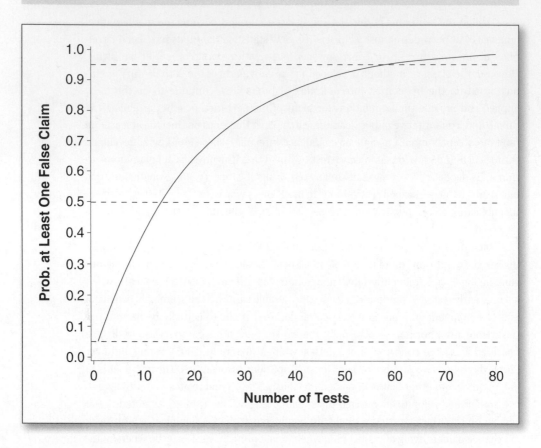

ADDITIONAL RESOURCES

Cook, T. D., & DeMets, D. L. (2008). *Introduction to statistical methods for clinical trials*. New York, NY: Chapman & Hall.

Freedman, D. A. (2009). *Statistical models: Theory and practice*. Cambridge, UK: Cambridge University Press.

Greenland, S. (1990). Randomization, statistics, and causal inference. *Epidemiology, 1*, 421–429.

REFERENCES

Cook, T. D., & DeMets, D. L. (2008). *Introduction to statistical methods for clinical trials*. New York, NY: Chapman & Hall.

Devlin, K. (2008). *The unfinished game*. New York, NY: Basic Books.

Fisher, R. A. (1925). *Statistical methods for research workers*. London, UK: Oliver & Boyd.

Fisher, R. A. (1966). *The design of experiments* (8th ed.). New York, NY: Hafner.

Freedman, D. A. (2009). *Statistical models: Theory and practice*. Cambridge, UK: Cambridge University Press.

Greenland, S. (1990). Randomization, statistics, and causal inference. *Epidemiology, 1*, 421–429.

Greenland, S. (2006). Bayesian perspectives for epidemiological research: I. Foundations and basic methods. *International Journal of Epidemiology, 35*, 765–775.

Greenland, S., & Robins, J. M. (1986). Identifiability, exchangeability, and epidemiological confounding. *International Journal of Epidemiology, 15*, 413–419.

Hernán, M. A., & Robins, J. M. (2012). *Causal inference*. New York, NY: Chapman & Hall.

Hulley, S. B., Cummings, S. R., Browner, W. S., Grady, D. G., & Newman, T. B. (2007). *Designing clinical research*. Philadelphia, PA: Lippincott.

Ioannidis, J. P. A. (2005). Contradicted and initially stronger effects in highly cited clinical research. *Journal of the American Medical Association, 294*, 218–228.

Kempthorne, O. (1979). Sampling inference, experimental inference, and observational inference. *Sankhya, 40*, 115–145.

Norman, G. R, & Streiner, D. L. (2008). *Biostatistics: The bare essentials* (3rd ed.). Hamilton, Ontario, Canada: B. C. Decker.

O'Brien, M. J., Halbert, C. H., Bixby, R., Pimentel, S., & Shea, J. A. (2010). Community health worker intervention to decrease cervical cancer disparities in Hispanic women. *Journal of General Internal Medicine, 25*, 1186–1192.

Peto, R. (1987). Why do we need systematic overviews of randomized trials? *Statistics in Medicine, 6*, 233–240.

Peto, R., Collins, R., & Gray, R. (1995). Large-scale randomized evidence: Large, simple trials and overviews of trials. *Journal of Clinical Epidemiology, 48*, 23–40.

Rao, D., Feldman, B. J., Fredericksen, R. J, Crane, P. K., Simoni, J. M., Kitahata, M. M., & Crane, H. M. (2012). A structural equation model of HIV-related stigma, depressive symptoms, and medical adherence. *AIDS Behavior, 16*, 711–716.

Reynolds, H. W., Toroitich-Ruto, C., Nasution, M., Beaston-Blaakman, A., & Janowitz, B. (2008). Effectiveness of training supervisors to improve reproductive health quality of care: A cluster-randomized trial in Kenya. *Health Policy and Planning, 23*, 56–66.

Rothman, K. J. (1990). Statistics in nonrandomized studies. *Epidemiology, 1*, 417–418.

Salsburg, D. (2001). *The lady tasting tea*. New York, NY: Henry Holt.

Senn, S. (1994). Testing for baseline balance in clinical trials. *Statistics in Medicine, 13*, 1715–1726.

Shumbusho, F., van Griensven, J., Lowrance, D., Turate, I., Weaver, M. A., Price, J., & Binagwaho, A. (2009). Task-shifting for scale-up of HIV care: Evaluation of nurse-centered antiretroviral treatment at rural health centers in Rwanda. *PLoS Medicine, 6*(10), e1000163.

Stewart, W. H. (2002). Groundhog Day: Cause and effect and the primary importance of the finite population induced by randomization. *Journal of Biopharmaceutical Statistics, 12*, 93–105.

Tukey, J. W. (1977). *Exploratory data analysis*. Reading, MA: Addison-Wesley.

Vadiakas, G., Oulis, C. J., Tsinidou, K., Mamai-Homata, E., & Polychronopoulou, A. (2011). Sociobehavioural factors influencing oral health of 12 and 15 year old Greek adolescents: A national pathfinder survey. *European Archives of Paediatric Dentistry, 12*, 139–145.

Young, S. S., & Karr, A. (2011). Deming, data, and observational studies: A process out of control and needing fixing. *Significance, 8*, 116–120.

NOTES

1. However, one should understand that random sampling and randomization are not the same thing; as will hopefully be clear from this section, their purposes and inference spaces differ.
2. We're only interested here in whether FitFad was better than placebo, on average.

3. For example, in "non-inferiority" tests, the null hypothesis states that groups differ by at least some prespecified margin; in this case, the hypothesis of no difference between groups is part of the alternative hypothesis.

4. That is, all possibilities are represented by either the null or alternative hypothesis, but never both.

5. Goodness-of-fit tests, used for validating models, are the sole exceptions to this rule.

6. Absence of evidence is not evidence of absence!

7. Some parameters require transformations, such as taking the logarithm of ratio parameters.

8 The Central Limit Theorem will typically apply for estimating any parameter as long as the sample size is sufficiently large, regardless of how the data themselves are distributed.

9. The appropriate value would be 1.96 for a 95% confidence interval.

10. An intent-to-treat approach is typically preferred for analyzing randomized trials in which all participants are analyzed according to randomized groups, regardless of treatment actually received.

11. The authors could have applied a method called Poisson regression, which is more appropriate than linear regression for modeling counts, but the results likely would have been very similar to those presented here given the large sample sizes.

12. Other sorts of mixed models, such as mixed logistic regression models for correlated dichotomous outcomes, are also available.

13. Although beyond the scope of this chapter, one should consider necessary assumptions before applying any statistical method.

14. Confounding as described here is impossible in properly randomized trials, although random imbalances of potential confounding factors are always possible (Senn, 1994). Confounding is a systematic bias that would persist across replications of a study, whereas random imbalances would not. Unfortunately, randomization of certain exposures (e.g., smoking) is either impossible or unethical.

19

Mixed Methods Research

Greg Guest and Paul Fleming

DEFINING MIXED METHODS

Mixing qualitative and quantitative data collection and analysis methods in public health research is not a recent phenomenon. For example, John Snow's foundational public health investigation of the London cholera epidemic in 1854 (detailed in Chapter 1) used and integrated multiple data sources to identify the Broad Street water pump as the source of the epidemic. Snow first used the quantitative data from the General Registries Office to determine the geographic distribution of deaths due to cholera in the Golden Square area of London (Brody, Rip, Vinten-Johansen, Paneth, & Rachman, 2000). Then, according to Snow's own account, he used qualitative interviews to zero in on the epidemic: "Families of the deceased persons informed me that they always sent to the pump in Broad Street, as they preferred the water to that of the pumps which were nearer" (Snow, 1854, p. 321). Snow's use of multiple data sources to answer different elements of his research question illustrates how varied data can help investigators reach swift and accurate conclusions.

Though Snow integrated qualitative and quantitative data in his study, it is uncommon to hear his cholera research described as "mixed methods." As a formally recognized field of inquiry, mixed methods has been around only since the late 1980s, when researchers began to operationalize data integration and develop mixed methods design typologies (see, e.g., Greene, Caracelli, & Graham, 1989; Morse, 1991). In the decades that have ensued, mixed methods research has become increasingly common and continues to expand, both theoretically and in practice. The field, while still in development, currently boasts a number of textbooks (Creswell & Plano Clark, 2011; Greene, 2007; Hesse-Biber, 2010; Morse & Niehaus, 2009; Teddlie & Tashakkori, 2009), two handbooks (Tashakkori & Teddlie, 2003, 2010), an annual international conference, and the flagship publication *Journal of Mixed Methods Research*.

Over the years, numerous definitions of mixed methods research have been posited.[1] These definitions vary in scope and detail, but virtually all refer to some form of integration of qualitative and quantitative research methods (for an exception, see Morse & Niehaus, 2009). Perhaps the most concise definition comes from Bergman (2008), who writes that mixed methods research is "the combination of at least one qualitative and at least one quantitative component in a single research project or program" (p. 1). We recognize that a host of varying definitions exist for what constitutes quantitative or qualitative data and that an entire body of literature focuses on the philosophy of information and data. For the purposes of this chapter, *qualitative* data refers to nonnumerical data—primarily text and images. Conversely, quantitative data are numerical in nature and can be in various forms—dichotomous, ordinal, and interval.

The basic premise behind using a mixed methods research design is that combining more than one type of data source provides a fuller understanding of a research problem than a single or mono-method approach. According to Creswell and Plano Clark (2011, p. 12) there are at least six potential advantages to integrating methodological approaches:

- The strengths of one approach offset the weaknesses of the other.
- Used properly, a combination of methods can provide more comprehensive and convincing evidence.
- Mixed methods research can answer certain research questions that a single method approach cannot.
- A mixed method study can encourage interdisciplinary collaboration.
- Mixed methods encourage the use of multiple worldviews/paradigms.
- Mixed methods research is "practical" in that it permits the usage of multiple techniques and approaches that best address the research question.

The same authors also make the case that there are six general types of research problems that benefit from integrating methodological approaches. These are research problems where a need exists:

- Because one data source may be insufficient to answer the research question.
- To explain initial results.
- To generalize exploratory findings.
- To enhance a study with a second method.
- To best employ a particular theoretical stance.
- To understand a research objective through multiple research phases. (Creswell & Plano Clark, 2011, pp. 7–11)

The overarching concept is that the integration of qualitative and quantitative components should provide some benefit to answering the research problem and to the overall research study. Therefore, it logically follows that if there is no benefit to using more than one type of method, there is probably no point in employing a mixed methods design. Many research questions in public health can be more than adequately answered with a mono-method approach (e.g., determining how many cases of tuberculosis were reported in Texas in 2012). In such cases, creating a more complicated (and typically larger) design is neither justified nor cost-efficient. This said, a majority of public health research questions are complex and can benefit from incorporating both qualitative and quantitative components in a research design.

MIXED METHODS NOTATION

Qual	Qualitative
Quan	Quantitative
UPPER CASE	Indicates that method is dominant in the study design and purpose (e.g., QUAL)
lower case	Indicates the less-dominant method in study (e.g., qual)
QUAL, QUAN	Comma indicates both methods equal in dominance
QUAL + QUAN	Plus sign indicates methods occur at the same time (i.e., concurrent design)
QUAL → quan	Arrow indicates methods occur in a sequence (i.e., sequential design) with the first noted method occurring chronologically before the latter
QUAN(qual)	The method in brackets is embedded within a larger design, with the non-bracketed method being dominant (i.e., embedded design)
QUAL→←QUAN	Methods are implemented in a recursive process (e.g., qual→quan→qual→quan)
QUAL→QUAN→ [QUAN + qual]	Mixed methods [QUAN + qual] is used within a single study/project within a series of studies
QUAN + QUAL =	Equal sign denotes purpose of integration in a concurrent design (e.g., convergence, divergence, explanation)

Source: Adapted from Creswell and Plano Clark (2011).

A BRIEF SUMMARY OF MIXED METHODS TYPOLOGIES

Various typologies have been developed by mixed methodologists to describe the different ways that qualitative and quantitative methods can fit into a research study. While many mixed methods typologies have been proposed over the years, we cover the more commonly referred to, and/or contemporary, typologies in use today. For brevity, the descriptions provided are at a summative level; most of the typologies we describe have multiple sublevels as well that are not presented in this chapter. For a more exhaustive, yet brief, description of typologies, readers should refer to the three-page table in Creswell and Plano Clark (2011, p. 56) that covers 15 typologies created by various mixed methods scholars.

One of the earlier, and simpler, typologies is David Morgan's (1998) four-quadrant system of classification (Table 19.1). Morgan uses both dimensions of temporality and method-emphasis (known as weighting) to distinguish four basic types of designs. *Temporality* refers to the sequence in time each method is used in the duration of the study, and *weighting* is simply which method the research team assigns priority according to their research questions (more details on these terms later). Per standard mixed methods notation (see text box), method emphasis is denoted by upper case for the primary method and lower case for the complementary method. Sequencing of each method relative to the other is indicated by an arrow.

Similar to Morgan, Morse and Niehaus (2009) use both relative weighting and temporal sequencing as defining features in their typology. However, Morse and Niehaus also extend beyond Morgan's typologies by adding dimensions of theoretical orientation and simultaneous timing (Table 19.2).

Table 19.1 Morgan's (1998) Four-Quadrant Typology

	Principal Method: Quantitative	Principal Method: Qualitative
Complementary Method: *Preliminary*	**Qualitative Preliminary** **qual→QUAN** e.g. – Focus groups used to develop survey domains and questions 1.	**Quantitative Preliminary** **quan→QUAL** e.g. – Use survey data to sample extreme cases for subsequent in-depth interview 2.
Complementary Method: *Follow-up*	**Qualitative Follow-up** **QUAN→qual** e.g. – In-depth interview data explain trends in survey data 3.	**Quantitative Follow-up** **QUAL→quan** e.g. – Survey used to assess prevalence of qualitatively derived themes within larger population 4.

Table 19.2   Morse and Niehaus's (2009) Eight Design Types

Design	Theoretical Orientation	Timing
QUAL → quan	Inductive	Sequential
QUAL → qual		
QUAN → qual	Deductive	
QUAN → quan		
QUAL + quan	Inductive	Simultaneous
QUAL + qual		
QUAN + qual	Deductive	
QUAN + quan		

As with Morgan, relative weighting is denoted by the type of letter case, and arrows signify sequential arrangement of the research components. Morse and Niehaus (2009) added a simultaneous timing component (denoted with a +) in which the two types of methods are conducted at the same time. The theoretical orientation describes the design as being primarily inductive or deductive. Another key distinction between Morse and Niehaus's model and other typologies is an implicitly different definition of mixed methods research. Their inclusion of qual/ qual and quan/quan designs diverge from the conventional definition of mixed methods—including Bergman's presented earlier—as the integration of *both* qualitative and quantitative data in a single research project.

Teddlie and Tashakkori's (2009) classification scheme, summarized into five "families" of designs (Table 19.3), is somewhat simpler than Morse and Niehaus's (2009) eight-design typology. As with the many other typologies, Teddlie and Tashakkori include a temporal dimension, distinguishing between parallel and sequential designs. Unique to their model is the inclusion of three other designs—conversion, multilevel, and fully integrated—which emphasize how data intersect. Another distinguishing feature is the absence of a weighting dimension.

The typology developed by Creswell and Plano Clark (2011) embodies the temporal elements of the other typologies, highlighting the difference between studies that integrate independent data types at the same time (convergent parallel) and sequential designs, in which interdependent datasets are chronologically arranged (Table 19.4).

Novel to Creswell and Plano Clark's (2011) typology, relative to others, are the embedded, transformative, and multiphase designs. Note that weighting also is a feature of the Creswell and Plano Clark typology, but is not explicit in the descriptions above.

Table 19.3 Teddlie and Tashakkori's (2009) Five Families of Mixed Methods Designs

Parallel
In these designs, mixing occurs in a parallel manner, either simultaneously or with some minimal time lapse; planned and implemented QUAL and QUAN phases answer related aspects of the same research question.

Sequential
In these designs, mixing occurs across chronological phases (QUAL, QUAN) of a study. Questions or procedures within one strand emerge from or depend on the previous strand, and research questions are related to one another, often evolving as the study unfolds.

Conversion
In these parallel designs, mixing occurs when one type of data is transformed and analyzed both qualitatively and quantitatively; this design answers related aspects of the same questions.

Multilevel
In these parallel or sequential designs, mixing occurs across multiple levels of analysis. QUAN and QUAL data from these different levels are analyzed and integrated to answer aspects of the same question or related questions.

Fully Integrated
In these designs, mixing occurs in an interactive manner at all stages of the study. At each stage, one approach affects the formulation of the other and multiple types of implementation processes occur.

Table 19.4 Creswell and Plano Clark's (2011) Six Major Design Types

Convergent Parallel
In this design the researcher uses concurrent timing to implement the quantitative and qualitative strands during the same phase of the research process, prioritizes the methods equally, keeps the strands independent during analysis, and mixes the results during the researcher's overall interpretation of the data.

Explanatory Sequential
In this two-phase design the research starts with the collection and analysis of quantitative data, followed by the collection and analysis of qualitative data to help explain the initial quantitative results.

Exploratory Sequential In this two-phase design the research starts with the collection and analysis of qualitative data, followed by the collection and analysis of quantitative data to test or generalize the initial qualitative findings.
Embedded In this design the researcher collects and analyzes both quantitative and qualitative data within a traditional quantitative or qualitative design to enhance the overall design in some way.
Transformative This is a design that the researcher shapes within a transformative theoretical framework seeking to address the needs of a specific population and to call for change.
Multiphase This design combines both sequential and concurrent strands, collected over a period of time, and the implementation of distinct projects or phases within an overall program of study.

According to the typology's creators, either qualitative or quantitative data can be primary or secondary in all of the designs except the convergent parallel, in which they are typically given the same weight.

Each of the typologies described above provide a framework to understand the different ways mixed methods research can be carried out. But like any framework seeking to simplify things, many real-life scenarios do not perfectly fit into the typologies described above, or into others not covered (Guest, 2013). Nonetheless, typologies provide a common vocabulary and a basic conceptual structure to help organize and describe designs and processes (Teddlie & Tashakkori, 2009, p. 139).

Below, we have extracted three common dimensions from the existing typologies that we feel are most useful in helping investigators think about, and plan for, method integration. These three dimensions—timing, weighting, and purpose—all refer to the integration of qualitative and quantitative datasets. We describe these and follow with practical examples to better explain their meaning and to illustrate their application.[2] As will be evident from the examples, these dimensions are all interrelated to a certain degree.

Timing

Timing of integration refers to how datasets are used chronologically and analytically with respect to each other. The two most common forms in this regard are sequential and concurrent (the latter also known as convergent or parallel) designs. Sequential designs are those in which integration occurs between chronological phases of a study, and in which data analysis procedures for one dataset type inform another type of dataset. In other words, the latter data collection and analysis procedures are dependent, in some way, on the previously existing dataset. In contrast, in a concurrent design, data collection and analysis are not dependent on each other and are integrated at the same time within an analysis.

Here we need to add a point of clarification regarding the research activity to which timing refers since multiple phases and activities occur over the course of a standard research study (planning, data collection, data analysis, interpretation, and write-up). So when we talk about integration occurring between chronological phases, or integrated at the same time, what do we mean? For the vast majority of mixed methods designs, timing of integration refers to the *use* of a dataset type relative to another. Using the example of sequential designs, findings from one dataset are used either to inform a subsequent data collection procedure (exploratory) or to explain and provide further insight to findings generated from another dataset (explanatory). Note that in the case of exploratory sequential designs, timing of a dataset's use coincides with data collection timing, since in order for one dataset to inform the other it must precede it chronologically. The same cannot be said of an explanatory sequential or concurrent design. If study instruments are well thought out, with their explicit objectives in mind, data collection in either of the two designs can occur either simultaneously or sequentially. It is *how* they are used and analyzed relative to each other that is important.

Weighting

Known also as *dominance*, weighting pertains to which methodological orientation (QUAL, QUAN) is given priority by the researchers in a mixed method study. It does not mean that the less dominant approach is not important to a study's objectives, but rather that it is not the central dataset in the study and will not get the starring role in the write-up of study findings. Note that weighting refers to relative dominance as anticipated and planned for in the initial research design. This can change throughout the course of the study. How research findings are ultimately presented will depend on a number of factors and may not coincide with the original plan (Guest, 2013).

Purpose

There can be multiple purposes behind collecting and integrating datasets. However, the three most common reasons are (1) providing information for subsequent data collection and analysis procedures (exploratory/formative design), (2) explaining the results of a previously analyzed dataset (explanatory design), and (3) comparing two datasets (concurrent/triangulation design) and interpreting whether data converge, diverge, or are contradictory.

INTEGRATING DATA

One of the lesser developed areas in mixed method research is the process of data integration.[3] Some basic frameworks for integrating data do exist, however, as illustrated in Table 19.5, which delineates the conceptual and procedural differences between sequential and concurrent designs. The sections immediately following Table 19.5 describe these types of integration in more detail.

Table 19.5   Basic Types of Data Integration

Type of Integration	Type of Design	Method of Integration	Point of Interface
Connecting	Sequential	One phase builds on the other	Between data analysis (phase 1) and data collection (phase 2)
Merging	Concurrent	Bring results together	After analysis of both quan and qual; can also be mixed in matrices or transformed and integrated in both the Results and Discussion sections

Exploratory Sequential Designs

One of the most common mixed methods designs is what Creswell and Plano Clark (2011) call the exploratory sequential, in which data collection from a prior phase informs a subsequent phase of a research study. And within this design, the qual→QUAN variation is by far the most widely used. In fact, using qualitative data to inform quantitative instruments and procedures is so widely used in survey instrument development that Morse and Niehaus (2009, p. 18) argue the procedure is not a true mixed methods design. For them, it is a standard part of instrument development and should be regarded as such. Nevertheless, given the widespread use of the design, we, along with others, feel it should be considered as a type of mixed method design.

Two important considerations in a qual→QUAN design to be considered are (1) the *degree* to which the QUAN component is informed by the qual and (2) the degree of rigor that is warranted, and feasible, for a given study. With respect to the former, a researcher, for example, may already have a solid survey instrument developed and just wish to qualitatively assess it for comprehensibility and cultural appropriateness for the study population, and then revise it based on the qualitative findings. On the other end of the spectrum, an investigator may not even know the most relevant topics to ask survey respondents about and so might use extensive qualitative research to come up with survey domains and questions. These are two very different endeavors; where a particular study falls on the continuum depends on the information already available about both the topic and the study population.

The second dimension—the degree of rigor/formality—can also be viewed on a continuum. On the less rigorous end, one may have time and/or resources only for what we call the "taxi driver test." This simple technique entails administering the instrument to easily accessible individuals from the general population (e.g., taxi drivers) and identifying any major problems with question content and wording. Conversely, more sophisticated and involved instrument development and pretesting techniques, such as cognitive interviewing

(Willis, 2004), are often necessary to test and revise a survey instrument. Where a study falls on the spectrum largely depends on study objectives, degree of rigor needed, and resources/time available. For a more detailed discussion on developing QUAN tools from qual data, we refer the reader to Onwuegbuzie, Bustamante, and Nelson (2010).

In the quan→QUAL variation of the exploratory sequential design, the most typical incarnation is using quantitative data to select participants for follow-up qualitative inquiry. Quantitative data in this case can be collected (through surveys, structured observation, or other quantitative techniques) or garnered from existing secondary sources. For example, we could choose the nth percentile of survey respondents on a variable of interest. The size of n in this case is predetermined by estimating how many individuals are necessary for follow-up study. These participants are then administered in-depth interviews, or participate in focus groups, on the topic (variable) of interest. This type of design is often used in what are sometimes called exemplar or deviant case studies. For example, if we want to know *qualitatively* what distinguishes the most frequent TV viewers from individuals who don't watch any TV, we can use a survey measure of TV viewing and then choose the most frequent viewers (highest fifth percentile) and the least frequent viewers (lowest fifth percentile) for follow-up qualitative inquiry.

Sometimes an investigator may be interested in only one group—defined by a key variable of interest—for follow-up. A study carried out by Steiner et al. (2007) exemplifies this latter approach. In a study seeking to understand why condoms fail, researchers first surveyed 314 Jamaican men to document the prevalence of condom failure, including breakage and slippage. From the quantitative data they selected 22 individuals with the highest reported failure rates (higher than 20%) and conducted in-depth interviews to understand the reasons for such high failure rates. The qualitative data collected from this group of interest revealed that unsuitable storage or exposure to heat, improper handling while putting on condoms, and incorrect use of lubricants all contributed to failure. While the quantitative findings in this study provided some information to answer the research question, the qualitative phase was more critical to explaining condom failure among the study population.

Secondary data can also be effectively used to sample individuals or other types of sampling units for a follow-up study. Using quantitative tax data, an investigator can identify the busiest (at least in terms of revenue) bars or restaurants in a community and subsequently choose certain locations for participant observation (see Chapter 15). The possibilities are almost infinite, limited only by the accessibility of data and the ability to identify and reach individual sampling units within a quantitative dataset.

Explanatory Sequential Designs

Explanatory sequential designs are less common than their exploratory counterparts, but are being used more and more frequently, and for good reason. The basic idea behind this design is that a subsequent dataset explains, at least to a certain degree, findings from another dataset previously analyzed within a study. In our view, it is these types of designs where the complementary nature of quantitative and qualitative data truly shines. Many of us have read purely quantitative articles that masterfully show how two or more variables are correlated. Yet when it comes to the discussion section, the authors must theorize (and sometimes merely speculate) on what this correlation means because the quantitative data do not provide any information on the *how* and *why* behind the association. Conversely, the status quo for qualitative research is to provide thick explanatory description of a phenomenon without indicating the variability of the findings within the larger study population. Sequential explanatory designs combine the strengths of each of the two method types to address their inherent shortcomings.

Qualitative Explains Quantitative

An example of an explanatory sequential analysis in public health—in which qualitative data were used to explain patterns observed in a quantitative dataset—can be found in Guest et al. (2008). The researchers wanted to document changes in sexual risk behavior among 400 participants in a clinical trial testing an HIV prevention product (a pill taken daily). In their analysis, the authors first analyzed quantitative data from a survey administered at 13 points in time throughout the trial, which showed changes in condom use over the course of the trial (Figure 19.1).

Their next task was to try to find the reasons behind the changes observed—an initial increase in unprotected sex after enrollment and then decline after the eighth

Figure 19.1 Rate of Unprotected Sex During Clinical Trial Enrollment

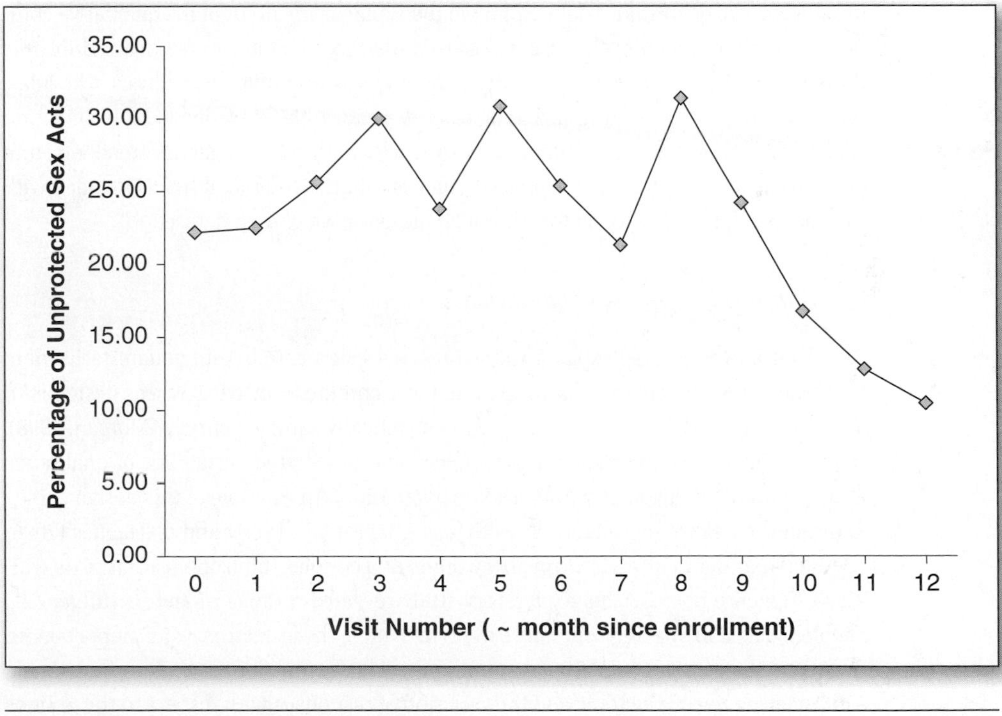

Source: Adapted from Guest et al. (2008).

visit. By looking for key words in the textual data derived from in-depth interviews with study participants, the researchers identified all of the instances in which the word *condom* was used, and looked for explanations of changes in condom use in each of those text segments. The qualitative data from this subsequent analysis documented several pathways explaining the patterns observed in the quantitative data, including increased access to condoms, perception of condom quality, and increased partner willingness to use condoms.

A study by Abildso, Zizzi, Gilleland, Thomas, and Bonner (2010) provides another example of an explanatory sequential study. The authors set out to evaluate the physical and psychosocial impact of a 12-week cognitive-behavioral weight management program and to identify factors associated with weight loss. Quantitative survey data were used to establish program completion rates and weight loss among participants ($N = 55$). Eleven of the participants were subsequently selected for in-depth interviews to identify potential mechanisms behind weight loss. Selection was based on survey results, and participants were recruited from each of the three dimensions of weight loss/completion rates. A subsequent thematic analysis of the in-depth interview data identified four major themes associated with degrees of program success: (a) fostering accountability, (b) balancing perceived effort and success, (c) redefining success, and (d) developing cognitive flexibility.

Note that not all examples of explanatory (or any mixed methods) designs need to be published in the same report. In a study on risk disinhibition conducted among participants in an HIV vaccine efficacy trial, quantitative and complementary qualitative results were published separately (Bartholow et al., 2005; Guest et al., 2005, respectively). The quantitative study documented the degree to which sexual behavior changed over the course of the 3-year trial, while the qualitative component helped explain the trajectories observed in the quantitative data. Although the explanatory intent of the qualitative component was embedded in the original research design, and data were collected for this purpose, logistical issues (independent analysis teams and different analysis schedules) prevented integration at the manuscript level. A disadvantage to a divided dissemination such as this is that readers may not read both articles and so do not get the broader picture of the research findings. An advantage, though, is that the additional space provided with two manuscripts allows for a more thorough presentation of each dataset.

Quantitative Informs Qualitative

Another form of the explanatory sequential design entails using quantitative data to further explain qualitative findings. The most common variation of this design is to follow up a qualitative analysis with a probabilistically sampled survey (Morgan, 1998). Here, the goal is to ascertain the prevalence, and associated variability, of qualitative findings among individuals within a study population. An example of this design can be found in the field of reproductive health (see Chapter 15). Lyerly and colleagues (2006) conducted in-depth interviews on how women and couples think about what to do with "extra" frozen embryos. This exploratory study revealed a range of factors influencing couples' decision making, but the extent to which these factors were important to women in the general population was unknown. The factors were, therefore, included in a national survey on the topic and the variation of responses with respect to the options was identified (Lyerly et al., 2010).

Hypothesis testing is only one possible objective of a qual → quan explanatory sequential design. In many cases a researcher may simply want to know, descriptively, how pervasive a particular perception, belief, or behavior is within a population. Themes derived from a qualitative inquiry among a small nonprobabilistic sample can be transformed into structured questions and administered to a larger probabilistic sample to assess the degree of variability within the larger population. In such a situation, description of the target population, not hypothesis testing, is the primary objective of the quantitative component.

Concurrent (Convergent or Parallel) Designs

The defining feature of a concurrent design is the relative independence of the datasets until *after* the analysis of each. All concurrent designs share the practice of conducting data analysis on each dataset separately and then integrating/mixing data sets once analysis of each is completed. Neither data nor analysis is dependent on the other.

Reasons for data integration in a concurrent design can differ. One common purpose can be generally classified as triangulation. *Triangulation* in the social, behavioral, and health sciences refers to using multiple sources, methods, or perspectives to address a research problem. As with all concurrent studies, in the triangulation design, qualitative and quantitative datasets are analyzed separately and integrated during the interpretation phase of the analysis, often in the Discussion section of a report. Integrating data from various sources enhances validity and minimizes the risk of a partial or inaccurate interpretation (Figure 19.2).

Figure 19.2   The Importance of Combining Data Sources

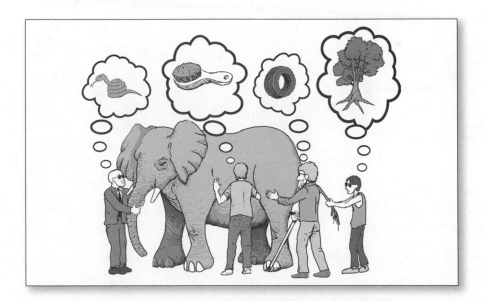

Source: Illustration by Mark Abramowsky. www.chromaticworkshop.com

During data integration, the analyst looks for evidence of convergence, divergence, or contradiction between the two datasets (recall the = notation in the earlier text box; this is the symbol that is used, at least by certain authors, to denote purpose of integration). An excellent example of this approach is Kawamura, Ivankova, Kohler, and Perumean-Chaney's (2009) study that looked at the association between social relationships and self-efficacy among radio listeners. The investigators administered structured surveys to 105 listeners of a particular radio program (a drama intended to motivate individuals to exercise) and generated a path analytic model based on structural equation modeling of the quantitative data. Eighteen participants were selected from the larger sample for in-depth interviews, which were subsequently analyzed using a grounded-theory approach. Resulting explanatory models from each dataset were then compared for areas of convergence and divergence. In their article, Kawamura et al. present a path analytic diagram depicting both qualitative and quantitative paths, and indicate the paths shared by both models (Figure 19.3).

According to the authors, "the major finding in this study is that there is a divergence in the findings based on the interpretation of the results of the path analysis and the grounded theory" (Kawamura et al., 2009, p. 99). Indeed, looking closely at the diagram, one can see only one path that exhibited (partial) convergence.

Figure 19.3   Working Integration Model

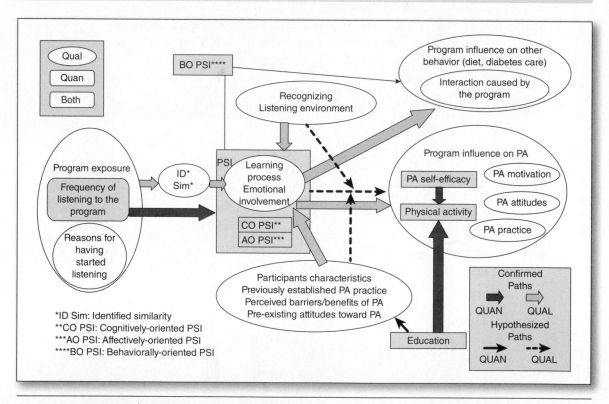

Source: Kawamura et al. (2009).

Note: PSI = parasocial interaction; PA = physical activity

The divergent outcome of the Kawamura et al. (2009) study is not an uncommon occurrence and presents one of the major challenges in a triangulated design. Convergent findings are clean and easy to explain: Findings are corroborated and have increased validity. But what do you do with divergent or contradictory results? They need to be explained. One possible, generic, explanation is that the observed disparity is a methodological artifact—that is, the difference in question wording and/or process of inquiry is responsible. A more thoughtful approach is to broaden or adjust one's theoretical perspective. Conflicting data can be the foundation for developing more sophisticated (and presumably more accurate) explanatory theories. In fact, Greene et al. (1989) point out that seeking divergence is an appropriate, and often informative, purpose for a concurrent design. The bottom line is that, whether intentionally sought or not, divergent findings need to be accounted for; researchers must be prepared for this possibility when planning and executing a triangulated concurrent design.

The concurrent design example above uses the most common type of data mixing in concurrent designs: analyzing qualitative and quantitative datasets separately, presenting them as independent datasets in the Results section, and integrating/mixing the findings in the Discussion. An alternate mixing strategy is described by Plano Clark, Garrett, and Leslie-Pelecky (2010). As shown in Table 19.6, key findings can be merged in such a way as to connect and present both sets of findings in one place. In this table, the two left columns contain quantitative data in the form of respondent category (professional discipline) and comparative measures on a key variable (skill improvement) that was part of an evaluation of a nontraditional graduate education program. Qualitative data are presented in the two columns to the right: one column shows key themes and the other illustrative quotes. Using this integrative method, the reader can see the qualitative and quantitative data alongside each other and look for convergence and/or divergence between groups and data collection methods. Note that the number of possible permutations of how data are presented in matrix form is virtually endless, and what a researcher ultimately chooses to highlight depends on the types of data available, the robustness of findings, and the intended purpose of the matrix and write-up.

Bryman also advocates using a matrix technique to combine findings in the Results section, arguing that presenting QUAL and QUAN data separately and limiting integration of the findings to the narrative in the discussion section is not an optimal form of mixing (Bryman, personal communication, 2010). Building on the work of Ritchie, Spencer, and O'Connor (2003), Bryman suggests using a matrix in which themes, instrument domains, or theoretical constructs (whichever best unifies the qualitative and quantitative datasets) constitute the rows, and qualitative and quantitative data points or summaries are listed in two separate columns and cross-referenced with each theme/construct. Fields in the qualitative or quantitative data columns can be either summaries (correlation coefficients, p-values, means, theme definitions, or frequencies) or raw data points (quotes, ratios). Note that more columns can be added to further summarize other aspects of integration. Table 19.7 provides a generic example of this type of mixing matrix.

Table 19.6 Example of Matrix Form of Data Mixing for Evaluation of a Nontraditional Graduate Education Program

Discipline	QUAN Comparisons "Improved Skills" M (SD)[a]	Most Prominent QUAL Themes About Benefits (% of statements)	Sample Quote
Biological Sciences (n = 6)	40.17 (3.06)[b, c]	Improved communication skills (30%)	It also let me translate very complicated concepts to children and it helped me work on my communication skills.
		Improved teaching skills (23%)	If I choose to go into academia I feel that my teaching skills have improved. My evaluations have been significantly more positive since working with [the program].
		Improved marketability (23%)	[The program] has made me a more marketable scientist. I believe it has enhanced my CV.
Physical sciences and engineering (n quan = 15; n qual = 13)	36.07 (4.11)[b]	Improved communication skills (37%)	Mostly, I learned a lot about communication. And it wasn't just about communicating with [teaching] students. I learned a lot about communicating with professionals.
		Camaraderie and friendship (22%)	I found the support of the other fellows to be very helpful on poor research days or weeks, since it often feels that the atmosphere is somewhat competitive within my own department.

Discipline	QUAN Comparisons "Improved Skills" M (SD)[a]	Most Prominent QUAL Themes About Benefits (% of statements)	Sample Quote
		Improved confidence (14%)	By gaining the ability to talk science with everyone, I am a more confident, coherent scientist in public and at work.
Mathematics (n quan = 14; n qual = 13)	34.79 (2.67)[c]	Improved teaching skills (39%)	One of the main goals of a PhD in mathematics is the betterment of one's teaching ability. I simply cannot say enough about the positive effect [of the program] with respect to my teaching.
		Improved marketability (23%)	Participating in [the program] has made me a more desirable candidate for a teaching position. I have heard that a credential such as this is highly desirable in the tenure-track job market.
		Working with people outside field (16%)	I was able to teach material and work with individuals outside my subject area. This will help me be more effective in interdepartmental collaboration in the future.

a = ANOVA test found a significant difference for the improved skills variable ($p = .011$).

b = Univariate post hoc comparisons found significant differences between biological sciences and physical sciences and engineering ($p = .048$).

c = Univariate post hoc comparisons found significant differences between biological sciences and mathematics ($p = .008$).

Source: Plano Clark et al. (2010).

Table 19.7 Generic Matrix Mixing Example

Theme/ Construct/ Domain	Method 1 (QUAN)	Method 2 (QUAL)	Method n	Relationship (e.g., convergence, divergence, explanation)	Interpretation/ Comments
Theme 1	Data	Data	Data		
Theme 2	Data	Data	Data		
Theme 3	Data	Data	Data		
Theme n	Data	Data	Data		

Another integrative method involves data transformation from one data type to another (a conversion design). This includes transforming qualitative data into quantitative data. A common form of a qual > quan transformation is presenting frequencies for thematic codes across a data set, as in the example in Table 19.8, which shows the most common themes pertaining to likes and dislikes about a vaginal microbicide among South African women. The table also plots these frequencies over four time points, reflecting four data collection points during the 6-month clinical trial in which participants were enrolled. The trial tested the safety and acceptability of the microbicidal gel in combination with a diaphragm for HIV prevention (Guest et al., 2007).

Table 19.8 Microbicide Acceptability Study: Frequency of Most Common Themes by Question, With Illustrative Quotes*

Theme	Month 1 (n = 110)	Month 3 (n = 106)	Month 5 (n = 97)	Month 6 (n = 100)
Likes About the Diaphragm and Gel				
Protection *I like it because I know that when I am using this method I am safe and nothing wrong will happen to me. (month 1)*	46	44	46	33
Ease of use/inconspicuous *I didn't feel it in the vagina. . . . it was like before I wasn't using the diaphragm, it was just the same. (month 5)*	19	12	21	24

Theme	Month 1 (n = 110)	Month 3 (n = 106)	Month 5 (n = 97)	Month 6 (n = 100)
Positive impact on sex *Penetration is also very easy and is no longer rough and every time after sex I always feel like I could have more. (month 3)*	12	11	4	11
Lubrication (of gel) *[T]he gel lubricates you and it even lubricates when you get dry during the intercourse so it helps a lot. (month 5)*	7	9	9	8
Dislikes About the Diaphragm and Gel				
Physical symptoms *What I don't like I am always wet in my vagina and I had a discharge, felt dizzy, and nauseous. (month 1)*	13	5	3	2
Partner disapproval *At first he said he couldn't penetrate me as he usually does and he doesn't feel comfortable with it. (month 1)*	7	0	0	3
Too wet/too much lubrication *When I am having sex with my partner, I become wet. I think this gel creates a lot of wetness. (month 1)*	4	4	3	0
Inconvenience *I have to insert the diaphragm whenever I want to have sex. (month 6)*	3	3	3	4
Smell of gel *The gel's smell was not good for me, it smelled bad. (month 6)*	1	0	1	3

*All frequencies in the cells refer to the number of unique interview participants expressing a theme.

Source: Guest et al. (2007).

Although calculating and presenting code frequencies is the most commonly employed form of qual to quan data transformation, note that a large number of other transformative methods have been developed and used, including code co-occurrence and graph-theoretic techniques (Bernard & Ryan, 2010; Guest, MacQueen, & Namey 2012; Guest & McLellan, 2003).

Similarly, quantitative data can be transformed into narratives or images and interpreted qualitatively. Common examples of quan to qual transformation are epidemic curves and social network diagrams, shown in Figure 19.4 and Chapter 14, respectively.

Figure 19.4   Epidemic Curve—Outbreak of Norovirus Gastroenteritis at a University Student Residence, Edmonton, Alberta, 2006

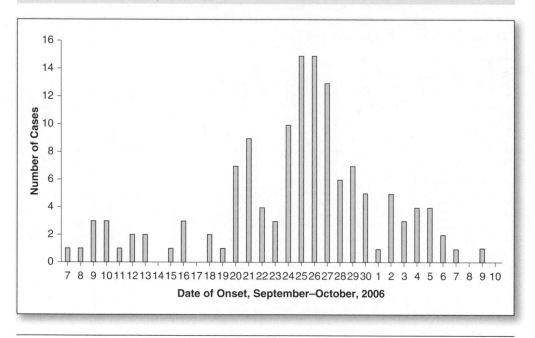

Source: Honish, Talbot, Dragon, and Utgoff (2008).

Q METHODOLOGY

Q methodology is a mixed method research technique that has been used to study a wide range of public health topics (Baker, Thompson, & Mannion, 2006; Cross, 2005; Simons, 2013). Developed by psychologist William Stephenson, the method is designed to study a collection of individual subjective viewpoints on a given topic and then identify common views across a group of individuals. The method comprises five basic steps.

1. A sample of statements is nonrandomly extracted from a summary body of text (known as the concourse). The body of text is derived from a series of interviews with individuals who are knowledgeable about the research topic. Selected statements are individually printed on small cards.

2. Each participant is then presented with the series of cards containing the statements (considered variables at this point).

3. The participant is then asked to rank the cards along a specified dimension (a Q sort).

4. Responses are then run through the Q method of factor analysis (in contrast to the most commonly used R method).

5. The Q factor analysis identifies correlations between subjects across a sample of variables and reduces the many individual participant viewpoints down to a few factors. These factors are interpreted as representing shared ways of thinking within a group or population.

A good example of the method's use is a study conducted by Shabila, Al-Tawil, Al-Hadithi, and Sondorp (2013). They used Q methodology to explore the range and diversity of viewpoints of primary health care providers toward the Iraqi health care system. Q-sort methodology revealed four distinct viewpoints among primary health care providers. One factor emphasized positive aspects of, and contentment with, the current system, while the other three factors highlighted the negative aspects. The diverse viewpoints identified by the researchers can subsequently be used to highlight ways in which the Iraqi health care system can be reformed.

On a final note, we wish to stress that in reality many mixed methods designs are more complex and variable than any of the existing typologies can adequately capture (Guest, 2013). More important, there is no "right" way of integrating data. The field of mixed methods is still evolving, and researchers should feel free and encouraged to be creative and develop new and interesting ways of integrating data. Several methodological journals publish innovative mixed methods articles and can be excellent sources of inspiration (see this chapter's Additional Resources for a list of journals). For those readers who seek general guidance in designing a mixed methods study, we provide a simple set of instructions in the Basic Steps text box.

BASIC STEPS IN DESIGNING A MIXED METHODS RESEARCH STUDY

1. State general research question/problem to be addressed.

2. Decide if a mixed methods approach is needed.
   - Be able to explicitly justify why you're using a mixed methods design and why each component is necessary.

3. List types of data to be collected and analyzed.

4. Choose mixed methods design(s): timing, weighting, and purpose.
   - Thoughtfully plan timing of both data collection and data integration at the onset. These are two different processes, and how they are timed has implications for how an analysis can be conducted.

5. Draw a schematic of your study, depicting how and when each component is related the others.
   a. Give a title to your study/model.
   b. Choose either horizontal or vertical layout.
   c. Draw boxes for quantitative and qualitative stages of data collection, analysis, and interpretation.
   d. Designate priority of quan and qual data (upper/lower case).
   e. Use single-headed arrows to show the flow of procedures.
   f. Specify procedures for each quantitative and qualitative data collection and analysis stage.
   g. Specify expected products or outcomes of each procedure.

6. Ensure your visual diagram is simple. Use concise language and fit on one page.

7. Review the design (and have others review it) to ensure that your data collection and analysis plan is the best possible, but feasible, approach for answering the research question.

MIXED METHODS IN PUBLIC HEALTH

In the field of public health, explicit mixed methods research designs are becoming increasingly common. In 2000, the PubMed database contained only 11 articles with "mixed method(s)" in the title or abstract (0.0021% of all articles catalogued). This number grew to 69 (0.0099% of titles) in 2005, and to 575 (0.0619% of titles) by 2010, representing a thirty-fold increase in a 10-year period.[4] The formal field of mixed methods is expanding in other ways as well. Some prominent funding organizations, such as the National Institutes of Health, have developed specific standards for reviewing mixed methods research (see, e.g., Creswell, Klassen, Plano Clark, & Smith, 2011).

Mixed methods research designs are currently utilized in almost every subfield of public health, some of which we've highlighted in the examples presented in earlier sections of this chapter (HIV prevention, obesity, mental health, gastroenterology, and reproductive health). Some other notable fields include health services research (Guthrie, Auerback, & Bindman, 2010), cancer research (Kubon, McClennen, Fitch, McAndrew, & Anderson, 2012), program evaluation (Carter, Callaghan, Khalil, & Morres, 2012), and environmental health (Corburn, 2002). The field of public health is so diverse that it would be impossible to give mixed methods examples from all subfields. Instead, below we describe some mixed methods studies that cover a range of different subfields of public health and that serve different research purposes.

Health Policy

One study from the field of health policy by Guthrie and colleagues (2010) sought to examine the impact of the California Medicaid pay-for-performance program on the quality of health care. Because the researchers wanted to understand both the *perceived* impact and the *actual* impact, they decided to use qualitative interviews for the former and a quantitative quality indicator for the latter (Healthcare Effectiveness Data and Information Set). The authors collected and analyzed data concurrently, but separately. Ultimately, these researchers were interested in comparing perceptions of the policy change to changes in quantitative quality indicators resulting from the new policy. They found no significant differences in quality indicators before and after the policy was implemented and therefore used the qualitative data to explain why. They found that the new policy failed to motivate health plans to invest new resources to improve the quality of care, and instead the plans simply shifted the focus of their previous efforts to better align with the quality indicators from the Healthcare Effectiveness Data and Information Set. Without the inclusion of the qualitative data in this investigation, Guthrie and colleagues would have been unable to discern why the policy failed to change quality of care in California.

Chronic Diseases

In another example, a research team in the United Kingdom employed a sequential mixed methods design to examine online health information seeking among older adults with chronic diseases (Mayoh, Bond, & Todres, 2012). The researchers first conducted a survey with members of chronic disease support groups. The responses to the survey questions, which included both open-ended and closed-ended questions, were analyzed to determine the most salient and common issues for this population when seeking health information online. The issues identified (including the experience of finding poor-quality health information online or the experience of sharing online health information with a health professional) became the framework for their subsequent qualitative interviews with adults over 60 who had sought health information online. One major finding was that although older adults with chronic disease are significantly less likely to seek health information online, a subpopulation of older adults confidently uses the Internet to find health information. By using a sequential design, the researchers were not only able to determine characteristics and prevalence of online health information seeking by older adults, but also to better understand *how* this population was finding and using this information.

Nutrition

Sometimes, public health researchers collect qualitative data to develop hypotheses for their analysis of quantitative data. Park et al. (2011) used in-depth interviews with Hispanic mothers in New York to examine their definition of, and access to, healthy foods. Then, using findings from these data, they developed hypotheses on the relationship between food consumption and access to healthy foods. Through the interviews, they found that Hispanic immigrant women often subscribed to views, similar to the "farm-to-table" and organic food movements, indicating that the fresher and more natural the food the healthier it was. For the quantitative portion, the researchers added questions to a survey designed to measure walking distance to fresh food markets (e.g., farmers markets, livestock markets) and to food stores (e.g., supermarkets). The women's food consumption patterns were then analyzed to determine to what extent their household's food consumption reflected the beliefs described in the qualitative interviews. The researchers found that households within walking access to farmers markets consumed more fruits and vegetables than those with walking access to only supermarkets. Without the qualitative findings, the researchers may have overlooked the importance of access to fresh food markets and instead focused only on access to supermarkets as other researchers have. This added perspective was gained by appropriately using a mixed methods design to develop and test new hypotheses.

Maternal and Child Health

With the overall goal to reduce maternal mortality, global health researchers Spangler and Bloom (2010) aimed to better understand the barriers and facilitators for low-income women's access to biomedical obstetric care in Tanzania. The researchers used quantitative data from a census of all pregnant women in the Kilombero Valley in Tanzania to explore patterns of obstetric care use and the influence of social status on use of care. The researchers then used the quantitative data to select women for qualitative interviews, based on who had given birth in the previous 6 months and several socio-economic variables. Spangler and Bloom weighted the qualitative and quantitative components equally and used the findings from one method to confirm findings of the other (triangulation). Additionally, they used qualitative findings to select variables of importance for their statistical models. In the end, they found that biomedical obstetric care use is predicted by ethnicity, household assets, and education, but that individual women have to balance material, social, and emotional costs with potential health benefits to determine whether they will seek care at a biomedical facility. Again, as with the example above, each method adds a different perspective. In this case, the quantitative data provide the overall trends for biomedical obstetric usage, but the qualitative data describe the nuanced decision making in which these women engage.

Epidemiological Surveillance

Epidemiological surveillance research is often considered the domain of quantitative researchers, but Monasta, Andersson, Lodegar, Theol, and Cockcroft (2008) demonstrate that a mixed methods approach can be important to ensuring accurate estimates for population statistics. Using Romá camps in Italy as a case study for epidemiological studies of small, dispersed minority populations, Monasta et al. used qualitative observational, interview, and focus group data to inform the development of a household questionnaire. Because Romá camps are both underserved and under-researched in Europe, the research team hoped to generate quality epidemiological data that the community could use to advocate for themselves. For the qualitative component, the researchers spent 1 month observing conditions in the Romá camps and interviewing key informants and community members to better understand the health of children in these camps. These qualitative data on household- and camp-related factors influencing children's health were integrated into a questionnaire on the prevalence of diarrhea and respiratory diseases among the camps' children. The researchers were able to obtain the camp children's prevalence statistics for diarrhea (15%) and having a cough (55%) within the past 15 days. Because the researchers felt there was a dearth of quantitative data on this population, they emphasized the survey component and used the qualitative data to ensure its cultural and contextual relevance for obtaining data in the camps.

CURRENT ISSUES AND FUTURE DIRECTIONS

In this chapter we have described some of the more common mixed methods design typologies. These do not represent the entire range of typologies, nor do all mixed methodologists agree on the importance of the three primary dimensions that we emphasize: timing, purpose, and weighting. We presented what we believe to be the most widely accepted and most practical aspects of the mixed methods design literature. We suggest that the reader view this chapter as a basic theoretical background which they can use to design studies and execute their own unique mixed methods analyses. Mixed methods designs can become an additional tool to answer complex research questions, and we hope this chapter has provided the foundation necessary to explore and apply this method. The public health studies described above are just a few examples of how public health researchers are using mixed methods to better understand important public health problems. Health is so strongly related to behavior, biology, and environment, and often the only way to understand such complexity is to use multiple data sources in the same study.

As we noted earlier, the field of mixed methods is rapidly growing. One of the areas still in development is data integration. Researchers are looking for (and in some cases finding) novel ways to integrate and present qualitative and quantitative data. Another area of both theoretical and practical expansion pertains to evaluative standards. Recently the National Institutes of Health commissioned scholars to write a set of guidelines to which reviewers of mixed methods research proposals can refer (Creswell et al., 2011). Other large research organizations, and scientific journals, may soon follow suit. Bryman (2006) discusses some potential directions in terms of evaluation criteria, as do Leech and Onwuegbuzie (2010), Mertens (2011), and O'Cathain, Murphy, and Nicholl (2008).

Another area for potential growth is in the types of data used in mixed methods research. When researchers talk about quantitative data, they are typically referring to secondary surveillance data or data collected through a structured survey. Likewise, qualitative data are generally conceptualized as being generated through in-depth interviews and focus groups, and to a lesser degree, participant observation. While these types of data are by far the most commonly employed in mixed methods designs, the potential for the incorporation of other types of data are virtually limitless. Some notable examples include free listing, decision modeling, visual data collection and analysis techniques, timelines, projective techniques, and personal diaries (Alaszewski, 2006; Bernard, 2012; de Munck & Sobo, 1998; Guest, Namey, & Mitchell, 2013).

Other methods that show promise for mixed methods include observation (Gillham, 2008), Geographic Information Systems (Chapter 21, this volume; Krieger, 2003; Ricketts, 2003), and social network analysis (Chapter 15, this volume; Valente, 2010). Larger research projects in public health also often collect biological data, which can be integrated with other data forms. MacQueen et al. (2007), for example, combined in-depth interview data with pregnancy data collected from participants in a randomized controlled trial in Nigeria, Cameroon, and Ghana. The trial was designed to test the efficacy of a drug in the context of HIV prevention among women at higher risk for HIV infection. Abnormally high pregnancy rates were observed among trial participants. MacQueen and colleagues employed qualitative interviews to better understand the reasons behind the elevated rates.

New technologies also offer researchers different data sources and the opportunity to use and integrate new qualitative and quantitative data collection and analysis methods. Online data sources are a good example. Facebook and Google are continually collecting large amounts of data on social interactions. For example, the U.S. Centers for Disease Control and Prevention (CDC) and Google recently collaborated on Google Flu Trends (www.google.org/flutrends). CDC and Google researchers found that the home location of a computer on which someone is conducting Google searches about influenza symptoms can accurately approximate the number of doctors' visits for flu symptoms in the same geographic location (Ginsberg et al. 2009). The take-home point here is that "data" can be defined as any information that informs a research question. Even household garbage has proven to be useful in social science and behavioral research (see, e.g., Rathje & Murphy, 2001). Be creative and open to novel sources of data and analyzing data in new ways. Nontraditional data sources and methods of analysis, as well as novel integration techniques, have the potential to provide public health with exciting new insights into the issues we have studied and will likely study for years to come.

ADDITIONAL RESOURCES

Books

Bergman, M. (Ed.). (2008). *Advances in mixed methods research.* Thousand Oaks, CA: Sage.

Creswell, J., & Plano Clark, V. (2011). *Designing and conducting mixed methods research* (2nd ed.). Thousand Oaks, CA: Sage.

Greene, J. (2007). *Mixed methods in social inquiry.* San Francisco, CA. Jossey-Bass.

Hesse-Biber, S. (2010). *Mixed methods research: Merging theory with practice.* New York, NY: Guilford Press.

Morgan, D. (2014). *Integrating qualitative and quantitative methods: A pragmatic approach.* Thousand Oaks, CA: Sage.

Morse, J., & Niehaus, L. (2009). *Mixed method design: Principles and procedures.* Walnut Creek, CA: Left Coast Press.

Onwuegbuzie, A., Slate, J., Leech, N., & Collins, K. (2012). *Mixed methods research: A step-by-step guide.* New York, NY: Routledge Academic.

Padgett, D. (2011). *Qualitative and mixed methods in public health.* Thousand Oaks, CA: Sage.

Ridenour C., & Newman, I. (2008). *Mixed methods research: Exploring the interactive continuum.* Carbondale: Southern Illinois University Press.

Tashakkori, A., & Teddlie, C. (Eds.). (2003). *Handbook of mixed methods in social and behavioral research.* Thousand Oaks, CA: Sage.

Tashakkori, A., & Teddlie, C. (Eds.). (2010). *Handbook of mixed methods in social and behavioral research* (2nd ed.). Thousand Oaks, CA: Sage.

Teddlie, C., & Tashakkori, A. (2009). *Foundations of mixed methods research: Integrating quantitative and qualitative approaches in the social and behavioral sciences.* Thousand Oaks, CA: Sage.

Methodological Journals

Field Methods

International Journal of Multiple Research Approaches

Journal of Mixed Methods Research

Qualitative Health Research

Quality and Quantity

REFERENCES

Abildso, C., Zizzi, S., Gilleland, D., Thomas, J., & Bonner, D. (2010). A mixed methods evaluation of a 12-week insurance-sponsored weight management program incorporating cognitive-behavioral counseling. *Journal of Mixed Methods Research, 4,* 278–294.

Alaszewski, A. (2006). *Using diaries for social research.* Thousand Oaks, CA: Sage.

Baker, R., Thompson, C., & Mannion, R. (2006). Q methodology in health economics. *Journal of Health Services and Research Policy, 11*(1), 38–45.

Bartholow, B., Buchbinder, S., Celum, C., Goli, V., Koblin, B., Para, M., . . . Mastro, T. (2005). HIV sexual risk behavior over 36 months of follow-up in the world's first HIV vaccine efficacy trial. *Journal of Acquired Immune Deficiency Syndrome, 39,* 90–101.

Bergman, M. (2008). Introduction: Whither mixed methods? In M. Bergman (Ed.), *Advances in mixed methods research* (pp. 1–7). Thousand Oaks, CA: Sage.

Bernard, H. (2012). *Social research methods: Qualitative and quantitative approaches* (2nd ed.). Thousand Oaks, CA: Sage.

Bernard, H., & Ryan, G. (2010). *Analyzing qualitative data: Systematic approaches.* Thousand Oaks, CA: Sage.

Brody, H., Rip, M. R., Vinten-Johansen, P., Paneth, N., & Rachman, S. (2000). Map-making and myth-making in Broad Street: The London cholera epidemic, 1854. *Lancet, 356,* 64–68.

Bryman, A. (2006). Paradigm peace and the implications for quality. *International Journal of Social Research Methodology, 9,* 111–126.

Carter, T., Callaghan, P., Khalil, E., & Morres, I. (2012). The effectiveness of a preferred intensity exercise programme on the mental health outcomes of young people with depression: A sequential mixed methods evaluation. *BMC Public Health, 12,* 187.

Corburn, J. (2002). Combining community-based research and local knowledge to confront asthma and subsistence-hazards in Greenpoint/Williamsburg, Brooklyn, New York. *Environmental Health Perspectives, 110,* 241–248.

Creswell, J. W., Klassen, A. C., Plano Clark, V. L., & Smith, K. C. (2011). *Best practices for mixed methods research in the health sciences.* Bethesda, MD: National Institutes of Health. Retrieved from http://obssr.od.nih.gov/mixed_methods_research

Creswell, J., & Plano Clark, V. (2011). *Designing and conducting mixed methods research* (2nd ed.). Thousand Oaks, CA: Sage.

Cross, R. (2005). Exploring attitudes: The case for Q methodology. *Health Education Research, 20,* 206–213.

de Munck, V., & Sobo, E. (Eds.). (1998). *Using methods in the field: A practical introduction and casebook.* Walnut Creek, CA: AtlaMira Press.

Gillham, B. (2008). *Observation techniques: Structured and unstructured.* London, UK: Continuum International.

Ginsberg, J., Mohebbi, M. H., Patel, R. S., Brammer, L., Smolinski, M. S., & Brilliant, L. (2009). Detecting influenza epidemics using search engine query data. *Nature, 457,* 1012–1014.

Greene, J. (2007). *Mixed methods in social inquiry.* San Francisco, CA: Jossey-Bass.

Greene, J. C., Caracelli, V. J., & Graham, W. F. (1989). Toward a conceptual framework for mixed-method evaluation design. *Educational Evaluation and Policy Analysis, 11,* 255–274.

Guest, G. (2013). Describing mixed methods research: An alternative to typologies. *Journal of Mixed Methods Research, 7,* 141–151.

Guest, G., Johnson, L., Burke, H., Rain-Taljaard, R., Severy, L., Von Mollendorf, C., & Van Damme, L. (2007). Changes in sexual behavior during a safety and feasibility trial of a microbicide/diaphragm combination: An integrated qualitative and quantitative analysis. *AIDS Education and Prevention, 19,* 310–320.

Guest, G., MacQueen, K., & Namey, E. (2012). *Applied thematic analysis.* Thousand Oaks, CA: Sage.

Guest, G., & McLellan, E. (2003). Distinguishing the trees from the forest: Applying cluster analysis to thematic qualitative data. *Field Methods, 15,* 186–201.

Guest, G., McLellan-Lemal, E., Matia, D., Pickard, R., Fuchs, J., McKirnan, D., & Neidig, J. (2005). HIV vaccine efficacy trial participation: Men-who-have-sex-with-men's experience of risk reduction counseling and perceptions of behavior change. *AIDS Care, 17,* 46–57.

Guest, G., Namey, E., & Mitchell, M. (2013). *Collecting qualitative data: A field manual for applied research.* Thousand Oaks, CA: Sage.

Guest, G., Shattuck, D., Johnson, L., Akumatey, B., Clarke, E., Chen, P., & MacQueen, K. (2008). Changes in sexual risk behavior among participants in a PrEP HIV prevention trial. *Sexually Transmitted Diseases, 35,* 1002–1008.

Guthrie, B., Auerback, G., & Bindman, A. B. (2010). Health plan competition for Medicaid enrollees based on performance does not improve quality of care. *Health Affairs, 29,* 1507–1516.

Hesse-Biber, S. (2010). *Mixed methods research: Merging theory with practice.* New York, NY: Guilford Press.

Honish, L., Talbot, J., Dragon, D., & Utgoff, D. (2008). Outbreak of norovirus gastroenteritis at a university student residence—Edmonton, Alberta, 2006. *Canada Communicable Disease Report, 34*(4), 1–7.

Kawamura, Y., Ivankova, N., Kohler, C., & Perumean-Chaney, S. (2009). Utilizing mixed methods to assess parasocial interaction of an entertainment-education program audience. *International Journal of Multiple Research Approaches, 3*(1), 88–104.

Krieger, N. (2003). Place, space, and health: GIS and epidemiology. *Epidemiology, 14,* 384–385.

Kubon, T. M, McClennen, J., Fitch, M. I., McAndrew, A., & Anderson, J. (2012). A mixed-methods cohort study to determine perceived patient benefit in providing custom breast prostheses. *Current Oncology, 19*(2), e43–e52.

Leech, N., & Onwuegbuzie, A. (2010). Guidelines for conducting and reporting mixed research in the field of counseling and beyond. *Journal of Counseling and Development, 68,* 61–70.

Lyerly, A. D., Steinhauser, K., Namey, E., Tulsky, J. A., Cook-Deegan, R., Sugarman, J., . . . Wallach, E. (2006). Factors that affect infertility patients' decisions about frozen embryos. *Fertility and Sterility, 85,* 1620–1630.

Lyerly, A. D., Steinhauser, K., Voils, C., Namey, E., Alexander, C., Bankowski, B., . . . Wallach, E. (2010). Fertility patients' preferences for frozen embryo disposition: Results of a multi-institutional U.S. survey. *Fertility and Sterility, 93,* 499–509.

MacQueen, K., Johnson, L., Alleman, P., Akumatey, B., Lawoyin, T., & Nyiama, T. (2007). Pregnancy prevention practices among women with multiple partners in an HIV prevention trial. *Journal of Acquired Immune Deficiency Syndrome, 46,* 32–38.

Mayoh, J., Bond, C. S., & Todres, L. (2012). An innovative mixed methods approach to studying the online health information seeking experiences of adults with Chronic Health Conditions. *Journal of Mixed Methods Research, 6,* 21–33.

Mertens, D. (2011). Publishing mixed methods research. *Journal of Mixed Methods Research, 5,* 3–6.

Monasta, L., Andersson, N., Lodegar, R. J., Theol, D., & Cockcroft, A. (2008). Minority health and small numbers epidemiology: A case study of living conditions and the health of children in 5 foreign Roma camps in Italy. *American Journal of Public Health, 98,* 2035–2041.

Morgan, D. (1998). Practical strategies for combining qualitative and quantitative methods: Applications to health research. *Qualitative Health Research, 8,* 362–376.

Morse, J. (1991). Approaches to qualitative-quantitative methodological triangulation. *Nursing Research, 40,* 120–123.

Morse, J., & Niehaus, L. (2009). *Mixed method design: Principles and procedures.* Walnut Creek, CA: Left Coast Press.

O'Cathain, A., Murphy, E., & Nicholl, J. (2008). The quality of mixed methods studies in health services research. *Journal of Health Services Research and Policy, 13,* 92–98.

Onwuegbuzie, A., Bustamante, R., & Nelson, J. (2010). Mixed research as a tool for developing quantitative instruments. *Journal of Mixed Methods Research, 4,* 56–78.

Park, Y., Quinn, J., Florez, K., Jacobson, J., Neckerman, K., & Rundle, A. (2011). Hispanic immigrant women's perspective on healthy foods and the New York City retail food environment: A mixed-methods study. *Social Science Medicine, 73*(1), 13–21.

Plano Clark, V., & Creswell, J. (2008). *The mixed methods reader.* Thousand Oaks, CA: Sage.

Plano Clark, V., Garrett, A., & Leslie-Pelecky, D. (2010). Applying three strategies for integrating quantitative and qualitative databases in a mixed methods study of a nontraditional graduate education program. *Field Methods, 22,* 154–174.

Rathje, W., & Murphy, C. (2001). *Rubbish! The archaeology of garbage.* Tucson: University of Arizona Press.

Ricketts, T. (2003). Geographic information systems and public health. *Annual Review of Public Health, 24,* 1–6.

Ritchie, J., Spencer, L., & O'Connor, W. (2003). Carrying out qualitative analysis. In J. Ritchie & J. Lewis (Eds.), *Qualitative research practice: A guide for social science students and researchers* (pp. 219–262). London, UK: Sage.

Shabila, N., Al-Tawil, N., Al-Hadithi, T., & Sondorp, E. (2013). The range and diversity of providers' viewpoints towards the Iraqi primary health care system: An exploration using Q-methodology. *BMC International Health and Human Rights, 13,* 18.

Simons, J. (2013). An introduction to Q methodology. *Nurse Researcher, 20*(3), 28–32.

Snow, J. (1854). The cholera near Golden-square, and at Deptford. *Medical Times Gazette, 9,* 321–322.

Spangler, S. A., & Bloom, S. S. (2010). Use of biomedical obstetric care in rural Tanzania: The role of social and material inequalities. *Social Science & Medicine, 71,* 760–768.

Steiner, M., Taylor, D., Hylton-Kong, T., Mehta, N., Figueroa, J., Bourne, D., . . . Behets, F. (2007). Decreased condom breakage and slippage rates after counseling men at a sexually transmitted infection clinic in Jamaica. *Contraception, 75,* 289–293.

Tashakkori, A., & Teddlie, C. (Eds.). (2003). *Handbook of mixed methods in social and behavioral research.* Thousand Oaks, CA. Sage.

Tashakkori, A., & Teddlie, C. (Eds.). (2010). *Handbook of mixed methods in social and behavioral research* (2nd ed.). Thousand Oaks, CA. Sage.

Teddlie, C., & Tashakkori, A. (2009). *Foundations of mixed methods research: Integrating quantitative and qualitative approaches in the social and behavioral sciences.* Thousand Oaks, CA. Sage.

Valente, T. (2010). *Social networks and health: Models, methods, and applications.* Oxford, UK: Oxford University Press.

Willis, G. (2004). *Cognitive interviewing: A tool for improving questionnaire design.* Thousand Oaks, CA: Sage.

NOTES

1. For a useful summary of some of these, see Tashakkori and Teddlie (2003, p. 711).
2. For more mixed methods examples, see Plano Clark and Creswell (2008). Part 2 of their reader contains nine illustrative studies.
3. For a summary of logistical and political barriers to integration, see Bryman (2006).
4. The amount of actual published mixed methods research in public health is much greater, however. Authors often do not explicitly label their mixed methods research as such.

IN FOCUS

Using Vignettes in Public Health Research

Paul Fleming and Michael Stalker

In research, vignettes are "short stories about hypothetical characters in hypothetical circumstances, to whose situation the interviewee is invited to respond" (Finch, 1987, p. 105). Participant responses can include perceptions, opinions, beliefs, attitudes, and behavioral or diagnostic predictions.

Vignettes are a mixed method technique used to approximate a real-world context in situations where observing or placing an individual in that actual context would not be possible, for either logistical or ethical reasons. The benefit of using vignettes as part of a data collection strategy—compared to context-absent forms of questioning—is that they present a more concrete and relatable context for participants to evaluate and respond to (Hughes & Huby, 2002). Since individuals' attitudes are often context-dependent and their decisions are based on various stimuli and cues, the presentation of contextual details in vignettes can elicit more valid responses (Finch, 1987).

Types of Vignette Research

Vignette-based research can be divided into three broad categories: exploratory, predictive, and experimental.

Exploratory

Exploratory studies, as detailed in Chapter 2, aim to better understand a given phenomenon and are often used to inform subsequent, more structured inquiry. In exploratory research, vignettes are utilized—in focus groups or in-depth interviews—to stimulate discussion about and conceptually explore a topic. The relatable context that vignettes provide can generate more targeted and meaningful responses than conventional qualitative techniques.

Thompson, Barbour, and Schwartz (2003), for example, utilized a vignette to prompt health professionals in focus groups and in-depth interviews to discuss their justifications for adhering to, or ignoring, patients' advance directives. Health professionals were presented with a fictional advance directive stating that should the patient experience "severe degenerative brain disease," the patient "should not be given active treatment such as antibiotics, ventilation, surgery, or blood transfusion" (p. 2). Then participants were presented with a detailed description of the patient, partially presented here:

> The patient is 78 years old. She lives in a residential home. Up until retirement she worked as a secretary to the headmaster of a private school. . . . The patient lives with dementia. She can walk and feed herself and needs some help with

dressing. She occasionally wanders at night. . . . One night, after a home outing, she comes down with a high fever. The doctor is called and examination shows that she has pneumonia. With antibiotic treatment she may make a full recovery, without it there is a significant chance she will die. (p. 2)

After reading the vignette, participants were asked to elaborate on what they would do next and why. If health professionals were asked simply how they respond to advance directives in the absence of a context, responses would have been relatively generic and more difficult to interpret. By using vignettes, Thompson and colleagues (2003) were able to mentally transport respondents to a situation and gain a more realistic and nuanced understanding of their opinions and decisions.

Predictive

Vignettes are also employed in a predictive capacity. In this context, respondents read a vignette and are then asked to respond to the vignette by choosing one of several structured responses. Responses can be opinions, attitudes, behavioral predictions, or any cognitive or behavioral element(s) of interest to a researcher. Variation of responses is then statistically described, and associations with independent variables are measured.

The British Social Attitudes survey, for example, is conducted every year in the United Kingdom to measure attitudes on health and other topics. The survey includes vignettes to help participants better conceptualize certain questions. For example, here is a question from the 2011 survey:

Suppose you were told by your GP [general practitioner] that you needed a hip replacement, as you were unable to walk unaided and the hip was causing you pain. How long do you think it would be reasonable to wait from the time your GP referred you to hospital before having an operation to replace your hip? (British Social Attitudes, 2010, p. 34)

Respondents were asked to answer in days, weeks, or months. The sentence prior to the question gave respondents contextual cues to better understand the situation and provide responses that are closer approximations of their true attitudes about waiting times. These data can then be analyzed to correlate tolerance for waiting times with demographic or other variables.

Experimental

Vignettes are commonly employed in an experimental capacity, wherein parts of a vignette are modified to produce multiple vignette versions. This design involves randomizing study participants to unique vignette versions, thereby minimizing threats to internal validity.

Experimental vignette designs are most often multifactorial, featuring a vignette with more than two factors (called dimensions) that the researcher manipulates. This produces multiple variations of the same vignette concept, differing only by selected factors of interest. Participants are randomized to read, and respond to, only one of the vignette variations (note: a single survey often includes multiple vignette concepts/questions). The benefit of this design, as with any experimental design, is that the influence of each factor (or independent variable) on a participant's response can be isolated.

The anatomy of a multifactorial vignette design consists of two primary elements: variables of interest (the vignette's dimensions) and the various permutations (or levels) of each dimension. A researcher might be interested in, for example, how patients' choices of medication are influenced by medication cost and packaging. Cost and packing are the two dimensions in this example. Cost might be divided into three levels: low, medium, and high. Packaging might contain only two levels: box or bottle. In this case, the vignette would have a total of six variations (three levels x two levels) and respondents would be randomly assigned to one of the six variations. Presenting multiple dimensions and levels in a single vignette variation allows for the analysis of interaction effects among dimensions and levels.

Research by St. Lawrence and colleagues (2004) provides an illustrative example of a factorial design. The authors set out to better understand physicians' treatment recommendations for sexually transmitted diseases (STDs). The researchers created a vignette with four dimensions: (1) patient's sex, (2) whether the patient described STD symptoms, (3) whether the patient reported having a sex partner diagnosed with an STD, and (4) whether the patient disclosed having high-risk sexual behavior. This vignette had four dimensions with two levels each, totaling 16 unique vignettes (2 x 2 x 2 x 2 = 16). One level from each of the four dimensions is shown here, followed by its alternative level in parentheses:

> You see a male [female] patient with acute non-purulent urethritis [no STD symptom mentioned]. You discover that the patient's sex partner was recently diagnosed with chlamydia [no information about partner(s)]. The patient also informs you of other recent high-risk sexual contacts [no information about high risk behavior]. (St. Lawrence et al., 2004, p. 1014)

A sample of 4,122 physicians was randomly assigned to receive 1 of the 16 vignettes and respond to questions rating the likelihood that they would take certain courses of action. Findings showed that physicians were more likely to use aggressive treatments for female patients than for male patients, and that factors indicating higher risk were all significant predictors of a physician's likelihood of using aggressive treatment options.

Developing Vignettes

Vignettes need to be plausible and relatable to respondents (Spalding & Phillips, 2007). Vignettes, and their corresponding questions and response options, also need to be constructed in such a way as to generate responses within a statistically acceptable range of variation. Failure to achieve either plausibility or adequate variability will result in poor validity and/or unusable data.

One of the simplest ways to develop vignettes is to transform relevant real-world scenarios into fictional narratives. Focus groups are also a good method to use for creating vignettes. Through iterative discussions, participants from the study population can provide salient details, dimensions, and levels that will be incorporated into the vignettes. Qualitative input into vignettes continues until stories and response categories are detailed and relevant enough (to the study population *and* the research objectives) to implement in survey form. Regardless of how the vignettes and response categories are developed, piloting the vignette instrument is critical to assess validity.

Additional Resources

Jenkins, N., Bloor, M., Fischer, J., Berney, L., & Neale, J. (2010). Putting it in context: The use of vignettes in qualitative interviewing. *Qualitative Research, 10*(2), 175–198.

Ludwick, R., & Zeller, R. (2001). The factorial survey: An experimental method to replicate real world problems. *Nursing Research, 50*(2), 129–133.

Rossi, P., & Nock, S. (1982). *Measuring social judgments: The factorial survey approach.* Beverly Hills, CA: Sage.

Wallander, L. (2009). 25 years of factorial surveys in sociology: A review. *Social Science Research, 38,* 505–520.

References

British Social Attitudes. (2010). Retrieved from http://www.natcen.ac.uk/series/british-social-attitudes

Finch, J. (1987). The vignette technique in survey research. *Sociology, 21*(1), 105–114.

Hughes, R., & Huby, M. (2002). The application of vignettes in social and nursing research. *Journal of Advanced Nursing, 37,* 382–386.

Spalding, N. J., & Phillips, T. (2007). Exploring the use of vignettes: From validity to trustworthiness. *Qualitative Health Research, 17,* 954–962.

St. Lawrence, J. S., Kuo, W. H., Hogben, M., Montano, D. E., Kasprzyk, D., & Phillips, W. R. (2004). STD care: Variations in clinical care associated with provider sex, patient sex, patients' self-reported symptoms or high-risk behaviors, partner STD history. *Social Science & Medicine, 59,* 1011–1018.

Thompson, T., Barbour, R., & Schwartz, L. (2003). Adherence to advance directives in critical care decision making: Vignette study. *BMJ, 327,* 1011.

20

Geographic Information Systems in Public Health

Candace Nykiforuk

Chapter 6 mentioned the epidemiological reliance on three categories of information to address public health issues: person, place, and time. **Geographic information systems** (GIS) offer tools and approaches to investigate and describe the second of these—the often overlooked place perspective. This chapter introduces GIS and its applications to public health.

A GIS combines mapping and statistical analysis to allow for the investigation of relationships between health and place and to present that information in a vivid, visual manner. Generally, a GIS is a computer-based system used for the integration and analysis of spatial data, which has the ability to generate extensive *relational databases* in order to examine statistical relationships that may occur across geographic areas. A **relational database** is a data storage model where sets of data organized in structured tables are linked to one another using unique identifier variables (i.e., employing the relational model).

A GIS comprises five key components: computer hardware, computer software, geographic and attribute data, a GIS analyst, and statistical methods for data modeling and analysis (Cromley & McLafferty, 2011). GIS software provides functions and tools designed to easily capture, store, update, manipulate, analyze, and display all forms of geographically referenced information (Riner, Cunningham, & Johnson, 2004).

A GIS database is similar to other relational databases, but also includes a database field that encodes the location of the variable on the surface of the earth using x,y coordinates. In other words, a GIS uses geo-referenced data to link a particular geographic area to other variables of interest, such as data on health outcomes, disease transmission, or health inequalities. This is how a GIS can be used to integrate spatial data with related qualitative or quantitative information (e.g., social, economic, political, health, or environmental conditions). These variables are listed as attributes of the spatial location in the relational database. Spatial analysis, or the analysis of geographically referenced variables, can then be used to identify and explore these variables of interest relative to location and then to create maps that display the geographic distributions of and relationships among those variables (see Figure 20.1). Some common types of public health questions that GIS are used to address are presented in the text box below.

Figure 20.1 Lifestyle and Risk Behavior, Adults in Hennepin County, Minnesota, 2010

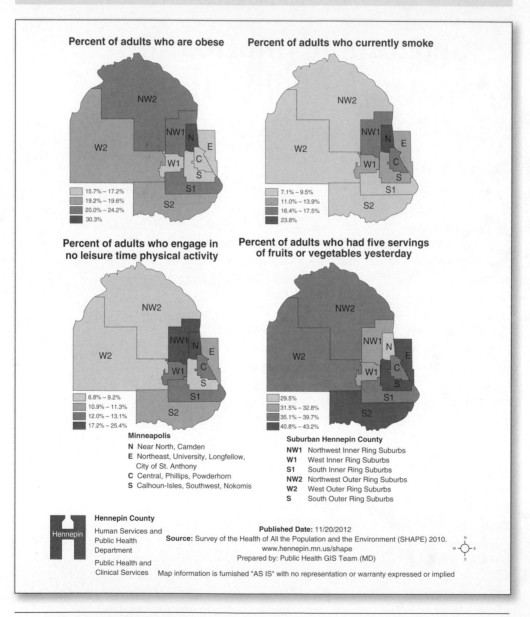

Source: Centers for Disease Control and Prevention.

TYPES OF PUBLIC HEALTH QUESTIONS ADDRESSED WITH GIS

Condition—what is occurring at a particular location
- What is the smoking rate at high schools in the low-income area of the city?

Location—where a behavior or outcome is occurring
- Where is the highest incidence of skin cancer in a country?

Trend—changes in a behavior or outcome at a particular location over time
- How has a disease spread across a region between year 1 and year 2?

Pattern—the spatial arrangement of a behavior or outcome
- Does incidence of a particular disease cluster in one or more areas?

Modeling—building scenarios to question what it would look like if a behavior or outcome occurred at a particular location over time
- How do asthma rates vary relative to different types and duration of environmental exposures?

GEOGRAPHIC INFORMATION SYSTEMS (GIS) IN PUBLIC HEALTH RESEARCH AND PRACTICE

Public health literature over the last few decades has recognized the value of understanding the context or environment of health issues when developing and implementing interventions. GIS have become a popular and valuable means to answer complex ecological questions in many public health arenas, including epidemiology, community medicine, environmental health, nursing, disease ecology, and health promotion, among others (Cromley & McLafferty, 2011; Foody, 2006; Goldman & Schmalz, 2000; McLafferty, 2003; Melnick & Fleming, 1999; Pearce, 2007; Riner et al., 2004).

Public health oriented GIS applications can be generally categorized into four predominant but interrelated themes: disease surveillance, risk analysis, health access and planning, and community health profiling (Nykiforuk & Flaman, 2011). This section provides an overview of each of these categories, with examples of research-generated maps cited for each category.

Disease Surveillance

Disease surveillance, one of the most longstanding uses of GIS in public health, is the tracking and synthesis of data on the incidence, prevalence, and spread of disease across place and time (Rushton, 2003). These applications systematically connect known epidemiologic data on disease with relevant, geographically referenced features in the physical and/or social environment. Figure 20.2 illustrates the use of GIS to characterize malaria risk data from an ongoing malaria incidence study that enrolled 300 participants under 6 years old; the data were used for planning malaria control and elimination programs in Bandiagara, Mali (Coulibaly et al., 2013).

Figure 20.2 Corrected Spatial Distribution of (A) the 300 Children Sampled and (B) the 296 Malaria Episodes Recorded Between June 2009 and May 2010 in Bandiagara

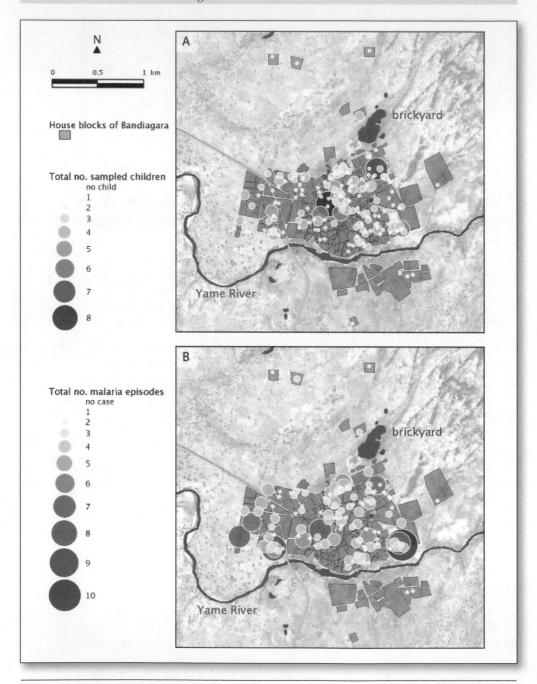

Source: Coulibaly et al. (2013).

Disease surveillance consists of two primary activities: disease mapping and disease modeling.

Disease Mapping

Many of the numerous disease mapping applications reported in the GIS literature involve either surveillance of disease incidence and prevalence to support control efforts or are dedicated to producing disease atlases that report the historical trends of the disease. Public health researchers have used GIS to examine everything from vector-borne illnesses to communicable diseases to cancer, in rural and urban areas of developed and developing nations worldwide. To this end, disease mapping is an effective public health tool for helping to prevent the spread of diseases, facilitating the development of interventions, evaluating health outcomes, appraising population risks, and summarizing and displaying health indicators (see, e.g., Horst & Coco, 2010; Nykiforuk & Flaman, 2008; Pedigo & Aldrich, 2011; Siffel, Strickland, Gardner, Kirby, & Correa, 2006; Vally et al., 2012).

Integration of disease mapping into routine or real-time health surveillance (Chapter 5) enhances rapid identification of unusual disease patterns or local disease outbreaks (Gosselin, Lebel, Rivest, & Douville-Fradet, 2005). It also provides opportunity for timely research into the disease, targeted intervention strategies, and a mechanism for collecting geographically referenced, time-oriented data for measuring the success of disease interventions such as the introduction of a vaccine. Simple mapping applications can be beneficial for summarizing and displaying health indicators in an intuitive way that can be utilized by healthcare providers, public health managers, and decision makers. Some of the more common uses include documenting health outcomes, assessing population risks, and planning intervention strategies (Sabesan & Raju, 2005).

Disease Modeling

Disease modeling takes the disease mapping application one step further to offer more comprehensive scenario-building features to inform future disease control (Vieira, Webster, Weinberg, & Aschengrau, 2008) and to generate predictive models that facilitate appropriate public health intervention (McKee, Shields, Jenkins, Zenilman, & Glass, 2000). Modeling and mapping of epidemiological data with geographic and environmental features is typically used to develop hypotheses about disease transmission. This can help health practitioners target immunization and screening initiatives and effectively allocate resources and personnel. Spatial analyses that identify patterns of disease can inform development of interventions to promote behavior change to offset social factors in disease risk and transmission.

The appeal of disease modeling applications lies in their flexible functionality. They can be employed to develop sophisticated spatial models based on identified risk or protective factors that, by extrapolation, can be used to predict disease risk over broad geographic areas where data may not be available. GIS applications systematically represent the spatial distribution of disease to allow exploration of statistical relationships between variables that may not be apparent using traditional tools and techniques. Additionally, modeling disease transmission along with socioeconomic factors can demonstrate how processes such as climate change interact with human rights to favor disease emergence (Winch, 1998). In this way, disease modeling can have a critical role in documenting the geography of social inequalities in public health and human rights.

Risk Analysis

Risk analysis often occurs in the domain of environmental health and is used to understand or mitigate the risk of exposure in relation to a factor of interest. This is achieved through *risk mapping* or *risk assessment*. This suite of GIS applications is also used for risk surveillance or monitoring, risk evaluation or vulnerability analysis, risk management, risk communication, and emergency planning. Typical risk analysis projects employing GIS examine exposure to hazardous waste or pollution, proximity to industrial sites or traffic, or residence in a locality with characteristics that may foster disease (e.g., landscapes favorable to disease vectors, poor social conditions, lack of access to health care; Bergquist, 2001; Brody, Peck, & Highfield, 2004; Caudeville et al., 2011; Weuve et al., 2012). An example is provided in Figure 20.3.

GIS-enhanced risk analysis can be information-intensive for scenario-building exercises. It encompasses data from secondary sources (i.e., administrative, census, environmental, or other data), primary data collected from field work or surveys, and remote sensing data collected via satellite or other data collection means not in direct contact with the object of interest. This intensity of information is necessary to facilitate risk modeling and prediction, and as such, it is often combined with disease modeling to estimate or evaluate environmental disease hazards for a given population or geographic area. The use of this GIS application helps researchers and practitioners to relate many different sources of environmental information to the places where people spend time in a simple, objective manner and to understand how that shapes the onset and spread of disease (Jarup, 2000). When done systematically over time, it also facilitates the creation of risk profiles that can enhance public health risk management.

Risk analysis via GIS can be used to help researchers identify locations of urgent need, increase the effectiveness of control efforts in targeted geographic areas, and generate information or design interventions that help to prevent the spread of outbreaks and epidemics over large areas and across populations. Used in this way, GIS applications have much to offer situational analysis and policy development. For example, the World Health Organization (WHO) uses GIS tools to map environmental health risks and to monitor the effects of disease control policies on the improvement of the environment and health in the population. WHO's Health Mapper system (http://gis.emro.who .int/PublicHealthMappingGIS/HealthMapper.aspx) has global mapping capability for infectious disease. This information is presented to facilitate management at the county or district level, with data on population distribution, environment, and basic health and social infrastructure that can be regularly monitored and updated using national health statistics and other important social or population data. GIS approaches for risk analysis can also be used for the effective communication of various health risks to the general public, whether related to environmental exposures, pollution, disease outbreaks, or vaccination strategies (Ali, Emch, Ashley, & Streatfield, 2001; Caudeville et al., 2011; Choi, Afzal, & Sattler, 2006; Maantay, 2002; Weuve et al., 2012).

Figure 20.3   Childhood Lead Poisoning Risk Analysis, Philadelphia

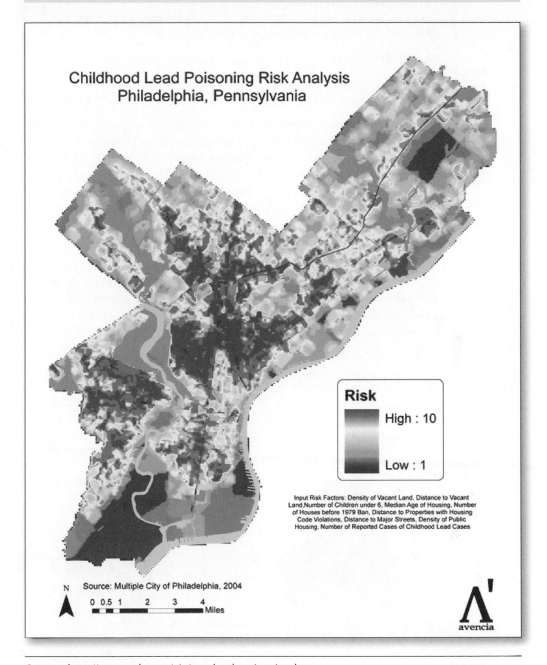

Source: http://www.cdc.gov/gis/mg_lead_poisoning.htm.

Health Access and Planning

GIS applications for health access and planning generally employ market segmentation and network analysis tools that support analysis of health services and delivery.

Health Access: a population's ability to use health services when needed (i.e., accessibility); typically describes relationships between service needs and characteristics of the service delivery system

Health Planning: planning for the purposes of improving health and accessibility of health services

Studies of geographic accessibility often assess specific populations' access to health services in a particular place or area over time in order to provide meaningful information for public health decision making (Cromley & McLafferty, 2011). These analyses can help decision makers improve allocation of resources based on identified needs and priorities, including when and where to locate health services or implement targeted public health initiatives. For example, consider the maps in Figure 20.4 documenting neighborhood-level disparities in access to prescription medication (Amstislavski, Matthews, Sheffield, Maroko, & Weedon, 2012).

Within the health access and planning cadre of GIS applications, we can also use *market segmentation* to create a general profile of how different segments of a population do or do not access a particular health service. This information can help public health managers and decision makers hypothesize about and investigate possible causes of inequitable use of services and then to target resources and tailor delivery to underserved groups that may have certain characteristics or needs.

Figure 20.4   Pharmacies and Selected SES Indicators by Community in New York City

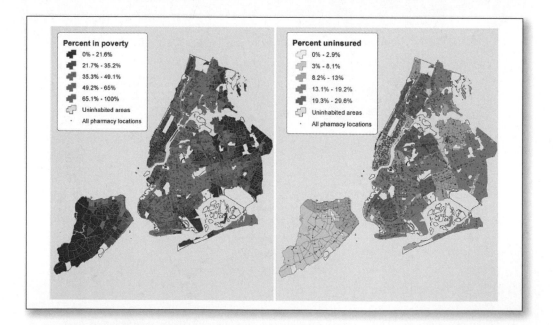

Source: Amstislavski et al. (2012).

The network of health services in a defined area (i.e., the physical location of various health services and the distance and ways to travel between them) is also a critical element for health access and planning GIS applications. *Network analysis* can be used to determine client catchment areas or to identify the proportion of the population in a given area with potential access to services within a defined network. GIS can be used to map, model, and communicate these types of analyses.

Market segmentation and network analysis come together in *market utilization* GIS applications, which are used to identify and characterize a population's realized access to services within a network or catchment area. Here, market utilization applications describe and analyze actual patterns of health service utilization, rather than modeling hypothetical uses. This can help public health practitioners identify and plan for service delivery to small geographic areas as well as specialized populations dispersed over larger areas. Further, mapped presentations of community needs relative to provision and utilization of health services can help ensure that future interventions, projects, and facilities limit overlap with current services and are located where there is a demand for services.

Community Health Profiling

Community health profiling is a rapidly emerging area of GIS. This category of applications generally involves compiling and mapping of social, structural, economic, and political information relative to the health of a population or community. Community profiles are built using variables that may influence well-being as well as specific health outcomes. Those variables may include, for example, sociodemographic factors, disease morbidity and mortality statistics, health behaviors, economic conditions, public health program availability, or coverage by local or higher-level legislation. Combined with the spatial location of infrastructure such as built environment features (e.g., roads, green spaces, churches, schools, grocery stores, hospitals and clinics, recreational facilities, public utilities), this research approach facilitates comprehensive and nuanced investigation of how community environments, or selected aspects thereof, shape opportunities and barriers for health—as well as their direct impact on health.

When created appropriately, community health profiles can be used by public health researchers for the purposes of

- generating hypotheses for obtaining more information to better serve the needs of a community,
- systematically observing and assessing relationships between the environment and health, and
- using evidence to inform subsequent public health planning and research (Basara & Yuan, 2008).

Profiling approaches can also be employed to improve access to health-related information by health professionals and to allow governments to engage diverse stakeholders in partnerships to improve community health. GIS has been used in this

Figure 20.5a Community Need by ZIP code in Western New York

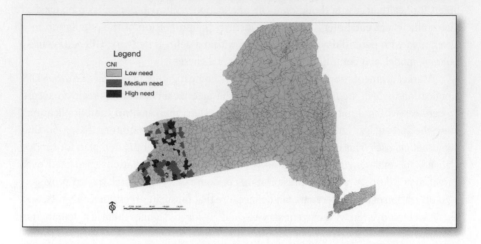

ZIP codes with darker tones had higher community needs. For this figure, only data from Western New York were entered. No data were entered or are shown for the rest of New York State.

Source: Caley (2004).

Figure 20.5b Locations of Different Types of Community Organizations in Selected ZIP Codes With Low, Medium, and High Community Need Scores

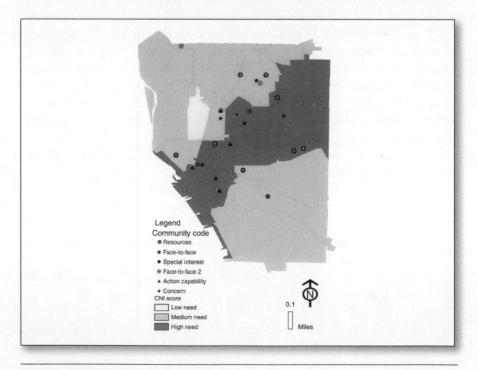

Source: Caley (2004).

capacity to support health needs assessment and problem solving, enhance community-level provision of health services, track common illnesses, develop and implement interventions, initiate strategic prevention activities, and inform healthy public policy (Horst & Coco, 2010; Moss & Schell, 2004; Nykiforuk & Flaman, 2011; Scotch & Parmanto, 2006; Scotch, Parmanto, Gadd, & Sharma, 2006). The maps provided in Figures 20.5a and 20.5b demonstrate how public health nurses could utilize GIS to design population-based community interventions (Caley, 2004).

Community health profiling approaches also permit sophisticated analyses of social determinants of health behavior and outcomes. For example, McLafferty (2003) documented the complex patterns of disadvantage related to the intersection of poor health outcomes and geographical barriers to health care with those based on class, race, and ethnicity.

The range of GIS applications described above were discussed as separate categories to illustrate various public health uses, but in practice these categories often overlap or are used in conjunction with one another to illuminate a particular health issue. Table 20.1 provides a few examples of these uses of GIS.

Table 20.1   Examples of Uses of GIS in Public Health

Research Topic	Focus	Sample Reference(s)
Walkability and neighborhood characteristics related to health behaviors and outcomes	Analyze environmental determinants of health-related behavior; address public health issues related to urban planning and community design	Hess & Russell (2012); Schopflocher et al. (2012); Wall et al. (2012)
Access to healthy and unhealthy foods, including assessment of food deserts	Inform both food security and obesity prevention efforts	McEntee & Agyeman (2010); Yamashita & Kunkel (2012)
Tobacco control	Document and analyze the locations and characteristics of tobacco billboards; assess marketing practices of the tobacco industry relative to the socioeconomic profiles of particular areas	Luke, Ribisl, Smith, & Sorg (2011); Ogneva-Himmelberger, Ross, Burdick, & Simpson (2010)
Injury prevention and control	Investigate spatial determinants of injury	N. Bell & Schuurman, (2010); Rinner, Moldofsky, Cusimano, Marshall, & Hernandez (2011)

PLANNING AND IMPLEMENTING GIS

This section outlines a basic protocol for planning and implementing GIS research. The protocol is a conceptual framework meant to guide the use of a GIS and, as such, does not include software-specific information. Rather, the steps provided are intended to support the user in making decisions about research using this tool—from conceptualizing the problem to gathering the data to executing the analysis—and then using maps appropriately to communicate the research findings. The maps created using GIS play many important roles, including as a critical starting point for research inquiry, a creative and flexible tool for hypothesis generation and testing, as well as one mode of sharing research findings with target audiences.

Basic Steps in GIS Research

Step 1: Conceptualizing the Research Question

The first step in planning a GIS study (as with any study) is to conceptualize a research question. The question will dictate the mapping and analysis approaches most appropriate for meaningfully addressing the research problem. As a general rule, any GIS-related research must be tied to geography and have to do with some aspect of place. There are five general types of research questions that a GIS can be used for; a particular research project may involve one or more of these types.

FIVE BASIC TYPES OF RESEARCH QUESTIONS FOR GIS PROJECTS

1. *What exists (or is occurring) at a specific location?* This is a descriptive question that is not trying to address why or how something exists, but focuses on what is or is not at a location of interest. For example, how many health providers are located in a low-income area of a city?

2. *Where should something be located?* This type of question determines ideal or inferior locations relative to a set of criteria that the researcher is interested in. For example, a social services organization may want to identify the best (or worst) places to locate a youth emergency shelter.

3. *What changes have occurred in a particular place over a period of time?* This can be an exploratory or explanatory question. From an exploratory perspective, the researcher is interested in identifying whether a change

occurred and to what extent within a particular time frame. For example, how have patterns of influenza rates in Canada changed in the last 10 years? In contrast, an explanatory perspective would examine the existence and scope of change along with other factors such as social, economic, or environmental conditions to attempt to reveal why a change may (or may not) have occurred. For example, how have patterns of influenza rates in Canada changed in the last 10 years relative to provincial immunization campaign efforts?

4. *Are there patterns in the geographic data? If so, what are they?* This is another question type that can be both exploratory and explanatory. For example, it may explore whether health outcomes are concentrated in particular areas (exploratory) and how those outcomes are relative to different degrees of an environmental exposures (explanatory); consider rates of childhood asthma and exposure to traffic-related air pollution near major roadways.

5. *What can be predicted if certain geographic or socio-environmental characteristics are changed?* This is a scenario-building or modeling question that can help researchers answer public health questions that will inform intervention development. For example, where should public health units be located on bus routes in order to be most accessible to a high-needs population? What might be the effect on air particulate exposures for residents living near a proposed location for an industrial plant?

To begin, we must determine what it is about the public health issue we want to investigate, how we will do that with the help of a GIS and its related analytical tools, and the geographic level at which we will analyze—and later display—the variables of interest. This will help dictate the mapping application chosen for the task. Given the recent emphasis of the public health community on knowledge translation and utilization (see Chapter 22), the researchers should consider the end uses of the findings that their GIS research will generate in the initial planning stage. Prior to mapping, we need (1) a clear understanding of the rationale for mapping (i.e., why we want to "see" a particular set of variables and how that will inform analysis); (2) a data analysis plan; and (3) the intended audience of the results being shared through the map(s), including a consideration of what might be most interesting to that audience, whether they are researchers, for use in hypothesis generation or testing, or an external audience such as local policymakers, health unit staff (e.g., to share results of the analysis), or both. This is a prime opportunity to ensure that we have all of the required data available as well as the appropriate tools and expertise to conduct the planned analyses.

Step 2: Data Decisions (Gathering the Data)

Once we have conceptualized the research question and rationale for mapping, and defined the data analysis and communication purposes of the project, we next need to identify the specific variables to be used and the sources of data for those variables. For example, if we are interested in examining health services utilization relative to a municipal population, we will require data sets that can provide information about health services, utilization rates, and census data. Decisions about which variables—and data sets—will be used for analysis and mapping are informed by whether we want to send a message about the number of people in a community irrespective of area or the relative population of the municipality when compared to others of different sizes. We can use a variable for raw population to denote the number of people living in an area, or the variable for population density may be used, which is a relative indicator of population as it represents the number of people per square kilometer.

The decision about which variables to use must be informed by the research question determined in Step 1, but may also include considerations of data quality, availability, and cost—either for the collection of primary data or for the procurement of secondary data. The timing of data collection and the level of aggregation should be consistent with the phenomena under investigation and, if using multiple data sources, should be congruent across data sets. We may select variables conceptually based on outcomes of interest relative to what is already known about a particular area or population in order to facilitate comparisons with others, or with different areas that are geographically proximal to, adjacent to, or otherwise comparable with (or of interest to) the reference area.

The size and shape of the geographic area to be investigated may also produce different results depending on the chosen political unit of study. Administrative boundaries can be used (e.g., county units, postal areas, census tracts), and these data are often available from government or private sources. Alternatively, GIS can be used to define neighborhoods via adjacency, the sharing of a common boundary, or, by proximity, the distance between areas. Geo-referenced "neighborhoods," defined on the basis of socio-economic (or other) variables, might be better geographic reference for GIS analyses than traditional administrative areas (Krieger, Waterman, Lemieux, Zierler, & Hogan, 2001; McElroy, Remington, Trentham-Dietz, Robert, & Newcomb, 2003), particularly in the case of small area analyses. This is because census tracts are recreated intermittently across census years, and ZIP codes (or postal codes) are sometimes redesignated or rebounded for mail delivery as municipalities evolve.

Similarly, if there are no formally defined boundaries that can be used for categorizing location data, a GIS can be used to divide the area into a number of arbitrary sectors to designate boundary lines that consider structural factors like residential patterns, planning eras, historical significance, major streets, and activity areas (see, e.g., Schopflocher et al., 2012; Zenilman et al., 2002). Methodological rigor requires that this process involve a priori operationalization of boundary definitions and representation of neighborhood clusters to the highest degree possible in order to minimize bias imposed by the GIS user.

Step 3: Data Preparation and Integration in a GIS Environment

In this step, all of the necessary data needed for the GIS analyses are compiled and integrated into the GIS. It may be necessary to prepare the nongeographic data for inclusion in the GIS by *geo-coding* the data set to the target geography (Rushton, 2009). As with other relational databases, additional data cleaning may be required to prepare nongeographic data for spatial analysis and mapping. It will be necessary to identify the area of interest and the level of aggregation to be mapped (e.g., country, state, region, city, neighborhood). Further, when adding boundary shape files of the area, we must also define a coordinate system to tell the software how the lines and polygons in the shape file relate to a geographic location.

> **Geo-coding:** Assigning geographic coordinates, typically latitude and longitude, to a location based on some other type of geographic information such as street address or ZIP code. It may involve techniques such as interpolating an address from a street network or assigning a point at the center of a designated land parcel (i.e., within a specific boundary).

In order to begin mapping, we must have all the data—both shape files (i.e., the base maps of the area) and attribute data (i.e., data about some characteristic about the location)—in the GIS software platform selected for use. This can be done in two ways: (1) the data can be manually entered into the attribute table associated with the base map, or (2) the data set can be imported and joined to the attribute table using a *common unique identifier*. A common unique identifier is a variable that includes a distinct value or string of characters for each row in the dataset and that commonly appears in different data sets. For example, Statistics Canada includes the variable *csduid*, a unique identifier for each census subdivision, in the attribute table of its census subdivision base maps as well as in the census data aggregated at the census subdivision level. This allows users to easily join—or link—the demographic data with the corresponding municipalities on the map in a GIS relational database. When we join data, missing data or broken links will prevent a successful linkage between data sets. Manual cleaning of the data in the data tables is necessary to repair these types of errors and join the data sets for mapping and analysis.

Once joined, attribute data can be represented on a map by adding thematic layers; each layer represents a different factor, such as health services locations, demographics (ethnicity, income, education, etc.), environmental conditions, health outcomes, or road networks.

Step 4: Selecting a Mapping and Analytic Approach

Once all data are cleaned and entered, we need to select a data visualization or mapping approach as well as our software. There are many software options for GIS mapping that range from very basic programs for viewing maps to very complex systems that can be used to create and manipulate many map layers and perform powerful mathematical operations. One consideration is whether the software employs vector or raster mapping approaches, or both. Vector mapping involves connecting a series of points and lines, while raster mapping uses polygons that represent bounded areas (see Figure 20.6).

Figure 20.6   Vector Versus Raster Approaches

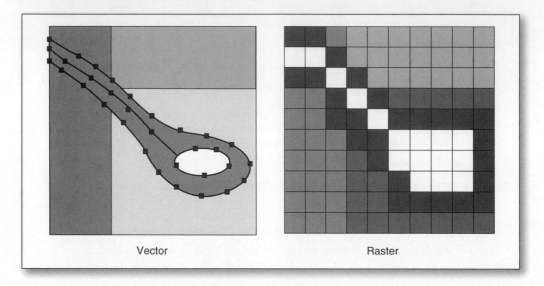

Vector   Raster

Source: Adapted from DiBiase (2014).

Major GIS Software Options

- ArcGIS (ESRI): www.esri.com
- MapInfo (Pitney Bowes): www.pitneybowes.ca
- Geomedia: www.intergraph.com
- Map3D: www.map3d.com

Examples of Software Options Linked to Other Analytical Software

- EpiMap module of EpiInfo (CDC): wwwn.cdc.gov/epiinfo
- SPSS Maps module and conversion utility of SPSS: www-01.ibm.com/software/analytics/spss
- SAS Maps in SAS: http://support.sas.com/rnd/datavisualization/maps/index.html
- STATA mapping application: www.stata.com

There are also many public domain, open source, and freeware GIS options available on the Internet.

The remainder of Step 4 involves data analysis and production of a series of maps to show potential patterns and statistical relationships in the data. A flowchart may help organize the data analysis steps relative to each research question. For example, will the analysis be limited to overlays of thematic data or include multivariate statistics (e.g., regressions) and spatial analysis? The answer to that question depends on the nature of the research questions posed for the study.

COMMON TYPES OF GIS ANALYSES

Exploratory Analysis: Allows the user to identify a phenomenon. Is there a spatial pattern?

Descriptive Analysis: Allows the user to describe a phenomenon. What is the nature of the spatial pattern? How has the pattern changed across place or over time?

Explanatory Analysis: Allows the user to explain a phenomenon. What causes the pattern to change? What was the relative contribution of different factors in causing the pattern to change?

Predictive Analysis: Allows the user to predict future occurrences or patterns of the phenomenon. What will the spatial pattern look like in the future? How will the spatial pattern be affected by a particular intervention?

The interpretation of output from a GIS analysis is directly related to the elements considered in the creation of the maps resulting from the data analysis. Maps generated from surveillance data can be generated as actual numbers, standardized rates, or mapped residuals of numbers compared with the population. There are several approaches for mapping data in a GIS platform. The most common way of analyzing patterns of health events using GIS is to create *choropleth maps* of the outcome of interest (e.g., disease incidence, prevalence rates).

Choropleth, or thematic, mapping is the display of the variation in a selected variable across space, for example, the distribution of disease cases across a health region. Choropleth maps display data values as a series of specific class intervals that are assigned a unique color, shade, or pattern so that differences in data ranges are visible by the variation of colors or pattern across the map (Figure 20.7).

The key consideration in the process is choice of intervals, as different interval schemes can change how the map looks and the message it sends. Data illustration may occur through presentation of gradients or different intervals of variable units through color, use of bar charts or pie charts superimposed on the map, dots to represent individual cases of the variable, or the use of unique values to describe nominal variables. The view or extent of the map can also be tailored to the topic and message of interest. In some cases a view of a zoomed area of map may be more informative than the full view of an area, or vice versa.

Figure 20.7   Choropleth Map of Obesity Rates in the United States, 2011

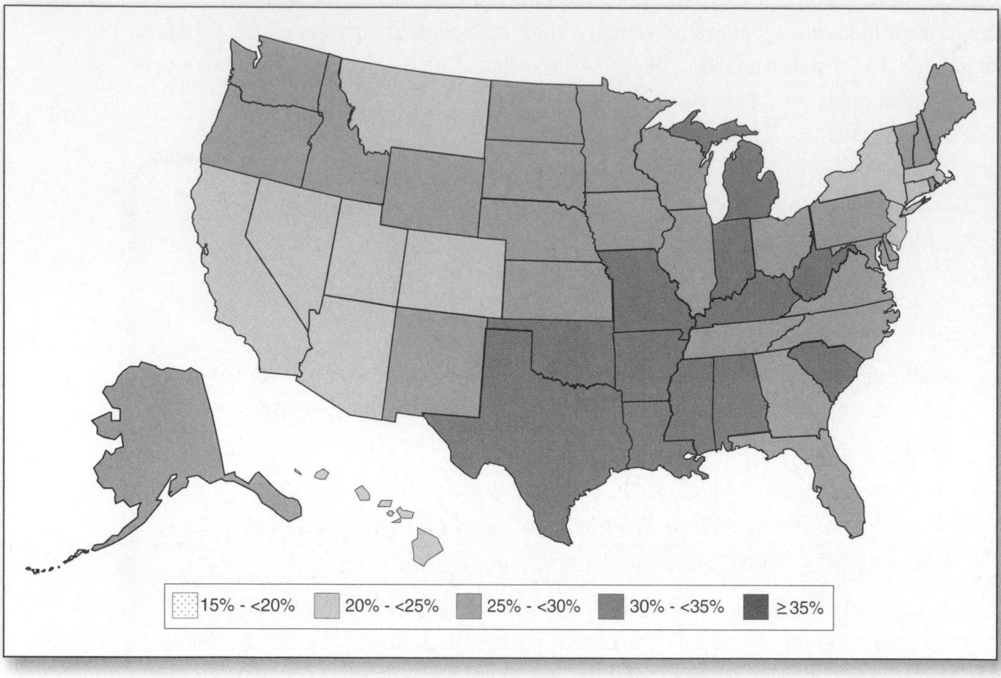

15% - <20%	20% - <25%	25% - <30%	30% - <35%	≥35%

Source: Centers for Disease Control and Prevention (2013).

Map sequences, or lag maps, can be used to study the spread of a variable across space and time, as in the instances of infectious disease or diffusion of a health program or policy. This involves generating a series of maps that are displayed side by side to show distributions of the variable of interest at different points in time. Map sequences can also be an animated series that actively illustrates continuous and dynamic change. The Centers for Disease Control and Prevention's NCHHSTP Atlas (www.cdc.gov/nchhstp/atlas) is an excellent example of a source for interactive maps and data queries that show spatial and temporal data for a range of communicable diseases.

Data queries are the use of a GIS to select areas of interest based on different combinations of variables in the dataset (e.g., neighborhoods in a municipality that have high-risk populations). This is an exploratory application that can be used to quickly identify places with a particular set of characteristics. For example, if we wanted to identify neighborhoods in a municipality with a high-risk population and poor access to health services, we would construct a data query based on the variables that make up the high-risk profile and the type(s) of health services of interest.

Step 5: Communicating Findings and Encouraging Feedback

This step involves data dissemination, or sharing the finalized maps with the target audience(s). Maps can be shared in a wide variety of ways—from traditional, static paper-based documents to interactive websites where users can access and manipulate the data to create maps to meet their own interests. Anticipating that different audiences will have different information needs, you will have to conceptualize and articulate the various messages you want your maps to communicate.

Methodological Techniques and Considerations

Utilization of GIS applications in public health is rapidly growing along with the increasing accessibility of practitioner-oriented training and publicly available, web-based GIS platforms. While appropriate use of GIS requires user training, expertise, and experience (particularly for more sophisticated applications), there remain a number of critical methodological issues that must be considered by any GIS user to ensure that the information presented on maps is done so in a valid, reliable, and meaningful way.

GIS and Spatial Analysis

Spatial analysis is a set of statistical techniques for analyzing data with geographic characteristics and provides the foundation for many GIS applications (see, e.g., Cromley & McLafferty, 2011; Gatrell & Loytonen, 2004; Rushton, 2003). Spatial analysis is concerned with the analysis of point patterns, surface analysis, and areal analysis. Point pattern analysis is used to identify patterns (e.g., clusters of disease incidence) in the spatial location of the phenomena under investigation and may involve testing hypotheses about the observed pattern of points. Surface analysis often involves spatial dependency, interpolation, and uncertainty measures to reconstruct a "surface" from which samples were measured (e.g., distribution of environmental hazard samples across an area to create a surface of relatively higher and lower risk). Areal analysis requires the delimitation of areas depicted by bounded polygons (e.g., a census subdivision) and population survey data such as census information or national health statistics. It involves data aggregation and statistical tests such as regression to investigate the distribution of a phenomenon across a population of interest.

> There are many accessible tools to implement spatial analysis techniques available in addition to ArcGIS Spatial Analyst, which is commonly used. For example, see the options listed on these websites:
>
> - www.spatialecology.com/htools/tooldesc.php
> - www.csiss.org/GISPopSci/research/tools/spatial.php
> - www.spatialanalysisonline.com

Spatial clusters

Spatial clusters are simply unusual concentrations of events such as disease cases. Exploratory analysis can identify event patterns, while confirmatory analysis can verify a suspected or preexisting pattern (Koch & Denike, 2001). Any analysis of spatial clusters must

- identify the number of cases relative to the population risk for the health event of interest;
- define the geographical extent or scale at which the clustering occurs; and
- articulate and implement statistically generated decision criteria for assessing how much clustering exists and at what level of statistical significance; these decision criteria must be generated using a probability distribution such as the Poisson distribution, which is used to model rare binary events in large populations, or through Monte Carlo simulation models, which can be used to yield a large number of random possible outcomes (Cromley & McLafferty, 2011).

There are many known challenges in spatial cluster analysis. The *small numbers problem* can arise when examining incidence or prevalence rates using spatial cluster analysis to compare data from areas that differ in population size or when a small geographic area is used. Because the calculated rates of disease for small areas vary more and are less reliable than those for large areas, a difference of one or two cases can greatly influence prevalence or incidence rates (Jon, 2001). This can be addressed through the use of smoothing techniques (see below), the use of statistical probability mapping where the statistical significance of rates are mapped rather than the rates themselves, or the inclusion of additional years of data in the analytic data set (Green, 2012). The Poisson distribution test can be used to assess statistical significance by measuring probability values that show the likelihood of the disease rate occurring given the normal rate of disease in the corresponding regional or national population (Cromley & McLafferty, 2011).

Smoothing techniques and spatial filtering

Smoothing techniques, such as Empirical Bayes smoothing, combine mapping and simple interval display of disease rates to adjust for variation relative to the size of the population on which they are based. Thus, these techniques can also be used to address the small area numbers problem. Disease rates are adjusted upward or downward (i.e., smoothed) according to the size of the population on which they are based. This pulls rates more toward the population base rate, making them less variable. Small area rates are smoothed more than large area rates to reflect differences in the reliability of rates linked to population size (Ranta & Penttinen, 2000).

Spatial filter models smooth point data to permit the calculation of values for central data points. Typically, the spatial filter technique involves placing a grid over the geographic area of interest, where each grid line intersection serves as the center of a circle. Disease rates are calculated for each circle in the series across the gridded areas to generate a continuous surface (Talbot, Kulldorff, Forand, & Haley, 2000). Spatial filtering techniques offer more precise approaches for modeling patterns of disease than smoothing techniques because they are not limited by the political boundaries of administratively defined areas.

Spatial autocorrelation and kernel estimation

Spatial autocorrelation is the degree to which there is spatial dependence of data values over space (Getis, 2008). Assessment of autocorrelation can be used to help test the significance of event clusters and is undertaken using measures such as Anselin's local indicators of spatial autocorrelation (LISA) or the G-statistic to measure the association between a value at a particular place and values for nearby or adjacent areas (Cromley & McLafferty, 2011).

Similarly, kernel estimation can be used to identify, explore, and display spatial patterns of health data by generating a continuous surface of point data through the density of events or cases (Koch & Denike, 2001; Robinson, 2000). There are several approaches for kernel estimation, each employing a different technique to identify locations of health event clusters. For example, one approach uses Monte Carlo procedures to simulate possible spatial patterns of health events within a fixed geographical population to create alternative maps of health events (Rushton & Lolonis, 1996). Another method examines only clusters that occur around cases, as opposed to those dispersed throughout a bounded area of interest. Kernel estimation can also be done utilizing a geographical analysis machine that involves testing for statistical significance of disease clusters and a spatial scan statistic which accounts for multiple testing (Cromley & McLafferty, 2011).

Kriging

Kriging depicts a discrete set of point measurements as a continuous surface while considering the distances between points and the spatial autocorrelation of measurements along those points (Briggs & Elliott, 1995). The mean is estimated from the best linear-weighted moving average. Kriging creates *risk contours* of point data to generate polygons that can be used for GIS-based analyses such as the *area-proportion technique* for population estimates from census data (Dent, Fowler, Kaplan, Zarus, & Henriques, 2000). This method is used to analyze disparate types of geo-referenced data by estimating values within a given polygon based on the values of polygons in another data layer. For example, it is possible to use kriging to estimate the number of people living in a selected contour based on the number of people living in census blocks in the same area in a target polygon. If a contour polygon crosses a number of census blocks, then a proportion of the area of the census blocks lying within the target polygon is used to compute the population numbers. Advantages of using kriging to develop risk contours are that it (1) provides a standard error for estimated grid point values that fall outside the range of known data values, making it possible to compute confidence intervals around predictions, and (2) models spatial dependence present in the data under analysis (Cromley & McLafferty, 2011).

Regression analysis

Regression analysis is a common suite of statistical techniques used to assess the relationship between variables (see Chapter 18). It includes many approaches for modeling relationships between a dependent variable and its covariates, or independent variables of interest. Common forms of regression analysis in geography include linear regression, logistic regression, multiple regression, and Poisson regression.

The statistical association between the variable of interest and independent (or predictor) variables can be estimated at the individual level, the ecological or environmental level, or multilevel, including both individual- and environmental-level data in the model (Pikhart et al., 1997). Logistic regression can be used at the individual level to examine the influence of selected variables on a health outcome of interest. At the eco-logical or environmental level, variation in the odds of the health outcome between different geographic areas can be modeled using the method of weighted least squares regression. Multilevel, or hierarchical, modeling is used to investigate health outcomes where cases at one level (e.g., individuals) are nested within units at a higher level (e.g., neighborhoods; Pickett & Pearl, 2001). Multilevel modeling assumes that cases within the same study area will be more alike than cases from different study areas, suggesting that it is important to carefully define the study areas at each level in the analysis.

Accessibility measures

Spatial analyses of accessibility of health services often examine the location of a given population relative to points of health service delivery and the distance between them. Adequate assessment of accessibility can be a complex endeavor requiring several different measures of access (Martin, Wrigley, Barnett, & Roderick, 2002). For example, distance may be operationalized as spherical distance (e.g., using latitude and longitude), Euclidean (straight-line, or linear) distance between two or more coordinate points, aerial distance (as the crow flies), total travel-time, or road-travel time (Ricketts, Savitz, Gesler, & Osborne, 1994). When examining movement of people from place to place, the distance measure(s) chosen should accurately reflect actual travel patterns and barriers. While Euclidean distance is often the default measure in a GIS, it may be more accurate to use the GIS to calculate distance or travel time along existing routes in a transporta-tion network. In this way, the user can assess differences by transportation mode and account for variations caused by peak flow periods.

Exposure measures

Isopleth maps can be used to portray an extensive number of data points as a surface (e.g., via kriging), much like a weather map. This can be particularly useful for illustrating regional differences in the case of small samples sizes, where region-level estimates of risk or exposure cannot be provided. Data analysis is not limited to administrative units such as municipalities, census tracts, or ZIP codes, but can still reveal variations in the data across a prescribed geographic area. Thus, isopleth maps, although not as commonly used as other mapping approaches, can be useful for mapping disease occurrence or risk of adverse health outcomes, especially at regional, state, or national levels where data limitations may make other analyses implausible (Bell, Hoskins, Pickle, & Wartenberg, 2006). Figure 20.8 provides an example of an isopleth map of SIDS mortality rates in North Carolina over time with a choropleth map of the same data for comparison.

Data treatment in GIS mapping

Different types of data are represented as layers, or themes, in GIS mapping. A GIS data layer is either a *vector* (i.e., data that occur as a set of points, lines, and polygons) or *raster* (i.e., grid-based data) file that contains attribute data such as demographics, health behaviors, mortality rates, environmental features, or road networks in a relational database. *Overlay* is the operation that allows the GIS user to present combinations of layers together to describe a geographic area's character-istics as well as the relationships between the variables of interest in that area. Map

Figure 20.8   Comparison of Isopleth (a) and Choropleth (b) Maps for Smoothed SIDS Mortality Rates of North Carolina

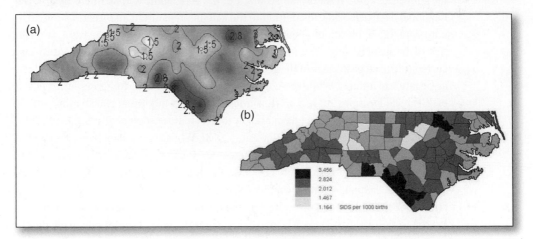

Source: Berke (2004).

operators, such as spatial statistics, can be applied to existing layers to create new layers and add new attributes to the spatial data (Contini, Bellezza, Christou, & Kirchsteiger, 2000).

Precision in data choices helps to ensure utility of the maps produced through GIS applications. As maps are produced to aid decision making by knowledge users in these domains, the development of a spatial database may be meaningless without a clear delineation of the goals for using that information for evidence-based decision making (Brooker & Michael, 2000). To mitigate misuse or misrepresentation of data in a GIS, it is important to create a log for metadata, which is a written, detailed description of the data used and their sources, including the geographic area(s) represented, who created the data set and when, and the intended use of the original data sets (Dent et al., 2000). Further, communication or involvement of knowledge users (e.g., through participatory GIS approaches) in the development and display of mapped information may enhance the uptake of the end product (Elwood, 2006).

Another potential issue is the *modifiable areal unit problem* wherein conclusions from GIS-based analyses may vary because the spatial area of interest is often selected based on administrative boundaries that are potentially not conducive to examining spatial patterns of disease or other health outcomes (Mitra & Buliung, 2012). To prevent this problem, the spatial unit selected for study should be meaningful to the issue of interest; large enough to be visible on a map, avoid small numbers, and protect the privacy of individuals and groups; small enough to reveal important spatial patterns; similar in size to other geographic areas to facilitate comparisons; and at a scale that is reflective of the underlying disease/health event process. In other words, the availability and resolution of GIS data should be consistent with the scale at which the health event of interest occurs.

Data accuracy

Ultimately, the capacity of a GIS to help the user generate meaningful information for knowledge users rests on the accuracy of the geographic and attribute data in the relational database. Thus, in addition to the careful preparation and treatment of attribute data, GIS applications should utilize accurate location data for the cases or facilities to be mapped (e.g., geo-coded address data, postal codes, x,y coordinates) and current digitized base maps of the geographic area of interest that permit analysis at the aggregation of interest. While geo-coding is a common technique for representing postal or ZIP code locations on a map (Rushton, 2009), it is often not effective in rural or remote areas where a single code may apply to a very large geographic area (Green, 2012; Hurley, Saunders, Nivas, Hertz, & Reynolds, 2003). While the availability and quality of maps at different aggregations or for different areas can vary substantially around the world, recent developments such as Google Earth and Google Street View are readily accessible in the public domain and have reduced barriers to access maps. But it is still critical for the GIS user to be aware that the quality of results from analysis is directly related to the quality of data and models used and the data assumptions made during data collection as well as in the data analysis and mapping stages.

Misrepresentation of data and other misuses of maps

Mark Monmonier's (1996) important book *How to Lie With Maps* is essential reading for anyone creating maps, working with GIS for data analysis, or using the information presented on a map. It is tremendously easy to create a bad map—whether intentionally or unintentionally—that fundamentally misrepresents the data presented and distorts the findings of data analysis (Rytkonen, 2004) or, at minimum, is confusing for map audiences (Parrott, Hopfer, Ghetian, & Lengerich, 2007). For example, different map projections or different aggregations or classifications of the same data can portray very different pictures of the same data in a geographic area (Monmonier, 1996). Color, graphics, and animation on a map can also be used to clarify or conceal data patterns across place or time. To help prevent misinterpretation of complex data presented in a GIS map, use detailed legends and supplemental text, where appropriate, recognizing that providing a legend does not make an otherwise bad map good.

GIS AND GLOBAL HEALTH

GIS has become an essential tool for public health research and practice on global health issues and in international settings. It is most often employed for its disease surveillance and health access and planning applications, the products of which target disease prevention, reduction of health disparities, and improved access to health and medical services. Remote sensing data, or data collected via satellite imagery or other remote sources, plays an essential role in GIS used in global health work (Dambach et al., 2012; Wang et al., 2013). For example, consider Dambach et al.'s (2009) work on risk mapping of malaria in the Nouna district of Burkina Faso. Here, remote sensing was used to collect data on areas of low and high risk for malaria based on environmental factors such as land cover conditions (Figure 20.9).

Figure 20.9   Land Cover Distribution in 500 m Buffer Zone Around the Villages of Sere (highest risk) and Dembelela (lowest risk), Land Cover Risk Within the Survey Region (pie diagram, same legend)

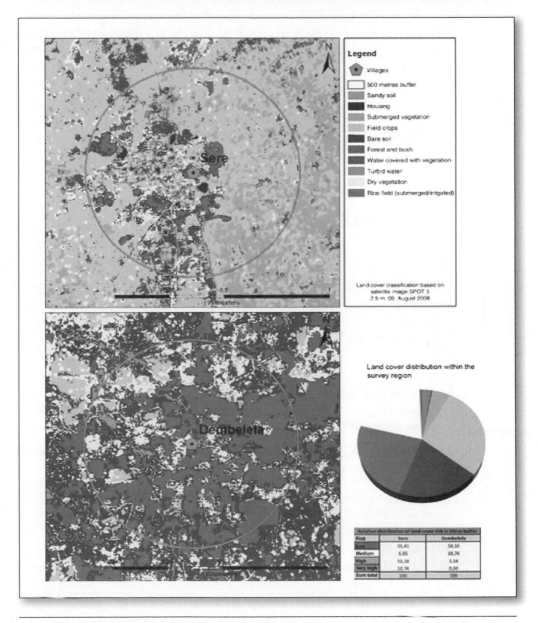

Source: Dambach et al. (2009).

Emerging public health concerns such as the impacts of climate change or the need for emergency planning for natural disasters or epidemics are other critical topics that can be informed by GIS methodologies. In addition to surveillance and monitoring capacities on a national or international scale, the use of GIS can offer public health officials the ability to effectively undertake real-time reporting to the public on both regular and emergency public health concerns. In these ways, GIS can be used to document, understand, and predict patterns in health and the effect on both residents (e.g., Yang et al., 2012) and travelers (e.g., Bauer & Puotinen, 2002) around the world.

Global health-related GIS work is conducted and shared by university-based units and private for-profit enterprise, and the WHO offers both static and interactive maps that portray the spatial distribution of public health issues—and a range of related factors—in developed and developing nations. For example, consider the WHO's Communicable Disease Global Atlas (http://apps.who.int/globalatlas), an interactive resource to create maps that illustrate social and environmental determinants of infectious disease transmission. Internationally oriented GIS applications allow public health surveillance and planning efforts to extend beyond geo-political or organizational boundaries to truly take on a global perspective of the factors influencing the delivery of public health as well as health outcomes across populations.

EXAMPLES OF INTERNATIONAL AND GLOBAL HEALTH GIS APPLICATIONS

- Centers for Disease Control and Prevention (United States): http://gis.cdc.gov
- Public Health Agency of Canada: http://204.187.39.30/surveillance/Maps.aspx
- Public Health Information Development Unit (Australia): www.publichealth.gov.au/interactive-mapping
- Public Health Observatories—Health Profiles Interactive (United Kingdom): www.apho.org.uk/default.aspx?QN=HP_INTERACTIVE2012
- WHO Global Health Observatory: www.who.int/gho/map_gallery/en
- HealthMap: http://healthmap.org/en

While many of the challenges of using GIS for global health are the same as the challenges of appropriate use of GIS in other public health domains, key issues specific to global health are those that make the conduct of public health research different in international or global settings. These settings are often low-resource environments, are in the developing world, and/or are in geographically remote locations. Thus, challenges typically involve (1) technology access barriers associated with Internet access, the costs of GIS software, and so on; (2) limits to the availability of data suitable for mapping or spatial analysis; (3) poor-quality data being presented on maps to seem rigorous and meaningful; and (4) low capacity among public health workers to properly analyze the information, increasing the likelihood of data misinterpretation (Fisher & Myers, 2011). Researchers and the GIS industry are currently exploring ways to make GIS technology more accessible to and well suited for those working in lower resource settings by offering reduced-cost GIS platforms, free and open-source GIS applications that do not require Internet access, or mobile or remote mapping systems that do not require continual linkage to a cellular or Internet network.

CURRENT ISSUES AND FUTURE DIRECTIONS

One long-standing issue in the GIS community concerns delineating and establishing political, economic, societal, and ethical accountability in the use of GIS. An example is how the use of GIS technology can simultaneously marginalize and empower the geographic area or population under exploration (Matthews, Moudon, & Daniel, 2009). Differential access to data, GIS software, and the results of GIS or spatial analyses can simultaneously create an opportunity for greater public participation in spatial decision making and exclude weaker or less powerful groups through selective or exclusive participation processes (Harris & Weiner, 1998).

The detailed, and potentially very precise, information that can result from the use of GIS technology to link, analyze, and share health, socioeconomic, environmental, and political data with a particular place can be a powerful aid for the public and decision makers to strengthen communities and improve health outcomes. However, this capacity for detail and precision can also adversely impact an individual's or group's privacy by revealing sensitive information or suggesting patterns or relationships in the data that may be misinterpreted by those unfamiliar with the community or issue. There are few ways to aggregate the data in a GIS platform to ensure privacy protection while maintaining the integrity of the spatial relationships in the data (Boulos, Curtis, & AbdelMalik, 2009). This is particularly concerning in a public health context where spatial data are linked with specific demographic or health information of individuals. Guidelines for responsible and ethical use of GIS across its multitude of public health applications should become systematized and institutionalized by the field to offset growing concerns as the technology continues to advance— in both technical capacity and potential user accessibility.

Emerging GIS technologies have created opportunities to broaden applications for public health in more creative and dynamic ways. For example, participatory GIS approaches adopt a community empowerment approach to actively involve community members in the generation and sharing of spatial information to support local action, advocacy, planning, and decision making (Elwood, 2006). Participatory GIS has been used with a range of public health, community development, and policy issues and often includes tools such as photography, sketch maps, or narratives that are more easily used and understood by community members (see, e.g., London, Zagofsky, Huang, & Saklar, 2011). Participatory GIS approaches facilitate the co-creation of knowledge by both the community and the researcher, and subsequently, meaningful identification of community priorities for public health action. When used in developing countries, participatory GIS can help to overcome social and structural barriers like availability of maps and infrastructure, cultural and social definitions of neighborhood boundaries, and engagement of community members in the uptake of health services.

Similarly, volunteered geographic information (VGI), or the use of web-based technologies and handheld devices, allows community members and the general public to contribute content to data sets for analysis and mapping (see, e.g., Langley, Messina, & Grady, 2013; Roche, Propeck-Zimmermann, & Mericskay, 2013). VGI offers researchers access to immediate and detailed local, experiential knowledge that is voluntarily provided by the user—often without the need for formal participant recruitment. While not yet a familiar tool in public health applications, this new direction is rapidly gaining popularity, particularly as more and more personal handheld devices such as smartphones and tablets come preloaded with simple-to-use geographic capabilities.

Inclusion of qualitative data (e.g., audio, photographs, videos, narratives) in analysis and products of GIS platforms is another developing area (see, e.g., Hawthorne & Kwan, 2012). For example, geographic definitions of community boundaries may be defined by the members that make up those communities. As such, community members' knowledge and perceptions of community can be essential to consider in local health needs assessments. This information is often obtained through quantitative surveys, but the depth and richness of the knowledge shared by community members through interviews, focus groups, or visual means may offer stronger documentation of their perceptions and health concerns.

The future of GIS in public health research is ripe for continued uptake of existing technologies and the development of new applications and techniques for addressing complex health issues worldwide. GIS is increasingly being used to inform public health intervention planning and program delivery, particularly in the arenas of sociophysical environment and community health (see, e.g., Elmore, Flanagan, Jones, & Heitgerd, 2010). Other recent examples from established areas of GIS application include identifying optimal settings for cancer prevention and control (Alcaraz, Kreuter, & Bryan, 2009); modeling the spread of disease in a pandemic outbreak (Aleman, Wibisono, & Schwartz, 2011); developing effective planning and decision-making platforms for community coalitions (Baum, Kendall, Muenchberger, Gudes, & Yigitcanlar, 2010); actively examining how social, economic, and political processes impact injury rates across geographic areas (Bell & Schuurman, 2010); and investigating adverse health effects associated with increases in temperatures and poor air quality (Merbitz, Buttstädt, Michael, Dott, & Schneider, 2012).

ADDITIONAL RESOURCES

Books

Craglia, M., & Maheswaran R. (2010). *GIS in public health practice*. Boca Raton, FL: CRC Press.
Cromley, E. K., & McLafferty, S. L. (2011). *GIS and public health* (2nd ed.). New York, NY: Guilford Press.
Fotheringham, A. S., & Rogerson, P. A. (2009). *The SAGE handbook of spatial analysis*. London, UK: Sage.
Shekhar, S., & Xiong, H. (Eds.). (2008). *Encyclopedia of GIS*. New York, NY: Springer.

Journals

Environmental Health Perspectives

Geospatial Health

Health & Place

International Journal of Geographical Information Science

International Journal of Health Geographics

Journal of Geographical Systems

Online Sources

Centers for Disease Control and Prevention: www.cdc.gov/gis

Geospatial Analysis: www.spatialanalysisonline.com

Measure Evaluation: www.cpc.unc.edu/measure/our-work/gis

Nykiforuk, C. I. J. (2012). Geographic information systems (annotated bibliography). In *Oxford bibliographies online: Public health.* Available from http://www.oxford bibliographies.com

WHO Global Health Observatory Map Gallery: http://gamapserver.who.int/ mapLibrary

WHO Health Mapper: http://gis.emro.who.int/PublicHealthMappingGIS/ HealthMapper.aspx

Select Examples of GIS Tools and Tutorials

ArcGIS Resources: http://resources.arcgis.com/en/home

ArcGIS Tutorials: http://help.arcgis.com/en/arcgisdesktop/10.0/help/index .html#//00v20000000t000000.htm

ESRI FAQ and Tutorials: www.esri.ca/en/faq-tutorials

GIS in Public Health Research—Harvard School of Public Health: www.hsph .harvard.edu/gis/arcgis-tips

GIS Lounge: www.gislounge.com/tutorials-in-gis

GISTutor: www.gistutor.com

GIS Tutorial 1: Basic Workbook; GIS Tutorial 2: Spatial Analysis; GIS Tutorial 3: Advanced Workbook: http://esripress.esri.com

GIS Tutorials and Exercises—Harvard College Library: http://hcl.harvard.edu/ libraries/maps/gis/tutorials.html

GIS Tutorials on YouTube: www.youtube.com/user/GISTutorials

Public Health Mapping and GIS—World Health Organization http://gis.emro.who .int/PublicHealthMappingGIS/HealthMapper.aspx

REFERENCES

Alcaraz, K. I., Kreuter, M. W., & Bryan, R. P. (2009). Use of GIS to identify optimal settings for cancer prevention and control in African American communities. *Preventive Medicine, 49*(1), 54–57.

Aleman, D. M., Wibisono, T. G., & Schwartz, B. (2011). A nonhomogeneous agent-based simulation approach to modeling the spread of disease in a pandemic outbreak. *Interfaces, 41*, 301–315.

Ali, M., Emch, M., Ashley, C., & Streatfield, P. K. (2001). Implementation of a medical geographic information system: Concepts and uses. *Journal of Health Population and Nutrition, 19*(2), 100–110.

Amstislavski, P., Matthews, A., Sheffield, S., Maroko, A. R., & Weedon, J. (2012). Medication deserts: Survey of neighborhood disparities in availability of prescription medications. *International Journal of Health Geographics, 11*(1), 1–13.

Basara, H. G., & Yuan, M. (2008). Community health assessment using self-organizing maps and geographic information systems. *International Journal of Health Geographics, 7*, 67.

Bauer, I. L., & Puotinen, M. E. (2002). Geographic information systems and travel health. *Journal of Travel Medicine, 9*, 308–314.

Baum, S., Kendall, E., Muenchberger, H., Gudes, O., & Yigitcanlar, T. (2010). Geographical information systems: An effective planning and decision-making platform for community health coalitions in Australia. *Health Information Management Journal, 39*(3), 28–33.

Bell, B. S., Hoskins, R., Pickle, L., & Wartenberg, D. (2006). Current practices in spatial analysis of cancer data: Mapping health statistics to inform policymakers and the public. *International Journal of Health Geographics, 5*(1), 49.

Bell, N., & Schuurman, N. (2010). GIS and injury prevention and control: History, challenges, and opportunities. *International Journal of Environmental Research and Public Health, 7*, 1002–1017.

Berke, O. (2004). Exploratory disease mapping: Kriging the spatial risk function from regional count data. *International Journal of Health Geographics, 3*, 18.

Bergquist, N. R. (2001). Vector-borne parasitic diseases: New trends in data collection and risk assessment. *Acta Tropica, 79*, 13–20.

Boulos, M. N. K., Curtis, A. J., & AbdelMalik, P. (2009). Musings on privacy issues in health research involving disaggregate geographic data about individuals. *International Journal of Health Geographics, 8*(1), 46.

Briggs, D., & Elliott, P. (1995). The use of geographical information systems in studies on environment and health. *World Health Statistics Quarterly, 48*, 85–94.

Brody, S. D., Peck, B. M., & Highfield, W. E. (2004). Examining localized patterns of air quality perception in Texas: A spatial and statistical analysis. *Risk Analysis, 24*, 1561–1574.

Brooker, S., & Michael, E. (2000). The potential of geographical information systems and remote sensing in the epidemiology and control of human helminth infections. *Advances in Parasitology, 47*, 245–288.

Caley, L. M. (2004). Using geographic information systems to design population-based interventions. *Public Health Nursing, 21*, 547–554.

Caudeville, J., Boudet, C., Denys, S., Bonnard, R., Govaert, G., & Cicolella, A. (2011). Characterization of environmental inequality in Picardie based on the linkage of multimedia exposure model and a geographic information system. *Environnement Risques & Santem, 10*, 485–494.

Centers for Disease Control and Prevention. (2013). Adult obesity facts. Retrieved from http://www.cdc.gov/obesity/data/adult.html

Choi, M., Afzal, B., & Sattler, B. (2006). Geographic information systems: A new tool for environmental health assessments. *Public Health Nursing, 23*, 381–391.

Contini, S., Bellezza, F., Christou, M. D., & Kirchsteiger, C. (2000). The use of geographic information systems in major accident risk assessment and management. *Journal of Hazardous Materials, 78*, 223–245.

Coulibaly, D., Rebaudet, S., Travassos, M., Tolo, Y., Laurens, M., Kone, A. K., . . . Doumbo, O. K. (2013). Spatio-temporal analysis of malaria within a transmission season in Bandiagara, Mali. *Malaria Journal, 12*(1), 82.

Cromley, E. K., & McLafferty, S. L. (2011). *GIS and public health* (2nd ed.). New York, NY: Guilford Press.

Dambach, P., Machault, V., Lacaux, J. P., Vignolles, C., Sié, A., & Sauerborn, R. (2012). Utilization of combined remote sensing techniques to detect environmental variables influencing malaria vector densities in rural West Africa. *International Journal of Health Geographics, 11*(1), 1–12.

Dambach, P., Sié, A., Lacaux, J. P., Vignolles, C., Machault, V., & Sauerborn, R. (2009). Using high spatial resolution remote sensing for risk mapping of malaria occurrence in the Nouna district, Burkina Faso. *Global Health Action, 2*, 10.

Dent, A. L., Fowler, D. A., Kaplan, B. M., Zarus, G. M., & Henriques, W. D. (2000). Using GIS to study the health impact of air emissions. *Drug and Chemical Toxicology, 23*, 161–178.

DiBiase, D. (2014). Integrating geographic data. In *Nature of Geographic Information*. Retrieved from https://www.e-education.psu.edu/natureofgeoinfo/book/export/html/1604

Elmore, K., Flanagan, B., Jones, N. F., & Heitgerd, J. L. (2010). Leveraging geospatial data, technology, and methods for improving the health of communities: Priorities and strategies from an expert panel convened by the CDC. *Journal of Community Health, 35*(2), 165–171.

Elwood, S. (2006). Critical issues in participatory GIS: Deconstructions, reconstructions, and new research directions. *Transactions in GIS, 10*, 693–708.

Fisher, R. P., & Myers, B. A. (2011). Free and simple GIS as appropriate for health mapping in a low resource setting: A case study in eastern Indonesia. *International Journal of Health Geographics, 10*, 15.

Foody, G. M. (2006). GIS: Health applications. *Progress in Physical Geography, 30*, 691–695.

Gatrell, A., & Loytonen, M. (2004). *GIS and health: GISDATA 6*. Philadelphia, PA: Taylor & Francis.

Getis, A. (2008). A history of the concept of spatial autocorrelation: A geographer's perspective. *Geographical Analysis, 40*, 297–309.

Goldman, K. D., & Schmalz, K. J. (2000). The gist of GIS (geographic information systems). *Health Promotion Practice, 1*, 11–14.

Gosselin, P., Lebel, G., Rivest, S., & Douville-Fradet, M. (2005). The Integrated System for Public Health Monitoring of West Nile Virus (ISPHM-WNV): A real-time GIS for surveillance and decision-making. *International Journal of Health Geographics, 4*(1), 21.

Green, C. (2012). Geographic information systems and public health: Benefits and challenges. *National Collaborating Centre for Infectious Disease, 37*, 1–12.

Harris, T., & Weiner, D. (1998). Empowerment, marginalization, and "community-integrated" GIS. *Cartography and Geographic Information Science, 25*(2), 67–76.

Hawthorne, T. L., & Kwan, M. P. (2012). Using GIS and perceived distance to understand the unequal geographies of healthcare in lower-income urban neighbourhoods. *Geographical Journal, 178*(1), 18–30.

Hess, D. B., & Russell, J. K. (2012). Influence of built environment and transportation access on body mass index of older adults: Survey results from Erie County, New York. *Transport Policy, 20*, 128–137.

Horst, M. A., & Coco, A. S. (2010). Observing the spread of common illnesses through a community: Using geographic information systems (GIS) for surveillance. *Journal of the American Board of Family Medicine, 23*(1), 32–41.

Hurley, S. E., Saunders, T. M., Nivas, R., Hertz, A., & Reynolds, P. (2003). Post office box addresses: A challenge for geographic information system-based studies. *Epidemiology, 14*, 386–391.

Jarup, L. (2000). The role of geographical studies in risk assessment. In P. Elliott, J. Wakefield, N. G. Best, & D. Briggs (Eds.), *Spatial epidemiology: Methods and applications* (pp. 415–433). Oxford, UK: Oxford University Press.

Jon, Z. (2001). Methods of mortality (incidence) rates interpretation assessment in small populations. *Central Europe Journal of Public Health, 9*, 14–21.

Koch, T., & Denike, K. (2001). GIS approaches to the problem of disease clusters: A brief commentary. *Social Science & Medicine, 52*, 1751–1754.

Krieger, N., Waterman, P., Lemieux, K., Zierler, S., & Hogan, J. W. (2001). On the wrong side of the tracts? Evaluating the accuracy of geocoding in public health research. *American Journal of Public Health, 91*, 1114–1116.

Langley, S. A., Messina, J. P., & Grady, S. C. (2013). Utilizing volunteered information for infectious disease surveillance. *International Journal of Applied Geospatial Research, 4*(2), 54–70.

London, J. K., Zagofsky, T. M., Huang, G., & Saklar, J. (2011). Collaboration, participation and technology: The San Joaquin Valley Cumulative Health Impacts Project. *Gateways: International Journal of Community Research and Engagement, 4*, 12–30.

Luke, D. A., Ribisl, K. M., Smith, C., & Sorg, A. A. (2011). Family Smoking Prevention and Tobacco Control Act: Banning outdoor tobacco advertising near schools and playgrounds. *American Journal of Preventive Medicine, 40*, 295–302.

Maantay, J. (2002). Mapping environmental injustices: Pitfalls and potential of geographic information systems in assessing environmental health and equity. *Environmental Health Perspectives, 110*(Suppl 2), 161–171.

Martin, D., Wrigley, H., Barnett, S., & Roderick, P. (2002). Increasing the sophistication of access measurement in a rural healthcare study. *Health & Place, 8*, 3–13.

Matthews, S. A., Moudon, A. V., & Daniel, M. (2009). Work group II: Using geographic information systems for enhancing research relevant to policy on diet, physical activity, and weight. *American Journal of Preventive Medicine, 36*(4S), S171–S176.

McElroy, J. A., Remington, P. L., Trentham-Dietz, A., Robert, S. A., & Newcomb, P. A. (2003). Geocoding addresses from a large population-based study: Lessons learned. *Epidemiology, 14*, 399–407.

McEntee, J., & Agyeman, J. (2010). Towards the development of a GIS method for identifying rural food deserts: Geographic access in Vermont, USA. *Applied Geography, 30*(1), 165–176.

McKee, K. T., Shields, T. M., Jenkins, P. R., Zenilman, J. M., & Glass, G. E. (2000). Application of a geographic information system to the tracking and control of an outbreak of Shigellosis. *Clinical Infectious Disease, 31*, 728–733.

McLafferty, S. (2003). GIS and healthcare. *Annual Review of Public Health, 24*, 25–42.

Melnick, A. L., & Fleming, D. W. (1999). Modern geographic information systems: Promise and pitfalls. *Journal of Public Health Management and Practice, 5*, 8–9.

Merbitz, H., Buttstädt, M., Michael, S., Dott, W., & Schneider, C. (2012). GIS-based identification of spatial variables enhancing heat and poor air quality in urban areas. *Applied Geography, 33*, 94–106.

Mitra, R., & Buliung, R. N. (2012). Built environment correlates of active school transportation: Neighborhood and the modifiable areal unit problem. *Journal of Transport Geography, 20*(1), 51–61.

Monmonier, M. (1996). *How to lie with maps* (2nd ed.). Chicago, IL: University of Chicago Press.

Moss, M. P., & Schell, M. C. (2004). GIS a scientific framework and methodological tool for nursing research. *Advances in Nursing Science, 27*(2), 150–159.

Nykiforuk, C. I. J., & Flaman, L. M. (2008). *Exploring the utilization of geographic information systems in health promotion and public health* (CHPS Document No. 08-001). Edmonton, Alberta, Canada: University of Alberta, School of Public Health, Centre for Health Promotion Studies.

Nykiforuk, C. I., & Flaman, L. M. (2011). Geographic information systems (GIS) for health promotion and public health: a review. *Health Promotion Practice, 12*(1), 63–73.

Ogneva-Himmelberger, Y., Ross, L., Burdick, W., & Simpson, S. A. (2010). Using geographic information systems to compare the density of stores selling tobacco and alcohol: Youth making an argument for increased regulation of the tobacco permitting process in Worcester, Massachusetts, USA. *Tobacco Control, 19,* 475–480.

Parrott, R., Hopfer, S., Ghetian, C., & Lengerich, E. (2007). Mapping as a visual health communication tool: Promises and dilemmas. *Health Communication, 22*(1), 13–24.

Pearce, J. (2007). Incorporating geographies of health into public policy debates: The GeoHealth Laboratory. *New Zealand Geographer, 63*(2), 149–153.

Pedigo, A., & Aldrich, T. (2011). Neighborhood disparities in stroke and myocardial infarction mortality: A GIS and spatial scan statistics approach. *BMC Public Health, 11*(1), 644.

Pickett, K. E., & Pearl, M. (2001). Multilevel analyses of neighbourhood socioeconomic context and health outcomes: A critical review. *Journal of Epidemiology and Community Health, 55*(2), 111–122.

Pikhart, H., Prikazsky, V., Bobak, M., Kriz, B., Celko, M., Danova, J., . . . Pretel, J. (1997). Association between ambient air concentrations of nitrogen dioxide and respiratory symptoms in children in Prague, Czech Republic. Preliminary results from the Czech part of the SAVIAH Study. Small area variation in air pollution and health. *Central Europe Journal of Public Health, 5,* 82–85.

Ranta, J., & Penttinen, A. (2000). Probabilistic small area risk assessment using GIS-based data: A case study on Finnish childhood diabetes. Geographic information systems. *Statistics in Medicine, 19,* 2345–2359.

Ricketts, T. C., Savitz, L. A., Gesler, W., & Osborne, D. N. (1994). *Geographic methods for health services research.* Lanham, MD: University Press of America.

Riner, M. E., Cunningham, C., & Johnson, A. (2004). Public health education and practice using geographic information system technology. *Public Health Nursing, 21*(1), 57–65.

Rinner, C., Moldofsky, B., Cusimano, M. D., Marshall, S., & Hernandez, T. (2011). Exploring the boundaries of web map services: The example of the online injury atlas for Ontario. *Transactions in GIS, 15*(2), 129–145.

Robinson, T. P. (2000). Spatial statistics and geographical information systems in epidemiology and public health. *Advances in Parasitology, 47,* 81–128.

Roche, S., Propeck-Zimmermann, E., & Mericskay, B. (2013). GeoWeb and crisis management: Issues and perspectives of volunteered geographic information. *GeoJournal, 78*(1), 21–40.

Rushton, G. (2003). Public health, GIS, and spatial analytic tools. *Annual Review of Public Health, 24*(1), 43–56.

Rushton, G. (2009). *Geocoding health data: The use of geographic codes in cancer prevention and control, research, and practice.* Boca Raton, FL: CRC Press.

Rushton, G., & Lolonis, P. (1996). Exploratory spatial analysis of birth defect rates in an urban population. *Statistics in Medicine, 15,* 717–726.

Rytkonen, M. J. (2004). Not all maps are equal: GIS and spatial analysis in epidemiology. *International Journal of Circumpolar Health, 63*(1), 9–24.

Sabesan, S., & Raju, K. H. K. (2005). GIS for rural health and sustainable development in India, with special reference to vector-borne diseases. *Current Science, 88,* 1749–1752.

Schopflocher, D., VanSpronsen, E., Spence, J. C., Vallianatos, H., Raine, K. D., Plotnikoff, R. C., & Nykiforuk, C. I. (2012). Creating neighbourhood groupings based on built environment features to facilitate health promotion activities. *Canadian Journal of Public Health, 103*(9), eS61–eS66.

Scotch, M., & Parmanto, B. (2006). Development of SOVAT: A numerical-spatial decision support system for community health assessment research. *International Journal of Medical Informatics, 75*, 771–784.

Scotch, M., Parmanto, B., Gadd, C. S., & Sharma, R. K. (2006). Exploring the role of GIS during community health assessment problem solving: Experiences of public health professionals. *International Journal of Health Geography, 5*, 39. Retrieved from http://www.pubmedcentral.nih.gov

Siffel, C., Strickland, M. J., Gardner, B. R., Kirby, R. S., & Correa, A. (2006). Role of geographic information systems in birth defects surveillance and research. *Birth Defects Research Part A: Clinical and Molecular Teratology, 76*, 825–833.

Talbot, T. O., Kulldorff, M., Forand, S. P., & Haley, V. B. (2000). Evaluation of spatial filters to create smoothed maps of health data. *Statistics in Medicine, 19*(1718), 2399–2408.

Vally, H., Peel, M., Dowse, G. K., Cameron, S., Codde, J. P., Hanigan, I., & Lindsay, M. D. (2012). Geographic information systems used to describe the link between the risk of Ross River virus infection and proximity to the Leschenault estuary, WA. *Australian and New Zealand Journal of Public Health, 36*, 229–235.

Vieira, V. M., Webster, T. F., Weinberg, J. M., & Aschengrau, A. (2008). Spatial-temporal analysis of breast cancer in upper Cape Cod, Massachusetts. *International Journal of Health Geographics, 7*(1), 46.

Wall, M. M., Larson, N. I., Forsyth, A., Van Riper, D. C., Graham, D. J., Story, M. T., & Neumark-Sztainer, D. (2012). Patterns of obesogenic neighborhood features and adolescent weight: A comparison of statistical approaches. *American Journal of Preventive Medicine, 42*(5), e65–e75.

Wang, Z., Liu, Y., Hu, M., Pan, X., Shi, J., Chen, F., . . . Christiani, D. C. (2013). Acute health impacts of airborne particles estimated from satellite remote sensing. *Environment International, 51*, 150–159.

Weuve, J., Puett, R. C., Schwartz, J., Yanosky, J. D., Laden, F., & Grodstein, F. (2012). Exposure to particulate air pollution and cognitive decline in older women. *Archives of Internal Medicine, 172*, 219–227.

Winch, P. (1998). Social and cultural responses to emerging vector-borne diseases. *Journal of Vector Ecology, 23*, 47–53.

Yamashita, T., & Kunkel, S. R. (2012). Geographic access to healthy and unhealthy foods for the older population in a US metropolitan area. *Journal of Applied Gerontology, 31*, 287–313.

Yang, K., LeJeune, J., Alsdorf, D., Lu, B., Shum, C. K., & Liang, S. (2012). Global distribution of outbreaks of water-associated infectious diseases. *PLoS Neglected Tropical Diseases, 6*(2), e1483.

Zenilman, J. M., Glass, G., Shields, T., Jenkins, P. R., Gaydos, J. C., & McKee, K. T. (2002). Geographic epidemiology of gonorrhea and chlamydia on a large military installation: Application of a GIS system. *Sexually Transmitted Infections, 78*(1), 40–44.

21

Public Health 2.0

Fresh Approaches to Old Problems

Hans C. Ossebaard and Lisette van Gemert-Pijnen

A s evidenced by the uses of GIS profiled in Chapter 20, technologies offer exciting new opportunities for public health research. This chapter explores the use of digital web-based and mobile media in communication and dissemination of public health information. We show how recent developments in information and communications technology (ICT) have gone beyond general use to play an important role in health science research.

A BRIEF HISTORY OF INFORMATION COMMUNICATIONS TECHNOLOGY AND THE WEB

Before we delve into the uses of ICT for public health, we briefly describe and situate the different technologies available. The changes to the web over the past 20 years or so have been fluid and dynamic, making it difficult to precisely define each stage (a common critique of web version terminology), but the summaries below provide a general idea of the technological and experiential differences.

Web 1.0

In the early years of the Internet, the period roughly from 1990 to 2000, the web was composed largely of HTML documents on stand-alone websites. This version of the Internet, termed Web 1.0, was essentially a digital Carthaginian library where documents were available at any hour, from any place with an Internet connection. The Web 1.0 user experience was rather passive: as with reading a book or listening to a lecture, the user was the passive recipient of information from an outside source in one-way communication.

Web 2.0

With the introduction of web applications such as JavaScript, XML, and their successors, the technology transitioned to the next stage, Web 2.0. This version of the web introduced an interactive dimension in a more decentralized environment. In Web 2.0, the user experience can include dialogue with both creators and other users of information or content, allowing anyone with a connection to participate in, and thus influence, the flow and content of communication. Online dialogue has endless applications, from Q&A sites, surveys, topical forums, and webinars to wiki information and the social media: Facebook, Twitter, LinkedIn, and other interactive sites. Web 2.0 users' ability to contribute content is a powerful tool of information dissemination with the potential to challenge, inform, and alter reality.

Related to this is the ability with Web 2.0 to enable a many-to-many flow of information instead of the simpler (often one way) one-to-one flow. Today's 2.0 technologies are ubiquitous, social, fashionable, and relatively cheap. And what's more, they are often in real time, with no special training necessary to use them. Because of their relative simplicity, they are generally compatible with cognitions, emotions, and behaviors of users. Most important, for users of 2.0 technologies, there is the opportunity to create value through social networking. They are able to add something—user-generated content—that represents new meaning and significance both individually and collectively. Such value may be monetary, or, as likely, it may be social, affective, moral, or informational (Osterwalder & Pigneur, 2010). When content (e.g., a photo, a song) with a single value (e.g., entertainment) is tagged with judgments, comments, or interpretations of other users, the original value is recharged and transformed into, for example, comparative choice information or recommendations.

Similarly, nonspecialist users also create value when they build new software with simple components, sharing knowledge and skills in an open source environment where anyone can participate, as opposed to conventional, expert-driven design. Popular access has been called "folksonomy," from *folk* and *taxonomy*, and describes the practice of classifying information by ordinary people. Users order content via tagging (social bookmarking) and the attribution of keywords to, for example, online content, websites, forum discussions, blog posts, and video. When such tags are shared, they add collective value and facilitate searching. Other examples of technologies for (co-)creating value are self-publishing platforms (e.g., blogs, microblogs, wikis, podcasts, video upload sites), social networking sites and virtual communities, and user-contributed sites (e.g., interactive news, web radio). The speed of growth and the large number of content users generate are striking features of Web 2.0 ICTs. This information revolution has touched all domains of life: economy, travel, education, art, journalism, safety, and politics, to name a few. Of particular interest to readers of this book, it affects medicine, health, health care, public health, and biomedical research, although the health sector has been relatively late to recognize the potential of ICTs.

Web 3.0

Even as Web 2.0 technology expands, new and more powerful changes are leading into the next stage, Web 3.0 (approximately 2010–present). These changes, primarily "under the hood" rather than geared at end-user interface, integrate small, fast, smart, and adaptable applications (apps) and structure data semantically to make them more easily retrievable for human or machine searches over worldwide data networks. In this stage, the *network of meanings*, where photo, video, text, and audio are interconnected, further enables new functions and new, tailored services such as the use of just one user-name/login for all apps. The most important contribution of intelligent 3.0 software is thought to be connecting, integrating, and analyzing different pieces of data from various sources into new meaningful information. Readers are referred to Chetty (2011) for more information on Web 3.0.

Given its predominance at the time of writing, and that most health applications of ICTs have used Web 2.0, in this chapter we focus on the more commonly used Web 2.0 technology.

ICT Terminology in Public Health

Where ICTs meet health we often speak of telemedicine, telecare, or eHealth (Figure 21.1). When the empowering, participatory, collaborative, or social aspects of health communication are emphasized, terms such as **Health 2.0**, participatory health, consumer health informatics, or medicine 2.0 are often used (Eysenbach, 2008). While the prefix *tele* implies (digital) distance and detachment between people, *2.0* is culturally associated with positive values, such as openness, transparency, sharing, cooperation, democracy, or empowerment. As is often the case in a new field of research, questions of definition continue to stimulate academic debate (Van de Belt, Engelen, Berben, & Schoonhoven, 2010).

Nonetheless, we find a substantial body of literature about the design, development, implementation, and evaluation of eHealth technologies for staying healthy, for decision making, for prescribing, for diagnosing, for curing, for monitoring and self-managing chronic disease or dealing with health issues. For example, in the area of coping with mental health problems, 2.0 technologies are known to add value (meaning, support, social comparison, skills) via social networking tools such as microblogs (like Twitter) or virtual environments (like Second Life). Practitioners generally agree that these **eHealth** technologies have the potential to help improve health processes and their safety, quality, and efficiency on a global scale.

When the focus moves from an individual, care/cure orientation to prevention and disease management in the wider population, we often speak of **ePublic Health**. This is

Figure 21.1 Concepts Commonly Associated With eHealth

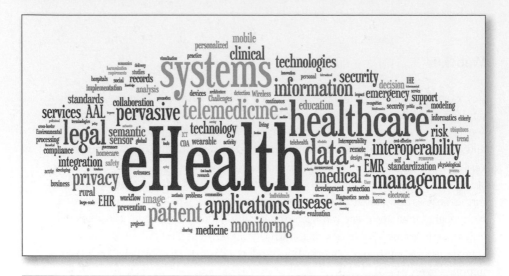

Source: Millar (2012).

in fact undefined territory. eHealth marketing, what some may consider ePublic Health, is the simplest example here. It refers to the use of emerging technologies and "new media" to improve the impact of health education and prevention, health promotion, health protection and communication campaigns, as well as research for the prevention of disease and injury. Health marketing often can be accomplished with Web 1.0 technology, such as dissemination of health information via a website created by experts to inform an audience, or marketing health services or products to a passive target group (Ossebaard, Van Gemert-Pijnen, & Seydel, 2012; Thackeray, Neiger, Smith, & Van Wagenen, 2012; Usher, 2012). But when public health interventions use principles of health technology at the Web 2.0 level, the term **Public Health 2.0** is often used. The 2.0 level is reached when there is opportunity for all stakeholders to actively take part in creating content and to collaborate on a health issue that concerns them.

Though beginning to take hold in public health practice, ePublic Health intervention is still in its early adoption stage. The seemingly boundless opportunities for 2.0 applications have led to an atmosphere of excitement, expectation, and hope with regard to what ICTs may achieve, not just in health, but in all domains of life (cf. Shirky, 2011). The breakthrough rate of new innovations is so high that consumers work to keep up with advancing technology, and researchers are challenged to design robust studies to verify passionate claims of success. This promising field of study needs more evidence to establish or refute the adoption and impact of ePublic Health interventions).

There are many definitions for **eHealth literacy**, but it is generally understood to refer to "the ability to seek, find, understand, and appraise health information from electronic sources and apply the knowledge gained to addressing or solving a health problem" (Norman & Skinner, 2006, para. 2). Because of the growing importance of eHealth interventions, an increasing body of literature is devoted to studying eHealth literacy.

These studies generally aim to measure the concept itself and the extent of technological literacy in the population, boost digital skills, and improve usability in order to reduce its contribution to health disparities.

Critiques of Public Health 2.0

2.0 health technologies are not immune to criticism. Skeptics cite the disagreement in defining terms such as Web 2.0 and (public) Health 2.0 (Hughes, Joshi, & Wareham, 2008). Since information, communication, and technology cut across all academic disciplines and health professions, the risk of fragmentation is clear. Inconsistent definitions limit comparison of research results, and doubt about the quality of online medical information is common. Though we have seen some successful attempts to control and maintain quality (such as the HON-code[1]), the far reaches of the online world make quality control an intricate and never-ending enterprise. Now that anyone can freely produce and disseminate medical content to anyone else, there is fear that amateur opinion may swallow expert fact. Cynics, playing on words, even speak of "loser-generated" content (Peterson, 2008).

Additionally, though use of the Internet and social networks is extensive in the Western world, some critics question whether the number of people actively using 2.0 features for health purposes is as high as proponents claim and note its limitation to specific subpopulations. Another common criticism is that eHealth technologies reproduce (health) disparities because of the digital divide and eHealth illiteracy. Other reservations concern the techno-utopianism sometimes found in enthusiastic publications, even in the academic press, as well as the negative effects of information overload (Gitlin, 2007), the lack of proper business models (Van Limburg et al., 2011), the lack of solid evidence for cost-effectiveness (Mistry, 2011), or the lack of knowledge concerning risks of eHealth technology (Institute of Medicine, 2012).

Other critics target social network companies that exploit voluntary labor by using content generated by worldwide participants to construct user profiles that are then sold to commercial marketers. Critics also cite the danger of permanent and pervasive surveillance of user behavior that they claim is taking place within and through social networks (Fuchs, 2011). They argue that collected data can easily be misused by authorities seeking to monitor and control dissenting citizens (Morozov, 2011). In spite of these reservations, we nevertheless believe that public health stands to benefit from 2.0 technologies.

PUBLIC HEALTH 2.0: RESEARCH AND PRACTICE

Why the urgency to adopt 2.0 technologies in public health? Today, healthcare delivery systems all over the world are in dire need of innovation (World Health Organization [WHO], 2010). Most countries face rising health care expenditures. Despite attempts to contain them, health care costs account for an ever-increasing share of the gross national incomes of most countries. Though health care is touted as sound investment, current health expenditures are basically unsustainable, especially in countries with rapidly aging populations, as in most Western countries and Japan. Increasing life expectancy coupled with decreasing birth rates has significant societal impacts. This means that not only will fewer and fewer have to produce the income for more and more, but also the need for health care—and the demand for more health professionals—will continue to increase. Demand is also changing with a parallel growth in age-related diseases and an increase in multi-morbid chronic diseases, while the threat of infectious diseases lurks in the background of today's post-antibiotic era.

Prevention, surveillance, and control are a matter of global concern. Epidemic and endemic disease, invisible and ever-present enemies, add to the urgency to invest in technology for the public's health. In short, the delivery of necessary care with fewer resources is a number-one political and practical challenge for most countries. It is no wonder that eHealth technologies have often been hailed as a panacea. The WHO's (2005) resolution WHA58.28 acknowledged eHealth's potential to enhance health systems and to improve the safety, quality, and efficiency of care. eHealth should, furthermore, increase health equity as a consequence of its ability to ease access to information and health services.

Despite its promise, however, successful realization of eHealth in daily practice lags behind expectations (KPMG, 2013). Studies confirm the complex nature of health care innovation and acknowledge that there is still little evidence that eHealth technologies influence health care (Black et al., 2011). Yet, changing socio-technological conditions favor eHealth. In most Western countries Internet access and connectivity are high and increasingly supported by newly built ICT infrastructures. Where Internet infrastructure is poor, which often is the case in low-resource countries, mobile technology is an effective alternative. Participation in social media is also increasing (Fox & Duggan, 2013). Older people are catching up and joining in, and consumer expectation, we predict, will be a major incentive for eHealth development.

Three Perspectives

To evaluate the impact of 2.0 technologies on the way we conduct public health research, we refer to three overlapping perspectives: human behavior, instrumental, and research and education. The first of these, *human behavior*, applies to the interaction of people with new health technologies. This perspective focuses on the extent to which information generated by 2.0 technology influences behavior online, as well as in ordinary life, if these can be differentiated.

Appropriate methodology to address questions about human behavior would use a mix of methods from social and behavioral sciences that measure emotional, cognitive, social, organizational, and behavioral factors.

The second perspective, *instrumental,* concerns the use of 2.0 technologies as tools to collect, analyze, and present data—as instruments, as defined in Chapter 2 and the In Focus section immediately following this chapter. The scope of study here is methodological, asking questions that lead to better tools for improved public health outcomes. For example, epidemiologists have applied an instrumental perspective on social media as a source and a tool to study infectious disease prevention, outbreak control, disaster response, syndromic surveillance, and social networks (Pervaiz, Pervaiz, Abdur Rehman,

Perspective 1—Human behavior: Research questions concerning human behavior and 2.0 technologies

- How do these technologies affect our relationships with others at home, at work, and at school?
- How could they be used to support healthy lifestyle habits and behavior modification, self-management of illness, disability, or chronic conditions?
- What risks do they represent for vulnerable groups, in terms of websites promoting, for example, anorexia, suicide, or drug abuse?
- What do they mean for our perception of health risks and the reliability of information?
- What do they imply for the innovation of public health organizations and their impact on effectiveness, quality, and efficiency of interventions?

Saif, 2012; St. Louis & Zorlu, 2012). It also is used to analyze *big data*, the massive amount of complex data that are automatically recorded and stored wherever digital transactions are made (Kamel Boulos, Sanfilippo, Corley, Wheeler, 2012; Sugawara et al., 2012). And virtual environments have been developed as a research tool for otherwise hard-to-study interventions. 2.0 technologies allow better visualization of data to enhance insight and analysis.

Questions such as these from an instrumental perspective require innovative interdisciplinary research methods that combine tools from statistics and computer sciences (e.g., web analytics, open source intelligence) with methods from the behavioral and health sciences.

Perspective 2—Instrumental: Research questions regarding data collection, analysis, and presentation via 2.0 technologies

- Could online search behavior predict a disease outbreak?
- Are social media useful channels for disseminating information on antibiotic resistance?
- Could they be used as a source and a tool for epidemic intelligence?
- What do anti-vaccination rumors on the Internet mean for a vaccination campaign?
- In what way can graphical, dynamic presentation enhance understanding?

The third perspective, *research and education,* leads us further into Web 2.0 technology for the practice of public health. Just as social networking via the Internet or mobile devices has improved collaboration among scientists worldwide, so too can it facilitate teaching and learning in health sciences. This perspective gives rise to new questions.

Perspective 3—Research and education: Research questions on ICTs enable cooperation and education via 2.0 technologies

- Is videoconferencing as effective as conventional meeting?
- How does distance learning technology affect study outcomes?
- Are webinars suitable for public health purposes?
- Are wikis a useful medium for academic cooperation?
- Does serious gaming enrich instruction and education?

Such issues have been studied with a combination of conventional social scientific methods and information technology that has inspired novel areas of development. Information science methods have been applied to computer learning and educational technology, virtual environments for blended learning, and instruction and training in public health. Serious gaming and other promising ways to enhance cooperation between scientists, citizens/patients, health institutions, and companies are also being explored.

Health Technology in Practice: Examples

In this section we illustrate the relevance of the three perspectives to public health research with examples from current practice. We caution, however, that development in this field moves rapidly; methods recommended today may be overtaken by new technological breakthroughs tomorrow.

Perspective 1: Human Behavior

One prominent example of health behavior and 2.0 technology is the use of social media in infectious disease prevention and to support new forms of risk communication in case of crises or emergencies (Centers for Disease Control and Prevention, 2013). Lyme borreliosis is an infectious tick-borne disease which, if left untreated, may cause serious, disabling symptoms. Van Velsen, Van Gemert-Pijnen, Nijland, Beaujean, and van Steenbergen (2012) report on the design and development of mobile technologies that target outdoor people at risk ("green" professionals, recreationists) to make them aware of possible risks of Lyme disease and related infections and to encourage them to avoid the vectors. Such applications (Figure 21.2) are typically not presented only in a one-way manner. They are designed for interactive web-based or mobile communication networks to deliver instruction and education at the right moment in the right format. Stakeholders and end users participate intensively in the design and development process.

Similar projects are conducted in the prevention and control of healthcare-associated, or nosocomial, infections. These infections are transmitted during medical care delivery in traditional hospital settings and long-term care facilities but also in

Figure 21.2   Public Health Apps

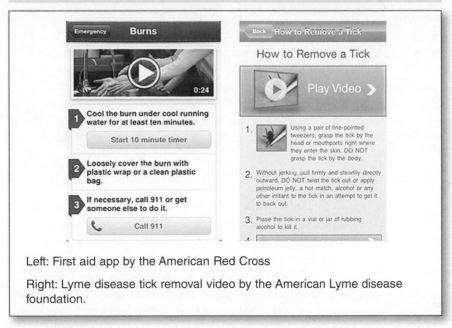

Left: First aid app by the American Red Cross

Right: Lyme disease tick removal video by the American Lyme disease foundation.

Source: American Red Cross/American Lyme Disease Foundation

outpatient care, rehabilitation centers, or community clinics. They are typically caused by organisms (viruses, bacteria, fungi) that have become resistant to antibiotics. They are largely preventable, because they are primarily caused by suboptimal adherence to prevention guidelines by both staff and patients. In the Dutch-German border area this public health threat has been tackled, for example, by implementing EurSafety Health-net,[2] a web-based environment to support the prevention of infection by superbugs such as MRSA (Jurek et al., 2013).[3] It is the first online information system to be based on human-computer interaction theories concerning how people search for and retrieve information in digital environments. The system and the Q&A content are adaptive to its users and based on international guidelines for MRSA prevention and local protocols for institutions and public health. A recent evaluation revealed that users' preferences are met and, more important, that using the tool reduced mistakes in infection prevention and control (Wentzel, De Jong, Karreman, & Van Gemert, 2012).

Another example is the development of an Internet-mediated screening facility for Hepatitis C virus (HCV) infection (www.heptest.nl/site/index.php?ndlang=en). The virus spreads mainly by blood-to-blood contact, for example, during unsafe physical procedures (transfusions, transplantations, tattooing, piercing), intravenous drug use, or unclean medical equipment. The virus harms the liver and ultimately leads to cirrhosis and other pathology. Though it can be treated, no vaccine is available, and many people with HCV remain undiagnosed. Ads in conventional mass media encouraged people at risk to complete an online questionnaire to assess their individual risk. Participants could request a free anonymous blood test and receive the outcome 1 week later under a personal login code. They were referred to medical services if indicated. This low-cost intervention proved to be an effective procedure for identifying undiagnosed HCV infection in the general population (Zuure et al., 2011).

A final illustration of how people interact with technology for public health is given by Catalani et al. (2012), who report on a community organizing project in the aftermath of the 2005 Hurricane Katrina disaster in New Orleans. Using the video-voice method people were trained to use video cameras to investigate, assess, and communicate issues of importance for them. The resulting movie, disseminated both offline (DVD) and online (YouTube), mobilized the community to take action on issues such as affordable housing, education, and economic development, all of which have a public health impact.

Perspective 2: Instrumental Issues

An interesting example of the second perspective, *instrumental* use of 2.0 technology, is infodemiology, which collects, analyzes, and presents public health data from the web. This approach, advanced by Eysenbach (2002, 2006, 2009), combines methods from epidemiology and informatics to investigate the distribution of health information on the Internet or within a population. Infodemiology may be used, for instance, to analyze queries in search engines or Internet navigation to predict outbreaks of infectious diseases or to monitor status updates in social media for disease surveillance (Bernardo et al., 2013). These technologies can also be used to detect disparities in the availability of health information. With specialized software, such data can be collected in real time to provide valuable information for public health prevention and promotion campaigns.

This was illustrated in 2009, when public health experts analyzed content produced through Twitter during the swine flu (H1N1) outbreak to investigate the usefulness of this social medium for public health messaging (Chew & Eysenbach, 2010). Similarly, Szomszor, Kostkova, and De Quincey (2011) analyzed millions of tweets (see Table 21.1) and demonstrated that microblogging can provide an indication of the spread of infection. They concluded that Twitter as a form of public self-report can detect epidemiological changes up to 1 week earlier than official surveillance reports filed by health practitioners.

Another innovative example of the use of 2.0 technologies as an instrument in research is the Real Names Discovery Pilot (Figure 21.3), where motivated individuals living with Parkinson's disease and Amyotrophic Lateral Sclerosis (ALS) cooperate with scientists and clinicians. These participants are recruited via patient communities, and "patients involved in the Pilot will agree to contribute their data in affiliation with their name and will be enthusiastic to play an active role on the project" (Bridge, n.d., para. 1). After working through a smart-informed consent tool, participants upload a range of qualitative, phenotypical, genomic, and other personal data. This information is made available through an open access, computational platform for public research. The project's goal is to create a large, longitudinal, multivariate dataset with which the original owners of the data (patients) can analyze the data in close collaboration with scientists. This form of "citizen science" may lead to a better and faster understanding of the determinants, diagnosis, and course of disease—and ultimately to improved treatment.

Table 21.1   Descriptions and Examples of Selected Content Categories Used to Analyze Tweets About H1N1

Content	Description	Example Tweets
Resource	Tweet contains H1N1 news, updates, or information. May be the title or summary of the linked article. Contents may or may not be factual.	"China Reports First Case of Swine Flu (New York Times): A 30-year-old man who flew from St. Louis to Chengdu is. http://tinyurl.com/ rdbhcg" "Ways To Prevent Flu http://tinyurl .com/r4l4cx #swineflu#h1n1"
Personal Experience	Twitter user mentions a direct (personal) or indirect (e.g., friend, family, co-worker) experience with the H1N1 virus or the social/ economic effects of H1N1.	"Swine flu panic almost stopped me from going to US, but now back from my trip and so happy I went:-))" "Oh we got a swine flu leaflet. Clearly the highlight of my day" "My sister has swine flu!"
Personal Opinion and Interest	Twitter user posts their opinion of the H1N1 virus/situation/news or expresses a need for or discovery of information. General H1N1 chatter or commentary.	"More people have died form Normal Flu than Swing flu, its just a media hoax, to take people's mind off the recession" "Currently looking up some info on H1N1" "Swine flu is scary!"
Jokes/Parody	Tweet contains H1N1 joke told via video, test, or photo; or a humourous opinion of H1N1 that does not refer to a personal experience.	"If you 're an expert on the swine flu, does that make you Fluent?"
Marketing	Tweet contains an advertisement for an H1N1-related product or service.	"Buy liquid vitamin C as featured in my video http://is.gd/y87r #health # h1n1"
Spam	Tweet is unrelated to H1N1	"musicmonday MM lamarodom Yom Kippur Polanski Jay-Z H1N1 Watch FREE online LATEST MOVIES at http://a.gd/b1586f"

Source: Chew and Eysenbach (2010).

Figure 21.3 Real Names Discovery Pilot Web Page

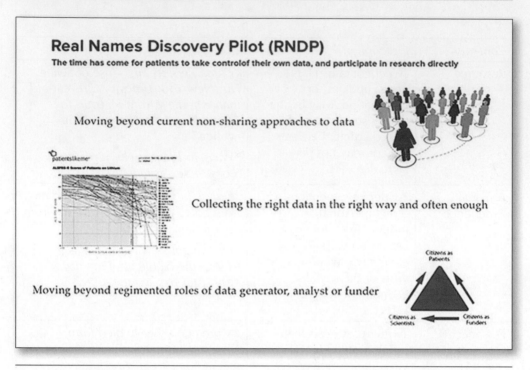

Source: SAGE Bionetworks.

Computational and creative developments in ICTs have also inspired a new and energetic area of research into visual imagery as it relates to health research and education (Friendly, 2007). Visual imagery is a powerful way to convey both abstract and concrete concepts. The earliest known maps—of space and earth—date back to 6200 B.C. (Tufte, 2001). One of the earliest examples of visualizing public health data is a surviving map of disease incidence of Valerie Seaman depicting an outbreak of yellow fever in New York City in 1790. As mentioned in the introduction to this book and shown in Chapter 6, perhaps the most famous historical example is John Snow's map of deaths from a cholera outbreak in London in 1854, showing spread of the disease in relation to the locations of public water pumps. The Public Health 2.0 equivalent uses graphical statistical techniques to visually represent quantitative data and transform them into useful information and knowledge. Data visualization and interactive (3D) infographics can reveal the content and structure of complex, multivariate population data and control or generate statistical assumptions. Most of all, and if applied well, they communicate clearly and effectively the outcomes of analysis, thereby engaging viewers and stimulating innovative ideas or new courses of action (Whitney, 2013). Figure 21.4, for instance, shows a graphical representation of another health disparity in London. The correspondence between life expectancy and neighborhood is expressed through an adapted map of the London Underground.

Figure 21.4   Infographic Relating Life Expectancies and Residential Areas

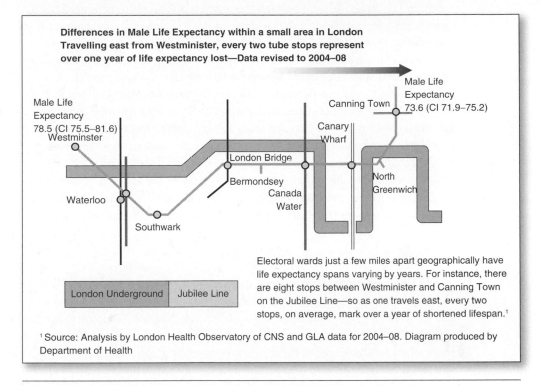

Source: Public Health England, Knowledge & Intelligence Team.

Another innovative example of Internet-based research is the Longitudinal Internet Studies for the Social Sciences (LISS) panel managed by CentERdata at Tilburg University, in The Netherlands. The LISS panel is a representative sample of Dutch individuals who participate in monthly online surveys. The panel is based on a true probability sample of households independently drawn from the population register since 2007 (Scherpenzeel & Das, 2011). Households that cannot otherwise participate are provided with a simple computer and an Internet connection. Every 2 years the panel's dropout participants are replaced with a fresh additional sample. In this way, the usual disadvantages of Internet panels, such as limited representativeness, are circumvented. Moreover, panel members are carefully and personally recruited and maintained. Persons not included in the original sample cannot participate, so people cannot sign up for the panel, as is the case for the opt-in or convenience panels. Panel members receive a financial incentive per half-hour of interview time. A longitudinal core study is fielded in the panel every year, covering a large variety of domains including work, education, housing, and leisure. For health studies, data may be enriched with objective measures collected by wireless devices such as weight scales or accelerometers. The LISS protocol has transformed survey design by using the Internet, wireless data transfer, and smart devices to record and report data with feedback of health behavior.[4] Thus, data collection, a costly and laborious stage in the research process, not only yields more information, but is faster, frequent, and more reliable. The huge historical database is accessible at no cost to academic researchers 4–6 months after data collection. The American Life Panel, managed by Rand Labor and Population and patterned after the CentERdata panel, provides a similar database for the American population (Rand Corporation, 1994–2013).

A final example of the instrumental use of 2.0 technology is a study by Metzger and Flanagin (2011) who investigated how these technologies could be used "to increase access to, enliven users' experiences with, and enrich the quality of the information available" (p. 45). Their work is based on the concept of the wisdom of the crowd, which posits that the aggregate of a set of proposed solutions from a collective of individuals will perform better than the majority of individual solutions (Surowiecki, 2004). This collective intelligence is consistent with the participative and collaborative features of 2.0 technologies. With regard to health information, and if certain conditions are present, it may result in reliable scientific information continuously supplemented with experiential input from a large number of users, thus making it more useful and credible in practice.

Perspective 3: Research and Education

The third perspective on the use of 2.0 technologies, *research and education*, focuses on scientific collaboration, training, and education in public health. This new and active area has interesting possibilities (Greenhow, 2009; Isaias, Ifenthaler, Sampson, & Spector, 2012). A wiki, for example, is a website where any authorized person may edit or add pages. Wikis are widely used in the academic community to foster collaboration. Some web-based technologies, such as wikis, are used for the management and implementation of multicenter studies, while others are used to recruit participants from social networks (crowdsourcing) or to facilitate academic open source publishing or knowledge transfer (Archambault et al., 2013).

An innovative public health example of employing such networks is the Dutch iSPEX experiment in which people measure the quantity of fine dust (aerosols) in the air with a camera add-on on their smartphones (http://ispex.nl/en). On a clear day, participants receive a text message to activate an app and turn their phone into a scientific instrument with which they measure characteristics of particulate matter in the air. Through this form of crowdsourcing, thousands of measurements at different locations are obtained, collected in a database, and combined with other data in order to assess atmospheric pollution in real-time.

Use of 2.0 technology in research and education is also a way to create simulated, virtual environments for blended (that is both offline and online) learning and other instruction and training in public health. So is augmented reality, which migrated from the aircraft and car industries to diverse applications in health and health care. It superimposes computer images, sensory input, or virtual objects onto the user's perception of the real world, in real-time 3D. Serious gaming is another form of an immersive learning environment. In a car simulator, drivers can artificially manipulate their alcohol-intake to experience what this does to their driving abilities and their perception. Researchers are also using 2.0 technology to study interventions that promote healthy food choices (Waterlander, Scarpa, Lentz, & Steenhuis, 2011). They designed a virtual supermarket to study food purchasing behavior of study participants in relation to their budget, pricing, labeling, and other product qualities (Figure 21.5). Participants feel that the application provides an environment resembling a real supermarket, while the researchers believe other kinds of health behavior can be studied in this highly controllable setting. Virtual behavior is assumed to be predictive of, and fairly comparable with, real behavior.

Figure 21.5   Shopping Cart in the Virtual Supermarket

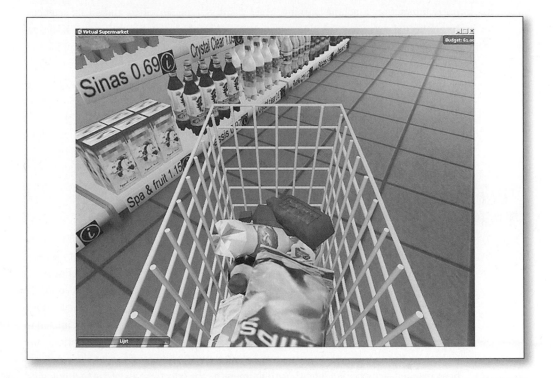

Source: Waterlander et al. (2011).

Games are used to train health care professionals in diagnostics, medical procedures, and patient monitoring, as well as for responding to epidemics and natural disasters. Gaming overlaps with the areas of e-learning and education technology, where forms of electronically supported learning and teaching are developed. The latter seeks to integrate social media into the curriculum to engage students and to enrich their learning experience (Kapp, LeMaster, Lyon, Zhang, & Hosokawa, 2009). The effectiveness of these technologies is evaluated using methods from social and educational sciences. The Great Flu (Ranj Serious Games, n.d.) is a serious game developed to teach users how a virus works and how to manage a worldwide outbreak of a new influenza virus before it turns into a pandemic. It also addresses dilemmas and choices that need to be made in the process. In an even more serious gaming project, Fischer, Jiang, and Moran (2012) studied and developed mixed reality games (MRGs) as a platform to explore scenarios in the real world that are hard to study in realistic settings, such as disaster response. These scenarios typically include groups of human, computational, and embodied agents (such as drones or robots) coordinating a response to a disaster such as an earthquake, a flood, a terrorist attack, or an epidemic outbreak. These *pervasive games* are developed with artists and designers and intended to study human-machine interactions "under stress" in order to support humans and agents in their need for agile teaming. Questions of motivation when faced with conflicting interests or trustworthiness of information from those involved are also addressed. This interdisciplinary research from human-computer interaction, machine learning, multi-agent systems, robotics, and social sciences has delivered several interesting pilots such as iZombie!, a product of the U.K.-based ORCHID project (www.orchid.ac.uk). Players in this MRG have to survive an epidemic outbreak of a Zombie virus, while other players act as infected Zombies whose motivation is to attack and kill noninfected players. While escaping these Zombies, players have to cooperate in teams to reach situational awareness and meet their objectives in a concerted action with all human and machine agents. Such a scenario may be fictional, but it is believed that it forms the basis for an attractive game to play while maintaining an analogue to real-world scenarios such as a virus outbreak.

CURRENT ISSUES IN PUBLIC HEALTH 2.0

What can we learn so far from these examples about the potential of new technologies for public health research? First, they illustrate how technological developments inspire people to use their intellectual and creative capacities to advance public health research. 2.0 technologies have expanded our methodological arsenal considerably. Second, as tools for study and to support collaboration, 2.0 technologies allow us to achieve more than we could before by facilitating, speeding up, and fostering the sharing of information. Third, we can observe that the field is currently developing. The expectations are as high as the investments, but the full potential of 2.0 technologies has likely not yet been reached—and the evidence base documenting the effectiveness of the technologies is still small. Though promising results have been reported, effectiveness needs to be substantiated through rigorous time-series studies and in both complex professional practice and ordinary daily life. This is what drives today's research in public health, and we foresee 2.0 technologies helping to better inform health policy and improve health outcomes in the near future.

A compelling example of the potential for use—and improved use—of Public Health 2.0 technologies comes from the National Institute for Public Health and the Environment (RIVM), an independent knowledge center funded by the Dutch government. Like the Centers for Disease Control and Prevention in the United States, RIVM is responsible, on a national level, for the prevention and control of infectious diseases, environmental health, population screening, consumer safety, and other public health related areas. In 2009, vaccination against the Human Papillomavirus (HPV) type 16/18, which can cause cervical cancer, was added to the Dutch national vaccination program, and a vaccination campaign was organized by the RIVM Center for Infectious Disease Control. In The Netherlands, the degree of vaccination among the general population is traditionally high. RIVM started out with a conventional campaign: Parents and their 13- to 16-year-old daughters received a written invitation to participate in the vaccination effort, together with an educational brochure that referred to a website. The tone of the messaging was factual and rational. Public uptake was relatively high, as expected, until traditional media (radio, TV, papers) reported unsubstantiated information about the vaccine that subsequently began to reverberate across online social media: the vaccine was supposedly unsafe; girls in other countries had died from it; the vaccine had not been properly tested; the Health Council could not be objective because of its alleged ties with the pharmaceutical industry. In short, these messages concluded that vaccination against HPV was one big state-experiment at the cost of innocent children. All of these news stories could be refuted: Evidence shows that worldwide millions of girls have been vaccinated with one of two available vaccines without adverse side effects. But anti-vaccination information continued to be distributed via websites, email chain letters, video uploads on YouTube, warnings on Internet forums, and so on. Other critics chimed in, adding fuel to the fire. They included scientists who doubted the cost-effectiveness of the campaign and religious leaders or parents who believed their abstinent daughters would not need a vaccine at all.

The RIVM-sponsored campaign's evaluation produced some interesting findings. According to those polled, the RIVM message had been too rational (e.g., x% chance for infection, x% chance for restless cells to develop, x% chance for these to become carcinomas, x% chance that you die from it) and at odds with a decision about vaccination that is much more complex. It also turned out that both mothers and daughters should be more central in the campaign, since mothers appeared to have a crucial role in the decision-making process. The (social) media they use could be utilized to include them. Finally, health professionals should be more involved to adequately respond to questions from the public and to convey expert consensus on the effectiveness of the vaccine beyond RIVM's institutional view.

These outcomes were implemented in the follow-up campaign, with the objective of helping people ground their decisions about vaccination in evidence-based information. The follow-up campaign addressed two central questions: Is the HPV vaccine useful, and is it safe? A new website published various opinions of medical experts, mothers, and daughters, including those still hesitating, or even refusing, vaccination. The website also provided a chat functionality with Q&A. The invitation mailed to homes now emphasized the mother-daughter conversation, and more time was given between receiving information and the invitation. General practitioners received a telephone script to facilitate consistent responses to parents' questions, and municipal public health organizations were intensely involved in the campaign. Finally, the social media were much more actively monitored and employed to keep abreast of the (anti-)vaccination buzz and to counter incorrect information, always explicitly on behalf of the RIVM. Several discussions were initiated on a multi-user chat community for girls, and traditional media were approached with information as well. The campaign turned out to be more effective than before.

This example shows

- how interactive social media can be employed to inform and communicate with both professionals and target groups;
- that information flows on the Internet and social media can be monitored and used for interventions and improvement of information and communication;
- the importance of collaboration in public health;
- that building skills, knowledge, and trust takes time; and
- that making mistakes is part of the valuable learning experience of new technologies.

Information and communication technologies have changed the classical information asymmetry in health (between sender and receiver, doctor and patient, producer and consumer, and so on) for good. For public health authorities, the new challenge is to remain a trusted medium in a chaotic media landscape. Experts entertain high hopes about the contribution of new information technologies to health and health care (Kreps & Neuhauser, 2010; Larson et al, 2013).

PUBLIC HEALTH 2.0 IN THE GLOBAL CONTEXT

Today's global health issues have been described extensively in the scientific literature. Their urgencies lie in the assumption that in the short term the health care system will be inaccessible to large parts of the population, or it will be too expensive to sustain with an acceptable quality of care. Faced with population aging, economic recession, consumerism, and changing demand due to a rise in multi-morbid chronic diseases, health care delivery is in dire need of innovation (WHO, 2010).

eHealth projects support public health services for the many socioeconomically deprived people living in remote rural areas, with poor infrastructure, often far from doctors, hospitals, or medical services. Such health services are usually village clinics run by nurse practitioners. Teleconsultations save transportation costs and enable point-of-care communication with health care professionals. In low-resource countries, evidence abounds that ePublic Health delivers health revenues when it comes to the prevention and control of HIV/AIDS and Malaria. An example of this is AIDS teledermatology. Over 90% of AIDS patients have skin problems, which are often the infection's first manifestation. Their nature and degree can allow diagnosis of the stage of HIV infection in an individual. In South Africa, a country with one of the world's highest HIV prevalence rates, teledermatology has resulted in skilled local management of many HIV-associated skin problems without referral (Colven, Shim, Brock, & Todd, 2011). Additionally, there are numerous examples of successful tele-education and telesurveillance programs involving health care workers in developing countries (Wynchank & Fortuin, 2011).

Similarly, scientific evidence has proven that mobile phone text messaging improves adherence to antiretroviral therapy and rates of viral suppression compared to standard care in Kenya (Horvath, Azman, Kennedy, & Rutherford, 2012). Mobile health (or mHealth) denotes the delivery of health services, information, and communication via mobile technologies such as mobile phones, personal digital assistants, tablets, and other wireless devices. mHealth is booming in developing countries as the shortage of health care workers, financial constraints, and high burdens of disease render traditional ways of health care unfeasible (Kayingo, 2012). While Internet infrastructure is often still under-developed, mobile phone access and use is high and rising. This provides opportunities for promoting good health and preventive measures, improving access to medical infor-mation for marginalized groups such as the disabled or those in rural areas, and exploring how mobile technology can provide assistance to health workers and users (Boakye, Scott, & Smyth, 2010). Many interesting and effective mHealth practices exist in diverse areas such as infectious disease control, pediatric mobile outpatient clinics, management of blood banks, or the quality of drinking water.

FUTURE DIRECTIONS

A Conceptual Model for the Design and Development of eHealth Technologies

The Dutch Center for eHealth Research and Disease Management developed a model based on an extensive literature review and empirical work (Van Gemert-Pijnen et al., 2011; Figure 21.6). Analysis of factors that influence the uptake and impact of eHealth technologies led to the conclusion that classic design approaches fall short in that most are technology driven. This means they do not sufficiently meet the needs of users and their social settings. Therefore, it is essential that eHealth technologies be developed with end users (WHO, 2010). A multidisciplinary approach is proposed, in which the values of all stakeholders and their respective contexts are accounted for. The model is further integrated with theoretical concepts from business modeling and human-centered design. This holistic approach is summarized in a roadmap that serves to improve, step by step, the design and development of eHealth technology with the ultimate goal of improving its uptake and impact. In this model, eHealth technology development transcends an instrumental, determinist, or functional approach of designing a technical product, service, or stand-alone device. The social dynamics and significance of eHealth technologies are recognized, as is their potential for improving health care. The model is published as a wiki and used in a range of research projects. The interaction between people, technology, and context forms the starting point for concrete innovations in health care and public health.

Research Into Persuasive Designs for eHealth Technologies

With regard to eHealth and Web 2.0 technology, the term *persuasive* refers to the capacity of technology to influence attitude and behavior (Fogg, 2003). It is currently used in eHealth development to understand the role of technology in changing behavior. One of the major challenges identified in the interaction of people with health

Figure 21.6 Conceptual Model for the Design and Development of eHealth Technologies

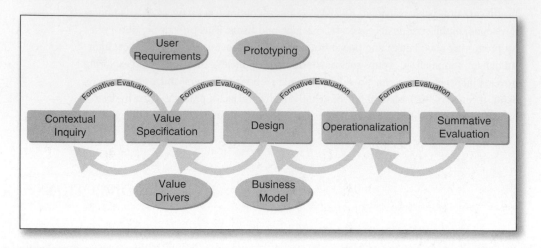

Source: van Limburg M, van Gemert-Pijnen JE, Nijland N, Ossebaard HC, Hendrix RMG, Seydel ER. Why Business Modeling is Crucial in the Development of eHealth Technologies. *J Med Internet Res 2011;13*(4):e124.

technology systems is non-adherence, or the tendency of participants to prematurely discontinue following an intervention protocol. As would be expected, if people drop out of a treatment or intervention, the intended effect diminishes. Low adherence affects adoption and impact of eHealth in general, and more research has been gradually devoted to this subject. Findings suggest that persuasive design may significantly improve adherence (Kelders, 2012).

Introduction and Management of eHealth Technologies

Another pressing issue is the management of innovation and change within organizations. Like other technologies, eHealth technology is not an amoral, value-free intervention. Just the thought of implementing eHealth provokes debate and discussion within health organizations. An international survey among health leaders revealed that suboptimal change management is perceived to be a major obstacle for implementation of eHealth (KPMG, 2013). The importance of social and psychological variables for technology adoption and innovation has been widely recognized since Everett Rogers (1962) published his foundational work on the diffusion of innovations. In eHealth, a business modeling approach is used to imbue the development of eHealth technology with value—anything that matters to anyone who is involved with it in real life. Through business modeling, technology is designed to match the values of different stakeholders so that they can connect with and make sense of it. This contributes to better uptake and a higher impact of health technology.

Ethical Considerations for eHealth and Public Health 2.0

All innovations generate new ethical issues. In the field of public health, the ethical issues around eHealth and Public Health 2.0 have not yet received much attention. A primary issue is the effect of technology on the patient-physician relationship, traditionally the basis of health care services (Bailey, 2011; Coeckelbergh, 2013). While eHealth is often promoted as a way to build empowerment and self-management, there are questions about whether the reduction of in-person contact between patient and physician will be suitable for everyone. eHealth can also be seen as enhancing patients' autonomy, yet technology may adversely affect people's autonomy if they cannot freely choose its application, if they cannot agree with its function, or if they believe their needs are not met.

And of course, privacy issues and the security of personal medical or health data are a recurring subject of concern (Ploug & HolmTake, 2013; Stein, Rump, Kretzschmar, & van Steenbergen, 2013). Remarkably, the risks of eHealth technologies are hardly a subject of academic interest. Though there is anecdotal evidence of the occurrence of harms at the levels of human functioning, organization, and technology, their magnitude is largely unknown (Ossebaard, Van Gemert-Pijnen, De Bruijn, & Geertsma, 2013). To ensure patient safety, quality of care, and sustainability, these risks need to be addressed with customary risk management procedures.

The Outlook for Public Health 2.0

Future directions start from today's developments. We observe promising work in the development of interactive games as tools for improving health behaviors ranging from healthy lifestyle habits and behavior modification, to self-management of illness and chronic conditions, to motivating and supporting physical activity. Games are also increasingly used to train health care professionals in methods for diagnosis, medical procedures, patient monitoring, and responding to epidemics and natural disasters. 2.0 technologies also enable participation of nonprofessionals in public health, which is an important development. Swan (2012) reviews several forms of citizen science in relation to crowdsourcing and Health 2.0, concluding that these kinds of initiatives grow rapidly and hold promise for things like understanding disease and drug response.

It is anticipated that participatory health initiatives and crowdsourced health research studies will pave the way to P4 medicine and public health genomics. *P4 medicine* is a term coined in 2003 by biologist Leroy Hood (Hood & Flores, 2012). He advances systems biology, big data, and patient-activated social networks whose combination will lead to a medicine that is Predictive, Personalized, Preventive, and Participatory. This would move medicine from a reactive to a proactive discipline where the ultimate objective is to maximize wellness for each individual, rather than to just treat disease. Public health genomics refers to a constituent part of this revolutionary development. It is defined as "a multidisciplinary field concerned with the effective and responsible translation of genome-based knowledge and technologies for the benefit of population health" (Burke, Khoury, Stewart, Zimmer, & Bellagio Group, 2006, p. 453). Genomics and cell and molecular biology will deeply impact public health practice and research in the near future (Zimmern & Khoury, 2012), and information sharing will be facilitated by 2.0 technologies. Individuals will be able to measure and track their own health as well, via the use of social media and online community networks.

These developments on the scientific and social levels are supported by high-speed developments in technology that enable knowledge grids in supercomputers to collect, analyze, and disseminate the exponentially growing amounts of data that are physically located on separate servers all over the world. This allows for new forms of academic collaboration and education through knowledge discovery methods such as data mining. *Data mining* is the automated scanning of large databases to discover meaningful patterns among data points. The limits of growth in computational power are not yet in sight and the impact of big data analysis for public health undoubtedly will be as revolutionary as it is for other societal domains (Mayer-Schonberger & Cukier, 2013).

In short, 2.0 technology has energized public health and created interest in

- health behavior and new consumer health technologies;
- new ways to collect, analyze, and present public health data; and
- novel forms of scientific collaboration, training, and education.

Technology is certainly an important driver of social change, especially as the Internet is explored as a tool for innovation on a global scale (cf. Sadowsky, 2012). Social media, for example, is expected to play a decisive role in strengthening health care systems (Finlayson, Hudson, & Ali, 2011). And to date, we have some evidence that 2.0 technologies may substantially contribute to solving global health challenges. There is certainly excitement about health applications of 2.0 technologies among a wide, supportive, and participative audience of professionals and lay people alike. But systematic technological changes take time, and attitudes change slowly. This is especially true in the health professions, where conservatism is inherently functional. In both developing and developed countries, the investment in eHealth increases as part of a process of social innovation. eHealth is a transitory concept in the progression toward embedded health technologies, *eHealth inside* as it were, but is helping to emphasize that information and communication are essential to improved health outcomes. How those outcomes are achieved, and the extent to which Web 2.0 technologies play a part in their accomplishment, will be determined over the next 10 years in the field.

ADDITIONAL RESOURCES

Centers for Disease Control—Crisis and Emergency Risk Communication: http://emergency.cdc.gov/cerc/pdf/CERC_2012edition.pdf

Data visualization: http://www.informationisbeautiful.net/

Digital Agenda for Europe—Living Healthy, Ageing Well: http://ec.europa.eu/digital-agenda/en/eHealth%20

Digital Methods Initiative: https://www.digitalmethods.net/Digitalmethods/WebHome

Google's Crisis Response: http://www.google.org/crisisresponse

The Internet of Things: http://en.wikipedia.org/wiki/Internet_of_Things

One Health: http://en.wikipedia.org/wiki/One_Health

PLoS Tech: http://blogs.plos.org/tech/about

Quantified Self: http://quantifiedself.com/

WHO eHealth: http://www.who.int/ehealth/programmes/en/index.html

Van Gemert-Pijnen, J. E. W. C., Peters, O., & Ossebaard, H. C. (2013). *Improving eHealth.* The Hague, Netherlands: Eleven.

REFERENCES

Archambault, P. M., van de Belt, T. H., Grajales, F. J., III, Faber, M. J., Kuziemsky, C. E., Gagnon, S., . . . Légaré, F. (2013). Wikis and collaborative writing applications in health care: A scoping review. *Journal of Medical Internet Research, 15*(10), e210.

Bailey, J. E. (2011). Does health information technology dehumanize health care? *American Medical Association Journal of Ethics, 13,* 181–185.

Bernardo, T.M., Rajic, A., Young, I., Robiadek, K., Pham, M.T., & Funk, J. A.(2013). Scoping review on search queries and social media for disease surveillance: A chronology of innovation. *J Med Internet Res 15*(7): e147 doi: 10.2196/jmir.2740

Black, A. D., Car, J., Pagliari, C., Anandan, C., Cresswell, K., Bokun, T., . . . Sheikh, A. (2011). The impact of eHealth on the quality and safety of health care: A systematic overview. *PLoS Med, 8*(1), e1000387.

Boakye, K., Scott, N., & Smyth, C. (2010). *Mobiles for development report 2010.* Retrieved from http://www.cto.int/wp-content/themes/solid/_layout/dc/ptojects/UNICEF%20Mobiles4Dev%20Report.pdf

Bridge. (n.d.). *Real names discovery pilot.* Retrieved from http://sagebridge.org/symptoms-conditions/real-names/rn-read-about

Burke, W., Khoury, M. J., Stewart, A., Zimmern, R. L., & Bellagio Group. (2006). The path from genome-based research to population health: Development of an international public health genomics network. *Genetics in Medicine, 8,* 451–458.

Catalani, C. E., Veneziale, A., Campbell, L., Herbst, S., Butler, B., Springgate, B., & Minkler, M. (2012). Videovoice: Community assessment in post-Katrina New Orleans. *Health Promotion Practice. 13*(1), 18–28.

Centers for Disease Control and Prevention. (2013). *Crisis and emergency risk communication (CERC).* Retrieved from http://emergency.cdc.gov/cerc/

Chetty L.-R. (2011). *Imagining Web 3.0.* Cape Town, South Africa: Big Red.

Chew, C., & Eysenbach, G. (2010). Pandemics in the age of Twitter: Content analysis of tweets during the 2009 H1N1 outbreak. *PLoS One, 5*(11), e14118.

Coeckelbergh M. (2013). E-care as craftsmanship: virtuous work, skilled engagement, and information technology in health care. *Med Health Care Philos.* 2013 Nov; 16(4): 807–16. doi: 10.1007/s11019-013-9463-7

Colven, R., Shim, M.-H., Brock, D., & Todd, G. (2011). Dermatological diagnostic acumen improves with use of a simple telemedicine system for underserved areas of South Africa. *Telemedicine Journal and E-Health, 17,* 363–369.

Eysenbach, G. (2002). Infodemiology: The epidemiology of (mis)information. *American Journal of Medicine, 113,* 763–765.

Eysenbach, G. (2006). Infodemiology: Tracking flu-related searches on the web for syndromic surveillance. *AMIA Annual Symposium Proceedings,* pp. 244–248.

Eysenbach, G. (2008). Medicine 2.0: Social networking, collaboration, participation, apomediation, and openness. *Journal of Medical Internet Research, 10*(3), e22. Retrieved from http://www.jmir.org

Eysenbach, G. (2009). Infodemiology and infoveillance: Framework for an emerging set of public health informatics methods to analyze search, communication and publication behavior. *Journal of Medical Internet Research, 11*(1), e11. Retrieved from http://www.jmir.org

Finlayson, A. E. T., Hudson, K. E. M., & Ali, F. R. (2011). *Use social media to strengthen health systems.* Retrieved from http://www.scidev.net/en/health/opinions/use-social-media-to-strengthen-health-systems.html

Fischer, J. E., Jiang, W., & Moran, S. (2012). AtomicOrchid: A mixed reality game to investigate coordination in disaster response. In M. Herrlich, R. Malaka, & M. Masuch (Eds.), *Entertainment Computing—ICEC 2012* (pp. 572–577). Berlin, Germany: Springer.

Fogg, B. J. (2003). *Persuasive technology: Using computers to change what we think and do.* San Francisco, CA: Morgan Kaufmann.

Fox, S., & Duggan, M., (2013). *Health online 2013.* Washington, DC: Pew Research Center, Internet and American Life Project. Retrieved from http://www.pewinternet.org/Reports/2013/Health-online.aspx

Friendly, M (2007). *DataVis.* Retrieved from http://www.datavis.ca

Fuchs, C. (2011). Web 2.0, presumption, and surveillance. *Surveillance & Society, 8,* 288–309.

Gitlin, T. (2007). Media unlimited: How the torrent of images and sounds overwhelms our lives (Rev. ed.). New York, NY: Metropolitan Books.

Greenhow, C. (2009). Social scholarship: Applying social networking technologies to research practices. *Knowledge Quest, 37*(4), 42–74.

Hood, L., & Flores, M. A. (2012). A personal view on systems medicine and the emergence of proactive P4 medicine: Predictive, preventive, personalized and participatory. *New Biotechnology, 29,* 613–624.

Horvath, T., Azman, H., Kennedy, G. E., & Rutherford, G. W. (2012). Mobile phone text messaging for promoting adherence to antiretroviral therapy in patients with HIV infection. *Cochrane Database of Systematic Reviews, 14*(3), CD009756.

Hughes, B., Joshi, I., & Wareham, J. (2008). Health 2.0 and medicine 2.0: Tensions and controversies in the field. *Journal of Medical Internet Research, 10*(3), e23.

Institute of Medicine. (2012). *Health IT and patient safety: Building safer systems for better care.* Washington, DC: National Academies Press.

Isaias, P., Ifenthaler, D., Sampson, D. G., & Spector, J. M. (Eds.). (2012). Towards learning and instruction in Web 3.0: Advances in cognitive and educational psychology. New York, NY: Springer.

Jurke, A., Köck, R., Becker, K., Thole, S., Hendrix, R., Rossen, J., Daniels-Haardt, I.,& Friedrich, A. W. (2013). Reduction of the nosocomial meticillin-resistant Staphylococcus aureus incidence density by a region-wide search and follow-strategy in forty German hospitals of the EUREGIO, 2009 to 2011. *Euro Surveill. 18*(36), pii=20579. Retrieved from http://www.euro surveillance.org/ViewArticle.aspx?

Kamel Boulos, M. N., Sanfilippo, A. P., Corley, C. D., & Wheeler, S. (2010). Social web mining and exploitation for serious applications: Technosocial predictive analytics and related technologies for public health, environmental and national security surveillance. *Computer Methods and Programs in Biomedicine, 100*(1), 16–23.

Kapp, J. M., LeMaster, J. W., Lyon, M. B., Zhang, B., & Hosokawa, M. C. (2009). Updating public health teaching methods in the era of social media. *Public Health Reports, 124*, 775–777.

Kayingo, G. (2012). Transforming global health with mobile technologies and social enterprises: Global health and innovation conference. *Yale Journal of Biology and Medicine, 85*, 425–427.

Kelders, S. M. (2012). *Understanding adherence to web-based interventions* (Unpublished PhD dissertation). University of Twente.

KPMG. (2013). *Accelerating innovation: The power of the crowd*. Retrieved from http://www.kpmg.com/ global/en/issuesandinsights/articlespublications/accelerating-innovation/pages/default.aspx

Kreps, G. L., & Neuhauser, L. (2010). New directions in eHealth communication: Opportunities and challenges. *Patient Education and Counseling, 78*, 329–336.

Larson, H. J., Smith, D., Paterson P., Cumming, M., Eckersberger, E., Freifeld C. C., Ghinai, I., Jarrett C., Paushter, L., Brownstein, J.S., Madoff, L.C. (2013). Measuring vaccine confidence: Analysis of data obtained by a media surveillance system used to analyse public concerns about vaccines *The Lancet Infectious Diseases, 13*(7), pp. 606–613. DOI: 10.1016/S1473-3099(13)70108-7

Mayer-Schonberger, V., & Cukier, K. (2013). *Big data: A revolution that will transform how we live, work, and think*. New York, NY: Eamon Dolan/Houghton Mifflin Harcourt.

Metzger, M. J., & Flanagin, A. J. (2011). Using Web 2.0 technologies to enhance evidence-based medical information. *Journal of Health Communication, 16*(Suppl 1), 45–58.

Millar, J. (2012, March 28). It's time to move beyond "eHealth" [Web log post]. Retrieved from http:// ethicstechnologyandsociety.wordpress.com/2012/03/28/its-time-to-move-beyond-ehealth/

Mistry, H. (2011). Systematic review of studies of the cost-effectiveness of telemedicine and telecare: Changes in the economic evidence over twenty years. *Journal of Telemedicine and Telecare 18*, 1–6.

Morozov, E. (2011). *The net delusion: The dark side of Internet freedom*. New York, NY: Public Affairs.

Norman, C. D., & Skinner, H. A. (2006). eHealth literacy: Essential skills for consumer health in a networked world. *Journal of Medical Internet Research, 8*(2), e9.

Ossebaard, H. C., Van Gemert-Pijnen, J. E. W. C., De Bruijn, A. C. P., & Geertsma, R. E. (2013). Magnitude of eHealth technology risks largely unknown: An exploratory study into the risks of information and communication technologies in healthcare. *International Journal on Advances in Systems and Measurements, 6*(1&2), 57–71.

Ossebaard, H. C., Van Gemert-Pijnen, J. E. W. C., & Seydel, E. R. (2012). Technology for transparency: The case of the Dutch national health portal. *Policy & Internet, 4*(2), 8.

Osterwalder, A., & Pigneur, Y. (2010). *Business model generation: A handbook for visionaries, game changers, and challengers*. Hoboken, NJ: Wiley.

Pervaiz, F., Pervaiz, M., Abdur Rehman, N., & Saif, U. (2012). FluBreaks: Early epidemic detection from Google Flu Trends. *Journal of Medical Internet Research, 14*(5), e125.

Peterson, S. M. (2008). Loser generated content: From participation to exploitation. *First Monday, 13*(3). Retrieved from http://journals.uic.edu/ojs/index.php/fm/index

Ploug, T. & Holm, S. (2013). Take not a musket to kill a butterfly—Ensuring the proportionality of measures used in disease control on the Internet. *Public Health Ethics* pht034, doi:10.1093/ phe/pht034

Rand Corporation. (1994–2013). *Welcome to the American Life Panel*. Retrieved from https://mmic-data.rand.org/alp/

Ranj Serious Games. (n.d.). *The great flu*. Retrieved from http://www.ranj.com/content/werk/the-great-flu

Rogers, E. M. (1962). *Diffusion of innovations*. New York, NY: Free Press.

Sadowsky, G. (Ed.). (2012). *Accelerating development using the web: Empowering poor and marginalized populations*. Retrieved from http://public.webfoundation.org/publications/accelerating-development/

Scherpenzeel, A. C., & Das, M. (2011). "True" longitudinal and probability-based Internet panels: Evidence from the Netherlands. In M. Das, P. Ester, & L. Kaczmirek (Eds.), *Social and behavioral research and the Internet: Advances in applied methods and research strategies* (pp. 77–104). Boca Raton, FL: Taylor & Francis.

Shirky, C. (2011). *Cognitive surplus: Creativity and generosity in a connected age.* London, UK: Penguin Press.

Stein, M.L., Rump, B.O., Kretzschmar, M.E.E. &. van Steenbergen, J.E. (2013). Social networking sites as a tool for contact tracing: Urge for ethical framework for normative guidance. *Public Health Ethics* phdoi:10.1093/phe/pht035

St. Louis, C., & Zorlu, G. (2012). Can Twitter predict disease outbreaks? *BMJ, 344,* e2353.

Sugawara, T., Ohkusa, Y., Ibuka, Y., Kawanohara, H., Taniguchi, K., & Okabe, N. (2012). Real-time prescription surveillance and its application to monitoring seasonal influenza activity in Japan. *Journal of Medical Internet Research, 14*(1), e14.

Surowiecki, J. (2004). *The wisdom of crowds.* New York, NY: Anchor Books.

Swan, M. (2012). Crowdsourced health research studies: An important emerging complement to clinical trials in the public health research ecosystem. *Journal of Medical Internet Research, 14*(2), e46.

Szomszor, M., Kostkova, P., & De Quincey, E. (2011). #swineflu: Twitter predicts swine flu outbreak in 2009. *Electronic Healthcare: Lecture Notes of the Institute for Computer Sciences, Social Informatics and Telecommunications Engineering, 69,* 18–26.

Thackeray, R., Neiger, B. L., Smith, A. K., & Van Wagenen, S. B. (2012). Adoption and use of social media among public health departments. *BMC Public Health, 26*(12), 242.

Tufte, E. R. (2001). *The visual display of quantitative information* (2nd ed.). Cheshire, CT: Graphics Press.

Usher, W. T. (2012). Australian health professionals' social media (Web 2.0) adoption trends: Early 21st century health care delivery and practice promotion. *Australian Journal of Primary Health, 18*(1), 31–41.

Van de Belt, T. H., Engelen, L. J. L. P. G., Berben, S. A. A., & Schoonhoven, L. (2010). Definition of Health 2.0 and Medicine 2.0: A systematic review. *Journal of Medical Internet Research, 12*(2), e18. Retrieved from http://www.jmir.org

Van Gemert-Pijnen, J. E. W. C., Nijland, N., Van Limburg, A. H. M., Ossebaard, H. C., Kelders, S. M., Eysenbach, G., & Seydel, E. R. (2011). A holistic framework to improve the uptake and impact of eHealth technologies. *Journal of Medical Internet Research, 13*(4), e111.

Van Limburg, A. H. M., Van Gemert-Pijnen, J. E. W. C., Nijland, N., Ossebaard, H. C., Hendrix, R. M. G., & Seydel, E. R. (2011). Why business modelling is crucial in the development of eHealth technologies. *Journal of Medical Internet Research, 13*(4), e124.

Van Velsen, L., Van Gemert-Pijnen, J. E. W. C., Nijland, N., Beaujean, D., & van Steenbergen, J. (2012). Personas: The linking pin in holistic design for eHealth. In J. E. W. C. Van Gemert-Pijnen, H. C. Ossebaard, A. Smedberg, S. Wynchank, & P. Giacomelli (Eds.), *Proceedings of the 4th International Conference on eHealth, Telemedicine, and Social Medicine eTELEMED 2012* (pp. 134–142). Washington, DC: IEEE Computer Society.

Waterlander, W. E., Scarpa, M., Lentz, D., & Steenhuis, I. H. M. (2011). The virtual supermarket: An innovative research tool to study consumer food purchasing behaviour. *BMC Public Health, 11,* 589.

Wentzel, J., De Jong, N., Karreman, J., & Van Gemert, L. (2012). Implementation of MRSA infection prevention and control measures: What works in practice? In C. Sudhakar (Ed.), *Infection control* (pp. 93–114). Rijeka, Croatia: InTech.

Whitney, H. (2013). *Data insights: New ways to visualize and make sense of data.* Waltham, MA: Morgan Kaufmann/Elsevier.

World Health Organization. (2005). Resolution WHA58.28. In *Fifty-eighth World Health Assembly, Geneva, 16–25 May 2005. Resolutions and decisions.* Geneva, Switzerland, Author. Retrieved from http://apps.who.int/gb/ebwha/pdf_files/WHA58-REC1/english/Resolutions.pdf

World Health Organization. (2010). *Medical devices: Managing the mismatch.* (Background Paper 6). Geneva, Switzerland: Author.

Wynchank, S., & Fortuin, J. (2011). Telenursing in Africa. In S. Khumar & H. Snooks (Eds.), *Telenursing.* New York, NY: Springer.

Zimmern, R. L., & Khoury, M. J. (2012). The impact of genomics on public health practice: The case for change. *Public Health Genomics, 15,* 118–124.

Zuure, F. R., Davidovich, U., Coutinho, R. A., Kok, G., Hoebe, C. J. P. A., Van Den Hoek, A., . . . Prins, M. (2011). Using mass media and the Internet as tools to diagnose hepatitis C infections in the general population. *American Journal of Preventive Medicine, 40,* 345–352.

NOTES

1. HON-code stands for Health On the Net code, an ethical standard with regard to the provision of online health information (www.hon.ch).
2. For more information, see www.eursafety.eu or www.infectionmanager.com.
3. Methicillin-resistant Staphylococcus aureus (MRSA) is a strain of staph bacteria that has become resistant to antibiotics commonly used to treat ordinary staph infections.
4. More information about the LISS panel can be found at www.lissdata.nl.

In Focus

Mobile Data Collection Techniques[1]

Mitesh Thakkar, Nikhil Wilmink, Rachna Nag Chowdhuri, and Sruthi Chandrasekaran

The rapidly increasing prevalence of mobile devices and networks opens up new opportunities to access **timely**, **detailed**, and **high-quality** data at relatively **low costs,** even from the remotest corners of the world. These data can be collected from large-scale census and household surveys or from tracking singular, iterative events, like the activities of a community nurse at the local health center.

Mobile technology will soon become a ubiquitous tool for data collection, as newer and cheaper technologies provide greater access and options. However, successful implementation of mobile data techniques requires intensive effort to change individual behaviors and organizational processes. Therefore, there must be a compelling need for timely, accurate, and actionable data to justify taking on these fundamental changes. As detailed in Chapter 21, there is a burgeoning field of mHealth for which the investment has been made. EpiSurveyor, for instance, is a free mobile phone- and web-based data collection system used in over 170 countries "for the collection of information regarding clinic supervision, vaccination coverage, or outbreak response, and it helps to identify and manage important public health issues including HIV/AIDS, malaria, and measles" (Royal Tropical Institute, n.d., para. 1). Having current data on outbreaks or services is essential for effective distribution of scarce resources. For data that are mainly used for record keeping and auditing, mobile data collection tools may not be necessary, or expedient.

How to Use Mobile Data Collection Tools

Mobile-based data collection requires four basic components (see IF Figure 2):

1. *Hardware devices*—to enter data into

   Mobile devices can range from "low-end" phones that can be used only for phone calls and SMS (text messaging) to specialized equipment such as biometric devices that can capture and transmit data.

   Add-on devices: Mobile devices such as smartphones can also be linked to add-on devices such as biometric sensors, barcode readers, NFC/RFID[2] chips to record data such as fingerprints, inventory tags, smart cards, and so on.

2. *Data collection software*—to control how data are entered into the device based on programmed formats and rules

   Data collection software is mainly required for smartphones, tablets, and notebooks, and it tends to be specific to the type of hardware device (e.g., Android phones, Windows notebooks). In some cases the software is built into the hardware (as with biometric terminals) or is not required (as with low-end phones for sending data via SMS or interactive voice response systems [IVRS]).

Data collection software can be (a) custom built, (b) licensed, or (c) subscribed to as a service/platform.

3. *Data transmission*—to transmit or transfer the field-level data to a remote location or a single central computer

Mobile networks allow data collected in the field to be transmitted via SMS, voice, and mobile Internet. With certain devices, like biometric sensors, data are transferred by physically hot-syncing cables to a computing device.

4. *Data aggregation and analysis*—to receive, collate, and analyze data

This can be done remotely through SMS/mobile Internet gateways on web servers with online databases or through hot-syncing on local computers using spreadsheets, databases, or statistical software.

IF Figure 2   Different Components of a Mobile-Based Data Collection System

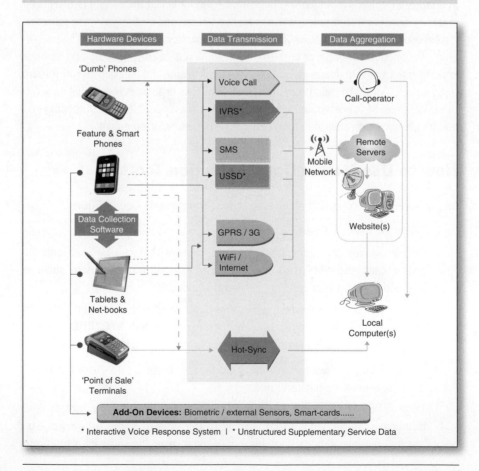

Source: Thakkar et al. (2013).

Selecting the Right Technology Tools

In practical terms, your options for selecting technology tools are limited to the following five combinations of the various technology components:

	Device	Software	Transmission	Aggregation
1	Low-end phones →	Not required	→ SMS →	Local/remote
2	Low-end phones →	Not required	→ USSD →	Remote
3	Low-end phones →	Not required	→ IVRS/Call →	Remote
4	Smartphones/tablets/ notebooks →	Required	→ GPRS/3G (mobile-net) →	Local/remote
5	Notebooks/PoS terminals →	Required	→ Hot-sync →	Local/remote

You can evaluate and select from these five options based on the criteria in IF Table 3.

IF Table 3 Technology Selection Criteria

Project Characteristics	Low-end phones + SMS	Low-end phones + USSD	Low-end phones + IVRS + Call	Smartphones + Internet	Notebook/PoS + Hot Sync
	1	**2**	**3**	**4**	**5**
Monitoring ongoing projects and staff	●	○	○	●	○
Carrying out large surveys				●	○
Verification/audit of field activities				●	○
Communication/outreach	●		○	○	
Provide real-time data to field staff	●	○	○	●	
Collect GIS/sensor/multimedia				●	
Real-time data analysis	●	○	○	●	
One-off activities	●	○	○		
Repeated ongoing activities	●	●	○	●	○

(Continued)

(Continued)

Varying ongoing activities	◉			◉	
Large number of internal staff	◉	○	○	◉	○
Mainly external respondents	◉	○	○		
Small number of internal staff	◉			◉	
Low set-up/hardware costs	◉		○		
Low running costs	◉			◉	○
Low literacy/numeracy of field staff			●		
Limited mobile network availability					◉
Limited mobile Internet availability	◉	○	○		○
Require non-Latin script			◉	◉	
Limited electricity/recharge for device	◉	◉	○	○	

● = Mandatory ◉ = Optimal ○ = Possible

Estimating Costs

A critical factor in deciding whether to switch from paper-based to mobile-based data collection is the cost-effectiveness of a mobile-based data collection system. This will vary from organization to organization, and from project to project. However, the common costs to consider relate to the four areas outlined earlier:

1. *Hardware costs*: Are your field staff full-time or part-time/contractual employees? How many field staff do you have? Is it better to purchase mobile devices for your staff or to incentivize them to use their own devices?

   If you purchase mobile phones/tablets, you can amortize hardware costs by assuming the devices' usable lifetime to be a minimum of 2 years and the breakage/loss rate to be around 5% over the 2-year period.

2. *Data transmission costs*: These are mainly recurring costs incurred by SMS, USSD, or mobile Internet (GPRS/3G) usage. In certain countries, you may also incur one-time set-up costs for dedicated services such as SMS short codes.

3. *Data aggregation costs*: These are recurrent costs that only apply if you use remote, web-based data aggregation and hosting. You or your technology vendor will need to subscribe to a server hosting (or cloud computing) service provider.

4. *Management costs*: The mobile system will require an internal or outsourced team to manage and support it. These costs will depend on the scale at which the mobile system is being implemented.

Case Study: Using Digital Data Collection in a Health Intervention

India has the highest incidence of tuberculosis (TB) in the world; every year nearly 2 million Indians develop TB and about 1,000 die. The national TB eradication strategy, in line with the World Health Organization's DOTS (Directly Observed Treatment–Short Course) method, requires a health worker to watch the TB patient take daily medications over a 6-month period. To prevent noncompliance and adequately implement and monitor this, mobile-based technology is being combined with a biometric system consisting of a fingerprint scanner connected to a computer and mobile phone.

J-PAL South Asia is conducting a randomized controlled trial evaluating the effect of introducing biometric technology in TB centers on health workers' attendance and patient compliance in four Indian states: Madhya Pradesh, Chhattisgarh, Orissa, and Delhi. Upon entering TB centers, health workers and patients identify themselves with a fingerprint scanner. The data are then sent by SMS several times per day to a server, and alerts and reminders are sent to health workers when noncompliance is detected.

To ensure compliance, J-PAL staff also monitor health workers through random spot checks. Mobile-based technology on Android phones is used to record if and at what time the health workers reach the center, whether the biometric device was used during treatment, and how many patients took their pills on a particular day. In addition to this monitoring, mobile data collection helps track patients in the evaluation sample in real time. Patient defaults on treatment are tracked digitally, triggering follow-up surveys.

This complicated operation would be extremely difficult without digitizing data collection. Mobile-based technology helps track patients and health workers in the study across the DOTS course and monitors attrition, which is crucial information for assessing the project's impact. The evaluation's field and survey activities are also planned based on these records, as surveyors visit the homes of patients at fixed periods in their treatment (which varies according to their enrollment date). In such cases mobile-based data collection tools allow for extra accountability measures such as sending photos with a time stamp of the surveyor in front of a TB center or the GPS coordinates of a patient's house when the patient receives treatment at home.

References

Royal Tropical Institute. (n.d.). *EpiSurveyor mobile health data collection.* Retrieved from http://mhealthinfo.org/project/episurveyor-mobile-health-data-collection

Thakkar, M., Floretta, J. Dhar, D., Wilmink, N., Sen, S., Keleher, N., . . . Shaughnessy, L. (2013). *Mobile-based technology for monitoring and evaluation.* New Delhi, India: Regional Centers for Learning on Evaluation and Results.

Notes

1. This section is an excerpt from Thakkar et al. (2013).
2. NFC = near field communication; RFID = radio frequency identification.

PART VI

Applying Research Findings

22

Enhancing Research Utilization

Jeffery C. Peterson and Angie M. Funaiole

R esearch can help address public health goals only when evidence-based interventions are shared by resource systems (e.g., researchers, trainers, consultants) with user systems (e.g., individuals, organizations, agencies, networks) that provide services in the field. Interventions also have to be successfully implemented to affect change (Kelly et al., 2000). The preceding sections in this book have discussed planning and implementing various types of public health research. In this section, the two chapters address the critical "what's next?" question and look into processes through which research findings are applied (or not) in public health practice. In this chapter, specifically, we discuss the field of research utilization (RU).

WHAT IS RESEARCH UTILIZATION?

Strauss, Tetroe, and Graham (2009) suggest there are more than 90 terms to describe the study of research utilization processes, though they prefer the term *knowledge translation* (KT) as an umbrella term. Another common term is *translational research* (Sofaer & Eyal, 2010); however, translational research means different things to different people. The most common distinction involves seeing this process in at least two distinctive blocks. The first, sometimes labeled T1, refers to the harnessing of knowledge from basic sciences to produce new drugs, devices, and treatment options for patients, while the second block (T2) refers to translating clinical research into everyday public health practice and decision making (Woolf, 2008).[1] Included in the scope of T2 are the following:

- Phase IV clinical trials, which may be aimed at reexamining the efficacy and safety of an approved drug, for example, in diverse populations (see Chapter 8)
- implementation science, which typically examines effective means of increasing uptake of research in particular settings (see Chapter 23)
- health services research, which investigates the health systems that deliver interventions (see Chapter 11)

Research utilization refers to the process in which knowledge, often in the form of research, is transformed from the findings of one or more studies into possible practice (Estabrooks, 1999). As we have noted elsewhere (Peterson, Rogers, Cunningham-Sabo, & Davis, 2007), we prefer the term *research utilization* to others such as *technology transfer* and *translational research*. Though these latter two terms have evolved to include a bidirectional process, they have been criticized to imply top-down models of information delivery and may still be criticized for overly focusing on the intent of the developer. This focus comes at the cost of end users and their reasons for using research-based practices and policies or, on the other hand, end-users' rejection of evidence-based knowledge and their continued use of current "habit-based" practice. Thus, we prefer *research* utilization to *knowledge* utilization because it helps us emphasize our focus on evidence-based practice, programs, and policies. And we prefer *utilization* to *transfer* or *translation* because of its emphasis on the point of view of user systems and not resource systems. Research utilization can refer to implementation and effectiveness evaluation of interventions or to the fields that contribute to the design of those interventions, including clinical epidemiology and evidence synthesis, communication theory, behavioral science, public policy, financing, organizational theory, informatics, and mixed methods/qualitative research (Woolf, 2008). In this chapter, we focus primarily on issues related to enhancing the utilization of research in population-based settings (T2) rather than clinical settings (T1). See Table 22.1 for definitions of key terms related to this discussion.

RESEARCH TO PRACTICE IN PUBLIC HEALTH

Historically, funding for T1 type translational research far overshadows funding for T2 type. Moses, Dorsey, Matheson, and Their (2005), for example, reported that in 2002 the $22.1 billion U.S. National Institutes of Health budget included $9.1 billion for applied and development research (T2) as opposed to $13.1 billion for basic (what some have called investigator- or curiosity-driven, T1) research. Only $787 million was spent on health services research, representing about 8% of the applied and developmental research budget and about 1.5% of biomedical research funding overall.

The research to practice gap is not unique to the field of public health (Bzdel, Wither, & Graham, 2004; Glaser, Abelson, & Garrison, 1983; Rynes, Bartunek, & Daft, 2001), but it is especially salient to the health sector, since considerable financial resources are dedicated to health research, with less than optimal returns. For example, the United States invested $140.5 billion on disability and disease research in 2010 but

Table 22.1   Definitions of Key Terms

Knowledge translation	"A dynamic and iterative process that includes the synthesis, dissemination, exchange and ethically sound application of knowledge to improve health, provide more effective health science and products, and strengthen the health care system." (Strauss, Tetroe, & Graham, 1999, p. 165)
Translational research	"Aims to carry across . . . the results of basic research into interventions that improve health." (Sofaer & Eyal, 2010, p. 19)
T1 translational research	"Bench-to-bedside enterprise of harnessing knowledge from basic sciences to produce new drugs, devices, and treatment options for patients." (Woolf, 2008, p. 211)
T2 translational research	Translating clinical research to everyday public health practice and decision-making (Woolf, 2008)
Health services research	Focuses on health systems that deliver interventions (Sofaer & Eyal, 2010)
Research utilization	A complete process in which knowledge, often in the form of research, is transformed from the findings of one or more studies into possible practice (Estabrooks, 1999)

ranked last among 16 industrialized nations in preventable deaths (Nolte & McKee, 2011; Trust for America's Health, 2010). Consider also that the combined resources devoted to agencies responsible for public health research and programs (i.e., CDC, SAMHSA, HRSA, and FDA) represent less than 4% of the entire U.S. Department of Health and Human Services budget (Trust for America's Health, 2013). Similarly, countries in the European Union combined allocate just 5% of total healthcare expenditures to public health research (University College London, 2011). Table 22.2 provides additional comparative statistics on health care spending per capita and investments in public health.

Table 22.2   Health Care Expenditure Comparisons Among the United States and Selected Other Western Countries

Country	Health Expenditure Per Capita ($)	% Health Expenditure Public Health and Prevention Services
United States	$8,233	3.4%
United Kingdom	$3,433	3.6%
Canada	$4,445	6.5%
Germany	$4,338	3.1%
New Zealand	$3,022	6.9%

Source: Adapted from Organization for Economic Co-operation and Development (2013).

The continual investment in disease treatment versus disease prevention is one explanation offered for why the United States lags behind other nations in health outcomes. The diagnosis and treatment of chronic diseases and conditions account for more than 75% of the nation's health care expenditures (Lambrew, 2007). Conversely, less than four cents of every dollar spent on health care is dedicated to public health prevention programs and policies (Lambrew, 2007; Partnership for Solutions, 2004). Increased prevalence of chronic diseases coupled with rising health care costs have driven recent activity in the public health arena to harness the collective capacity of various entities (e.g., government agencies, academic institutions, health care professionals, public health practitioners) to generate prevention research that yields evidence-based practices that can be translated into improved health outcomes (Centers for Disease Control and Prevention [CDC], 2009, Green, Ottoson, Garcia, & Hiatt, 2009).

Recognizing the aforementioned funding imbalance, leading public health agencies, such as the CDC, are initiating actions to encourage the utilization of prevention research in public health practice. The CDC's commitment to translating evidence-based research to practice is demonstrated through the establishment and funding of 37 Prevention Research Centers (PRCs) across the United States, each of which is charged with conducting prevention research with the explicit intent of using findings to inform public health practices and policy.

Workforce development opportunities are also available to public health practitioners (CDC, 2012a). The CDC has published case studies to document the public health work conducted nationwide at PRCs in areas such as nutrition, obesity, HIV prevention, and violence prevention (CDC, 2012b). Further, the Agency for Healthcare Research and Quality is funded through an allocation from the U.S. Congress to enhance public health research utilization.

The increasing perceived importance of adopting evidence-based research into public health practice is also reflected in the most recent iteration of the U.S. government's health objectives. One aim of Healthy People 2020, for example, is to "engage multiple sectors to take actions to strengthen policies and improve practices that are driven by the best available evidence and knowledge" (U.S. Department of Health and Human Services, 2012). Recognition of the research-to-practice gap is not limited to the United States. The World Health Organization (2006) cites bridging this gap as one of the most critical challenges to public health for the 21st century.

TYPES OF RESEARCH UTILIZATION

Before describing RU practices and processes, we first describe three primary ways in which research may be utilized: symbolically, instrumentally, and conceptually (Pelz, 1978, Weiss, 1979). As will be clear from the following section, not all research utilization is created equal. It is important for individuals across all levels of the RU process to be aware of this fact and to plan accordingly.

Symbolic Use

Symbolic use refers to situations in which research findings, or selected elements of research findings, that support existing behavior are utilized to legitimize habit-based practice while other findings are ignored. For example, practitioners may conduct evaluation research in the hope that the results will confirm, legitimate, and sustain their habit-based practice. When results are not what they expected, they "use" the parts of the research that apply to their situation (and their point of view) while rejecting the parts that do not.

There is evidence indicating this type of research utilization is somewhat common, especially in translation of research to policy. For instance, Lavis and colleagues (2002) found that available research in health services was used in at least one stage of decision making in only four of eight cases they investigated, while research was utilized in all the policymaking stages of only one of the eight cases. Supporting this study is evidence indicating that ineffective programs are often about as likely to continue as are effective programs (Shadish, Cook, & Leviton, 1991) and that the more rigorously program effects are measured, the fewer effects are found (Hornik, 2002).

Instrumental Use

Instrumental use occurs when the process designated in the translation of findings to practice is followed as specifically intended and outlined in the research development phase. In other words, research is used, perhaps with intended slight variations, as it was designed to be used. However, this can be difficult to do. An accepted wisdom exists that there is a tension between "fidelity" and "adaptation" of science-based interventions (Backer, 2001) that revolves around the following:

- the goal of developing universal health practices, policies, and programs
- the need to implement these with fidelity (or while staying true) to their rigorous design
- the necessity of utilizing practices and policies that are responsive, appropriate, and sensitive to the needs of local communities (Castro, Barrera, & Martinez, 2004)

Adapt too little and communities may reject practices and policies as a "bad fit." Adapt too much and risk violating the "core" principles of the research that led to its evaluation as science or research based.

Conceptual Use

Conceptual use of research is the adaptation of practice or policy, based on previous research, but with significant deviations from the original research indications. To make research findings useful, some level of adaptation must occur for a program to be successful in a particular context (Resnicow, Baranowski, Ahluwalia, & Braithwaite, 1999). For instance, a nutrition program validated among urban White middle-class youth that advocates for five-a-day consumption of fruits and vegetables will likely have to be culturally adapted for impoverished urban communities where access to fresh produce is problematic. Notwithstanding, when adaptation leads to the violation of core or essential principles, it can be said that research has been used conceptually or as a starting point for current practice.

COMMON BARRIERS TO RESEARCH UTILIZATION

Glasgow and Emmons (2007) outline 32 barriers to the dissemination of evidence-based interventions that include characteristics of the intervention itself as well as the situations and contexts of the user system. Strauss and colleagues (2009) cite over 250 distinct barriers to knowledge utilization! The barriers we briefly introduce here represent what we believe are some of the broader conceptual factors that inhibit research utilization.

Differing Worldviews

A primary factor contributing to limited instrumental utilization, or the unchecked use of conceptual and symbolic use of research by public health practitioners, is their concern about the replicability and applicability of research findings to real-world settings. This stems from the distinct traditions that influence how academicians and practitioners approach their work. Practitioners are typically embedded within communities and possess local knowledge of health priorities as well as an awareness of community conditions that act as assets or barriers to health. As a result, practitioners must be sensitive to the extent to which knowledge is perceived as relevant and suitable to their respective communities. Researchers approach their work from a more rigid methodological standpoint. Studies are theory driven and aim to address a particular research question(s). Adhering to established research protocols is essential to the generation of valid findings. Although researchers produce knowledge for uptake by potential users (e.g., public health practitioners), the degree to which the findings are replicable and transferable (external validity) is generally secondary to efforts to establish a causal relationship (internal validity; Glasgow, Lichtenstein, & Marcus, 2003; Green et al., 2009). The aforementioned descriptions are consistent with the delineation between efficacy and effectiveness research described in Chapter 16. As a result of the differing priorities between the two, intended users of research findings are challenged to translate evidence-based findings from efficacy research into practices that are compatible with community settings.

Ineffectual Information Dissemination

Ineffectual information dissemination is another factor associated with the research-to-practice gap. Successful research typically culminates with publications in academic journals and presentations at academic conferences. Accordingly, research findings are presented in a manner to appeal to academic peers since they are primarily vetted in academic circles. This well-established practice limits the viability and accessibility of data to external audiences. In particular, public health practitioners may have little or no exposure to data that can guide public health decision-making processes and practices.

Differing Timelines/Schedules

An additional but related challenge lies within the duration of the academic research cycle. Systematic inquiry into particular health topics can take several months or even years. Although these processes may result in important empirical evidence to support public health practice, it is incompatible with the manner in which public health practitioners typically operate. For instance, the prolonged time frame is impractical for practitioners who are expected to be responsive to emergent situations (e.g., disease outbreak). Green and colleagues (2009) suggest it may take as many as 17 years for a paltry 14% return on investment in the case of turning original research into public health practice.

SMOKING AND PUBLIC HEALTH POLICY: THE LONG AND WINDING ROAD TO RU

German physician Fritz Lickint was among the first in the medical establishment to recognize the link between smoking and lung cancer in 1929 (Witschi, 2001). The evidence base supporting this link was not established, though, until multiple case-control and cohort studies, initiated in the 1950s, began to publish findings. The most notable of these is the British Doctors Study, which provided the first solid epidemiological evidence of the link between lung cancer and smoking (Doll & Hill, 1956). Controversies about the initial findings ensued, and issued from the research community (e.g., Fisher, 1959), policymakers, and (primarily) the tobacco industry and its lobbyists. Many, essentially redundant, case-control studies of smoking and lung cancer followed the initial studies to bolster the evidence base and disarm criticisms. It wasn't until 1964 that the Surgeon General of the United States recommended smokers should stop smoking.

Opposition from the tobacco industry, and their powerful lobbyists, continued unabated for the next half century, resulting in numerous costly and lengthy legal battles (see Derthick, 2011, for an engaging account of this history). Even today, with the knowledge that the most common cause of lung cancer is long-term exposure to tobacco smoke, and that smoking causes 85% of lung cancers (Horn, Pao, & Johnson, 2012; Merck, 2013), utilization of the enormous evidence base varies significantly. In the United States, smoking laws vary widely among states and municipalities, from almost no regulations at all, to smoking bans specific to indoor areas, to bans including certain outdoor areas. At the time of writing (June 2013), after 60 years of evidence generation, 10 states still do not have general statewide bans on smoking in non-government-owned spaces (Alabama, Alaska, Kentucky, Mississippi, Missouri, Oklahoma, South Carolina, Texas, West Virginia, and Wyoming).

(Continued)

(Continued)

Equally large variability in tobacco policy exists between countries worldwide. One example is legislation pertaining to packaging and advertising of tobacco products. Some countries require no health warnings. Others require what is called "plain packaging," that is, the removal of enticing branding details. At another level are written warnings on the side of cigarette packages, as seen in the United States:

> SURGEON GENERAL'S WARNING: Smoking Causes Lung Cancer, Heart Disease, Emphysema, and May Complicate Pregnancy.

Other countries require larger, and more prominent, placement of warnings. Below is an example from Turkey (the text translates to "smoking kills"). The warning is required to cover at least 30% of the package front.

> **Sigara**
> **İçmek**
> **öldürür**

Australia and Canada (among other countries) have adopted even more stringent packaging regulations, requiring the front of packages to contain graphic photographs alongside written warnings:

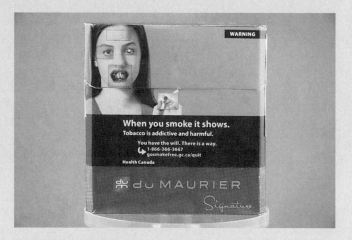

Photo by Steve Ward.

RESEARCH UTILIZATION OF CONCEPTUAL FRAMEWORKS

Despite the barriers described above, progress has been made toward reducing the research-to-practice gap. At the conceptual level, several models have been developed to better understand and communicate about the RU process (e.g., Stetler, 2001; White, Leske, & Pearcy, 1995). Davis, Peterson, Helfrich, and Cunningham-Sabo (2007), for example, provide a five-stage framework for planning and implementing research utilization (Figure 22.1). The model is founded on diffusion of innovations (DOI) theory and research (Rogers, 2003). According to DOI theory, *diffusion* is the process by which a product or service that is perceived to be new (the *innovation*) is communicated over time to and among the members of a community or social system. Typically, DOI focuses on understanding the real and perceived characteristics of an innovation (see the Appendix) as well as the social networks through which information about an innovation spreads.

Stage 0: Research Development

Stage 0 of the model refers to the research development process. Almost all research, at least in the field of public health, is designed and intended to be useful in some capacity. Yet not all research is conducted with a specific application in mind. And even in cases where the applied goal of a research project is explicitly outlined, an explicit plan or strategy for dissemination and utilization is often absent.

Stage 1: Dissemination

Stage 1 encompasses dissemination of findings, including the choice of dissemination strategy, the vehicle for dissemination, and the appropriateness of the targeted audience. Dissemination in this context is planned communication rather than passive spread of an innovation. Dissemination activities center on making information about research-informed innovations accessible.

Stage 2: Intent to Adopt

Stage 2 entails the adoption and implementation of an innovation. Activities include setting an agenda (e.g., prioritizing the issue/innovation) and matching innovations with a social system's needs, resources, and perspectives. According to the model, agenda setting and matching activities precede the decision to adopt an innovation. Adoption occurs between Stages 2 and 3.

Figure 22.1 Stages of the Research Utilization Model

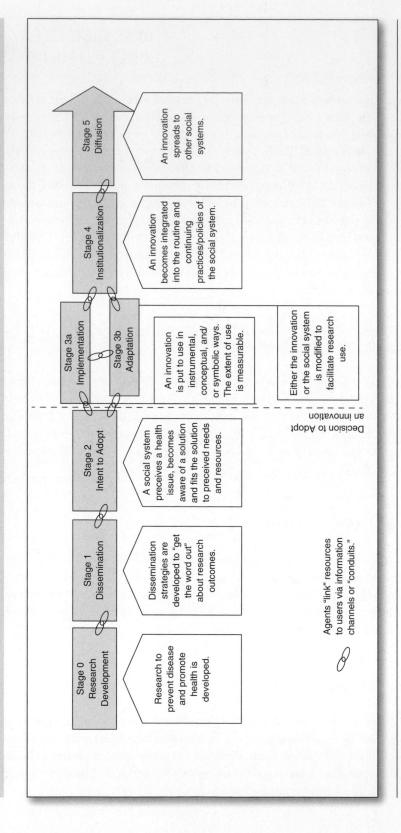

Source: Davis et al. (2007).

Stage 3a: Implementation

Typically, decisions to adopt an innovation are made concurrently with decisions about its implementation. Decisions may be based on factors such as the type and level of use of research, practices, and policies. The concepts of adaptation, fidelity, and reinvention play a key role in these decisions. Balancing adaptation and fidelity is a dynamic process in which the need for an innovation to adhere to the evidence base of the original innovation is weighed against the need for local adaptation.

Stage 3b: Adaptation

Over time, an innovation, the social system into which it is introduced, or both may change or be modified to facilitate use of the innovation. Thus, the perceived fit between the innovation and social system resources that led to the decision to adopt needs to be reexamined and adjustments made as necessary.

Stage 4: Institutionalization

Institutionalization is the process whereby an innovation becomes integrated into existing programs, practices, and policies of the social system into which it was introduced. Institutionalization is the degree to which the results of research are incorporated into the activities of a community, school, or other system (Goodman & Steckler, 1989). This concept has also been called *sustainability* (Altman, 1995).

Stage 5: Diffusion

In the final stage of Davis et al.'s (2007) model, an innovation is replicated or diffused to another social system. It becomes routine or standard practice in a broader social network. Diffusion can be spontaneous and is usually achieved through interpersonal contact, whereas replication is planned with specific aims. Both, however, result in an extension of research activities beyond the original efforts.

ENHANCING RESEARCH UTILIZATION

In addition to the development and validation of conceptual models, like the one described above, research utilization scholars and practitioners have also made progress with respect to documenting key factors that affect the potential success of RU efforts. In this section we discuss the more complex of these concepts and present a summary of additional strategies to bridge the research-to-practice gap (Table 22.3).

Compatibility

A vast DOI research literature illustrates how ensuring a few key characteristics of a research-based innovation enhances its potential for use. Here, we elaborate on the issue of compatibility or *fit* of a research-based innovation in the context of a user system and current programs, practices, or policies. To begin, we believe that in the initial research development process, practices, programs, and policies should be designed with the understanding that they not only will be, but *should be* modified/adapted *by intended users*. Rogers (2003), in his discussion of the reinvention of innovations, discusses the fact that some designers of public health practices, policies, and programs may look unfavorably on adaptations and thus structure new ideas or practices in such a way as to be difficult to modify (consider the use of proprietary software or rigid practice guidelines with highly interdependent components, for example). However, Castro et al. (2004) remind us that some form of adaptation, especially as related to cultural adaptation, is a pervasive practice, having emerged from recent emphasis on community-based participation in program planning, evaluation, and research implementation (Minkler & Wallerstein, 2003). Though issues remain regarding dynamic definitions of culture, participation, and even what counts as research, community involvement in shaping interventions should be the rule rather than the exception (Peterson, 2010).

Here are some suggestions for how to encourage adaptation while ensuring fidelity:

- Identify the core and superficial elements of the research to be utilized.
- Consider the option of "modularizing" research.
- Conceptualize adaptation as a process rather than a one-time event.

An example by Kelly et al. (2004) illustrates nicely the identification of core elements. The authors conducted a randomized trial to test the effectiveness of transferring a research-based HIV prevention intervention via an interactive, distance-learning computer training curriculum with individualized distance consultation among nongovernmental organizations (NGOs) in 78 countries. Kelly et al. chose the popular opinion leader (POL) model for dissemination of the community-level intervention. Core elements of this model include

- the use of ethnography to identify large numbers of opinion leaders,
- training POLs to deliver theory-based messages that personally endorse and instill positive attitudes about safer behavior,
- encouraging POLs to deliver these messages to friends and acquaintances in everyday conversations.

The project began with an initial assessment of whether core elements of the POL model already existed among the potential adopting agencies. After potential adopters received training, postcurriculum consultation continued for 6 months, during which time questions were asked and answered regarding how to culturally tailor the intervention for local use.

As a result of the consultants' decision to not pressure organizations to adopt the intervention but instead to follow a provider-centered approach to help each NGO achieve its own goals, there were mixed results. On one hand, significantly more NGOs in the experimental condition than in control developed a new HIV prevention program based on the model that was disseminated, incorporated POL core elements into an existing program, or otherwise modified an existing program based on the disseminated model. On the other hand, Kelly et al. (2004) report that most NGOs did not adopt the dissemination intervention in its entirety and that their use of core elements was selective. Thus, this example serves as evidence of the generalizations that (1) higher degrees of adaptation lead to faster and more sustained utilization of research, (2) it is necessary to clearly and proactively identify core elements of an intervention lest it become impossible to manage the fidelity/adaptation tension (Backer, 2001), and (3) making core elements available for utilization in modular form in *a la carte* fashion increases the likelihood of research utilization (though potentially in conceptual or symbolic form).

Kelly and colleagues' (2004) case further supports the need to view research utilization as a process and not a single-point-in-time decision. Cunningham-Sabo and colleagues (2007) reviewed 86 articles meeting the criteria of peer-reviewed studies that explicitly described how evidence-based disease prevention and health promotion research was disseminated or used for practice or policy. The study found that nearly two thirds of these studies focused solely on describing effective means for either (1) promoting one-way dissemination strategies that focused on creating awareness of research, (2) measuring the intent to adopt by a user system's promise to use research at some future point, or (3) the actual adoption of research, which we defined as the official decision to adopt research-based policies or practices without description of how that research was routinely used over time.

Though a third of the studies described how the research was implemented, only 5 of the 86 described how the research was adapted for use, and 4 focused on institutionalization, or the long-term use of research in a user system's routine practices and policies. To summarize, research utilization was not complete when user systems became aware of efficacious and effective research, or when they decided to "try out" the research in a limited way. Effective research utilization is a process of resourcing user systems but also subsequently nurturing a customized process of fitting the research to local circumstances for sustained use.

Identifying and Engaging Linking Agents

To this point, we have focused primarily on facets of the research to be used that can be addressed in development and design—is it research based or habit based? Is it easy to modify or not? Can bits and pieces of it be used, or must it be used in its entirety? This is important when we realize that much of what enhances or inhibits research utilization happens *after* the initial decision to adopt a research-based innovation.

At this point, we shift focus to the importance of *linking agents* on the research utilization process. These individuals serve as a bridge or liaison between resource systems and user systems. They may be constituents of a linking system (Davis et al., 2007) and can be representatives of the user system, resource system, or objective third parties interested in research utilization (Dijkstra, de Vries, & Parcel, 1993). Linking agents' primary advantage is that they have sufficient knowledge about the research-based innovation as well as knowledge about the culture of the adopting social system, including the local language. Two dimensions of credibility are essential for linking agents. The first is technical expertise with respect to the innovation. Trustworthiness is another key dimension of credibility. For example, in "Indian Country" in the United States (and many indigenous communities around the globe), there is a history of mistrust of health providers that is attributed to past research abuses. In these communities, the use of community health workers can be problematic if these linking agents are seen to be constituents of the resource system rather than trustworthy members of the community or as objective third parties (Peterson, 2010).

Nevertheless, in practice the most common linking agents have been community health workers, also commonly known as lay health workers (LHWs), or *promotores* in Spanish-speaking communities. Evidence for the usefulness of these linking agents is promising. For example, in a review of the effect of using lay health workers to improve mother and child health and to help people with infectious diseases, the Cochrane Collaboration concluded that LHWs are beneficial in efforts to increase uptake of immunization and breastfeeding, improve tuberculosis treatment outcomes, and reduce child morbidity and mortality (Lewin et al., 2010).

Table 22.3 Summary of Strategies to Enhance Research Utilization

Plan for RU early in the research design	Plan and budget for dissemination activities beyond publication of journal articles. Activities can include postresearch stakeholder workshops and individual meetings with key individuals. Create actionable research documents written in nonacademic language.
Design flexible processes and practices	Design research-based processes, programs, policies, and practices to be modified/adapted/tailored by the intended users. This speeds up adoption and enhances long-term use.
Acknowledge flexibility of use	Do not be surprised if research is used, but in ways that were not originally intended. Research utilization is not a point-in-time phenomenon but an often lengthy, negotiated process.
Recognize when core elements are transgressed	Flexibility is important, but recognize that adapted/modified processes, programs, policies, and practices may no longer be evidence based. Plan to conduct efficacy trials for these second-generation innovations that transgress core elements of the original research-tested product or process.

Involvement of qualified individuals	Involve qualified individuals from resource, user, and/or interested third-party systems to help facilitate research utilization. Involve these individuals "upstream" or as early on in the process as is feasible. However, keep in mind that qualification may rest on perceived trustworthiness as well as subject-matter expertise.
Plan for and encourage dialogue among a broad range of stakeholders	Acknowledge that research utilization is a long, negotiated process that can be enhanced by broad stakeholder participation—and therefore there will be conflict. Plan on designing and implementing processes that encourage feedback and dialogue but that also serve as a platform for resolving disagreements.
Employ a participatory approach	Focus on user systems, not as consumers to be persuaded, won over, or converted, but as partners in a process of addressing a community-identified need, studying community problems and issues, and engaging in the development of programs that improve health.
Engage "champions"	Identify key individuals who have the passion, social connections, and authority to promote research findings, particularly over the long term.
Develop tools to facilitate implementation	Tools, such as job aids, can help individuals understand and adhere to new policies and procedures.

RESEARCH UTILIZATION AND GLOBAL HEALTH

Our discussion on enhancing research utilization to this point has focused, if briefly, on factors related to the innovation (fidelity vs. adaptation) and the individuals (our discussion of linking agents), but has so far left out discussion of the more structural features that affect the use of research. These are prominent within research utilization efforts in global health. If the more efficient use of research is an important topic in the United States, it is even more crucial worldwide when we take into consideration the greater disparity between the availability of life-saving research-based interventions and the impact of these interventions on improving public health. Jones and colleagues (2003) argue, for instance, that two thirds of child deaths can be prevented with existing but underutilized interventions that are feasible to use internationally. Data reveal that 14,000 people in sub-Saharan Africa and South Asia die daily from HIV, malaria, and diarrheal disease, despite available prevention and treatment options for these diseases in developed countries (Madon, Hofman, Kupfer, & Glass, 2007).

Lack of cultural appropriateness and cost-effectiveness have been cited as two of the most common stumbling blocks in research utilization in the global context, but as Madon et al. (2007, p. 1728) observe, a "bewildering constellation of social constraints and health threats" exist for less developed regions of the world. These include, but are no means limited to, limited knowledge of preventive health practices; sporadic access to basic quality health care; structural issues related to the underfinanced, under-regulated nature of health systems; inadequate sanitation infrastructure; and exposure to environmental contaminants.

Given the difficulties involved in addressing even the simplest of structural issues, research utilization in the global context has typically taken the form of community health information campaigns. However, research on knowledge gap theory (Viswanath & Finnegan, 2002) and diffusion of innovations (Rogers, 2003) suggests that these information-focused interventions typically increase the gaps between the health rich and the health poor rather than mitigating them. In short, individuals from higher socioeconomic strata gain greater preventive knowledge from health information campaigns compared to their lower socioeconomic counterparts (Dutta, 2008). The case is even more pronounced in the gap between women and men (Shefner-Rogers, Rao, Rogers, & Wayangankar, 1998).

To combat the issue of information campaigns inadvertently increasing health disparities, campaigns should be targeted toward linking agents further "upstream" in the decision-making process. However, rather than this dissemination- or translation-oriented approach, we suggest a more user-oriented point of view that involves community engagement in the research utilization process. Thus, we turn to our discussion of current issues and future directions to community-based, culturally centered, and participatory research approaches.

CURRENT ISSUES AND FUTURE DIRECTIONS

Green et al. (2009, p. 166) argue that the most salient question for the future of research utilization might not be how to make practice more science based, but rather "how can we make science more practice-based?" To address this question, we highlight, with our own modifications, four of Green and colleagues' broad principles required to move scientific practice toward a more participatory or community-engaged process (see also Chapter 4).

1. A health research agenda should be dictated by the needs of patients and affected populations. This includes the local community's point of view regarding the characterization and prioritization of issues—which community resources can be mobilized to address issues and how—and the degree to which implementation can be considered a success.

2. Research utilization strategies must not consider contextual and implementation issues in communities as merely barriers to be overcome. Strategies should also incorporate what Green and colleagues (2009) call *accountability systems*. This means, in our view, encouraging feedback and dialogue between resource systems and users.

3. The research agenda should dictate research methodologies rather than the other way around. In the case of participatory research, this might mean, for

example, utilizing qualitative or mixed methods in both process and outcome evaluation (Chapters 15 and 19, respectively) in order to more fully engage community capabilities and increase both the internal and external validity of the research itself.

4. The level of funding for research utilization strategies should be proportionate to the magnitude of the task. Additionally, to be truly participatory, interventions should attempt to equitably fund resource, linking, and user systems alike.

Culturally adapting interventions in the United States and in global health contexts can encourage initial adoption of an innovation. Cultural adaptation can also help adopters institutionalize or make sustained use of a practice, policy, or program over time, by facilitating buy-in through community participation in the research process (Peterson & Gubrium, 2011). The goal of culturally tailored research, then, is to identify underlying cultural dimensions that may be incorporated successfully into the delivery of local health interventions, programs, and messaging (Dutta, 2008). Cultural sensitivity in the tailoring process has two dimensions: surface and deep structure. Surface structure refers to attempts to infuse health interventions with superficial characteristics of a target population, such as language, food, and music. Deep structure refers to attempts to design programs with respect to core cultural values and environmental, social, and historical factors that affect specific health behaviors (Resnicow et al., 1999).

This latter, deep-structure perspective is echoed by Dutta (2008), who proposes a culture-centered approach that incorporates culture at a deeper and more salient structural level. The culture-centered framework is rooted in community-defined and -prioritized health issues. Salient local issues are generated by asking questions such as "What does it mean to be healthy in your community?" and "What is stopping you from realizing that vision?" The active role of the affected community is then engaged in answering those questions and developing health applications.

As noted in the In Focus section, "Community-Based Participatory Research" (after Chapter 4), many public health research studies and programs use community advisory boards/committees (CABs/CACs) to represent a community throughout the research process. Though clearly there are many advantages to the enhancement of research utilization by having a powerful, credible, and active CAB, there are negative aspects, too (Peterson, 2010). If CABs are populated by "the usual suspects," this may promote the rise of a "volunteer sector elite" and the promotion of a narrow community point of view. Such was the critique leveled at the implementation of the World Health Organization's Healthy City Initiative in the United Kingdom (Jewkes & Murcott, 1998). Further, CABs can be used symbolically to suggest full community participation when sometimes this participation can be nominal and sporadic. Long-term research utilization can be compromised if these (potential) issues are not addressed.

We suggest that CABs consider recruiting broad representation and create and maintain structures and processes to engage with various communities-within-communities in order to address conflicts, contradictions, and changing circumstances. This would be an example of an element of an accountability system that encourages dialogue, as mentioned earlier—one that privileges the point of view of the community and utilizes it as a partnership. Less engaged use of CABs can backfire and cause research to be rejected if participants realize they are being made to feel a part of, but are not really part of, a participatory process (see the Cambodia TDF example in Chapter 4). It is an example of a symbolic or political use of community input rather than instrumental use of it as a partnership mechanism.

We agree with Maurana, Wolff, Beck, and Simpson (2001) that the future of enhanced and successful research utilization should focus on user systems, not as consumers to be persuaded, won over, or converted, but as real partners in the process of addressing community needs, studying community issues, and developing health programs.

ADDITIONAL RESOURCES

Internet

Agency for Health Research and Quality (latest information on translating research into practice): www.ahrq.gov/health-care-information/topics/topic-translating-research-into-practice.html

FHI 360 (*Eight Strategies for Research to Practice*, well-written and practical document outlining specific strategies): http://www.fhi360.org/sites/default/files/media/documents/eight-strategies-for-research-to-practice.pdf

University of Alberta, Knowledge Utilization Studies Program (comprehensive listing of research/knowledge utilization bibliographies and databases): www.uofaweb.ualberta.ca/kusp/bibliographies-databases.cfm

Journal Articles

Bero, L. A., Grilli, R., Grimshaw, J. M., Harvey, E., Oxman, D., & Thomson, M. A. (1998). Closing the gap between research and practice: An overview of systematic reviews of interventions to promote the implementation of research findings. *British Medical Journal, 317,* 465–468.

Hemsley-Brown, J. V. (2004). Facilitating research utilization: A cross-sector review of research evidence. *International Journal of Public Sector Management, 17,* 534–553.

REFERENCES

Altman, D. G. (1995). Sustaining interventions in community systems: On the relationship between researchers and communities. *Health Psychology, 14,* 526–536.

Backer, T. E. (2001). *Finding the balance program fidelity and adaption in substance abuse prevention: A state of the art review.* Washington, DC: Substance Abuse and Mental Health Services Administration. Retrieved from http://sshs.promoteprevent.org/resources/finding-balance-program-fidelity-and-adaptation-substance-abuse-prevention

Bzdel, L., Wither, C., & Graham, P. (2004). *KU resource guide.* Retrieved from http://www.kusp.ualberta.ca/en/Resources/KUResourceGuide.aspx

Castro, F. G., Barrera, M., Jr., & Martinez, C. R. (2004). The cultural adaptation of prevention interventions: Resolving tensions between fidelity and fit. *Prevention Science, 5,* 41–45.

Centers for Disease Control and Prevention. (2009). *The power of prevention: Chronic disease . . . the public health challenge of the 21st century.* Atlanta, GA: Author. Retrieved from http://www.cdc.gov/chronicdisease/pdf/2009-Power-of-Prevention.pdf

Centers for Disease Control and Prevention. (2012a). *Prevention Research Centers: Fast facts about PRCs.* Retrieved from http://www.cdc.gov/prc/about-prc-program/fast-facts.htm

Centers for Disease Control and Prevention. (2012b). *Prevention Research Centers: Prevention strategies.* Retrieved from http://www.cdc.gov/prc/prevention-strategies/index.htm

Cunningham-Sabo, L., Carpenter, W. R., Peterson, J., Anderson, L., Savitz, L., & Davis, S. (2007). Utilization of prevention research: Searching for evidence. *American Journal of Preventive Medicine, 33*(1), S9–S20.

Davis, S. M., Peterson, J. C., Helfrich, C. D., & Cunningham-Sabo, L. (2007). Introduction and conceptual model for utilization of prevention research. *American Journal of Preventive Medicine, 33*(1S), S1–S5.

Derthick, M. (2011). *Up in smoke: From legislation to litigation in tobacco politics* (3rd ed.). Washington, DC: CQ Press.

Dijkstra, M., de Vries, H., & Parcel, G. S. (1993). The linkage approach applied to a school-based smoking prevention program in The Netherlands. *Journal of School Health, 63,* 339–342.

Doll, R., & Hill, A. (1956). Lung cancer and other causes of death in relation to smoking. *British Medical Journal, 2,* 1071–1081.

Dutta, M. J. (2008). *Communicating health: A culture centered approach.* Cambridge, UK: Polity Press.

Estabrooks, C. A. (1999). The conceptual structure of research utilization. *Research in Nursing & Health, 22,* 203–216.

Fisher R. (1959). Cigarettes and cancer. *Centennial Review, 1959,* 60–66.

Glaser, E. M., Abelson, H. H., & Garrison, K. N. (1983). *Putting knowledge to use: Facilitating the diffusion of knowledge and the implementation of planned change.* San Francisco, CA: Jossey-Bass.

Glasgow, R. E., & Emmons, K. M. (2007). How can we increase translation of research into practice? Types of evidence needed. *Annual Review of Public Health, 28,* 413–433.

Glasgow, R. E., Lichtenstein, E., & Marcus, A. C. (2003). Why don't we see more translation of health promotion research to practice? Rethinking the efficacy-to-effectiveness transition. *American Journal of Public Health, 93,* 1261–1267.

Goodman, R. M., & Steckler A. (1989). A model for the institutionalization of health promotion programs. *Family and Community Health, 11,* 63–78.

Green, L. W., Ottoson, J. M., Garcia, C., & Hiatt, R. A. (2009). Diffusion theory and knowledge dissemination utilization, and integration in public health. *Annual Review of Public Health, 30,* 151–174.

Hiatt, R. A. (2010). The epicenter of translational science. *American Journal of Epidemiology, 172,* 525–527.

Horn, L., Pao, W., & Johnson, D. (2012). Neoplasms of the lung. In D. Longo, A. Fauci, D. Kasper, S. Hauser, J. Jameson, & J. Loscalzo (Eds.), *Harrison's principles of internal medicine* (18th ed., pp. 737–753). New York, NY: McGraw-Hill.

Hornik, R. C. (2002). Public health communication: Making sense of contradictory evidence. In R. C. Hornik (Ed.), *Public health communication: Evidence for behavior change* (pp. 1–22). Mahwah, NJ: Lawrence Erlbaum.

Jewkes, R., & Murcott, A. (1998). Community representatives: Representing the "community"? *Social Science & Medicine, 46,* 843–858.

Jones, G., Steketee, R. W., Black, R. F., Bhutta, Z. A., Morris, S .S., & Bellagio Child Survival Group. (2003). How many child deaths can we prevent this year? *Lancet, 362,* 65–71.

Kelly, J. A., Somlai, A. M., Benotsch, E. G., McAuliffe, T. L., Amirkhanian, Y. A., Brown, K. D., . . . Opgenorth, K. M. (2004). Distance communication transfer of HIV prevention interventions to service providers. *Science, 305,* 1953–1954.

Kelly, J. A., Somlai, A. M., DiFranceisco, W. J., Otto-Salaj, L. L., McAuliffe, T. L., Hackl, K. L., & Rompa, D. (2000). Bridging the gap between the science and service of HIV prevention: Transferring effective research-based HIV prevention interventions to community AIDS service providers. *American Journal of Public Health, 90,* 1082–1088.

Lambrew, J. M. (2007). *A wellness trust to prioritize disease prevention.* Washington, DC: Brookings Institution. Retrieved from http://www.brookings.edu/research/papers/2007/04/useconomics-lambrew

Lavis, J. N., Ross, S. E., Hurley, J. E. Hohennadel, J. M., Stoddart, G. L., Woodward, C. A., & Abelson, J. (2002). Examining the role of health services research in public policymaking. *Milbank Quarterly, 80*(1), 125–154.

Lewin, S., Munabi-Babigumira, S., Glenton, C., Daniels, K., Bosch-Capblanch, X., van Wyk, B. E., . . . Scheel, I. B. (2010). Lay health workers in primary and community health care for maternal and child health and the management of infectious diseases. *Cochrane Database of Systematic Reviews, 3,* CD004015.

Madon, T., Hofman, K. J., Kupfer, L., & Glass, R. I. (2007). Implementation science. *Science, 318,* 1728–1729.

Maurana, C. A., Wolff, M., Beck, B., & Simpson, D. E. (2001). Working with our communities: Moving from service to scholarship in the health professions. *Education for Health, 14,* 207–220.

Merck. (2013). Lung carcinoma. In *The Merck Manual for Health Care Professionals.* Retrieved from http://www.merckmanuals.com/professional/pulmonary_disorders/tumors_of_the_lungs/lung_carcinoma.html

Minkler, M., & Wallerstein, N. (2003). *Community based participatory research for health.* San Francisco, CA: Jossey-Bass.

Moses, H., III, Dorsey, E. R., Matheson, D. H., & Their, S. O. (2005). Financial anatomy of biomedical research. *Journal of the American Medical Association, 294,* 1333–1342.

Nolte, E., & McKee, M. (2011). Variations in amenable mortality—Trends in 16 high income nations. *Health Policy, 103*(1), 47–52.

Organization for Economic Co-operation and Development. (2013). Health status. Retrieved from http://stats.oecd.org/index.aspx?DataSetCode=HEALTH_STAT

Partnership for Solutions. (2004). *Chronic conditions: Making the case for ongoing care.* Retrieved from http://www.rwjf.org/pr/product.jsp?id=14685

Pelz, D. C. (1978). Some expanded perspectives on use of social science in public policy. In M. Yinger & S. J. Cutler (Eds.), *Major social issues: A multidisciplinary view* (pp. 346–357). New York, NY: Free Press.

Peterson, J. C. (2010). CBPR in Indian Country: Tensions and implications for health communication. *Health Communication, 25*(1), 50–60.

Peterson, J. C., & Gubrium, A. (2011). Old wine in new bottles? The positioning of participation in 17 NIH funded CBPR projects. *Health Communication, 26,* 724–734.

Peterson, J. C., Rogers, E. M., Cunningham-Sabo, L., & Davis, S. M. (2007). A framework for research utilization applied to seven case studies. *American Journal of Preventive Medicine, 33*(Suppl 1), S21–S34.

Resnicow, K., Baranowski, T., Ahluwalia, J. S., & Braithwaite, R. L. (1999). Cultural sensitivity in public health: Defined and demystified. *Ethnicity & Disease, 9,* 10–21.

Rogers, E. M. (2003). *Diffusion of Innovations* (5th ed.). New York, NY: Free Press.

Rynes, S. L., Bartunek, J. M., & Daft, R. L. (2001). Across the great divide: Knowledge creation and transfer between practitioners and academics. *Academy of Management Journal, 44*, 340–355.

Shadish, W. R., Cook, T. D., & Leviton, L. C. (1991). *Foundation of program evaluation: Theories of practice*. Newbury Park, CA: Sage.

Shefner-Rogers, C., Rao, N., Rogers, E. M., & Wayangankar, A. (1998). The empowerment of women dairy farmers in India. *Journal of Applied Communication Research, 26*, 319–337.

Sofaer, N., & Eyal, N. (2010). The diverse ethics of translational research. *American Journal of Bioethics, 10*(8), 19–30.

Stetler, C. (2001). Updating the Stetler model of research utilization to facilitate evidence-based practice. *Nursing Outlook, 49*, 272–279.

Strauss, S. E., Tetroe, J., & Graham, I. (2009). Defining knowledge translation. *Canadian Medical Association Journal, 181*, 3–4.

Trust for America's Health. (2010). *Ten top priorities for prevention: Promoting disease prevention*. Retrieved from http://www.healthyamericans.org/assets/files/TFAH%202010Top10Priorities DiseasePrevention.pdf

Trust for America's Health. (2013). *A healthier America 2013: Strategies to move from sick care to health care in four years*. Retrieved from http://healthyamericans.org/report/104/

U.S. Department of Health and Human Services. (2012). Introducing *healthy people* 2020. Retrieved from http://www.healthypeople.gov/2020/about/default.aspx

University College London, Department of Epidemiology and Public Health. (2011). *STEPS report: Public health research—Europe's future*. Retrieved from http://www.steps-ph.eu/steps_report/

Viswanath, K., & Finnegan, J. R. (2002). Reflections on community health campaigns: Secular trends and the capacity to effect change. In R. Hornik (Ed.), *Public health communication* (pp. 289–313). Mahwah, NJ: Lawrence Erlbaum.

Weiss, C. H. (1979). The many meanings of research utilization. *Public Administration Review, 39*, 426–431.

White, J. M., Leske, J. S., & Pearcy, J. M. (1995). Models and processes of research utilization. *Nursing Clinics of North America, 30*, 409–420.

Witschi, H. (2001). A short history of lung cancer. *Toxicological Sciences, 64*(1), 4–6.

Woolf, S. H. (2008). The meaning of translational research and why it matters. *Journal of the American Medical Association, 299*, 211–213.

World Health Organization. (2006). *Bridging the "know-do" gap*. Retrieved from http://www.who.int/kms/WHO_EIP_KMS_2006_2.pdf

NOTE

1. Note that while some scholars would go further by splitting T2 into T3 and T4 categories, others have questioned the utility of these distinctions (see Hiatt, 2010).

23

Implementation Science

Identifying the Path From Innovation to Impact

Temina Madon

Implementation science is perhaps one of the most recent innovations in public health research, and it is emblematic of the shift in modern science toward greater complexity and cross-disciplinary collaboration. This new field of inquiry has arisen in response to the so-called know-do gap: After decades of rigorous research in public health and medicine, there are thousands of biomedical and behavioral interventions with demonstrated impact on health outcomes. These are often tested at pilot scale, using scientific methods for evaluation—including randomized controlled trials (RCTs), the gold standard in medicine. Yet when practitioners try to implement these interventions under naturalistic, real-world conditions, it is often difficult to achieve expected health outcomes. Not surprisingly, the environment for public health delivery is more complex and heterogeneous than the controlled conditions of a research study; as a result, highly efficacious interventions often prove ineffective in the field.

An example is the persistent failure to achieve universal childhood immunization in low- and middle-income countries, particularly in India and Nigeria. Although recommended vaccines (e.g., for diphtheria, pertussis, and tetanus) are made available through UNICEF and the World Health Organization, in 2011 more than 22 million children failed to receive a full course of routine vaccinations within their first year of life (Centers for Disease Control and Prevention, 2012). Barriers to implementation include lack of maternal knowledge about the benefits of immunization (Owais, Hanif, Siddiqui, Agha, & Zaidi, 2012) as well as distribution and supply chain failures and difficulties accessing children in remote areas and conflict zones.

To improve the translation of new evidence and technologies into better health outcomes, public health researchers have established the discipline of implementation science. **Implementation science** (IS) comprises a set of theories and scientific methods that can be applied to maximize the take-up and impact of proven interventions, such as routine immunizations, preventive cancer screenings, or antenatal care. As an initial step, IS researchers are beginning to gather a body of empirical data to describe why evidence sometimes fails to be adopted, how environmental or contextual factors affect an intervention's impact, and how variability in the implementation of an evidence-based practice (including variation in fidelity, scale, or intensity of the intervention) affects targeted health outcomes. Over time, advances in this area of research will yield novel strategies for implementing health-related programs and policies. Ultimately, this will help to narrow the profound gap between our stock of proven health interventions and our ability to improve health at scale.

IS has early roots in political science and public policy (Elmore, 1979), where it has been applied to understand and optimize the implementation of new social and economic policies. In the context of public health, it is being used to expose facilitators of, and barriers to, successful implementation of health programs (Yamey, 2012). It is also being applied to develop novel promotion and delivery strategies that enhance program impacts.

It is important to note that implementation science (also known as implementation research) does not simply seek to increase the take-up of research findings or promote the replicability of proven interventions; ultimately, the goal must be to improve health outcomes. Sometimes, this requires modification of a proven intervention to suit local constraints or the integration of two complementary interventions to capture synergies.

Over the span of just a few years, the field of IS has been defined and redefined by a number of thought leaders, and review articles have been published in numerous journals (Eccles & Mittman, 2006; Madon, Hofman, Kupfer, & Glass, 2007; Proctor, Powell, Baumann, Hamilton, & Santens, 2012). Yet like many emerging fields, the discipline lacks a clear scientific consensus: What are the priority research questions in implementation science? Which approaches generate the most reliable and applicable new knowledge?

Part of the challenge in defining a research agenda is that IS draws insights and techniques from a range of disciplines, including economics, management science, social psychology, behavioral science, and applied mathematics. Each discipline comes with its own techniques, norms, and jargon. In such cases, it can be useful to explore how a new field differs from more established disciplines. Here, implementation science is considered in relation to health services research (discussed in Chapter 11), health systems research, and operations research (see Table 23.1).

Health services research (HSR) is most similar to IS, in that it focuses on the determinants of accessing and using health services; it also examines strategies for enhancing service delivery through improvements in care quality and efficiency. This field of research can result in generalizable knowledge, for example, through multisite effectiveness trials that evaluate the scale-up of disease management protocols across different contexts and settings (Lemmens et al., 2011; see also Chapter 16). However, HSR tends to be provider and patient oriented (Institute of Medicine [IOM], 1979), and it primarily examines interventions in the personal health care setting.

In contrast, IS extends beyond the health sector to include workplace or school-based programs, environmental policies, and poverty-reduction initiatives that target health outcomes. It can also be used to examine the diverse structural and social factors (e.g., employment conditions, social stigma, gender norms) that influence the impacts of health interventions in the "real world."

Table 23.1 Comparison of IS With Other Fields of Public Health Research

Field	Focus of Analysis	Focus of Observation	Common Approaches	Applicability
Health services research (IOM, 1994)	Delivery, accessibility, utilization, cost, and quality of personal health services	Patients, providers	Observational, formative, interventional	Studies the determinants of health service quality within specific contexts. External validity can be established through multisite intervention trials.
Health systems research (National Library of Medicine [NLM], 2009)	Organization, performance, financing, and workforce of public health and personal health care delivery systems	Providers, clinics or hospitals, insurance providers	Observational, secondary data analysis	Usually highly context specific. Can apply more generally if contextual factors are well identified.
Operations research (Utley, 2012)	Maximization of targeted outcomes in the context of limited resources	Provider organizations, insurance providers, firms in the medical supply chain	Mathematical modeling, statistical analysis	Usually highly context specific. Can apply more generally if model assumptions are valid.
Implementation science	Delivery, accessibility, utilization, and cost of evidence-based programs in real-world settings	Communities, patients, care providers, insurers, employers, schools	Observational, formative, interventional	Studies drivers of health outcomes for real-world implementation of proven interventions. External validity can be established through multisite intervention trials.

STUDIES IN HEALTH SERVICES RESEARCH

A recent study examined the cost-efficiency of primary care services when delivered by a physician practicing alone, compared to a nurse practitioner working with a supervising physician (Liu & D'Aunno, 2012). Researchers constructed a series of mathematical models that describe the process of primary care service delivery, using model parameters informed by the literature (including data on provider salaries, productivity, and referral rates). The models predicted that a physician plus a supervised nurse would be optimally cost-efficient when the nurse practitioner is allocated at least 38% to 47% of the clinic's overall workload. Otherwise, the solo physician practice is most cost-efficient (although it is less productive, with longer patient wait times). This model was designed as a planning tool to assist clinics in the management of staffing and personnel policies.

Another recent study in HSR evaluates the adjustment of health insurance benefits by a major U.S. employer in 2009. Using administrative data, the researchers found that eliminating the co-pay for a common cholesterol-lowering statin can result in improved adherence to treatment among at-risk patients (Choudhry et al., 2010). Studies like these can be valuable in guiding the design of public insurance and public health programs.

If health services research focuses on the micro-level interactions of patients, clinics, and care providers, health systems research resides at the macro level, examining the system-level properties of institutions that deliver health care, including the design, financing, and performance of public health agencies. Systems-level research does not typically focus on specific diseases or interventions (NLM, 2009). Rather, it examines the supply of health services, including factors like physical infrastructure, workforce, and governance (Sanders & Haines, 2006). It often focuses on measurement of health system properties (Handler, Issel, & Turnock, 2001) rather than health outcomes.

An example is the development of tools and methods to measure the emergency preparedness of public health agencies. A recent study in this area (Nelson, Lurie, & Wasserman, 2007) presents a conceptual framework for assessing preparedness, including critical inputs, quality standards, and performance thresholds for agencies tasked with emergency response. This study, like many in the field of health systems research, relies primarily on models, observational data, and secondary data analysis. Indeed, it is difficult to imagine an experiment that empirically measures "preparedness" for a public health emergency, given that we cannot control the timing or location of emergencies.

Overall, health systems research can be extremely context specific and difficult to generalize, particularly for studies conducted at a national level (in which the number of observable units is typically quite small). As a result, health systems research may be less germane to implementation science. Nevertheless, it can be useful as formative research, for example, by identifying institutions, trends, or actors that may influence the adoption of evidence within health systems.

Operations research (OR) is a set of tools with roots in the mathematical sciences, statistics, and computer science that has been applied broadly to the study of health services and, to a lesser extent, health systems. The analytic methods associated with OR have also been applied to problems in financial, environmental, transportation, and organizational decision making. In the arena of public health, OR has come to focus on specific aspects of health programs or systems, such as efficient resource allocation or supply chain management. The aim of OR is to maximize performance given resource constraints, using mathematical models to represent specific health care processes.

OR is often used by health services researchers, as in the primary care cost-efficiency example described earlier (Liu & D'unno, 2012). It tends to focus on small, tractable systems, generating solutions that are applicable to the particular processes being studied. Given the complexity of public health interventions—and the paucity of empirical data to explain how real-world implementation of an intervention varies across contexts—the use of this approach by implementation scientists has been somewhat limited to date (Utley, 2012).

In summary, IS draws on methods and concepts from HSR, health systems research, and OR—including qualitative and formative research, mathematical modeling, and even randomized evaluation (or effectiveness trials). However, IS has a relatively sharper focus: It examines the adoption or practice of evidence-based interventions by individuals, communities, and institutions. The ultimate goal is to uncover behavioral, social, or institutional strategies for program implementation that facilitate health impact. In this sense, IS is a subdiscipline of health services research. Yet it is broader in scope, as it also applies to evidence-based practices that are implemented through schools, employers, and other institutions that can affect health.

PRACTICAL GUIDANCE

How does the adoption of evidence vary across time, environments, and implementation agents? How should we modify the elements of an evidence-based practice to improve its effectiveness in a new context? Answering these questions requires empirical data collection across a broad range of interventions and settings, as well as the development and validation of theoretical and mathematical models that describe implementation processes. It also requires the design and rigorous testing of implementation strategies or alternatives that improve health.

This section provides an overview of implementation research design and methods. In brief, the study of implementation starts with the observation of current public health practice, including the extent to which implementing agents (e.g., clinicians, school health officials, community-based organizations) and beneficiaries (e.g., patients, parents, employers) are adopting specific research evidence. These observations, once classified and quantified, can be described as *implementation variables*. As a next step, researchers often search for correlations between implementation variables and health outcomes, which may reveal important relationships or mechanisms.

Observations can be further formalized through the development of models, or theories of change, that describe the plausible causal links between implementation variables and public health outcomes. These models can take the form of conceptual frameworks, or they can be further specified using mathematical expressions. Both classes of models can be used to pinpoint performance-limiting steps along the causal chain; this results in problem identification and hypothesis generation. Armed with a clear hypothesis of how a practice influences health outcomes, novel strategies can be designed to improve the performance of interventions in real-world settings.

The next step is to design and rigorously evaluate the effectiveness of implementation strategies, using experimental and quasi-experimental research designs. Rigorous evaluation allows us to test specific hypotheses, validate our theories of change, and refine our models and assumptions. Ultimately, proven implementation strategies should be scaled up, with continued monitoring to track performance and health status against expected outcomes. In this way, the research cycle begins again, with the collection of observational data (see Figure 23.1).

Figure 23.1   Cycle of Implementation Science Applied to an Evidence-Based Intervention

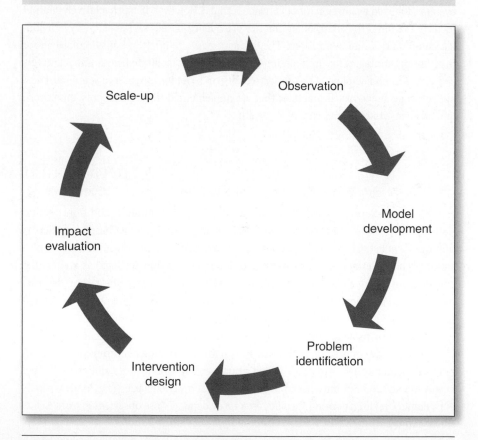

Source: Adapted from Allotey, Reidpath, Ghalib, Pagnoni, and Skelly (2008).

VIEWING IMPLEMENTATION SCIENCE THROUGH AN ECONOMIC LENS

In formulating an implementation research question, it is useful to begin with a systems-level analysis of the intervention being delivered and the environment into which it is being introduced. This assessment can consider the implementers of the intervention, the beneficiaries, the resource inputs, and the array of institutions and factors in the environment that affect outcomes—including, for example, local food vendors, employers, public transit systems, and religious beliefs.

In the economics literature, implementers and beneficiaries are often modeled as the *supply* side and the *demand* side, respectively, in the "market" for health (Eichler & Levine, 2009). Improvements in health can be seen as goods that increase an individual's utility or productivity (Drummond, 2005). Health can further be viewed as a good that is jointly produced by patients and clinicians or by communities and public health agents (Scott, Solomon, & McGowan, 2001). Accordingly, the market for health can be influenced by the behavior of patients and clinicians as well as the institutions that deliver health care (e.g., clinics, hospitals, public health agencies). It can also be influenced by other markets—such as the markets for food, jobs, housing, or financial services.

The market model serves as a useful conceptual framework for implementation science because it allows us to access a rich body of research from the economics literature. Indeed, behavioral economists and other economists have intensively studied the adoption of novel technologies and improved practices, both by individuals and by communities or firms.

For example, consider the case in which physicians are found to bias the delivery of patient services, favoring services that are easiest to deliver or most profitable. This can be modeled as a supply-side problem in the delivery of evidence-based public health services. Further, it falls within a class of principal-agent problems, in which physician incentives are poorly aligned with patient preferences and public health priorities. To address this problem, economists have developed pay-for-performance contracting mechanisms that incentivize health workers to deliver more of the highest-impact, most evidence-based services. A quasi-experimental evaluation of this approach was implemented by health clinics in Rwanda (Basinga et al., 2011). For half of the clinics, the government tied reimbursement for services to the quality of physician care, with "premiums" placed on priority services like prenatal care visits, referrals of pregnant women for institutional delivery, and the full round of routine child immunizations. The other clinics received direct payment for services, without incentives for the priority interventions. Researchers found that the pay-for-performance strategy improved the quality and appropriateness of care provided to mothers.

(Continued)

(Continued)

Strategies that specifically target the demand side (i.e., consumers or beneficiaries) include computer- or mobile phone–based reminders to improve patient adherence to treatment as well as incentives like conditional cash transfers, which reward patients' use of preventive health services (Eichler & Levine, 2009). In this sense, implementation science is the study of how to promote adoption of best practices on both the supply side and the demand side of the public health system.

As an example of a more complex intervention, consider opt-out cervical cancer screening, which has been proposed as a strategy for improving health outcomes in resource-constrained communities (Dim, Nwagha, Ezegwui, & Dim, 2009). The opt-out approach addresses important behavioral problems on the patient (demand) side, such as a woman's tendency to procrastinate or the stigma she experiences in accessing reproductive health care. It also addresses behavioral issues on the provider (supply) side, such as the weak incentives for private health workers to deliver high-quality preventive services. Furthermore, it can address structural factors that prevent the take-up of services, such as the high costs of transport to clinics or the inflexible work hours that low-wage patients might face. The opt-out implementation strategy ensures that physicians automatically provide patients with a service at the initial consultation (rather than calling them back for a follow-up visit).

Observational Methods: Associating Implementation Variables With Outcomes

Improving the real-world outcomes of a proven intervention might start with evidence that the intervention, as currently implemented, is not generating expected results. For example, suppose that staff working in the intensive care units of 40 hospitals have been trained to implement specific infection control guidelines. In a pilot study at one hospital, these guidelines were effective in reducing nosocomial infections. Yet after staff members in the 40 hospitals have been trained, rates of infection among hospitalized patients have declined only in select facilities, with the majority showing no change. To document and explore this trend, we draw on observational methods—such as cross-sectional analysis, panel data sets (cohorts), interrupted time series analysis, and case studies.

For most observational studies, both quantitative and qualitative observations will be collected, in the form of outcomes data (e.g., patient infection rates) as well as demographic data (e.g., characteristics of hospital staff) and process indicators (e.g., number of trainings delivered). In our infection control example (adapted from de Vos et al., 2010), we might conduct a survey of hospital staff to assess their knowledge, current practice, motivations, time use, and work load. We might also capture facilities-level data, such as stocks of essential medical supplies, staffing levels, and the socioeconomic status of households in hospital catchment areas. All of these measures represent potential determinants of guideline implementation. We can then look for relationships between nosocomial infection rates (the outcome) and our implementation variables. This is known as cross-sectional analysis, and it is used to identify statistically significant correlations between independent variables and outcomes of interest. This approach presents a snapshot of the implementation process at a single point in time. (While the focus of these activities is quantitative, qualitative data [see Chapter 15] are essential for building a richer understanding of potential implementation failures or successes. Shadowing or other observational activities could be employed to validate self-reported practices and work load.)

As another example of this approach, suppose that a gym franchise is offering its members a monetary incentive to complete a new, evidence-based weight loss regimen. Some of the gyms choose to offer high-powered incentives, for example, a cash payment of $100 per unit of weight lost. Others offer weaker incentives, such as a letter of recognition for those completing the regimen. We can track gym members' completion of the regimen—and even measure body mass index (BMI)—after the program has begun. We want to assess the extent to which a change in BMI is correlated with the intensity of the incentive offered. We can search for trends in the data by regressing the outcome of interest (in this case, participants' BMI) against the variation in implementation (e.g., the intensity of the incentive delivered). We might control for participant age, gender, and weight at baseline. As appropriate, we might stratify our data by gym or neighborhood characteristics to explore heterogeneity in our results.

In this example, the intensity of the incentive does not vary randomly across program participants, since each gym in the franchise sets its own incentive. So we cannot demonstrate causal links between the incentives and the gym members' health or exercise outcomes. However, we can identify correlations, at a single point in time, that may be indicative of the success or failure of the incentives approach.

Cohort studies and panel data sets (Chapter 7) are a different class of observational techniques that allow us to track implementation indicators over time and correlate trends in performance with changes in targeted outcomes. These techniques allow us to explore how an implementation strategy might influence health outcomes over time. In such studies, it is important to document the extent to which an intervention is implemented with fidelity across time; conversely, it is essential to observe variations in implementation across implementing agents and time periods. This can be ascertained by collecting process indicator data.

EXAMPLES OF PROCESS INDICATORS

In observing the implementation of an evidence-based intervention, it is important to identify the key steps in the process and define indicators at each stage. Indicators should be measurements that are reliable, accurate, and meaningful (Zeller & Carmines, 1980).

In some cases, process indicator data might already exist in the form of administrative records, routine census or surveillance data, or large-scale surveys. For example, health clinics may maintain administrative data on nurses' hours worked, productivity, and pay. Facilities are likely to maintain detailed records on the stocking and dispensing of supplies. National health agencies may collect nationally representative data on household knowledge or adoption of public health practices, for example, through Demographic and Health Surveys.

Interrupted time series (ITS) analysis is another approach used to track outcomes over time. This approach is applicable only when the onset of an intervention occurs rapidly, generating a clearly associated discontinuity (or step change) in outcomes. Unfortunately, a systematic review suggests that ITS analyses published in the public health literature often suffer from inappropriate analysis and weak control for bias (Ramsay, Matowe, Grilli, Grimshaw, & Thomas, 2003). Nevertheless, it can be an effective tool for assessing implementation strategies, when applied appropriately.

EXAMPLE OF AN INTERRUPTED TIME SERIES ANALYSIS

In Australia, a media campaign to reduce skin cancer was developed to deliver preventive health messages to the public over a fixed period of time (Del Mar, Green, & Battistutta, 1997). Researchers sought to determine whether the campaign had an impact on the number of skin lesions removed by doctors and whether this affected the thickness of excised melanomas. Because the start and end dates of the media campaigns were cleanly defined, data could be collected at multiple intervals, both before and after the intervention. The study reported significant increases in the numbers of excisions performed during the campaign periods, relative to noncampaign periods. However, there was no change in the proportion of excised lesions that were found to be malignant. This is an example of a strategy that stimulates demand for preventive health services, resulting in enhanced implementation of screening practices.

Observational methods form the basis for identifying potential implementation facilitators and barriers; however, none of these approaches can causally link an implementation strategy with long-term outcomes and impacts. This is a weakness of observational methods, and one that is often overlooked by policymakers (who frequently assign the same credibility to observational studies that they assign to randomized trials). Observational research can, however, help the researcher generate new hypotheses about why the adoption of evidence fails in some contexts. These hypotheses, in turn, serve as the foundation for logic models (or theories of change) that link implementation with health outcomes.

Theoretical Models: Drawing Concepts From Multiple Disciplines

Theoretical models in the field of implementation research seek to elaborate the causal chain between specific strategies for program implementation and beneficiaries' health outcomes. In general, theoretical models rely on extensive empirical data, both for design and for validation. Given the scarcity of empirical data currently available to implementation scientists, there is an imperative to draw on other literatures when developing new theoretical models.

A recent example is a theoretical model explaining the variability in adaptation of proven HIV prevention interventions by community-based organizations (Bowen et al., 2010). This study sought to answer a basic research question: Why do some implementing organizations adapt a proven intervention (as opposed to implementing with fidelity)? What features of the organization predict the likelihood of adaptation?

The research team drew on principles of information diffusion theory and the theory of policy determinants to develop a model predicting the level of intervention adaptation by program managers (see Figure 23.2). The researchers subjected this model to a preliminary test, using data from a cross-sectional study of 63 HIV program managers implementing five different evidence-based interventions. They found that the most relevant determinants of program adaptation included the intervention's perceived compatibility with existing organizational practices as well as the anticipated advantages of the evidence-based intervention (over internally developed interventions). While this model does not directly focus on the health outcomes resulting from intervention adaptation, it does explore a facet of program implementation that is likely to affect health outcomes.

Design and Evaluation of Implementation Strategies: Proving What Works and Why

Once researchers have developed a model that links intervention performance with health outcomes, it is possible to identify potential bottlenecks or barriers to health

Figure 23.2   Theoretical Model to Explain Program Adaptation

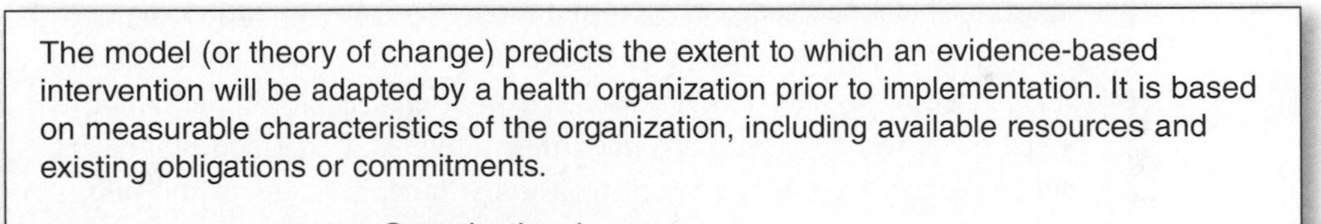

The model (or theory of change) predicts the extent to which an evidence-based intervention will be adapted by a health organization prior to implementation. It is based on measurable characteristics of the organization, including available resources and existing obligations or commitments.

Source: Adapted from Bowen et al. (2010).

impact. Next, we can design and test novel implementation strategies to overcome or relax these barriers. Strategies may be based on existing evidence from other fields and contexts, or they may be completely novel, representing a departure from existing approaches.

Experimental trials are the most reliable method for evaluating a novel implementation strategy. This approach—which measures outcomes for those exposed to a novel implementation strategy, relative to those exposed to "business as usual"—is based on the RCT methods prevalent in the medical literature. As covered in Chapter 8, randomized trials control for factors that are unrelated to the implementation strategy that could, in principle, affect health outcomes. Some researchers claim that RCTs cannot be used in real-world contexts; however, as detailed in Chapter 16, public health researchers and social scientists have successfully adapted the approach in recent years to accommodate the operational constraints of complex program implementations in the field (Banerjee & Duflo, 2009). In the case of public health, studies of real-world impact are known as *effectiveness trials*; among social scientists, they are called *impact evaluations*.

A few other nonrandomized, but highly rigorous, methods have been developed in recent years. Called quasi-experimental methods, these approaches enable the researcher to identify a causal link between implementation strategy and outcome by constructing a credible comparison group against which to compare the treatment group. The most common techniques include regression discontinuity design, difference-in-difference analysis, and propensity score matching.

EXAMPLE OF A RANDOMIZED CONTROLLED TRIAL

A strategy to improve the delivery of routine childhood immunizations in Rajasthan, India, succeeded in improving vaccination rates by addressing both supply- and demand-side implementation barriers (Banerjee, Duflo, Glennerster, & Kothari, 2010). The strategy offered a pay-for-performance bonus to nurses, delivered only when they attended a specified number of immunization camps held in rural Rajasthan. Random audits of the nurses were performed to confirm attendance at the camps. This component of the program addressed the problem of health worker absenteeism, a common challenge in developing countries that makes health services less reliable (and therefore more costly to potential beneficiaries).

In tandem, the program offered a small incentive (either a 1kg bag of lentils or a set of dishes) to mothers who brought their children to the camps for vaccination. The intervention was randomized at the village level, with a random selection of villages benefiting from the two program components. The combined intervention, offered in villages where both health worker incentives and incentives for mothers were offered, yielded a 38% increase in immunization for children 1–3 years old relative to the controls.

The regression discontinuity research design approximates the random assignment of individuals to treatment and control. However, this approach applies only for cases in which the intervention being evaluated is assigned to individuals or households according to a sharp, well-enforced eligibility criterion. By comparing those individuals immediately above the eligibility threshold with those immediately below, it is possible to simulate a randomized controlled trial (Linden & Adams, 2012). An example is the impact of a novel medical insurance program for low-income households in the republic of Georgia (Bauhoff, Hotchkiss, & Smith, 2010). Households with incomes just exceeding the eligibility threshold (identified through a proxy means test) were compared with those just qualifying for the program, controlling for average household age, gender, and level of assets. To confirm that the two groups actually approximated random assignment, the authors checked a series of demographic variables to verify that they were well balanced at baseline. Outcome measures were then compared across the treatment and control groups, including health service utilization and chronic disease management (which did not change with intervention) as well as out-of-pocket health expenditures, which were significantly less for those in the intervention group.

The remaining two methods, difference-in-difference analysis and propensity score matching, are highly sensitive to problems of selection bias and omitted variables. This compromises the ability to infer causality between inputs and expected outcomes. However, when appropriately applied—or mixed with other research designs—these approaches can generate credible inferences.

ADDRESSING HEALTH DISPARITIES

Because IS research links variation in the delivery of care with variation in health outcomes, it is a particularly useful tool for identifying the drivers of health disparities—particularly where there are demonstrated gaps in the adoption of evidence. Indeed, the methods described in this chapter can be used to tease apart the aspects of interventions or implementation strategies that are responsible for health disparities. IS can also be used to design variations of existing interventions that are tailored for communities and individuals experiencing suboptimal health outcomes. For example, a public health agency might target specialized technical assistance to clinics in low-income neighborhoods (Pallin, Sullivan, Espinola, Landman, & Camargo, 2011) in order to speed the use of technologies with demonstrated impact on the quality of care.

IMPLEMENTATION SCIENCE IN GLOBAL HEALTH

Many of the citations and examples offered in this chapter are from studies conducted in low-resource settings and in low- and middle-income countries. This is perhaps unsurprising: Improvements in implementation efficiency can stretch scarce health care dollars by enhancing health outcomes at small marginal cost. Indeed, many of the advances in implementation science have been made in the context of global health. However, some of these studies are carried out by behavioral economists and development economists; as a result, they may not appear in the public health literature.

An important consideration in conducting implementation research in general, particularly in international settings, is the role of context. Implementation strategies may be highly context specific; this argues for the central involvement of local researchers familiar with local norms and culture. Implementation scientists working in international settings will benefit from equal partnership with local collaborators.

CURRENT ISSUES

Given that IS is a relatively new field of inquiry, there are many issues being considered by those within and outside the community. One concern is the replicability of implementation strategies: How important or relevant are the context, local environment, or recruiting strategies of an intervention? Is it really possible to generate broadly applicable implementation strategies (like pay-for-performance or opt-out services)? Some behavioral scientists and organizational theorists argue that there are universal principles (e.g., from the psychology literature) that guide the adoption of evidence by individuals. Nevertheless, there is a clear need for replication of existing work, across different settings and intervention types.

Another current issue is the role of implementation science in comparative cost-effectiveness research. The latter is currently a priority for public sector health funding agencies. In the context of limited resources for health, there will always be demand to find lower-cost, more efficient means of implementing evidence-based practices. However, this requires careful collection of costing data whenever a novel implementation strategy is tested (see Chapter 10). As in medicine, the collection of data on costs (including the costs of provider or beneficiary time) is rarely included in a study's design, although this is gradually changing.

For the most part, both observational and evaluative studies in implementation science rely on outcomes and process indicators that are self-reported by subjects. A shortcoming of this approach is that subjects may modify their survey responses, or even change their health habits over time, in reaction to the "intervention" of interviewing. This phenomenon, known as the Hawthorne effect, can alter the results of observational and experimental studies and should be monitored where feasible (Zwane et al., 2011). To address this issue, there is increasing interest in using sensors, mobile phone data, and other direct measurements of individuals' behavior, rather than relying on self-reports as a proxy for outcomes.

The ultimate goal of implementation science is to improve health outcomes. Most of the methods used in this field are derived from other disciplines, such as epidemiology, economics, and ethnography, and are described in detail in other chapters in this book. What is novel is the application of these methods to a new set of questions. And while some implementation studies will measure the fidelity of an intervention's implementation, or the intermediate outcomes of an implementation strategy, or even the costs of alternative approaches, it is always useful to connect back to health impacts, recognizing that this is the goal of any public health research.

ADDITIONAL RESOURCES

There two excellent, practical guides, to implementing a rigorous impact evaluation, which includes examples of survey questionnaires, research budgets, and report templates:

Gertler, P. J., Martinez, S., Premand, P., Rawlings, L. B., & Vermeersch, C. M. J. (2010). *Impact evaluation in practice*. Washington, DC: World Bank. Retrieved from http://documents.worldbank. org/curated/en/2011/01/13871146/impact-evaluation-practice

Glennerster R. & Takavarasha K. (2013) Running randomized evaluations: a practical guide. Princeton, NJ: Princeton University Press.

The websites associated with each book offer guidance and videos explaining how to design an evaluation; collect, store, and analyze evaluation data; and monitor program performance during and after the evaluation: http://go.worldbank.org/IT69C5OGL0

The U.S. National Institutes of Health maintains a website on implementation research in health: http://obssr.od.nih.gov/scientific_areas/translation/dissemination_and_ implementation/index.aspx

For a comprehensive review of program implementation, and its interaction with program outcomes, see:

Durlak, J. A., & DuPre, E. P. (2008). Implementation matters: A review of research on the influence of implementation on program outcomes and the factors affecting implementation. *American Journal of Community Psychology, 41*, 327–350.

REFERENCES

Allotey, P., Reidpath, D. D., Ghalib, H., Pagnoni, F., & Skelly, W. C. (2008). Efficacious, effective, and embedded interventions: Implementation research in infectious disease control. *BMC Public Health, 8*, 343.

Banerjee, A. V., & Duflo, E. (2009). The experimental approach to development economics. *Annual Review of Economics, 1*(1), 151–178.

Banerjee, A. V., Duflo, E., Glennerster, R., & Kothari, D. (2010). Improving immunisation coverage in rural India: Clustered randomised controlled evaluation of immunisation campaigns with and without incentives. *BMJ, 340*, c2220.

Basinga, P., Gertler, P. J., Binagwaho, A., Soucat, A. L. B., Sturdy, J., & Vermeersch, C. M. J. (2011). Effect on maternal and child health services in Rwanda of payment to primary health-care providers for performance: An impact evaluation. *Lancet, 377*, 1421–1428.

Bauhoff, S., Hotchkiss, D. R., & Smith, O. (2010). The impact of medical insurance for the poor in Georgia: A regression discontinuity approach. *Health Economics, 20*, 1362–1378.

Bowen, S. A., Saunders, R. P., Richter, D. L., Hussey, J., Elder, K., & Lindley, L. (2010). Assessing levels of adaptation during implementation of evidence-based interventions: Introducing the Rogers-Rütten framework. *Health Education and Behavior, 37*, 815–830.

Centers for Disease Control and Prevention. (2012). Global routine vaccination coverage, 2011. *Morbidity and Mortality Weekly Report, 61*, 883–885.

Choudhry, N. K., Fischer, M. A., Avorn, J., Schneeweiss. S., Solomon, D. H., Berman, C., . . . Shrank, W. H. (2010). At Pitney Bowes, value-based insurance design cut copayments and increased drug adherence. *Health Affairs (Millwood), 29*, 1995–2001.

de Vos, M. L., van der Veer, S. N., Graafmans, W. C., de Keizer, N. F., Jager, K. J., Westert, G. P., & van der Voort, P. H. (2010). Implementing quality indicators in intensive care units: Exploring barriers to and facilitators of behaviour change. *Implementation Science, 5*, 52.

Del Mar, C. B., Green, A. C., & Battistutta, D. (1997). Do public media campaigns designed to increase skin cancer awareness result in increased skin excision rates? *Australian and New Zealand Journal of Public Health, 21,* 751–754.

Dim, C. C., Nwagha, U. I., Ezegwui, H. U., & Dim, N. R. (2009). The need to incorporate routine cervical cancer counselling and screening in the management of women at the outpatient clinics in Nigeria. *Journal of Obstetrics and Gynaecology, 29,* 754–756.

Drummond, M. F. (2005). *Methods for the economic evaluation of health care programmes.* Oxford, UK: Oxford University Press.

Eccles, M. P., & Mittman, B. S. (2006). Welcome to *Implementation Science. Implementation Science, 1,* 1.

Eichler, R., & Levine, R. (2009). *Performance incentives for global health: Potential and pitfalls.* Washington, DC: Center for Global Development.

Elmore, R. F. (1979). Backward mapping: Implementation research and policy decisions. *Political Science Quarterly, 94,* 601–616.

Handler, A., Issel, M., & Turnock, B. (2001). A conceptual framework to measure performance of the public health system. *American Journal of Public Health, 91,* 1235–1239.

Institute of Medicine. (1979). *Health services research.* Washington, DC: National Academy of Sciences.

Institute of Medicine. (1994). *Health services research: Opportunities for an expanding field of inquiry—An interim statement.* Washington, DC: National Academy of Sciences.

Lemmens, K. M., Rutten-Van Mölken, M. P., Cramm, J. M., Huijsman, R., Bal, R. A., & Nieboer, A. P. (2011). Evaluation of a large scale implementation of disease management programmes in various Dutch regions: A study protocol. *BMC Health Services Research, 11,* 6.

Linden, A., & Adams, J. L. (2012). Combining the regression discontinuity design and propensity score-based weighting to improve causal inference in program evaluation. *Journal of Evaluation in Clinical Practice, 18,* 317–325.

Liu, N., & D'Aunno, T. (2012). The productivity and cost-efficiency of models for involving nurse practitioners in primary care: A perspective from queueing analysis. *Health Services Research, 47,* 594–613.

Madon, T., Hofman, K. J., Kupfer, L., & Glass, R. I. (2007). Public health: Implementation science. *Science, 318,* 1728–1729.

National Library of Medicine. (2009) *Recent and future trends in public health workforce research.* Bethesda, MD: Author.

Nelson, C., Lurie, N., & Wasserman, J. (2007). Assessing public health emergency preparedness: Concepts, tools, and challenges. *Annual Review of Public Health, 28,* 1–18.

Owais, A., Hanif, B., Siddiqui, A. R., Agha, A., & Zaidi, A. K. (2011). Does improving maternal knowledge of vaccines impact infant immunization rates? A community-based randomized-controlled trial in Karachi, Pakistan. *BMC Public Health, 11,* 239.

Pallin, D. J., Sullivan, A. F., Espinola, J. A., Landman, A. B., & Camargo, C. A., Jr. (2011). Increasing adoption of computerized provider order entry, and persistent regional disparities, in US emergency departments. *Annals of Emergency Medicine, 58,* 543–550.e3.

Proctor, E. K., Powell, B. J., Baumann, A. A., Hamilton, A. M., & Santens, R. L. (2012). Writing implementation research grant proposals: Ten key ingredients. *Implementation Science, 7*(1), 96.

Ramsay, C. R., Matowe, L., Grilli, R., Grimshaw, J. M., & Thomas, R. E. (2003). Interrupted time series designs in health technology assessment: Lessons from two systematic reviews of behavior change strategies. *International Journal of Technology Assessment in Health Care, 19,* 613–623.

Sanders, D., & Haines, A. (2006). Implementation research is needed to achieve international health goals. *PLoS Medicine, 3*(6), e186.

Scott, R. D., Solomon, S. L., & McGowan, J. E. (2001). Applying economic principles to health care. *Emerging Infectious Diseases, 7,* 282–285.

Utley, M. (2012). Editorial. *Operations Research for Health Care, 1*(1), iv–v.

Yamey, G. M. (2012). What are the barriers to scaling up health interventions in low and middle income countries? A qualitative study of academic leaders in implementation science. *Global Health, 8,* 11.

Zeller, R. A., & Carmines, E. G. (1980). *Measurement in the social sciences: The link between theory and data.* Cambridge, UK: Cambridge University Press.

Zwane, A. P., Zinman, J., Van Dusen, E., Pariente, W., Null, C., Miguel, E., . . . Banerjee, A. (2011). Being surveyed can change later behavior and related parameter estimates. *Proceedings of the National Academy of Sciences of the United States of America, 108,* 1821–1826.

Appendix

Theories and Models in Public Health Research

C hapter Two discusses the use of conceptual models and theory in guiding the development and implementation of research designs. In this Appendix we describe some commonly employed models and theories in public health. Our coverage is by no means exhaustive, as public health researchers utilize theories and models—some more esoteric than others—from a number of different disciplines. We have attempted to include the major models and theories that public health texts discuss, although, for obvious reasons, our treatment of the topic in the pages that follow is more cursory.

Before getting started, it is essential to point out the distinction between a *theory* and a *model*. The definitions below are derived from the National Cancer Institute's (2012) *Theory at a Glance: A Guide for Health Promotion Practice*. A key difference between the two is that theories are intended to explain phenomena. Models, in contrast, are typically used to frame and represent processes—not explain them—and are often employed to develop a study's design and methodological procedures.

Theory

- An integrated set of propositions that serves as an explanation for a phenomenon
- Introduced after a phenomenon has already revealed a systematic set of uniformities
- A systematic arrangement of fundamental principles that provide a basis for explaining certain happenings of life

Examples: Social Cognitive Theory, Theory of Planned Behavior

Model

- A subclass of a theory, it provides a plan for investigating and/or addressing a phenomenon
- Does not attempt to explain the processes underlying learning, but only to represent them
- Provides the vehicle for applying theories

Examples: Health Belief Model, Trans-theoretical Model

Models and theories are often characterized by the level of analysis to which they apply: individual, interpersonal, social/community, or multiple. Which theory/model you elect for developing or framing a study or explaining study findings will depend on the research objectives as well as the unit of observation analysis embodied in your research. We, therefore, categorize them according to their level of abstraction. In order of coverage, we include the following:

Trans-theoretical Model

Health Belief Model

Information, Motivation & Behavioral Skills Model

Locus of Control Theory

Rational Choice Theory

Conservation of Resources Theory

Elaboration Likelihood Model of Persuasion

Theory of Reasoned Action

Theory of Planned Behavior

Precaution Adoption Process Model

Protection Motivation Theory

Social Learning Theory

Social Network Theory

Gender Theory

Community Coalition Action Theory

Natural Helper Model

Diffusion of Innovations Theory

Communication Theory

Symbolic Interaction Theory

Theory of Triadic Influence

Interactive Domain Model

Social-Ecological Model

Behavioral Ecological Model

INDIVIDUAL LEVEL

Trans-theoretical Model

The Trans-theoretical Model of behavioral change is a well-known, and commonly utilized, model in public health. The model posits that an individual's readiness to change or attempt to change toward healthier behaviors can be categorized into one of five stages

(stages of change): Precontemplation, Contemplation, Preparation, Action, and Maintenance (Figure A.1). Note that there is an unofficial sixth stage referred to as the Relapse stage in which an individual reverts to unhealthy behaviors.

The idea is to use the model to identify an individual's stage of change with

Figure A.1 Trans-theoretical Model

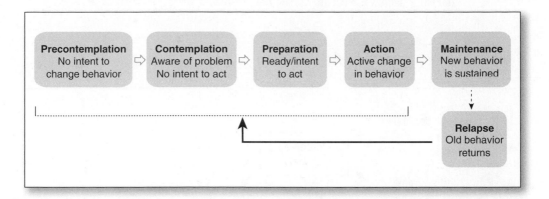

respect to a particular behavior and then move him or her toward the next stage and, ultimately, the maintenance stage where health-protective behavior is sustained. The Trans-theoretical Model, developed by Prochaska and DiClemente (1983), has been widely applied to diverse public health problems, including domestic violence, HIV prevention, and child abuse (Prochaska & Prochaska, 2009).

Health Belief Model (HBM)

The Health Belief Model is one of the best known social cognition models and is commonly used in public health research and practice. The HBM is a health behavior change model that was developed by Rosenstock (1966) to study and promote the use of health services. The revised model (Rosenstock, Strecher, & Becker, 1988) hypothesizes that health-related behaviors depend on six factors (Figure A.2):

An individual's perceived susceptibility to a health problem

The perceived severity of that problem

Perceived benefits of healthier behavior to reduce vulnerability to the problem

Perceived barriers to engaging in the healthy behavior

Sufficient cues to action, to motivate actual behavior

Self-efficacy, or one's belief in his or her ability to successfully perform the healthy behavior

For example, a patient is told by his doctor that he is at particularly high risk for a heart attack and is told to go on a low-fat diet. If the patient believes the risk to be serious (1, 2) and that a leaner diet will reduce this risk (3), he will adopt this behavior if (a) there are no or few perceived barriers to acting (changing his diet; 4), (b) sufficient cues to act exist (5), and (c) he feels that he can successfully adhere to the new diet (6).

The Health Belief Model has been applied to a broad range of preventive health behaviors, sick role behaviors (e.g., compliance with recommended medical regimens), and clinic/facility use (Conner & Norman, 1996).

Figure A.2   Health Belief Model

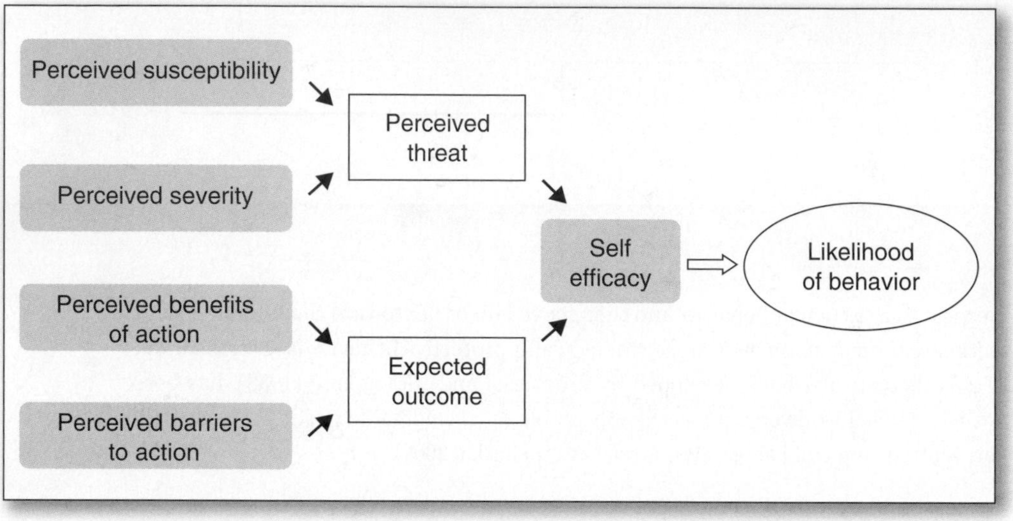

Information, Motivation, and Behavioral Skills (IMB) Model

The IMB model was originally developed as a basis for understanding HIV risk and prevention across multiple populations (Fisher & Fisher, 1992; Fisher, Fisher, Bryan, & Misovich, 2002). The model includes three primary dimensions (Figure A.3). The *information* dimension is cognitive in nature and refers to an individual's knowledge regarding the health risk and corresponding behavior change. *Motivation* is an emotive component and pertains to an individual's attitude toward positive health behavior and capitalizing on existing support systems to enhance motivation. The third component is *behavioral skills*, which refers to an individual's self-efficacy and ability to engage in a particular healthy behavior. In the context of HIV prevention, information might refer to knowledge about HIV transmission and how to reduce risk of transmission. Motivation may derive from, for example, knowing someone who recently died of AIDS, triggering a feeling of being personally at risk, heightening motivation to engage in some form of preventive action. Behavioral skills in this context could include knowing how to use condoms properly or learning how to negotiate safe sex (or no sex) with a partner.

Figure A.3 Information, Motivation, and Behavioral Skills Model

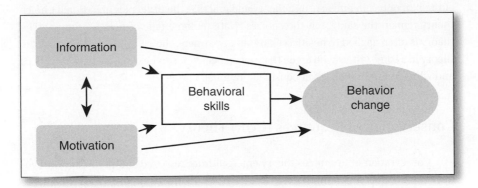

Although originally developed for HIV prevention, the IMB model has been subsequently used in other areas of public health, such as promoting contraception (Bryan, Fisher, Fisher, & Murray, 1993; Shattuck et al., 2011) and self breast examination (Misovich, Martinez, Fisher, Bryan, & Catapano, 2006).

Locus of Control (LOC) Theory

The LOC theory derives from personality psychology and refers to the extent to which individuals believe that they can control events that affect them (Rotter, 1954). In this theory, a person's locus can be conceptualized as either internal (individuals believe they control their life) or external (they believe that their life is controlled by environmental factors beyond their control). In public health, the LOC theory has been refined to form the Health Locus of Control theory (Wallston & Wallston, 1978), which focuses on health behavior. External beliefs are premised on the notion that one's health outcome is under the control of others (e.g., medical professionals) or is determined by fate, luck, or chance. Internal beliefs characterize one's health condition as being the direct result of one's own actions.

Internal locus of control has been associated with a variety of positive health behaviors such as reduced likelihood of depression (van Dijk, Dijkshoorn, van Dijk, Cremer, & Agyemang, 2013), returning to work after back pain (S. Richard, Dionne, & Nouwen, 2011), resilience following spinal cord injury (Kilic, Dorstyn, & Guiver, 2013), and coping with chronic disease (Janowski, Kurpas, Kusz, Mroczek, & Jedynak, 2013).

Various psychometric scales have been developed to measure locus of control, with the Duttweiler (1984) Internal Control Index being one of the most popular. A Health Locus of Control scale, developed and validated by the theory's progenitors, is also available and has been applied to public health research and practice (Wallston, Wallston, Kaplan, & Maides, 1976).

Rational Choice Theory

Rational Choice theory is a social-economic theory based on the premise that economics play a large role in human behavior (Gilboa, 2010). The theory posits that people make choices so as to maximize advantage and minimize cost. Behavior is a consequence of an individual's cost-benefit analysis, which leads to a "rational" decision. The decision is based on what an individual perceives will render the most benefit to him or her. In public health theory and practice, the principles of Rational Choice theory remain the same, but the choices relate to some type of health behavior. The theory is often applied to health seeking, and treatment choice, behavior. Note that the theory has some critics who argue that not all behavior can be explained by economics and what an external observer considers "rational."

Conservation of Resources (COR) Theory

Conservation of Resources theory emerged from resource and psychosocial theories of stress and human motivation (Hobfoll, 1989, 1998). A key postulate of the theory is that both *personal* resources (e.g., self-efficacy, expectations) and social resources (e.g., emotional support, social networks) help mitigate the potential negative impact of stressful life events. According to the theory, stress stems from the combined effect of the subjective perception of an event—in as much as it exceeds available resources—and the actual environmental circumstances that threaten or cause depletion of an individual's resources. COR theory has been used as an explanatory model for organizational stress in health systems (Glebocka & Lisowska, 2007; Halbesleben & Rathert, 2008) as well as depression (Holahan, Moos, Holahan, & Cronkite, 1999).

Elaboration Likelihood Model (ELM) of Persuasion

The Elaboration Likelihood Model describes how people choose to process and manage information they encounter (Petty & Cacioppo, 1981). The ELM is based on the concept that attitudes guide decisions and other behaviors, and that persuasion is a primary source of attitudes. The model specifically focuses on persuasion and asserts that there are two routes to persuasion: a central route and a peripheral route (Figure A.4). Central route processing is systematic; an individual internally weighs the logical merits of a message that is intended to persuade. The peripheral processing route is more experiential in nature; in this context an individual might be unmotivated and/or unable to elaborate on the logical merits of a message.

A key variable in this process, therefore, is involvement—that is, the extent to which an individual is willing and able to think about the position advocated in the message. The propensity for involvement is represented by the concept of *elaboration likelihood*, the probability that an individual will engage in effortful thought when exposed to a given message. Elaboration involves cognitive processes such as evaluation, critical judgment, and inferential judgment. When elaboration is high, the central persuasive route is operational.

Another defining element of the ELM is motivation. Even though individuals may have the ability to contemplate the arguments of a message, their level of motivation determines the extent to which they will actually do so. The model suggests that as motivation and ability to engage in effortful elaboration decrease, peripheral cues become more important in the persuasion process. Peripheral cues are sources of information, or cognitive cues, external to the message.

A central argument of ELM is that changes in attitude that result from central route processing will be more persistent, will be better predictors of behavior, and will be more resistant to counter-persuasion than are attitude changes that result from exposure to peripheral cues. Not surprisingly, the ELM has primarily been used in public health communication.

Figure A.4 Elaboration Likelihood Model of Persuasion

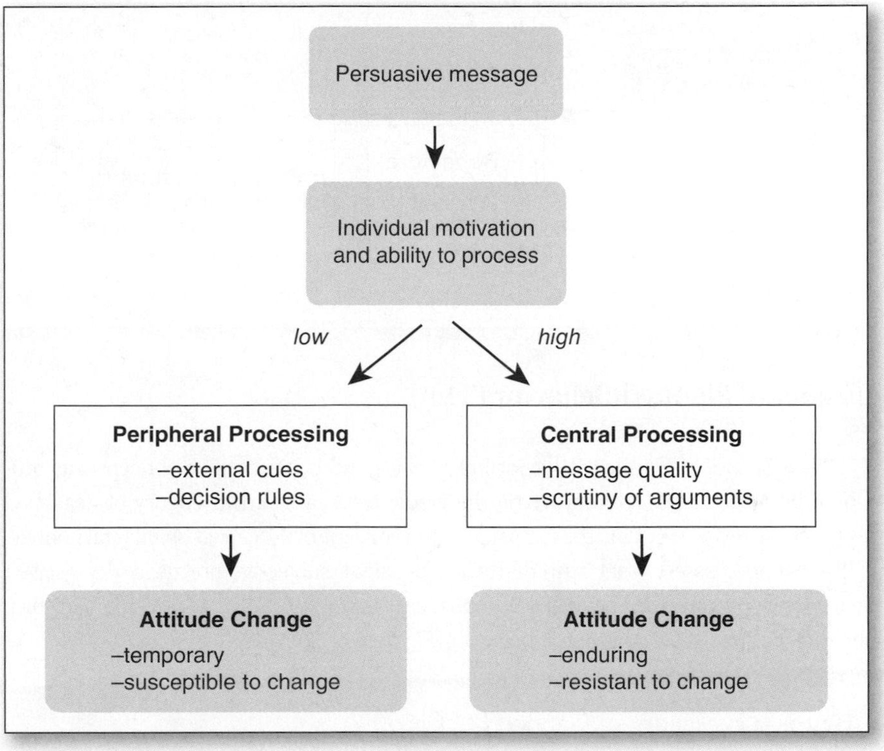

Source: Wilson (2007).

Theory of Reasoned Action (TRA)

The Theory of Reasoned Action (Ajzen & Fishbein, 1980; Fishbein & Ajzen, 1975) is one of the most popular theories in public health research and practice. It comprises three general constructs: behavioral intention (BI), attitude (A), and subjective norm (SN; Figure A.5). TRA suggests that a person's behavioral intention depends on his or her attitude about the behavior and subjective norms (BI = A + SN) and that behavioral intention predicts actual behavior.

Miller (2005) defines each of these three components of the theory as follows:

Attitudes: the sum of beliefs about a particular behavior weighted by evaluations of these beliefs

Subjective norms: the influence of people in one's social environment on his or her behavioral intentions; the beliefs of people, weighted by the importance of one's attributes to each of these beliefs, will influence behavioral intention

Behavioral intention: a function of both attitudes toward a behavior and subjective norms

Figure A.5   Theory of Reasoned Action

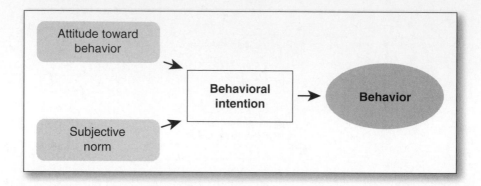

Theory of Planned Behavior (TPB)

The Theory of Planned Behavior links beliefs and behavior. The concept was proposed by Ajzen (1991) to improve on the predictive power of the Theory of Reasoned Action. The revision entails the inclusion of the concept of perceived behavioral control. TPB, therefore, asserts that attitude toward behavior, subjective norms, and perceived behavioral control together shape an individual's behavioral intentions, which, in turn, are directly related to subsequent behavior (Figure A.6).

Figure A.6   Theory of Planned Behavior

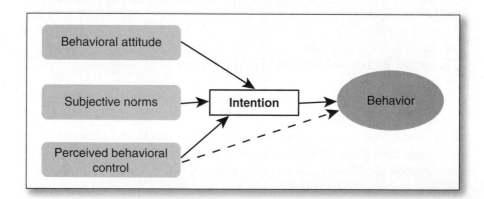

According to various studies, TPB has improved the predictability of intention in various fields of public health, including condom use (Fishbein, Albarracin, Johnson, & Muellerieile, 2001) and use of dietary supplements (Conner, Kirk, Cade, & Barrett, 2003).

Precaution Adoption Process Model (PAPM)

The Precaution Adoption Process Model is sequential in design, based on seven distinct stages moving from lack of awareness to adoption and/or maintenance of a health behavior (Weinstein, Sandman, & Blalock, 2008; Figure A.7).

Figure A.7   Precaution Adoption Process Model

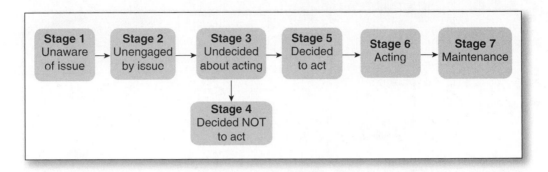

In the first stage of the model, an individual may be unaware of a hazard or health issue. The individual may become aware of the issue but remain unengaged by it (Stage 2). In Stage 3, the individual must decide whether to act with respect to the issue. The outcome of that decision leads to either Stage 4, deciding not to act, or Stage 5, deciding to act. The next two stages are acting and then maintaining that action. According to the PAPM, as individuals pass through the stages they must experience each stage in sequence. People may move backward from some later stages to earlier ones, but once they have completed the first two stages of the model it's not possible to return to them (that is, one can't move from awareness to unawareness).

The PAPM is similar in many respects to the Trans-theoretical Model. A key difference between the two models is that the Trans-theoretical Model offers insight into persistent unhealthy behaviors such as substance abuse. The PAPM better addresses hazards that have recently been recognized or precautions that are newly available.

Although the PAPM is a relatively new model, it has been applied to a range of health behaviors, including osteoporosis prevention, colorectal cancer screening, mammography, hepatitis B vaccination, and home testing for radon gas (Weinstein et al., 2008).

Protection Motivation Theory (PMT)

The Protection Motivation Theory proposes that people protect themselves based on four factors: perceived severity of a threatening event, perceived probability of the occurrence (susceptibility), perceived efficacy of a given preventive behavior (will it remove the threat?), and belief in one's ability to execute the preventive behavior, or self-efficacy (Rogers, 1975; Rogers & Prentice-Dunn, 1997). The first two of these factors make up what is called the *threat appraisal*, while the latter two factors combine to create the *coping appraisal* (Figure A.8).

Figure A.8 Protection Motivation Theory

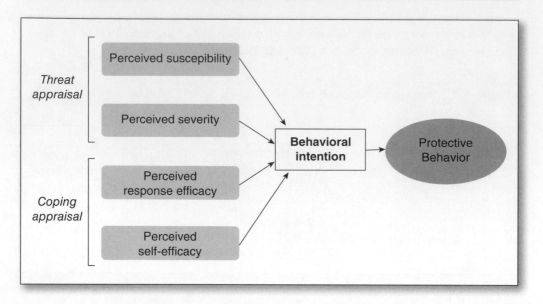

The PMT has been employed in more than 20 different health-related fields to study intentions and behavior (Grindley, Zizzi, & Nasypany, 2008).

INTERPERSONAL LEVEL

Social Learning Theory (SLT)

Social Learning Theory is a type of social-cognitive theory that was developed by Bandura (1977) to merge Cognitive Theory with Stimulus-Response Learning Theory to create a more inclusive explanation of human behavior. The basic premise behind SLT is that people learn within a social context. Learning is primarily facilitated through observation of one's surrounding environment and modeling the behavior of others, particularly influential people. According to the theory, a given behavior will be continued or ceased depending on whether or not it is reinforced (behavior that is "rewarded" is positively reinforced, while behavior that is "punished" is negatively reinforced).

Social learning theory further proposes that observational learning can occur in relation to three models:

1. *Live model:* An actual person whom the individual observes engages in a behavior.

2. *Verbal instruction:* A person describes the desired behavior in detail and instructs the individual how to engage in the behavior and encourages him or her to do so.

3. *Symbolic:* Modeling occurs by means of the media, including movies, television, Internet, literature, and radio. This latter type of modeling is also the driving force behind the Media Effects Model, which posits that mass media influences health behavior.

Social Network Theory (SNT)

Social Network Theory asserts that the structure and nature of relationships around an individual, group, or organization affect beliefs and/or behaviors. The axiom of the social network approach is that behavior is investigated within the context of the properties of *relations* between and within individuals (or other units within a network) instead of the properties of individuals themselves. It is a relational approach.

Social Network Theory views social relationships in terms of nodes and ties. Nodes represent individual actors within the networks, and ties the relationships between the actors. The power of SNT stems from its focus on relationships rather than individual units. For more about SNT, and its use in public health, refer to Chapter 14 in this volume.

Gender Theory

A wide variety of gender theories exist, and many are used in public health research. Such a large and diverse range of theories prohibits full coverage of these theories in a single appendix. In the context of public health, however, they all share a common premise: that a culture or society's view of gender—what it means to be a man or a woman—and the nature of relationships between men and women are central facets in health behavior and outcomes. Gender Theory is of particular relevance in global health and in countries where gender inequality is exceptionally prevalent and culturally embedded (Öhman, 2008).

Two illustrative examples of Gender Theory's applicability to public health are Gender Role Theory (Eagly, 1987) and the Theory of Gender and Power (Connell, 1987). The former views the differentially constructed social roles assigned to men and women as the root of sex-differentiated social behavior. The Theory of Gender and Power is also a social structural theory, but focuses more specifically on the concepts of sexual inequality and power imbalances between men and women. It postulates that three major social structures characterize relationships between men and women: the sexual division of labor, the sexual division of power, and the structure of cathexis (emotional context and significance).

Various scales have been developed to measure constructs related to gender. A compendium of some of these scales can be found at www.c-changeprogram.org/content/gender-scales-compendium/index.html.

COMMUNITY LEVEL

Community Coalition Action Theory (CCAT)

Butterfoss and Kegler (2002) developed the Community Coalition Action Theory (Figure A.9), a variation of the Inter-Organizational Relations (IOR) Theory. The basic premise underlying the CCAT is that a community coalition—a structured arrangement between individuals and organizations within a community—works together toward common goals and objectives. According to the theory, a coalition has a *lead agency* or *convener group* which agrees to manage and support financially the coalition. Coalitions are formal, multipurpose in scope, and often composed of long-term alliances that work locally or regionally. A community coalition works together on a regular basis to solve emergent and ongoing social and health problems within a community or region and to track progress of existing community-level programs. Butterfoss and Kegler argue that success of the coalition is more likely when the lead agency enrolls members of the community to help build and maintain trust throughout the community.

Figure A.9 The Community Coalition Action Theory Process

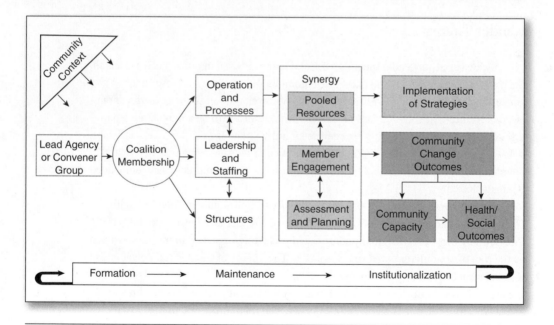

Source: Adapted from Butterfoss (2007).

Natural Helper Model (NHM)

The Natural Helper Model is a community-based approach designed to enhance the ability of individuals to help others through their own personal social networks

(Tessaro et al., 2000). Key individuals within the community's social network—*natural helpers*—are recruited to provide support to fellow community members (Bergstrom, 1982). Natural helpers are typically respected and trusted among their community peers and recognized for their listening skills and responsiveness to the needs of others, as well as the ability to demonstrate control over their own life circumstances (Bishop, Earp, Eng, & Lynch, 2002). Natural helpers provide a viable approach to health programs (Bergstrom, 1982), whether it is short- or long-term action in response to community health needs (DeBate & Plescia, 2005).

The goal of the NHM is to promote individual health behavior change by improving the health, particularly of a friend, family member, or acquaintance (Bishop et al., 2002), who usually shares the same values. The NHM enhances the cultural relevance of health promotion programs and allows information about health promotion to be diffused through general conversation and through the development of group activities. The model helps enhance healthier social norms and promotes systems change.

Another type of helper in the NHM is the lay health advisor (LHA), which is similar to the natural helper but exhibits a greater level knowledge with respect to health and resources (Bishop et al., 2002). Another difference is that LHAs may operate as paid workers and may or may not be part of a targeted community. Rather, they are likely to be selected based on criteria set forth by the governing agency, not community members (Scott, 2009). The natural helper model provides a community-based system of care and social support designed to complement, not replace, formal healthcare services (DeBate & Plescia, 2005).

Diffusion of Innovations (DOI) Theory

Diffusion of Innovation Theory, developed by Everett Rogers in 1962, is one of the most widely used theories in public health, with a textbook in its fifth edition (Rogers, 2003). The central tenet of the theory is that adoption of a new idea, behavior, or product (*innovation*) does not occur as a single step, but rather is the result of a process whereby a few select members of a community or population first adopt the innovation. The innovation then *diffuses* throughout the community/population through a series of social and behavioral processes. According to the theory, there are five adopter categories, with the majority of individuals falling in the third and fourth categories (Figure A.10):

1. *Innovators*: Innovators are the first to try an innovation. They are generally risk takers, and as such little, if anything, needs to be done to appeal to this population. A key aspect of their personality is to seek out and experience new things.

2. *Early adopters*: This group generally represents opinion leaders who enjoy leadership roles and embrace opportunities for change. They are aware of the need for change, and open to it, but will likely need guidance and instruction as to how to best implement change.

3. *Early majority*: This group will adopt change before the average person, but they are typically not leaders, and they require evidence that the innovation works before actually adopting it. To convince this group of adoption, one might use strategies such as success stories and evidence of the innovation's effectiveness.

4. *Late majority*: This group of people is not quite the last to adopt change, but they will adopt an innovation only after it has been tried, and approved, by the majority. Appealing to this group often entails providing information about how many other people have tried, and successfully used, the innovation.

5. *Laggards*: Exceptionally conservative by nature, laggards are skeptical of change and the hardest group to bring on board with respect to innovative ideas and products. Strategies to convince this population to change include statistical evidence, fear tactics, and social pressure from adopters.

Figure A.10   Categories of Adopters Within the General Population

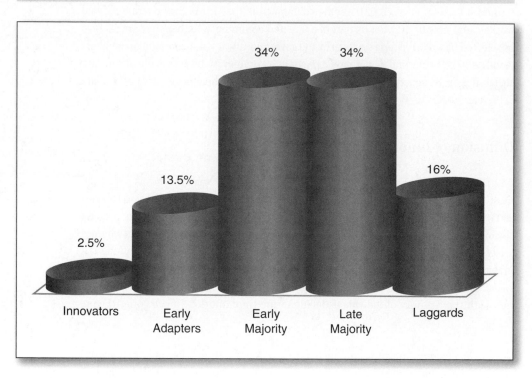

Source: Adapted from E. Rogers (1962).

The stages by which any one person adopts an innovation, and through which diffusion is achieved, include *awareness* of the need for an innovation, *decision* to adopt (or reject) the innovation, *initial use* of the innovation to test it, and *continued use* of the innovation. The theory asserts that five primary factors influence adoption, with some factors playing more of a role than others, depending on the category of an adopter:

1. *Relative advantage*: The degree to which an innovation is seen as advantageous over what it replaces

2. *Compatibility*: How congruent the innovation is with the values and lives of the target population

3. *Complexity*: How difficult the innovation is to understand and/or use

4. *Triability*: The extent to which an innovation can be experienced or tested prior to a commitment to adopt

5. *Observability*: The degree to which an innovation shows concrete and observable results

In public health, DOI Theory is often used to accelerate the adoption of public health programs and diffusion of products within a social system.

Communication Theory

The fundamental premise of Communication Theory is that communication permeates all levels of human experience and is, therefore, essential to understanding human behavior and how to change it. As with Gender Theory, no single communication theory exists that encompasses all aspects of communication. Gerbner (1985), however, provides a useful grouping of the study of communication into three categories:

1. *Semiotics*: The study of signs and symbols and how they combine to convey meaning in different social contexts

2. *Media effects*: The study of behavior and interaction through exposure to messages

3. *Message production*: The study of the large-scale organization of communications through social institutions and systems (mass media, political organizations, government, advocacy groups)

In public health, the application of Communication Theory is often observed in the context of health education and promotion, and involves creating communication programs or activities and subsequently measuring their effect on health behavior. Programs can target, and effects on behavior can be measured at, various levels of interaction: *intrapersonal* (individuals' processing of information), *interpersonal* (how two individuals influence one another), *group* (communication dynamics among many individuals), *organizational* (communication in the context of organizations such as hospitals, schools, or public health agencies), and *community/society* (social and cultural dimensions of communication).

Community-based approaches to public health gained credence during the last quarter of the 20th century, in recognition of the need to change health behavior at multiple levels of human experience. Not surprisingly, the majority of theories and models of health behavior change include a communication component, whether implicit or explicit.

MULTILEVEL APPROACHES

Symbolic Interaction Theory (SIT)

Symbolic Interaction Theory is a framework for understanding how individuals interact with each other and within society through the meanings of *symbols*, including both verbal and nonverbal responses. It is an individual's interaction with others and the environment and his or her interpretation of these interactions that are essential. According to Charon (2009), SIT is composed of five main concepts:

1. The human being must be understood as a social person. Interaction between individuals is the basic unit of study.

2. The human being must be understood as a thinking being. Human action is not only interaction among individuals but also interaction within the individual. We are, to our very core, thinking animals, always conversing with ourselves as we interact with others.

3. Humans define the situation and environment in which they exist and act. An environment exists, but it is our definition of it that is important. Definition results from ongoing social interaction and thinking.

4. The cause of human action is the result of what is occurring in our present situation. Social interaction, thinking, and definition of the situation that takes place in the present are what matter most.

5. Human beings are viewed as active beings in relation to their environment, as opposed to being passive in relation to their surroundings.

Theory of Triadic Influence (TTI)

The TTI proposes that variables of behavioral influence can be arranged by three tiered *streams* of causation:

6. *Individual*: Biological and personality characteristics of an individual that contribute to one's self-efficacy regarding specific behaviors

7. *Social*: The social situation/context that contribute to social normative beliefs about specific behaviors

8. *Environmental*: Sociocultural and macro-environmental factors that contribute to attitudes toward specific behaviors

Each of these streams of influence is composed of variables that are defined based on their causal proximity to behavior (Figure A.11). Intentions, for example, have direct effects on behavior and are causally proximal or immediate. Other variables, such as one's motivation to comply with or please others, are mediated through other variables (e.g., social normative beliefs) and are more causally distal. These three streams merge to form an individual's behavioral intentions, which in turn affect the likelihood of enacting a particular behavior.

Figure A.11 Theory of Triadic Influence

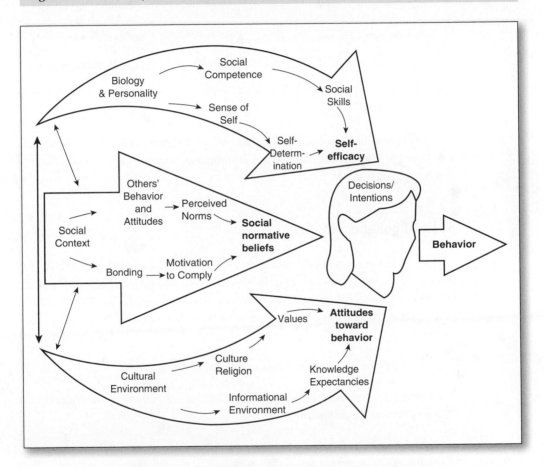

Source: Bella, Wells, and Merritt (2009).

Interactive Domain Model (IDM)

The Interactive Domain Model is a reflexive set of best practices within health promotion (Kahan & Goodstadt, 2001). The underlying premise of the IDM is that the quality and value of health promotion efforts depend on the presence and magnitude of four primary processes:

Awareness: We must be aware of a health problem in order to act on it.

Discussion: Talking openly about an issue with others enhances what we can do about it.

Clarity: If we are unclear about who the problem affects, which factors influence it, and possibilities for dealing with it, we won't address it effectively.

Reflection: If we don't reflect on our thoughts, knowledge, and activities related to the issue, we won't improve in our efforts to address it.

The conceptual model itself is based on three interactive domains:

Underpinnings: For example, theory, values, beliefs, goals, and evidence

Understanding of the environment: Vision, health analysis, organizational analysis

Practice: Processes/activities related to health issues, research and evaluation, and organizational issues

All of these interactive domains operate within a broader environmental context, which, in the IDM, include the physical environment, socioeconomic structures, and psychological conditions.

Social-Ecological Model

Socio-ecological models of behavior were developed to better understand the dynamic relationships among various levels of intervention and the effect on individual behavior and health outcomes (McElroy, Bibeau, Steckler, & Glanz, 1988; Stokols, 1996). Health status and behavior are viewed as being determined by the combination of five factors:

Public policy: Local, state, national, and global laws and policies

Community: Relationships among organizations, institutions, and informational networks within defined boundaries

Institutional: Social institutions with organizational characteristics and formal (and informal) rules and regulations for operations

Interpersonal processes and primary groups: Formal and informal social networks and social support systems, including family, work group, and friendship networks

Intrapersonal: Characteristics of the individual, such as knowledge, attitudes, behavior, self-concept, skills, and developmental history

These factors are often depicted as being related to one another in a nested manner, as depicted in Figure A.12. For an excellent review of ecological models in health, see L. Richard, Gauvin, and Raine (2011).

Figure A.12 Social-Ecological Model

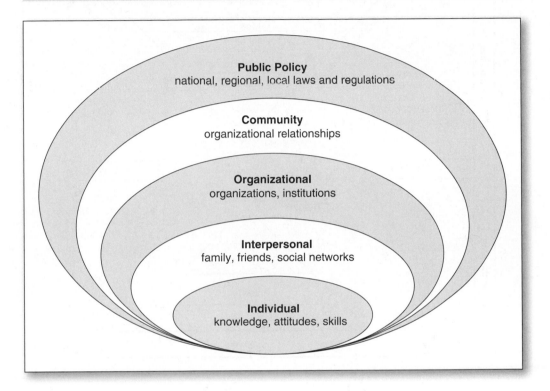

Behavioral Ecological Model (BEM)

The BEM builds on other ecological models by adding learning principles from the field of psychology—classical conditioning, operant conditioning, and social learning theories—as well as individual biological factors (Hovell, Wahlgren, & Adams, 2009; Hovell, Wahlgren, & Gehrman, 2002). The BEM equally stresses the individual and the social/environmental context in which an individual acts (Figure A.13). The internal and external components are viewed as hierarchies of interacting variables. The BEM assumes an interaction among both physical and social factors to explain health behavior. A key characteristic of the model is the notion that all of these factors are continuously shaping behavior and that change in an individual's behavior is a direct function of the degree of reinforcement.

Figure A.13 Behavioral Ecological Model

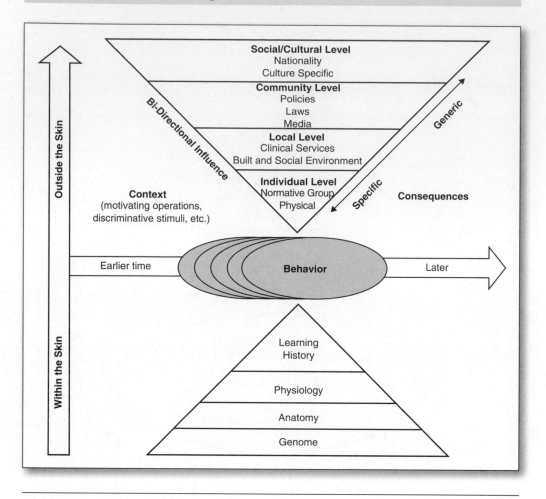

Source: Adapted from Hovell et al. (2002).

SUMMARY

Not all public health programs, interventions, and research derive from, or are supported by, the above theories. In some cases, a program developer or researcher will need to go beyond these theories and models and look at a more granular level in a specific academic subfield for guidance. Given its focus on understanding human behavior, it's no surprise that psychology is commonly mined by public health practitioners and researchers for theories to explain health behavior. But other fields such as sociology, social work, anthropology, and communications, among others, are ripe with theory. We borrowed theories, for example, from anthropology and psychology—Cultural Consensus Theory (Romney, Batchelder, & Weller, 1986) and Self-Categorization Theory (Turner,

Hogg, Oakes, Reicher, & Wetherell, 1987), respectively—to develop hypotheses for a methodological study. The take-home point is that you don't need to restrict yourself to the theories and models in this Appendix, or in other textbooks, if they aren't relevant to your study design. Dig into the literature and be creative.

ADDITIONAL RESOURCES

DiClemente, R., Crosby, R., & Kegler, M. (Eds.). (2009). *Emerging theories in health promotion practice and research* (2nd ed.), San Francisco, CA: Jossey-Bass.

DiClemente, R., Salazar, L.,, & Crosby, R. (2011). *Health behavior theory for public health: Principles, foundations and applications.* Burlington, MA: Jones & Bartlett Learning.

Edberg, M. (2007). *Essentials of health behavior: Social and behavioral theory in public health.* Sudbury, MA: Jones & Bartlett.

Glanz, K., Rimer, B., & Viswanath, K. (2008). *Health behavior and health education: Theory, research, and practice* (4th ed.). San Francisco, CA: Jossey-Bass.

Munro, S., Lewin, S., Swart, T., & Volmink, J. (2007). A review of health behaviour theories: How useful are these for developing interventions to promote long-term medication adherence for TB and HIV/AIDS? *BMC Public Health, 7,* 104.

Simons-Morton, B., McLeroy, K., & Wendel, M. (2011). *Behavior theory in health promotion practice and research.* Burlington, MA: Jones & Bartlett Learning.

REFERENCES

Ajzen, I. (1991). The theory of planned behavior. *Organizational Behavior and Human Decision Processes, 50,* 179–211.

Ajzen, I., & Fishbein, M. (1980). *Understanding attitudes and predicting social behavior.* Englewood Cliffs, NJ: Prentice Hall.

Bandura, A. (1977). *Social learning theory.* Englewood Cliffs, NJ: Prentice Hall.

Bella, C., Wells, S., & Merritt, L. (2009). Integrating cultural competency and empirically-based practices in child welfare services: A model based on community psychiatry field principles of health. *Children and Youth Services Review, 31,* 1206–1213.

Bergstrom, D. (1982). Collaborating with natural helpers for delivery of rural mental health services. *Journal of Rural Community Psychology, 3*(2), 5–26.

Bernardo, T.M., Rajic, A., Young, I., Robiadek, K., Pham, M.T., & Funk, J. A.(2013). Scoping review on search queries and social media for disease surveillance: A chronology of innovation. *J Med Internet Res 15*(7): e147 doi: 10.2196/jmir.2740

Bishop, C., Earp, J. A., Eng, E., & Lynch, K. S. (2002). Implementing a natural helper lay health advisor program: Lessons learned from unplanned events. *Health Promotion Practice, 3,* 233–244.

Bryan, A. D., Fisher, J. D., Fisher, W. A., & Murray, D. M. (1993). Unwanted teenage pregnancies: Incidence interpretation, intervention. *Applied Prevention Psychology, 2,* 101–113.

Butterfoss, F. (2007). *Coalitions and partnerships in community health.* San Francisco, CA: Jossey-Bass.

Butterfoss, F., & Kegler, M. (2002). Toward a comprehensive understanding of community coalitions: Moving from practice to theory. In R. J. DiClemente, R. A. Crosby, & M. C. Kegler (Eds.), *Emerging theories in health promotion practice and research strategies for improving public health* (pp. 157–193). San Francisco, CA: Jossey-Bass.

Charon, J. (2009). *Symbolic interactionism: An introduction, an interpretation, an integration* (10th ed.). Englewood Cliffs, NJ: Prentice Hall.

Connell, R. (1987). *Gender and power.* Cambridge, UK: Cambridge University Press.

Conner, M., Kirk, S., Cade, J., & Barrett, J. (2003). Environmental influences: Actors influencing a woman's decision to use dietary supplements. *Journal of Nutrition, 133,* 1978.

Conner, M., & Norman, P. (Eds.). (1996). *Predicting health behaviour: Search and practice with social cognition models.* Ballmore, UK: Open University Press.

DeBate, R., & Plescia, M. (2005). I could live other places, but this is where I want to be: Support for natural helper initiatives. *International Quarterly of Community Health Education, 23,* 327–339.

Duttweiler, P. C. (1984). The Internal Control Index: A newly developed measure of locus of control. *Educational and Psychological Measurement, 44,* 209–221.

Eagly, A. (1987). *Sex differences in social behavior: A social role interpretation.* Hillsdale, NJ: Lawrence Erlbaum.

Fishbein, M., & Ajzen, I. (1975). *Belief, attitude, intention, and behavior: An introduction to theory and research.* Reading, MA: Addison-Wesley.

Fishbein, M., Albarracin, D., Johnson, B., & Muellerieile, P. (2001). Theories of reasoned action and planned behavior as models of condom use: A meta-analysis. *Psychological Bulletin, 127,* 142–161.

Fisher, J. D., & Fisher, W. A. (1992). Changing AIDS-risk behavior. *Psychological Bulletin, 111,* 455–474.

Fisher, J. D., Fisher, W. A., Bryan, A. D., & Misovich, S. J. (2002). Information-motivation-behavioral skills model-based HIV risk behavior change intervention for inner-city high school youth. *Health Psychology, 21*(2), 177–186.

Gerbner, G. (1985). Field definitions: Communication theory. In *1984–85 U.S. directory of graduate programs.* Princeton, NJ: Educational Testing Service.

Gilboa, I. (2010). *Rational choice.* Cambridge, MA: MIT Press.

Glebocka, A., & Lisowska, E. (2007). Professional burnout and stress among Polish physicians explained by the Hobfoll resources theory. *Journal of Physiology and Pharmacology, 58,* 243–252.

Grindley, E., Zizzi, S., & Nasypany, A. (2008). Use of protection motivation theory, affect, and barriers to understand and predict adherence to outpatient rehabilitation. *Physical Therapy, 88,* 1529–1540.

Halbesleben, J., & Rathert, C. (2008). Linking physician burnout and patient outcomes: Exploring the dyadic relationship between physicians and patients. *Health Care Management Review, 33,* 29–39.

Hobfoll, S. (1989). Conservation of resources: A new attempt at conceptualizing stress. *American Psychologist, 44,* 513–524.

Hobfoll, S. (1998). *Stress, culture, and community.* New York, NY: Plenum Press.

Holahan, C. J., Moos, R. H., Holahan, C. K., & Cronkite, R. C. (1999). Resource loss, resource gain, and depressive symptoms: A 10-year model. *Journal of Personality and Social Psychology, 77,* 620–630.

Hovell, M., Wahlgren, D., & Adams, M. (2009). The logical and empirical basis for the behavioral ecological model. In R. J. DiClemente, R. Crosby, & M. Kegler, (Eds.), *New and emerging theories in health promotion practice and research* (2nd ed., pp. 415–449). San Francisco, CA: Jossey-Bass.

Hovell, M., Wahlgren, D., & Gehrman, C. (2002). The behavioral ecological model: Integrating public health and behavioral science. In R. J. DiClemente, R. Crosby, & M. Kegler (Eds.), *New and emerging theories in health promotion practice and research* (pp. 347–385). San Francisco, CA: Jossey-Bass.

Janowski, K., Kurpas, D., Kusz, J., Mroczek, B., & Jedynak, T. (2013). Health-related behavior, profile of health locus of control and acceptance of illness in patients suffering from chronic somatic diseases. *PLoS One, 8*(5), e63920.

Kahan, B., & Goodstadt, M. (2001). The interactive domain model of best practices in health promotion: Developing and implementing a best practices approach to health promotion. *Health Promotion Practice, 2,* 43–67.

Kilic, S., Dorstyn, D., & Guiver, G. (2013). Examining factors that contribute to the process of resilience following spinal cord injury. *Spinal Cord, 51,* 553–557.

McElroy, K., Bibeau, D., Steckler, A., & Glanz, K. (1988). An ecological perspective on health promotion programs. *Health Education Quarterly, 15,* 351–377.

Miller, K. (2005). *Communications theories: Perspectives, processes, and contexts.* New York, NY: McGraw-Hill.

Misovich, S. J., Martinez, T., Fisher, J. D., Bryan, A., & Catapano, N. (2006). Predicting breast self-examination: A test of the information-motivation-behavioral skills model. *Journal of Applied Social Psychology, 33* 775–790.

National Cancer Institute. (2012). *Theory at a glance: A guide for health promotion practice.* Bethesda, MD: Author.

Öhman, A. (2008). Global public health and gender theory: The need for integration. *Scandinavian Journal of Public Health, 36,* 449–451.

Petty, R., & Cacioppo, J. (1981). Attitudes and persuasion: Classic and contemporary approaches. Dubuque, IA: William C. Brown.

Prochaska, J. O., & DiClemente, C. C. (1983). Stages and processes of self-change of smoking: Toward an integrative model of change. *Journal of Consulting and Clinical Psychology, 51,* 390–395.

Prochaska, J. O., & Prochaska, J. M. (2009). Change (stages of). In S. J. Lopez (Ed.), *The encyclopedia of positive psychology.* Oxford, UK: Wiley-Blackwell.

Richard, S., Dionne, C., & Nouwen, A. (2011). Self-efficacy and health locus of control: Relationship to occupational disability among workers with back pain. *Journal of Occupational Rehabilitation, 21,* 421–430.

Richard, L., Gauvin, L., & Raine, K. (2011). Ecological models revisited: Their uses and evolution in health promotion over two decades. *Annual Review of Public Health, 32,* 307–326.

Rogers, E. (1962). *Diffusion of innovations.* Glencoe, IL: Free Press.

Rogers, E. (2003). *Diffusion of innovations* (5th ed.). New York, NY: Free Press.

Rogers, R. (1975). A protection motivation theory of fear appeals and attitude change. *Journal of Psychology, 91,* 93–114.

Rogers, R., & Prentice-Dunn, S. (1997). *Protection motivation theory.* New York, NY: Plenum.

Romney, A., Batchelder, W., & Weller, S. (1986). Culture as consensus: A theory of culture and informant accuracy. *American Anthropologist, 88,* 313–38.

Rosenstock, I. (1966). Why people use health services. *Milbank Memorial Fund Quarterly, 44,* 94–124.

Rosenstock, I., Strecher, V., & Becker, M. (1988). Social learning theory and the health belief model. *Health Education Quarterly, 15,* 175–183.

Rotter, J. B. (1954). *Social learning and clinical psychology.* New York, NY: Prentice Hall.

Scott, T. N. (2009). Utilization of the natural helper model in health promotion targeting African American men. *Journal of Holistic Nursing, 27,* 282–292.

Shattuck, D., Kerner, B., Gilles, K., Hartmann, M., Ng'ombe, T., & Guest, G. (2011). Encouraging contraceptive uptake by motivating men to communicate about family planning: The Malawi Male Motivator Project. *American Journal of Public Health, 101,* 1089–1095.

Stokols, D. (1996). Translating social ecological theory into guidelines for community health promotion. *American Journal of Health Promotion, 10,* 282–298.

Tessaro, I. A., Taylor, S., Belton, L., Campbell, M. K., Benedict, S., Kelsey, K., & DeVellis, B. (2000). Adapting a natural (lay) helpers model of change for worksite health promotion for women. *Health Education Research, 15*, 603–614.

Turner, J., Hogg, M., Oakes, P., Reicher, S., & Wetherell, M. (Eds.). (1987). *Rediscovering the social group: A self-categorization theory.* Oxford, UK: Basil Blackwell.

van Dijk, T., Dijkshoorn, H., van Dijk, A., Cremer, S., & Agyemang, C. (2013). Multidimensional health locus of control and depressive symptoms in the multi-ethnic population of the Netherlands. *Social Psychiatry and Psychiatric Epidemiology.* Advance online publication. doi:10.1007/s00127-013-0678-y

Wallston, B. S., & Wallston, K. A. (1978). Locus of control and health: A review of the literature. *Health Education Monographs, 6,* 107–117.

Wallston, B., Wallston, K., Kaplan, G., & Maides, S. (1976). Development and validation of the Health Locus of Control (HLC) scale. *Journal of Consulting and Clinical Psychology, 44,* 580–585.

Weinstein, N., Sandman, P., & Blalock, S. (2008). The precaution adoption process model. In K. Glanz, B. Rimer, & K. Viswanath (Eds.), *Health behavior and health education* (4th ed., pp. 123–148). San Francisco, CA: Jossey-Bass.

Wilson, B. (2007). Designing media messages about health and nutrition: What strategies are most effective? *Journal of Nutrition Education and Behavior, 39,* S13–S19.

AUTHOR INDEX

SUBJECT INDEX